T·H·E

·FAT· COUNTER

THIRD EDITION

Revised and Updated

Annette B. Natow, Ph.D., R.D., and Jo-Ann Heslin M.A., R.D.

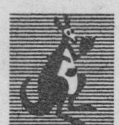

POCKET BOOKS

New York   London   Toronto   Sydney   Tokyo   Singapore

An *Original* Publication of POCKET BOOKS

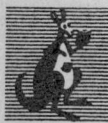

POCKET BOOKS, a division of Simon & Schuster Inc.
1230 Avenue of the Americas, New York, NY 10020

ISBN: 0-671-78335-1

First Pocket Books printing of this revised edition October 1995

10 9 8 7 6 5 4 3 2 1

POCKET and colophon are registered trademarks of
Simon & Schuster Inc.

Cover design by Tom McKeveny

Printed in the U.S.A.

T·H·E

·FAT· COUNTER

Health and nutrition experts agree that Americans eat too much fat: 34% of all our calories come from fat. The Department of Health and Human Services recommends "reducing dietary fat intake to an average of 30% of calories or less, and average saturated fat intake to less than 10% of calories among people aged two and older."

In its 1994 Trends report, the Food Marketing Institute noted that the top nutritional concern of American consumers is the amount of fat in their food: 59% of consumers now focus on fat, more than twice the number in 1988. Americans know that they eat more fat than is good for them, and they want to do something about it. Now it's easy to watch your fat intake—and protect your health—with the more than 19,000 handy alphabetical items listed in this all-new, revised and updated edition of THE FAT COUNTER.

―――――――

ANNETTE B. NATOW, Ph.D., R.D., and JO-ANN HESLIN, M.A., R.D., are the authors of eighteen books on nutrition, including The Antioxidant Vitamin Counter, The Cholesterol Counter, The Diabetes Carbohydrate and Calorie Counter, The Fast-Food Nutrition Counter, The Fat Attack Plan, The Iron Counter, The Pregnancy Nutrition Counter, The Sodium Counter, and The Supermarket Nutrition Counter. Both are former faculty members of Adelphi University and State University of New York, Downstate Medical Center. They are editors of the Journal of Nutrition for the Elderly, serve as editorial board members for the Environmental Nutrition Newsletter, and are frequent contributors to magazines and journals.

Books by Annette B. Natow and Jo-Ann Heslin

The Antioxidant Vitamin Counter
The Cholesterol Counter
The Diabetes Carbohydrate and Calorie Counter
The Fast-Food Nutrition Counter
The Fat Attack Plan
The Fat Counter
The Iron Counter
Megadoses
No-Nonsense Nutrition for Kids
The Pocket Encyclopedia of Nutrition
The Pregnancy Nutrition Counter
The Sodium Counter
The Supermarket Nutrition Counter

Published by POCKET BOOKS

To our families who support us through every project:
Harry, Allen, Irene, Sarah, Meryl, Laura, Marty,
George, Emily, Steven, Joseph, Kristen and Karen.

ACKNOWLEDGMENTS

Without the tireless cooperation of Steven and Stephen, *The Fat Counter* would never have been completed. A special thanks to our editor, Julie Rubenstein, and our agent, Nancy Trichter.

Our thanks also go to all the food manufacturers who graciously shared their data.

"Too much fat is a disadvantage . . . laying the foundation for troubles with the heart."

"Foods very high in fuel value, i.e., fats and dishes containing much fat, should be avoided."

Mary Swartz Rose, Ph.D.
Feeding the Family
The Macmillan Company, 1919

CONTENTS

CONTENTS

SOURCES OF DATA

Values in this counter have been obtained from the Composition of Foods, United States Department of Agriculture, Agricultural Handbooks: No. 8-1, Dairy and Egg Products; No. 8-2, Spices and Herbs; No. 8-3, Baby Foods; No. 8-4, Fats and Oils; No. 8-5, Poultry Products; No. 8-6, Soups, Sauces and Gravies; No. 8-7, Sausages and Luncheon Meats; No. 8-8, Breakfast Cereals; No. 8-9, Fruits and Fruit Juices; No. 8-10, Pork Products; No. 8-11, Vegetables and Vegetable Products; No. 8-12, Nut and Seed Products; No. 8-13, Beef Products; No. 8-14, Beverages; No. 8-15, Finfish and Shellfish Products; No. 8-16, Legumes and Legume Products; No. 8-17, Lamb, Veal and Game Products; No. 8-19, Snacks and Sweets; No. 8-20, Cereal Grains and Pasta; No. 8-21, Fast Foods; Supplements 1989, 1990, 1991.

Nutritive Value of Foods, United States Department of Agriculture, Home and Garden Bulletin No. 72.

J. Davies and J. Dickerson, *Nutrient Content of Food Portions*. Cambridge, UK: The Royal Society of Chemistry, 1991.

G. A. Leveille, M. E. Zabik, K. J. Morgan, *Nutrients in Foods*. Cambridge, MA: The Nutrition Guild, 1983.

Souci, Fachmann, Kraut, *Food Composition and Nutrition Tables*. Stuttgart: Wissenschaftliche Verlagsgesellschaft MbH, 1989.

Information from food labels, manufacturers and processors. The values are based on research conducted prior to 1995. Manufacturer's ingredients are subject to change, so current values may vary from those listed in the book.

INTRODUCTION

Americans know that they eat more fat than is good for them and they want to do something about it. In fact, the American Dietetic Association's Center for Nutrition and Dietetics Consumer Hotline reports receiving more questions on fat than any other issue.

In spite of this we still eat too much fat. Thirty-four percent of total calories in the average American diet comes from fat, down from 42 percent in the mid-sixties but still above the 30 percent goal. Saturated fat makes up 12 percent of calories, down from 16 percent in the mid-sixties but still one and a half times the recommended level of 8 percent of calories.

The experts all agree, less fat is better:

> Thirty-eight health organizations ranging from the American Heart Association to the American Medical Association recommend limiting the number of calories from fat to no more than 30 percent of the daily diet.
>
> National Heart, Lung and Blood Institute,
> National Institutes of Health

> ". . . the primary priority for dietary change is the recommendation to reduce intake of total fats."
>
> C. Everett Koop,
> Surgeon General's Report on Nutrition
> and Health

"Reduce dietary fat intake to an average of 30 percent of calories or less, and average saturated fat intake to less than 10 percent of calories among people aged two and older."

Healthy People 2000,
Department of Health and Human Services

The Women's Health Trial found that it's easier to meet health goals on a lowfat diet, rather than a low-calorie diet.

Fred Hutchinson Cancer Research Center

"Researchers have found that you can lose weight simply by reducing the amount of fat you eat."

Division of Nutritional Sciences,
Cornell University

And consumers are getting the message. In its 1994 Trends report the Food Marketing Institute noted that the top nutritional concern of American consumers is the amount of fat in their food. Fifty-nine percent of consumers now focus on fat, more than twice the number in 1988.

TOO MUCH IS NOT SAFE

High-fat diets are unhealthy. Almost three fourths of the two million Americans who die annually die from diseases linked to our high-fat diet.

Eating too much fat increases the risk for:

HEART ATTACK—Each year, Americans have more than one and a half million heart attacks resulting in more than half a million deaths.

STROKE—Americans have one half million each year; many result in death or disability.

CANCER—Studies suggest that high fat intake increases risk for breast, colon and prostate cancers.

OVERWEIGHT—Diets high in fat lead to overweight more easily than do diets high in proteins or carbohydrates. High-fat diets make you fatter faster.

GALLBLADDER DISEASE—Overweight people with high-fat diets have a greater risk of gallbladder problems.

OSTEOARTHRITIS—High-fat diets cause overweight, which places more strain on the joints.

HEARING LOSS—Studies suggest that as people age, high fat and high cholesterol intakes coupled with high blood pressure can lead to hearing loss.

GOUT—A high-fat diet aggravates gout (joint inflammation).

DIABETES—A high-fat diet causes overweight, which increases the risk for diabetes. It also complicates treatment for existing cases of diabetes.

FAT FACTS

Most foods contain fat. Some have more, some less, few have none. Some fat can be easily seen—butter, margarine, salad oils and the fat on your steak or chop. Much of the fat you eat can't be seen—invisible fat—in meat, milk, egg yolks, olives, walnuts, cakes, pies, cookies and candy. Whether you can see the fat or not, it adds up quickly.

FAT FACT #1 *Everyone should be eating less fat.* Americans eat too much fat. More than one third of all the calories we eat are from fat! Experts agree that we should be eating much less—no more than 30 percent of our calories should come from fat. Some experts state that less than 30 percent would be even better.

FAT FACT #2 *Fat makes you fatter faster.* The fat we eat turns into body fat much easier than the other things we eat. Fat calories make us fatter than calories from protein, sugar or starch. A lower fat diet is helpful in weight loss.

FAT FACT #3 *Fat comes in three forms*—saturated, polyunsaturated and monounsaturated.

There are different kinds of fats, identified by the types of fatty acids they contain. They can be saturated, polyunsaturated or monounsaturated. Most foods contain all three of these fats. Some foods have more of one type than another. For example, beef has a lot more saturated fat, margarine a lot of polyunsaturated fat, and olive oil is high in monounsaturated fat.

Saturated Fat

If you leave a stick of butter on the kitchen counter all day it will soften but it won't melt. Butter is high in saturated fats. Saturated fat is solid at room temperature.

Research shows that eating a lot of saturated fats raises blood cholesterol levels. People with higher blood cholesterol levels are more likely to have a heart attack. Recently it has been found that not all saturated fats raise cholesterol. Even though that is true, foods we eat never contain only one type of saturated fat. All fats in foods are mixtures of fats. Foods often contain some saturated fats that raise cholesterol and other saturated fats that may not. That makes it difficult to translate these studies into food recommendations. *The best advice: eat less total fat.*

Fat Fact

Saturated fat has been shown to be a factor in cancer of the ovaries. A recent study suggests that eating 10 grams of saturated fat a day may raise a woman's risk of ovarian cancer by 20 percent. The good news is that lowering fat intake by 10 grams a day reduces risk by 20 percent.

FOODS HIGH IN SATURATED FATS

Bacon	Hot dogs
Beef	Ice cream
Butter	Lamb
Cheese	Lunch meats
Chicken	Palm kernel oil
Chocolate	Palm oil
Coconut	Pork
Coconut oil	Sausage
Cream	Sour cream
Duck	Veal
Fish	Whipped cream
Half and half	Whole milk

Polyunsaturated Fat

Corn oil left out on the kitchen counter will not become solid. It doesn't even solidify in the refrigerator. Polyunsaturated fats are liquid at room temperature. These fats may help lower cholesterol levels in the blood. Research suggests that too much polyunsaturated fat may not be good. High intake may cause gallbladder disease, depress the immune system and put you at greater risk for some cancers. *The best advice: eat less total fat.*

FOODS HIGH IN POLYUNSATURATED FATS

Bluefish	Salmon
Corn oil	Sesame oil
Cottonseed oil	Soft margarine
Herring	Soybean oil
Mackerel	Sunflower oil
Mayonnaise	Tuna
Rainbow trout	Walnut oil
Sablefish	Walnuts
Safflower oil	Wheat germ
Salad dressing	Whitefish

Monounsaturated Fat

Olive oil left out on the kitchen counter never becomes solid. In the refrigerator olive oil gets cloudy as it becomes partly solid. Monounsaturated fat stays liquid at room temperature but becomes partly solid when chilled. You have been hearing more about monounsaturated fats lately as part of the Mediterranean diet. Research shows these fats may help lower blood cholesterol. This sounds good, but too much of any fat is not good for you. *The best advice: eat less total fat.*

FOODS HIGH IN MONOUNSATURATED FAT

Almonds	Peanut butter
Canola oil	Peanut oil
Cashews	Peanuts
Chicken fat	Pignoli (pine nuts)
Filberts (hazelnuts)	Pistachio nuts
Macadamia nuts	Sesame oil
Olive oil	Soybean oil
Olives	Soybean oil margarine

Trans Fatty Acids

When liquid oils are hardened to make margarine and solid shortening, some of the unsaturated fats become trans fatty acids which, like saturated fats, can raise blood cholesterol. In the ingredients list on food labels these hardened oils are called "partially hydrogenated" or "hydrogenated vegetable oils." Research suggests that eating trans fatty acids increases risk of heart disease in the same way that eating saturated fats does. Many experts do not agree with this and recommend waiting for more conclusive evidence.

In the meantime, you can choose tub margarines, which have fewer trans fatty acids, or liquid squeeze margarines, which do not contain any trans fatty acids at all. If a food is low fat, there won't be enough trans fatty acids to worry about. So again, *the best advice is to use less of all fats because the less fat you eat, the fewer trans fatty acids you will eat.*

CHOOSING LOW-FAT FOODS

Choosing the Best Fats

Once in a while everyone feels like having toast with butter or margarine. In most homes you find butter, margarine and some kind of cooking oil. Even low-fat recipes may call for some oil or shortening. There are things you should remember to help you choose the best fats.

When selecting a margarine, choose one with a liquid oil as the first ingredient. Avoid margarines with tropical oils such as palm oil and palm kernel oil. Soft tub margarines or liquid squeeze types are often highest in polyunsaturates. For example, if liquid sunflower oil is the first ingredient, this would be a highly polyunsaturated margarine. Using moderate amounts of this or a similar margarine would be a good choice.

Butter blends are a combination of margarine and some butter. Blends have less saturated fat than butter but more saturated fat than margarine.

A good all-purpose cooking oil is tasteless and fries without smoking. Corn, safflower, sunflower, soybean and cottonseed are all highly polyunsaturated oils. Olive, canola and peanut oils are high in polyunsaturates and monounsaturates. All are good choices.

Choosing Low-Fat Proteins

1. Choose skim or lowfat milk and lowfat or nonfat yogurt. Use skim-milk cheese, reduced-fat or fat-free cheese. On occasions when you eat regular cheese, limit the portion.

2. Use lowfat or nonfat yogurt, reduced-fat or fat-free sour cream in place of regular sour cream.

3. Choose the leanest cuts of meat; remove all visible fat before cooking.

4. Choose lean or extra-lean ground beef that has as little fat as possible. Supermarkets often label the ground beef with the percentage of fat; sometimes it is as low as 10 percent or less. Ground poultry is a good substitute for ground meat. It is usually, but not always, lower in fat. Check the label.

5. Roast, broil or grill meats on a rack so that fat drips off during cooking. When making soups, stews or sauces, skim fat off the top.

6. Avoid turkey and turkey breasts that are "self-basted." The basting usually adds more fat.

7. Poultry skin is high in fat. You can cook poultry with it's skin on but remove it before eating.

8. All fish contain less fat than most cuts of meat. Very lean fish choices are: cod, scrod, flounder, halibut, pollock, sole and haddock. Shellfish like shrimp, lobster, scallops and crab are low in fat too.

9. Choose tuna canned in water. Tuna is a low-fat fish but when it is canned in oil, this adds seven times more fat than tuna canned in water.

10. Choose poached, steamed or broiled fish instead of breaded, battered or fried.

FAT FACT

To have healthy low-fat meals, fill three quarters of your plate with high–complex-carbohydrate foods like rice, bulgur and other grains, pasta, potatoes, vegetables, fruits and bread. Have lean meat, poultry or fish on the other quarter of your plate.

Ten Steps to Lower Your Fat Intake

1. Choose skim or lowfat milk, evaporated skim milk, lowfat or nonfat yogurt and reduced-fat or fat-free cheese. Look for the words: skim, 1% fat, 2% fat, fat-free, nonfat.
Beware: Cheeses labeled "made with partially skim milk" may contain almost as much fat as regular cheese.

2. Choose lean meats trimmed of all visible fat and poultry without skin. Look for ground meat and poultry labeled "lean" or "extra lean" or lowfat ground beef that contains fiber fillers like oat bran and carrageenan.
Beware: Meat, poultry and fish contain invisible fat. Limit

portion size to 4 ounces, about the size of the palm of your hand.

3. Choose lean fish like cod, scrod, haddock and halibut. When using fatty fish like salmon, bluefish or mackerel, remove the skin and all visible fat.

Beware: Canned fish packed in oil is high in fat. Choose fish canned in water, broth, mustard or tomato sauce.

4. Roast, broil, grill, bake or poach meat, poultry and fish so no extra fat is added. During cooking, fat drips off—discard it.

Beware: When you add breadcrumbs or cereal to ground meat for meat loaf or hamburgers, the crumbs act like a blotter, soaking up fat instead of allowing it to drip off.

5. Use honey, all-fruit preserves, jelly or jam as a spread on toast and bread instead of butter, margarine or regular cream cheese—good taste and no fat.

6. Sour cream as a topping for baked potatoes is a lower fat choice than butter, but plain, lowfat or nonfat yogurt is even better. Use butter flavor sprinkles or fat-free sour cream.

7. Use lowfat milk in tea or coffee instead of half and half, cream or nondairy creamers (whiteners). It gives beverages the same flavor but less fat.

8. Dress your salad with lemon juice, herb-flavored vinegar or fat-free dressings instead of regular oil-based salad dressing.

9. Sweet rolls, donuts and Danish pastries are high-fat snacks. Try cinnamon raisin bread or bagels for a low-fat sweet treat.

10. Use cooking spray to oil pans and sauté foods.

These suggestions are just a beginning. To reduce the total amount of fat you eat you have to learn how to recognize fat when you see it and even when you don't see it. It's not always easy. *The Fat Counter* will help.

FINDING FAT IN FOODS

Doesn't everybody need some fat?

Yes, you do need a small amount of fat. Fat is part of every cell in your body. It is used to make hormones, cushion bones and body organs, and insulate the body to help maintain normal temperature. Food fats carry fat soluble vitamins A, D, E and K. Fats stay in the stomach longer, making you feel full, so you don't get hungry as quickly.

Finding Food Fats

Most fruits and vegetables have little or no fat. There are a few exceptions like avocadoes and olives (see page 10 and page 353).

Dried peas and beans are all pretty low in fat. Soybeans have a little more fat than other beans (see page 511). All nuts and seeds, including coconut and peanuts, have a lot of fat. These are examples of hidden fat.

Grains like oats, rice, wheat, rye and barley contain little fat. Cereals, breads and pasta made from grains are usually low in fat. Exceptions are some regular granola-type cereals, cookies, pies, sweet rolls and cakes. You can tell how much fat is in a cookie by how soft it is. The softer the cookie, the more fat it has. Judge your cookies by breaking them in half; a cookie that bends instead of breaking is higher in fat. Place a croissant, muffin or Danish on a napkin for a few minutes. If a grease ring forms, it's high in fat.

People think of animal foods like meat, milk, cheese,

eggs, poultry and fish as good protein foods. While this is true, it is also true that all animal foods contain fat. In fact, an ounce of lean meat has the same amount of calories from protein as from fat. In fatty meats like spare ribs, there may be twice as many calories from fat as from protein. Meats like bacon should really be thought of as fat not meat. The fat in one slice of bacon is equal to the fat in a pat of butter.

Reading Labels

There's a lot of information on labels but sometimes it can be confusing. When you want to know more about a food, look at the list of ingredients. Packaged foods must list ingredients. The first ingredient listed is the main one in the food. If it is fat, this is a high-fat food. But even if fat is the second or third ingredient listed, the food is fairly high in fat.

LABEL LINGO

Fat-free: Less than ½ gram of fat in a serving

Lowfat: Three grams or less of fat in a serving (except for milk, which can contain 5 grams)

Lean: Meat, poultry, seafood or packaged meals with less than 10 grams of fat, less than 4 grams of saturated fat and less than 95 milligrams of cholesterol in a 3½-ounce serving

Extra lean: Meat, poultry, seafood or packaged meals with less than 5 grams of fat, 2 grams of saturated fat and 95 milligrams of cholesterol in a 3½-ounce serving

Light or Lite: One-third fewer calories or 50 percent less fat than in the original, higher calorie, higher fat version

Fats on labels can appear as any of the following:

Animal fats	Margarine
(lard, suet, chicken fat)	Monoglycerides
Butter	Oil
Cocoa butter	Partially hydrogenated fat
Cheese	Partially hydrogenated oil
Cream	Shortening
Diglycerides	Vegetable fat
Fat	Vegetable oil
Hydrogenated fat	Whole milk
Hydrogenated oil	

When Is Fat Not a Fat?

In spite of the fact that high-fat foods make us fat and are not healthy, we love fatty foods. Fried foods, cakes, pies, cookies, butter and ice cream are often named as favorites. This is where fat substitutes come in. They give reduced-fat or fat-free products the texture and mouth feel of higher fat foods with less fat and usually fewer calories. By replacing all or part of the fat in processed foods, they may offer us healthier choices.

Some ingredients that are used as fat substitutes also have other functions in food. Some of these have been used for years, others have been developed more recently. Many of these substitutes are natural, like carrageenan, which is found in seaweed. Others are snythetic, often made from ordinary foods like eggs, milk and corn. The synthetic fat substitutes require more testing than the natural substances before they are approved for use in food by the Food and Drug Administration.

You'll see fat substitutes as ingredients in frozen desserts, margarine, baked goods, puddings, salad dressings, sauces and other foods. Some commonly used fat substitutes are:

Carrageenan
Cellulose
Dextrins
Gelatin
Maltodextrin
Modified food starch

Pectin
Polydextrose
Starch
Whey protein
Xanthum

Food experts, including The American Dietetic Association, support the use of fat substitutes for some of the fat in foods when they are used as part of a healthy diet. While fat replacers can make lower-fat eating more enjoyable, they should not be used as an excuse for eating too many desserts or as a green light to eat more high-fat foods because "you have saved so many calories with the fat replacers."

Finding Fat Calories in Food

Fat calories make you fatter faster. The food fat we eat is easily turned into body fat. You can limit fat calories by counting fat grams.

Nutrition labels can help you find out how much fat is in a food. Fat is listed in grams.

1 gram of fat = 9 calories

For example, 1 ounce of corn chips has 155 calories and 9 grams of fat.

9 grams of fat × 9 calories = 81 fat calories

More than one half of the calories in corn chips comes from fat.

Fat foods have a lot of calories. One teaspoon of fat has 45 calories. A teaspoon of protein, sugar or starch has only 20 calories.

Another example: 1 ounce of pretzels has 120 calories and 1 gram of fat.

1 gram of fat $\times$ 9 calories = 9 fat calories

Less than one tenth of the calories in pretzels comes from fat. Pretzels are a good snack choice: less fat, less fat calories, less fattening for you.

How Much Fat Should You Eat?

Americans eat too much fat. Not too long ago, the average American got over 40 percent of his calories from fat. We now eat less. But still, we get a whopping 34 percent of our calories from fat. Experts agree we should be eating much less.

The American Heart Association, the American Cancer Society, the American Health Foundation and the National Institutes of Health all recommend lowering fat intake. Americans should eat no more than 30 percent fat calories each day.

That's a good suggestion. How do you do it? The question is, How many grams of fat can you eat and still limit your fat intake to no more than 30 percent of your calories? It's easy to find out.

STEP 1. *Find out how many calories you eat each day.* If you maintain the same weight, you are probably eating:

13 calories per pound, if you are not very active
15 calories per pound, if you are moderately active
17 calories per pound, if you are very active
20 calories per pound, if you are extremely active

For example, if you weigh 145 pounds and are moderately active you need 2175 calories per day (145 pounds $\times$ 15 calories = 2175 calories). Round that number to 2200 calories. You need 2200 calories per day to maintain your weight.

If you are overweight, estimate your desirable weight and multiply that by the appropriate number of calories per pound. For example, if you would like to weight 130 pounds and are not very active, estimate your calorie needs as follows:

130 pounds × 13 calories per pound = 1690 calories

Round answer to 1700 Calories

STEP 2. *Find out how many of grams of fat you should be eating each day.* In Step 1 you found out how many calories you need each day. Find the number of calories you need each day in the list below. Next to it is the maximum grams of fat allowed for the day. This amount will confine your fat intake to less than 30 percent of your total calories for the day.

For example, if you need 1800 calories each day, you should be eating no more than 60 grams of fat per day.

STEP 3. *Find out how many grams of saturated fat you should be eating each day.* In Step 1 you found out how many calories you need each day. Find the number of calories you need each day on the list below. On the same line is the maximum grams of saturated fat allowed for the day. This amount will keep your saturated fat intake at less than 10 percent of your total calories for the day.

MAXIMUM GRAMS OF FAT AND SATURATED FAT ALLOWED

Calories	Grams of Fat	Grams of Saturated Fat
1200	40 —	13
1300	43	14
1400	47	16
1500	50	17
1600	53	18
1700	57	19
1800	60	20
1900	63	21
2000	67	22
2100	70	23
2200	73	24
2300	77 —Dad	26
2400	80	27
2500	83	28
2600	87	29
2700	90	30
2800	93	31
2900	97	32
3000	100	33

Now that you know how many grams of fat you should be eating each day, it's time to count up your fat.

COUNT UP YOUR FAT

We often eat on the run and pick foods high in fat. By the end of the day, we've eaten too much fat. You know you shouldn't be eating so much fat. You want to cut back. *The Fat Counter* will help you do it. Now it's simple to find out the amount of fat in all the foods you are eating.

Let's look at a typical day. Are the food choices familiar? Let's see how much fat this sample day has in it.

FAT COUNTING
A SAMPLE DAY OF HIGH-FAT FOOD CHOICES

	FAT GRAMS	SAT. FAT GRAMS	TOTAL CALORIES
BREAKFAST			
Orange juice (1 cup)	1	tr	110
French toast (1 slice)	7	2	151
Butter (1 pat)	4	3	36
Maple syrup (2 tbsp)	0	0	122
Pork sausage (1 link)	4	1	48
Coffee &	0	0	4
Half & half (2 tbsp)	4	2	40
LUNCH			
Cheeseburger w/ bun	15	6	320
Catsup (1 tbsp)	tr	tr	16
French fries (10 strips)	4	2	111
Diet cola (12 oz)	0	0	2
SNACK			
Jelly donut	16	4	289
Coffee &	0	0	4
Half & half (2 tbsp)	4	2	40
DINNER			
Flank steak, broiled (3 oz)	11	5	292
Baked potato (5 oz) &	tr	tr	145
Sour cream (2 tbsp)	6	4	52
Tossed salad &	0	0	16
French dressing (1 tbsp)	6	2	67
Pound cake (1 slice)	5	1	120
Tea &	0	0	0
Sugar (1 tsp)	0	0	16
TV SNACK			
Rich vanilla ice cream (½ cup)	12	8	175
TOTAL	99	42	2176

To determine your total fat calories for the day multiply the number of grams of fat by 9 (calories per gram of fat):

99 grams of fat × 9 calories = 891 fat calories

To determine the *percentage* of calories from fat, divide the total *fat* calories by the total calories for the day:

891 fat calories ÷ 2176 = 41% fat (rounded)

To find the number of *saturated* fat calories, multiply the number of grams of saturated fat by 9 (calories per gram of fat). Saturated fat calories should total no more than 10 percent of your total calories for the day. In the Sample Day of High-Fat Food Choices shown, 10 percent of the total calories for the day equals 218 saturated fat calories.

42 grams of saturated fat × 9 calories = 378

This is too much fat and saturated fat for one day: 41 percent of the day's calories came from fat, and well over 10 percent of the day's calories came from saturated fat. Now you can see how easy it is to eat too much fat.

TIME-SAVER: There's no need to count saturated fat every day. Keeping track of *total* fat is more important. Check your saturated fat intake once in a while. You'll find that when you eat less total fat, you automatically eat less saturated fat.

NOTE: In this and the following sample, as throughout *The Fat Counter,* the number of fat grams in each food has been rounded to the nearest whole number.

FAT COUNTING
A SAMPLE DAY OF WISE FOOD CHOICES

	FAT GRAMS	SAT. FAT GRAMS	TOTAL CALORIES
BREAKFAST			
Orange juice (1 cup)	1	tr	110
All-bran cereal (½ cup) &	1	tr	76
Lowfat milk (½ cup)	tr	tr	43
Toast (1 slice) &	1	tr	67
Strawberry jam (2 tsp)	0	0	46
Coffee &	0	0	4
Skim milk (2 tbsp)	0	0	11
LUNCH			
Hamburger w/ bun	12	4	275
Catsup (1 tbsp)	tr	tr	16
French fries (10 strips)	4	2	111
Diet cola (12 oz)	0	0	2
SNACK			
Pear	1	tr	98
DINNER			
Flank steak, broiled (3 oz)	11	5	292
Baked potato &	tr	0	145
Plain nonfat yogurt (2 tbsp)	0	0	16
Tossed salad &	0	0	16
Reduced-calorie Italian dressing (2 tbsp)	4	tr	32
Angelfood cake (1 slice)	tr	tr	129
Tea &	0	0	0
Sugar (1 tsp)	0	0	16
TV SNACK			
Light vanilla ice cream (½ cup)	3	2	92
TOTAL	38	13	1597

Now, determine the number of fat calories, the percentage of fat and the number of saturated fat calories.

38 grams of fat $\times$ 9 calories $=$ 342 fat calories

Remember, the percentage of calories from fat is determined by dividing the calories from fat by the number of total calories.

342 fat calories $\div$ 1597 total calories $=$ 21% fat (rounded)

Multiply the number of grams of saturated fat by 9 (calories per gram of fat) to determine the number of saturated fat calories, which should total no more than 10 percent of the total calories for the day. In this sample day, this figure is 160 saturated fat calories.

13 grams of saturated fat $\times$ 9 calories $=$ 117 saturated fat calories

These wise food choices show a much healthier intake of fat for the day. When you cut down on grams of fat, you cut down on calories too. In this sample day, fat calories are only 21 percent of the total.

TIME-SAVER: There's no need to count saturated fat every day. Keeping track of total fat is more important. Check your saturated fat intake once in a while. You'll find that when you eat less total fat, you automatically eat less saturated fat.

Now it's your turn to count your fat. Note everything you eat today, then look up the fat and saturated fat (if you wish) in each food and see how much fat you've eaten today. While you're at it, jot down the calories too.

FAT COUNTING
A SAMPLE WORKSHEET

FOOD	FAT GRAMS	SAT. FAT GRAMS	TOTAL CALORIES
BREAKFAST			
SNACK			
LUNCH			
SNACK			
DINNER			
SNACK			
TOTAL			

Now it's time for the calculations.

_____ grams of fat × 9 calories = _____ fat calories

Calories from fat divided by total calories equals the percentage of calories from fat.

_____ fat calories ÷ _____ total calories = _____%

Grams of saturated fat times 9 calories (per gram) gives you saturated fat calories, which should total no more than 10 percent of total calories for the day.

___ grams of saturated fat × 9 calories = ___ saturated fat calories

10% of _____ (total calories) = _____

Did you eat more than 30 percent fat today? Did you eat more than 10 percent saturated fat? If you did, you're eating too much fat and saturated fat. Turn back to page xxxiii, "Maximum Grams of Fat and Saturated Fat Allowed."

Start right now to make lower fat food choices.

USING YOUR FAT COUNTER

This book lists the fat, saturated fat and calorie content of over 19,000 foods. Now, with this information about fat values at your fingertips, you will find it easy to follow a lowfat diet.

Before *The Fat Counter* it was impossible to compare so many foods at one time. When you want to pick a lowfat cookie, look up the cookie category, page 166. Fresh foods like meat, chicken, fish and cheese do not usually have a label. The same goes for take-out items like potato salad, coleslaw, ice cream or foods bought at the bakery. How can you tell how much fat there is in a burger or taco that you enjoy at the local fast-food restaurant? *The Fat Counter* lists them all!

The Fat Counter is divided into two main sections. Part I, Brand-Name and Generic Foods, lists foods alphabetically. In each group, you will find brand-name foods listed first in alphabetical order, followed by an alphabetical listing of generic foods. Large categories are divided into subcategories—canned, fresh, frozen, ready-to-use—to make it easier to find what you are looking for.

If you want to know how much fat is in the hamburger you are having for lunch, look under HAMBURGER, where you will find all kinds of hamburgers listed; or, if you are making a homemade hamburger, look under ROLL, where you will find the hamburger roll listed alphabetically, and under BEEF, where you will find a cooked chopped-beef patty. For foods like FRENCH TOAST, HONEY or SALAD DRESSING, simply look for the specific food alphabetically in the complete listing. For example, FRENCH TOAST is found on page 243, listed alphabetically between FRENCH FRIES and FROG'S LEGS. Two slices have 8 grams of fat and 2 grams of saturated fat.

If you are eating at home, simply look up the individual foods you are eating and total the fat and saturated fat for the entire meal. For example, your dinner may consist of:

	FAT (GRAMS)	SATURATED FAT (GRAMS)
rib lamb chops, broiled	50	22
Broccoli Cuts in Cheese Sauce (Green Giant)	3	tr
Minute Microwave French Pilaf (General Foods)	3	2
cheese cake	18	9
glass of white wine	0	0
TOTAL FOR THE MEAL	74	33

If you are eating out, most food categories will have a take-out subcategory. Items found in the take-out subcategory will help you estimate the fat and calories in similar restaurant or take-out menu items. For example, if you order tuna salad, look under TUNA DISHES on page 541.

Most foods are listed alphabetically. But in some cases,

foods are grouped by category. For example, all pasta dishes, like spaghetti and meat balls, lasagna and fettuccini are found under the category PASTA DINNERS.

Other group categories include:

DINNER (page 215): includes all frozen dinners by brand name

ICE CREAM AND FROZEN DESSERTS (page 281): includes all dairy and nondairy ice cream and frozen novelties

LIQUOR/LIQUEUR (page 311): includes all alcoholic beverages except wine or beer

LUNCHEON MEATS/COLD CUTS (page 313): includes all sandwich meats except chicken, ham and turkey

NUTRITIONAL SUPPLEMENTS (page 344): includes all meal replacers, diet bars and diet drinks

ORIENTAL FOOD (page 357): includes all Oriental-type foods

SPANISH FOOD (page 515): includes all Mexican-type foods

Part II, Restaurant, Take-Out and Fast-Food Chains, contains an alphabetical listing of 60 popular chains, such as BURGER KING, DOMINO'S PIZZA, TACO BELL and WENDY'S. Fast foods are listed alphabetically under the chain's name. For example, a Big Mac is listed on page 621 under McDONALD'S.

We have tried to include all foods for which fat values are known. There will be some foods, however, that are not listed in *The Fat Counter* because the fat values are not available for that particular food.

When you can't locate your favorite brand, look at other similar foods. You will probably find a brand-name food, a generic product or a home recipe that is like your favorite food. For example, you find that your favorite brand of vanilla yogurt is not listed. Look at the different vanilla yogurts listed on page 574. From these entries you can quickly determine that vanilla yogurt has from 0 to 7 grams of fat in a serving. You can then assume that your favorite brand has a comparable amount.

With *The Fat Counter* as your guide, you will never again wonder how much fat is in the food you eat. You will always be able to tell if a food is high in fat, moderate in fat or low in fat. Your goal is to pick low-fat foods each time you eat.

DEFINITIONS

as prep (as prepared): refers to food that has been prepared according to package directions

cooked: refers to food cooked without the addition of fat (oil, butter, margarine, etc.); steaming, poaching, broiling and dry roasting are examples of this type of preparation

generic: describes a food without a brand name

home recipe: describes homemade dishes; those included can be used as a guide to the fat and calorie values of similar products you may prepare or take-out food you buy ready-to-eat

lean and fat: describes meat with some fat on its edges that is not cut away before cooking, or poultry prepared with skin and fat as purchased

lean only: lean portion, trimmed of all visible fat

shelf stable: refers to prepared products found on the supermarket shelf that are ready to be eaten or cooked and do not require refrigeration

take-out: describes prepared dishes that you purchase ready-to-eat; those included serve as a guide to the fat and calorie values of similar products you may purchase

trace (tr): value used when a food contains less than one calorie or less than one gram of saturated fat or total fat

ABBREVIATIONS

ave	=	average	pt	=	pint
diam	=	diameter	qt	=	quart
frzn	=	frozen	reg	=	regular
g	=	gram	sm	=	small
in	=	inch	sq	=	square
lb	=	pound	tbsp	=	tablespoon
lg	=	large	tr	=	trace
med	=	medium	tsp	=	teaspoon
mg	=	milligram	w/	=	with
oz	=	ounce	w/o	=	without
pkg	=	package	<	=	less than
prep	=	prepared			

EQUIVALENT MEASURES

Dry

3 teaspoons	=	1 tablespoon
4 tablespoons	=	¼ cup
8 tablespoons	=	½ cup
12 tablespoons	=	¾ cup
16 tablespoons	=	1 cup
1000 milligrams	=	1 gram
28 grams	=	1 ounce
4 ounces	=	¼ pound
8 ounces	=	½ pound
12 ounces	=	¾ pound
16 ounces	=	1 pound

Liquid

2 tablespoons	=	1 ounce
2 ounces	=	¼ cup
4 ounces	=	½ cup
6 ounces	=	¾ cup
8 ounces	=	1 cup
2 cups	=	1 pint
4 cups	=	1 quart

FAT FACT

If you are an average weight, moderately active adult and want a quick benchmark for total fat grams each day, simply divide your weight in half.

FAT FACT

Saturated fat should equal no more than 10 percent of your total fat intake. For example, if you weigh 120 pounds, you should eat no more than 60 grams of fat per day (120 ÷ 2) and no more than 6 grams of saturated fat (10 percent of 60).

NOTES

Throughout the Counter portion of this book, SAT. FAT in the column headings indicates the *saturated* fat content, and FAT indicates the *total* fat content.

Discrepancies in figures are due to rounding, product reformulation and reevaluation.

ALL FAT AND SATURATED FAT VALUES OF FOODS ARE GIVEN IN GRAMS (g).

ALL FAT AND SATURATED FAT VALUES OF FOODS HAVE BEEN ROUNDED TO THE NEAREST WHOLE NUMBER

— indicates data not available

PART 1

Brand-Name and
Generic Foods

FOOD	PORTION	CALS.	SAT. FAT	FAT
ABALONE				
fresh fried	3 oz	161	1	6
raw	3 oz	89	tr	1
ACEROLA				
acerola	1 fruit	2	—	tr
juice	1 cup	51	—	1
ADZUKI BEANS				
CANNED				
sweetened	1 cup	702	—	tr
DRIED				
cooked	1 cup	294	—	tr
READY-TO-USE				
yokan, sliced	3¼ in slices	112	—	tr
AKEE				
fresh	3.5 oz	223	—	20
ALE				
(see BEER AND ALE, AND MALT)				
ALFALFA				
sprouts	1 cup	40	tr	tr
sprouts	1 tbsp	1	tr	tr
ALLIGATOR				
tail, cooked	3.5 oz	143	—	3
ALLSPICE				
ground	1 tsp	5	tr	tr
ALMONDS				
Almond Butter (Erewhon)	1 tbsp (16g)	90	—	8
Almond Butter Natural Raw (Hain)	2 tbsp	190	2	18
Almond Butter Toasted (Hain)	2 tbsp	220	2	19
Almonds (Beer Nuts)	1 pkg (1 oz)	180	—	14
Almonds (Planters)	1 oz	170	2	15
Blanched Slivered (Dole)	1 oz	170	—	14
Blanched Whole (Dole)	1 oz	170	—	14
Chopped Natural (Dole)	1 oz	170	—	14
Honey Roasted (Planters)	1 oz	170	1	13
Nutella	1 tbsp (0.5 oz)	85	—	5
Sliced (Planters)	1 oz	170	2	15

FOOD	PORTION	CALS.	SAT. FAT	FAT
Sliced Natural (Dole)	1 oz	170	—	14
Slivered (Planters)	1 oz	170	2	15
Smoked (Lance)	1 pkg (0.7 oz)	120	1	11
Whole Natural (Dole)	1 oz	170	—	14
almond butter, honey & cinnamon	1 tbsp	96	1	8
almond butter w/ salt	1 tbsp	101	1	9
almond butter w/o salt	1 tbsp	101	1	10
almond meal	1 oz	116	tr	5
almond paste	1 oz	127	1	8
dried, blanched	1 oz	166	1	15
dried, unblanched	1 oz	167	1	15
dry roasted, unblanched	1 oz	167	1	15
dry roasted, unblanched, salted	1 oz	167	1	15
oil roasted, blanched	1 oz	174	2	16
oil roasted, blanched, salted	1 oz	174	2	16
oil roasted, unblanched	1 oz	176	2	16
toasted, unblanched	1 oz	167	1	14

AMARANTH
(*see also* CEREAL, COOKIES)

FOOD	PORTION	CALS.	SAT. FAT	FAT
Amaranth Cereal w/ Bananas (Health Valley)	½ cup	110	—	2
Amaranth Crunch w/ Raisins (Health Valley)	¼ cup	110	—	3
Amaranth Flakes 100% Organic (Health Valley)	½ cup (1 oz)	90	—	tr
Fast Menu Amaranth w/ Garden Vegetables (Health Valley)	7.5 oz	140	—	3
Seeds (Arrowhead)	¼ cup (1.6 oz)	170	1	2
cooked	½ cup	59	tr	tr
uncooked	½ cup	366	2	6

ANASAZI BEANS
DRIED

FOOD	PORTION	CALS.	SAT. FAT	FAT
Arrowhead	¼ cup (1.5 oz)	150	0	1
Bean Cuisine	½ cup	115	—	1

ANCHOVY
CANNED

FOOD	PORTION	CALS.	SAT. FAT	FAT
in oil	5	42	tr	2
in oil	1 can (1.6 oz)	95	1	4

FOOD	PORTION	CALS.	SAT. FAT	FAT
FRESH				
raw	3 oz	62	1	4
fillets	3 (0.4 oz)	21	—	1
ANGLERFISH				
raw	3.5 oz	72	—	1
ANISE				
seed	1 tsp	7	—	tr
ANTELOPE				
roasted	3 oz	127	1	2
APPLE				
CANNED				
Escalloped Apples (White House)	4 oz	120	0	0
Fried Apples (Luck's)	8 oz	190	—	0
Sliced (White House)	4 oz	55	0	0
Spiced Apple Rings (White House)	1 ring	25	0	0
sliced, sweetened	1 cup	136	tr	1
DRIED				
Mariani	¼ cup	150	—	0
cooked w/ sugar	½ cup	116	tr	tr
cooked w/o sugar	½ cup	172	tr	tr
rings	10	155	tr	tr
FRESH				
Dole	1	80	—	1
apple	1	81	tr	tr
w/o skin, sliced	1 cup	62	tr	tr
w/o skin, sliced & cooked	1 cup	91	tr	tr
w/o skin, sliced & microwaved	1 cup	96	tr	tr
FROZEN				
Apple Fritters (Mrs. Paul's)	2	270	—	9
Escalloped (Stouffer's)	1 cup (6 oz)	180	—	3
sliced w/o sugar	½ cup	41	tr	tr
JUICE				
Apple & Eve	6 fl oz	80	0	0
Apple & Eve Cider	6 fl oz	80	0	0
Apple & Eve Nothin' But Juice	6 fl oz	78	0	0
Bruce Lite	½ cup	88	0	0
Hi-C Jammin' Apple	8 fl oz	130	0	0

FOOD	PORTION	CALS.	SAT. FAT	FAT
Juice Works	6 oz	100	—	0
Minute Maid				
Box	8.45 fl oz	120	0	0
Frozen	8 fl oz	110	0	0
Juices To Go	1 bottle (10 fl oz)	110	0	0
Juices To Go	1 bottle (16 fl oz)	140	0	0
Juices To Go Apple	1 can (11.5 fl oz)	160	0	0
Naturals	8 fl oz	110	0	0
Mott's from Concentrate, as prep	8 fl oz	120	0	0
Mott's Fruit Basket Apple Juice Cocktail, as prep	8 fl oz	120	0	0
Mott's Natural	8 fl oz	120	0	0
Ocean Spray	8 fl oz	110	0	0
Odwalla Live Apple	8 fl oz	140	0	0
Red Cheek from Concentrate	8 fl oz	120	0	0
Red Cheek Natural	8 fl oz	120	0	0
S&W 100% Unsweetened	6 oz	85	0	0
Seneca Clarified frzn, as prep	8 fl oz	120	0	0
Seneca Granny Smith frzn, as prep	8 fl oz	120	0	0
Seneca Natural frzn, as prep	8 fl oz	120	0	0
Sippin Pak 100% Pure	8.45 fl oz	110	0	0
Sipps Apple	8.45 oz	130	—	0
Tree Top	6 oz	90	0	0
Cider	6 oz	90	0	0
Cider frzn, as prep	6 oz	90	0	0
frzn, as prep	6 oz	90	0	0
Sparkling Juice	6 oz	90	0	0
Unfiltered	6 oz	90	0	0
Unfiltered frzn, as prep	6 oz	90	0	0
w/ Vitamin C	6 oz	90	0	0
Tropicana				
Season's Best	1 bottle (10 fl oz)	140	0	0
Season's Best	1 bottle (7 fl oz)	100	0	0
Season's Best	1 can (11.5 fl oz)	160	0	0
Season's Best	1 container (10 fl oz)	140	0	0
Season's Best	1 container (6 fl oz)	80	0	0
Season's Best	1 container (8 fl oz)	110	0	0
Season's Best	(8 fl oz)	110	0	0

FOOD	PORTION	CALS.	SAT. FAT	FAT
Veryfine 100%	8 oz	107	0	0
White House	6 oz	90	0	0
apple	1 cup	116	tr	tr
frzn, as prep	1 cup	111	tr	tr
frzn, not prep	6 oz	349	tr	1

APPLESAUCE
JARRED
Mott's

FOOD	PORTION	CALS.	SAT. FAT	FAT
Chunky	5 oz	110	0	0
Cinnamon	5 oz	120	0	0
Mott's Fruit Snacks Apple Spice	4 oz	70	0	0
Fruit Snacks Cinnamon	4 oz	90	0	0
Fruit Snacks Strawberry	4 oz	80	0	0
Fruit Snacks Sweetened	4 oz	90	0	0
Sweetened	5 oz	110	0	0
S&W				
Diet	½ cup	55	0	0
Gravenstein Sweetened	½ cup	90	0	0
Gravenstein Unsweetened	½ cup	55	0	0
Sweetened	½ cup	55	0	0
Unsweetened	½ cup	25	—	2
Seneca				
Cinnamon	½ cup	100	0	0
Golden Delicious	½ cup	100	0	0
McIntosh	½ cup	100	0	0
Natural	½ cup	60	0	0
Regular	½ cup	100	0	0
Tree Top Cinnamon	½ cup	80	0	0
Tree Top Natural	½ cup	60	0	0
Tree Top Original	½ cup	80	0	0
White House				
Chunky	4 oz	800	0	0
Cinnamon	4 oz	100	0	0
Natural Packed w/ Apple Juice	4 oz	60	0	0
Regular	4 oz	80	0	0
Unsweetened	4 oz	50	0	0
sweetened	½ cup	97	tr	tr
unsweetened	½ cup	53	tr	tr

FOOD	PORTION	CALS.	SAT. FAT	FAT

APRICOTS
CANNED

FOOD	PORTION	CALS.	SAT. FAT	FAT
Halves, Diet (S&W)	½ cup	35	0	0
Halves Unpeeled in Heavy Syrup (S&W)	½ cup	110	0	0
Halves Unpeeled Lite (Libby)	½ cup (4.4 oz)	60	0	0
Halves Unsweetened (S&W)	½ cup	35	0	0
Whole Peeled, Diet (S&W)	½ cup	28	0	0
Whole Peeled in Heavy Syrup (S&W)	½ cup	100	0	0
halves, heavy syrup pack w/ skin	1 cup (9.1 oz)	214	tr	tr
halves, water pack w/ skin	1 cup (8.5 oz)	65	tr	tr
halves, water pack w/o skin	1 cup (8 oz)	51	tr	tr
heavy syrup w/ skin	3 halves	70	tr	tr
juice pack w/ skin	3 halves	40	tr	tr
light syrup w/ skin	3 halves	54	tr	tr
puree juice pack w/ skin	1 cup (8.7 oz)	119	tr	tr
puree from heavy syrup w/ skin	¾ cup (9.1 oz)	214	tr	tr
puree from light pack w/ skin	¾ cup (8.9 oz)	160	tr	tr
puree from water pack w/ skin	¾ cup (8.5 oz)	65	tr	tr
water pack w/ skin	3 halves	22	tr	tr
water pack w/o skin	4 halves	20	tr	tr
DRIED				
Mariani	¼ cup	140	—	0
halves	10	83	tr	tr
halves, cooked w/o sugar	½ cup	106	tr	tr
FRESH				
apricots	3	51	tr	tr
FROZEN				
sweetened	½ cup	119	tr	tr
JUICE				
Kern's Nectar	6 oz	110	0	0
Libby Nectar	1 can (11.5 fl oz)	220	0	0
S&W Nectar	6 oz	35	0	0
nectar	1 cup	141	tr	tr

FOOD	PORTION	CALS.	SAT. FAT	FAT
ARROWHEAD				
fresh, boiled	1 med (⅓ oz)	9	—	tr
ARROWROOT				
flour	1 cup	457	tr	tr
ARTICHOKE				
CANNED				
Hearts Marinated (S&W)	½ cup	225	—	26
FRESH				
Dole	1 lg	23	—	tr
boiled	1 med (4 oz)	60	tr	tr
hearts, cooked	½ cup	42	tr	tr
jerusalem, raw, sliced	½ cup	57	0	tr
FROZEN				
Hearts Deluxe (Birds Eye)	½ cup	30	0	0
cooked	1 pkg (9 oz)	108	tr	1
ARUGULA				
raw	½ cup	2	—	tr
ASPARAGUS				
CANNED				
Cut Spears (Owatonna)	½ cup	20	—	0
Points Water Pack (S&W)	½ cup	17	0	0
Seneca	½ cup	20	0	0
Spears Colossal Fancy (S&W)	½ cup	20	0	0
Spears Fancy (S&W)	½ cup	18	0	0
spears	½ cup	24	tr	1
FRESH				
Dole	5 spears	18	—	0
cooked	½ cup	22	tr	tr
cooked	4 spears	14	tr	tr
raw	½ cup	16	tr	tr
raw	4 spears	14	tr	tr
FROZEN				
Big Valley	5–6 spears (3 oz)	20	0	0
Cut (Birds Eye)	½ cup	23	0	tr
Harvest Fresh Cuts (Green Giant)	½ cup	25	0	0
Spears (Birds Eye)	½ cup	25	0	0
cooked	4 spears	17	tr	tr
cooked	1 pkg (10 oz)	82	tr	1

FOOD	PORTION	CALS.	SAT. FAT	FAT

AVOCADO
FRESH
FOOD	PORTION	CALS.	SAT. FAT	FAT
California Avocado	½	153	—	14
California Avocado, mashed	1 cup	407	—	36
avocado	1	324	5	31
puree	1 cup	370	6	35

BABY FOOD
Nutritional guidelines for infants are different from those recommended for older children and adults. Check with a pediatrician for advice on feeding children under the age of two.

BAKED SELECTIONS
Gerber
FOOD	PORTION	CALS.	SAT. FAT	FAT
Chunky Animal Cookies	2 (0.5 oz)	60	—	2
Chunky Biter Biscuits	1 (0.4 oz)	50	—	1
Chunky Zwieback Toast	2 (0.5 oz)	70	—	2
Graduates Animal Crackers Cinnamon	2 (0.2 oz)	30	—	1
Graduates Arrowroot Cookies	2 (0.4 oz)	50	—	2
Graduates Pretzels	2 (0.4 oz)	45	0	0

CEREAL
Beech-Nut
FOOD	PORTION	CALS.	SAT. FAT	FAT
Stage 1 Barley	½ oz	60	0	0
Stage 1 Oatmeal	½ oz	60	—	2
Stage 1 Oatmeal & Apples	1 jar (4 oz)	70	0	0
Stage 1 Rice	½ oz	60	0	0
Stage 2 Mixed	½ oz	50	—	1
Stage 2 Mixed & Apples	1 jar (4 oz)	70	0	0
Stage 2 Oatmeal & Chiquita Bananas	½ oz	60	—	1
Stage 2 Rice & Apples	1 jar (4 oz)	70	0	0
Stage 2 Rice & Chiquita Bananas	½ oz	60	0	0
Stage 2 Rice & Golden Delicious Apples	½ oz	60	0	0
Brown Rice 100% Organic Health Valley	1 tbsp (0.5 oz)	60	—	1

Earth's Best
FOOD	PORTION	CALS.	SAT. FAT	FAT
Brown Rice	5 tbsp (0.5 oz)	60	—	0
Mixed Grain	5 tbsp (0.5 oz)	60	—	0

FOOD	PORTION	CALS.	SAT. FAT	FAT
Peach, Oatmeal, Banana	1 jar (4.5 fl oz)	60	—	0
Prunes & Oatmeal	1 jar (4.5 fl oz)	100	—	0
Gerber				
1st Foods Barley	4 tbsp (0.5 oz)	60	—	1
1st Foods Oatmeal	4 tbsp (0.5 oz)	50	—	1
1st Foods Rice	4 tbsp (0.5 oz)	60	—	1
2nd Foods High Protein	4 tbsp (0.5 oz)	50	—	1
2nd Foods Mixed	4 tbsp (0.5 oz)	60	—	1
2nd Foods Mixed	4 tbsp (0.5 oz)	60	—	1
2nd Foods Mixed With Applesauce & Bananas	1 jar (4 oz)	90	—	1
2nd Foods Mixed With Banana	4 tbsp (0.5 oz)	60	—	1
2nd Foods Oatmeal With Applesauce & Bananas	1 jar (4 oz)	90	—	1
2nd Foods Oatmeal With Banana	4 tbsp (0.5 oz)	60	—	1
2nd Foods Rice With Applesauce & Bananas	1 jar (4 oz)	90	0	0
2nd Foods Rice With Bananas	4 tbsp (0.5 oz)	60	—	1
3rd Foods Mixed With Applesauce & Bananas	1 jar (6 oz)	140	—	1
3rd Foods Oatmeal With Applesauce & Bananas	1 jar (6 oz)	140	—	1
3rd Foods Rice With Mixed Fruit	1 jar (6 oz)	130	—	0
Tropical Foods Corn Cereal	4 tbsp (0.5 oz)	60	—	1
Tropical Foods Rice With Mango	4 tbsp (0.5 oz)	50	0	0
Health Valley Sprouted Baby Cereal 100% Organic	1 tbsp (0.5 oz)	60	—	1
DESSERT				
Beech-Nut				
Stage 2 Apple & Strawberry Dessert	1 jar (4 oz)	100	0	0

FOOD	PORTION	CALS.	SAT. FAT	FAT
Beech-Nut *(cont.)*				
Stage 2 Apple Yogurt Dessert	1 jar (4 oz)	100	—	1
Stage 2 Apple, Peach & Strawberry Dessert	1 jar (4 oz)	100	0	0
Stage 2 Banana Pineapple Dessert	1 jar (4 oz)	100	0	0
Stage 2 Banana Pudding (Spanish label)	1 jar (4 oz)	110	0	0
Stage 2 Banana Yogurt Dessert	1 jar (4 oz)	120	—	2
Stage 2 Cottage Cheese With Pears Dessert	1 jar (4 oz)	120	—	1
Stage 2 Dutch Apple Dessert	1 jar (4 oz)	100	0	0
Stage 2 Flan de Banana	1 jar (4 oz)	110	0	0
Stage 2 Flan de Vanilla	1 jar (4 oz)	120	—	3
Stage 2 Fruit Dessert	1 jar (4 oz)	80	0	0
Stage 2 Frutas Islenas Dessert	1 jar (4 oz)	100	0	0
Stage 2 Guava Tropical Fruit Dessert	1 jar (4 oz)	90	0	0
Stage 2 Mango Tropical Fruit Dessert	1 jar (4 oz)	110	0	0
Stage 2 Mixed Fruit Yogurt Dessert	1 jar (4 oz)	100	0	0
Stage 2 Papaya Tropical Fruit Dessert	1 jar (4 oz)	100	0	0
Stage 2 Vanilla Custard Pudding	1 jar (4 oz)	120	—	3
Stage 3 Cottage Cheese With Pears	1 jar (6 oz)	180	—	2
Stage 3 Fruit Dessert	1 jar (6 oz)	120	0	0
Stage 3 Mixed Fruit Yogurt Dessert	1 jar (6 oz)	170	0	0
Stage 3 Vanilla Custard Pudding	1 jar (6 oz)	190	—	6
Gerber				
2nd Foods Banana Apple Dessert	1 jar (4 oz)	80	0	0
2nd Foods Banana Yogurt Dessert	1 jar (4 oz)	90	0	0
2nd Foods Cherry Vanilla Pudding	1 jar (4 oz)	80	0	0

FOOD	PORTION	CALS.	SAT. FAT	FAT
2nd Foods Dutch Apple	1 jar (4 oz)	100	—	2
2nd Foods Fruit Dessert	1 jar (4 oz)	100	0	0
2nd Foods Hawaiian Delight	1 jar (4 oz)	90	0	0
2nd Foods Mixed Fruit Yogurt Dessert	1 jar (4 oz)	90	0	0
2nd Foods Peach Cobbler	1 jar (4 oz)	90	0	0
2nd Foods Peach Yogurt Dessert	1 jar (4 oz)	90	0	0
2nd Foods Vanilla Custard Pudding	1 jar (4 oz)	100	—	1
3rd Foods Dutch Apple	1 jar (6 oz)	130	—	2
3rd Foods Fruit Dessert	1 jar (6 oz)	120	0	0
3rd Foods Hawaiian Delight	1 jar (6 oz)	150	0	0
3rd Foods Peach Cobbler	1 jar (6 oz)	130	0	0
3rd Foods Vanilla Custard Pudding	1 jar (6 oz)	150	—	2
Tropical Foods Banana Vanilla Dessert	1 jar (4 oz)	100	—	1
Tropical Foods Guava With Tapioca	1 jar (4 oz)	80	0	0
Tropical Foods Mango Banana Passion Fruit	1 jar (4 oz)	80	0	0
Tropical Foods Mango With Tapioca	1 jar (4 oz)	80	0	0
Tropical Foods Papaya Pineapple Dessert	1 jar (4 oz)	90	0	0
Tropical Foods Papaya With Tapioca	1 jar (4 oz)	70	0	0
Tropical Foods Peaches Mango	1 jar (4 oz)	80	0	0
Tropical Foods Pineapple Banana Dessert	1 jar (4 oz)	90	0	0
Tropical Foods Tropical Fruit Medley	1 jar (4 oz)	70	0	0
DINNER				
Beech-Nut				
Stage 2 Beef & Egg Noodle	1 jar (4 oz)	100	—	6
Stage 2 Beef Supreme	1 jar (4 oz)	130	—	9
Stage 2 Chicken & Rice	1 jar (4 oz)	80	—	3

FOOD	PORTION	CALS.	SAT. FAT	FAT
Beech-Nut *(cont.)*				
Stage 2 Chicken Noodle	1 jar (4 oz)	70	—	4
Stage 2 Chicken Soup	1 jar (4 oz)	90	—	4
Stage 2 Turkey Supreme	1 jar (4 oz)	90	—	4
Stage 2 Vegetable Chicken	1 jar (4 oz)	80	—	4
Stage 2 Vegetable Ham	1 jar (4 oz)	80	—	3
Stage 2 Vegetable Lamb	1 jar (4 oz)	80	—	3
Stage 2 Vegetable Beef	1 jar (4 oz)	80	—	4
Stage 3 Beef & Egg Noodle	1 jar (6 oz)	130	—	6
Stage 3 Chicken Noodle	1 jar (6 oz)	110	—	4
Stage 3 Macaroni & Beef	1 jar (6 oz)	130	—	6
Stage 3 Spaghetti & Beef	1 jar (6 oz)	130	—	6
Stage 3 Turkey Rice	1 jar (6 oz)	100	—	3
Stage 3 Vegetable Chicken	1 jar (6 oz)	110	—	4
Stage 3 Vegetable Beef	1 jar (6 oz)	130	—	6
Table Time Chicken & Stars	1 bowl (6 oz)	150	—	6
Table Time Macaroni & Cheese	1 bowl (6 oz)	200	—	12
Table Time Seashells In Tomato Sauce	1 bowl (6 oz)	150	—	4
Table Time Spaghetti Rings In Meat Sauce	1 bowl (6 oz)	160	—	6
Table Time Turkey Stew With Rice	1 bowl (6 oz)	150	—	4
Table Time Vegetable Stew With Beef	1 bowl (6 oz)	110	—	3
Vegetables Stage 2 Turkey Rice	1 jar (4 oz)	70	—	3
Earth's Best				
Corn, Rice & Cheese Dinner	1 jar (4.5 fl oz)	120	—	5
Macaroni & Cheese	1 jar (4.5 oz)	100	—	4
Pasta Dinner	1 jar (4.5 fl oz)	90	—	3
Potato & Green Bean Dinner	1 jar (4.5 fl oz)	100	—	3
Rice & Lentil Dinner	1 jar (4.5 fl oz)	80	—	2
Summer Vegetable Dinner	1 jar (4.5 oz)	90	—	3

FOOD	PORTION	CALS.	SAT. FAT	FAT
Gerber				
2nd Foods Apples & Chicken	1 jar (4 oz)	70	—	2
2nd Foods Apples & Ham	1 jar (4 oz)	70	—	1
2nd Foods Apples & Turkey	1 jar (4 oz)	80	—	2
2nd Foods Beef Egg Noodle	1 jar (4 oz)	80	—	3
2nd Foods Broccoli & Chicken	1 jar (4 oz)	50	—	2
2nd Foods Carrots & Beef	1 jar (4 oz)	70	—	3
2nd Foods Chicken Noodle	1 jar (4 oz)	70	—	2
2nd Foods Green Beans & Turkey	1 jar (4 oz)	70	—	2
2nd Foods Macaroni Cheese	1 jar (4 oz)	80	—	3
2nd Foods Macaroni Tomato Beef	1 jar (4 oz)	70	—	2
2nd Foods Turkey Rice	1 jar (4 oz)	70	—	3
2nd Foods Vegetable Bacon	1 jar (4 oz)	90	—	5
2nd Foods Vegetable Beef	1 jar (4 oz)	70	—	3
2nd Foods Vegetable Chicken	1 jar (4 oz)	70	—	2
2nd Foods Vegetable Ham	1 jar (4 oz)	70	—	3
2nd Foods Vegetable Turkey	1 jar (4 oz)	60	—	2
3rd Foods Beef Egg Noodle	1 jar (6 oz)	110	—	4
3rd Foods Chicken Noodle	1 jar (6 oz)	100	—	3
3rd Foods Macaroni Tomato Beef	1 jar (6 oz)	110	—	2
3rd Foods Spaghetti Tomato Sauce Beef	1 jar (6 oz)	120	—	3
3rd Foods Turkey Rice	1 jar (6 oz)	100	—	3
3rd Foods Vegetable Beef	1 jar (6 oz)	120	—	4
3rd Foods Vegetable Chicken	1 jar (6 oz)	100	—	3

FOOD	PORTION	CALS.	SAT. FAT	FAT
Gerber *(cont.)*				
3rd Foods Vegetable Ham	1 jar (6 oz)	110	—	4
3rd Foods Vegetable Turkey	1 jar (6 oz)	100	—	3
3rd Foods Vegetable Bacon	1 jar (6 oz)	130	—	6
Chunky Homestyle Noodles & Beef	1 jar (6 oz)	150	—	6
Chunky Macaroni Alphabets With Beef & Sauce	1 jar (6.3 oz)	140	—	4
Chunky Noodles & Chicken With Carrots & Peas	1 jar (6 oz)	110	—	3
Chunky Rice With Beef & Tomato Sauce	1 jar (6.3 oz)	140	—	4
Chunky Saucy Rice With Chicken	1 jar (6 oz)	120	—	3
Chunky Spaghetti Tomato Sauce Beef	1 jar (6.3 oz)	150	—	4
Chunky Vegetables & Beef	1 jar (6.3 oz)	130	—	5
Chunky Vegetables & Chicken	1 jar (6.3 oz)	140	—	5
Chunky Vegetables & Ham	1 jar (6.3 oz)	130	—	5
Chunky Vegetables & Turkey	1 jar (6.3 oz)	110	—	3
Graduates Chicken Stew With Noodles	1 bowl (6 oz)	120	—	4
Graduates Macaroni And Beef In Sauce	1 bowl (6 oz)	150	—	4
Graduates Spaghetti With Mini Meatballs & Sauce	1 bowl (6 oz)	160	—	5
Graduates Tomato Sauce With Beef Ravioli	1 bowl (6 oz)	170	—	4
Graduates Tomato Sauce With Cheese Ravioli	1 bowl (6 oz)	170	—	4
Graduates Turkey Stew With Rice	1 bowl (6 oz)	100	—	2

FOOD	PORTION	CALS.	SAT. FAT	FAT
Graduates Vegetable Stew With Beef	1 bowl (6 oz)	130	—	3
Tropical Foods Beans & Rice	1 jar (4 oz)	60	—	2
Tropical Foods Chicken & Rice	1 jar (4 oz)	60	—	2
FRUIT				
Beech-Nut				
Stage 1 Applesauce Golden Delicious	1 jar (2.5 oz)	50	0	0
Stage 1 Applesauce Golden Delicious	1 jar (4 oz)	70	0	0
Stage 1 Bananas Chiquita	1 jar (2.5 oz)	70	0	0
Stage 1 Bananas Chiquita	1 jar (4 oz)	110	0	0
Stage 1 Chiquita Bananas With Pears & Apples	1 jar (4 oz)	90	0	0
Stage 1 Peaches Yellow Cling	1 jar (2.5 oz)	45	0	0
Stage 1 Peaches Yellow Cling	1 jar (4 oz)	70	0	0
Stage 1 Pears Bartlett	1 jar (2.5 oz)	50	0	0
Stage 1 Pears Bartlett	1 jar (4 oz)	70	0	0
Stage 2 Apples & Apricots	1 jar (4 oz)	70	0	0
Stage 2 Apples & Bananas	1 jar (4 oz)	60	0	0
Stage 2 Apples & Blueberries	1 jar (4 oz)	70	0	0
Stage 2 Apples & Cherries	1 jar (4 oz)	80	0	0
Stage 2 Apples & Pears	1 jar (4 oz)	80	0	0
Stage 2 Apples, Pears & Bananas	1 jar (4 oz)	90	0	0
Stage 2 Apricots With Pears & Apples	1 jar (4 oz)	90	0	0
Stage 2 Bartlett Pears & Pineapple	1 jar (4 oz)	70	0	0
Stage 2 Peaches & Bananas	1 jar (4 oz)	70	0	0
Stage 2 Plums With Apples & Rice	1 jar (4 oz)	90	0	0

FOOD	PORTION	CALS.	SAT. FAT	FAT
Beech-Nut *(cont.)*				
Stage 2 Prunes With Pears	1 jar (4 oz)	110	0	0
Stage 3 Apples & Bananas	1 jar (6 oz)	90	0	0
Stage 3 Apples & Cherries	1 jar (6 oz)	110	0	0
Stage 3 Applesauce	1 jar (6 oz)	100	0	0
Stage 3 Apricots With Pears & Apples	1 jar (6 oz)	130	0	0
Stage 3 Bananas Chiquita	1 jar (6 oz)	160	0	0
Stage 3 Peaches	1 jar (6 oz)	100	0	0
Stage 3 Pears Bartlett	1 jar (6 oz)	110	0	0
Earth's Best				
Apples	1 jar (4.5 oz)	70	0	0
Apples & Apricots	1 jar (4.5 fl oz)	70	—	0
Apples & Blueberries	1 jar (4.5 fl oz)	70	—	0
Apples & Plums	1 jar (4.5 fl oz)	70	—	0
Bananas	1 jar (4.5 oz)	90	0	0
Pear	1 jar (4.5 fl oz)	60	—	0
Plums, Bananas & Rice	1 jar (4.5 fl oz)	90	—	1
Gerber				
1st Foods Applesauce	1 jar (2.5 oz)	25	0	0
1st Foods Bananas	1 jar (2.5 oz)	70	0	0
1st Foods Peaches	1 jar (2.5 oz)	30	0	0
1st Foods Pears	1 jar (2.5 oz)	40	0	0
1st Foods Prunes	1 jar (2.5 oz)	70	0	0
2nd Foods Apple Blueberry	1 jar (4 oz)	50	0	0
2nd Foods Applesauce	1 jar (4 oz)	60	0	0
2nd Foods Applesauce Apricot	1 jar (4 oz)	60	0	0
2nd Foods Apricots With Tapioca	1 jar (4 oz)	80	0	0
2nd Foods Banana With Pineapple And Tapioca	1 jar (4 oz)	60	0	0
2nd Foods Banana With Tapioca	1 jar (4 oz)	90	0	0
2nd Foods Peaches	1 jar (4 oz)	70	0	0
2nd Foods Pear Pineapple	1 jar (4 oz)	60	0	0
2nd Foods Pears	1 jar (4 oz)	60	0	0

FOOD	PORTION	CALS.	SAT. FAT	FAT
2nd Foods Plums With Tapioca	1 jar (4 oz)	80	0	0
2nd Foods Prunes With Tapioca	1 jar (4 oz)	90	0	0
JUICE				
Beech-Nut				
Stage 1 Apple	4 fl oz	60	0	0
Stage 1 Pear	4 fl oz	60	0	0
Stage 1 White Grape	4 fl oz	100	0	0
Stage 2 Apple Banana	4 fl oz	70	0	0
Stage 2 Apple Cherry	4 fl oz	70	0	0
Stage 2 Apple Cranberry	4 fl oz	60	0	0
Stage 2 Apple Grape	4 fl oz	70	0	0
Stage 2 Juice Plus Grape	4 fl oz	100	0	0
Stage 2 Mango Nectar (Spanish label)	4 fl oz	80	0	0
Stage 2 Mixed Fruit	4 fl oz	70	0	0
Stage 2 Papaya Nectar (Spanish label)	4 fl oz	80	0	0
Stage 2 Tropical Blend	4 fl oz	90	0	0
Stage 2 Tropical Blend Nectar (Spanish label)	4 fl oz	90	0	0
Stage 3 Orange	4 fl oz	60	0	0
Earth's Best				
Apple	1 bottle (4.2 fl oz)	60	—	0
Apple Banana	1 bottle (4.2 fl oz)	60	—	0
Apple Grape	1 bottle (4.2 fl oz)	60	0	0
Apples & Bananas	1 jar (4.5 fl oz)	80	0	0
Pear	1 bottle (4.2 fl oz)	60	—	0
Gerber				
1st Foods Apple	4 fl oz	60	0	0
1st Foods Pear	4 fl oz	60	0	0
1st Foods Red Grape	4 fl oz	80	0	0
1st Foods White Grape	4 fl oz	80	0	0
2nd Foods Apple Banana	4 fl oz	60	0	0
2nd Foods Apple Cherry	4 fl oz	60	0	0
2nd Foods Apple Grape	4 fl oz	60	0	0
2nd Foods Apple Peach	4 fl oz	60	0	0
2nd Foods Apple Plum	4 fl oz	60	0	0
2nd Foods Apple Prune	4 fl oz	60	0	0
2nd Foods Apple With Yogurt	4 fl oz	100	—	2
2nd Foods Banana With Yogurt	4 fl oz	110	—	2

FOOD	PORTION	CALS.	SAT. FAT	FAT
Gerber *(cont.)*				
2nd Foods Mixed Fruit	4 fl oz	60	0	0
2nd Foods Mixed Fruit With Yogurt	4 fl oz	100	—	2
2nd Foods Orange	4 fl oz	60	0	0
2nd Foods Pear Peach With Yogurt	4 fl oz	90	—	1
3rd Foods Apple Carrot	4 fl oz	50	0	0
3rd Foods Apple Sweet Potato	4 fl oz	60	0	0
3rd Foods Orange Carrot	4 fl oz	50	0	0
3rd Foods Pineapple Carrot	4 fl oz	60	0	0
Graduates Apple	4 fl oz	80	0	0
Graduates Apple Banana	4 fl oz	90	0	0
Graduates Apple Cherry	4 fl oz	80	0	0
Graduates Apple Grape	4 fl oz	90	0	0
Tropical Foods Guava With Mixed Fruit	4 fl oz	70	0	0
Tropical Foods Mango With Mixed Fruit	4 fl oz	70	0	0
Tropical Foods Papaya With Mixed Fruit	4 fl oz	70	0	0
MEAT				
Beech-Nut				
Stage 1 Beef And Broth	1 jar (2.5 oz)	90	—	6
Stage 1 Chicken And Broth	1 jar (2.5 oz)	70	—	3
Stage 1 Lamb And Broth	1 jar (2.5 oz)	60	—	3
Stage 1 Turkey And Broth	1 jar (2.5 oz)	90	—	6
Stage 1 Veal And Broth	1 jar (2.5 oz)	60	—	2
Gerber				
2nd Foods Beef	1 jar (2.5 oz)	80	—	4
2nd Foods Chicken	1 jar (2.5 oz)	90	—	6
2nd Foods Egg Yolks	1 jar (2.5 oz)	130	—	11
2nd Foods Ham	1 jar (2.5 oz)	90	—	6
2nd Foods Lamb	1 jar (2.5 oz)	80	—	4
2nd Foods Turkey	1 jar (2.5 oz)	80	—	5
2nd Foods Veal	1 jar (2.5 oz)	70	—	4
3rd Foods Beef	1 jar (2.5 oz)	80	—	4
3rd Foods Chicken	1 jar (2.5 oz)	90	—	6

FOOD	PORTION	CALS.	SAT. FAT	FAT
3rd Foods Ham	1 jar (2.5 oz)	90	—	6
3rd Foods Turkey	1 jar (2.5 oz)	90	—	5
3rd Foods Veal	1 jar (2.5 oz)	80	—	4
Graduates Chicken Sticks	1 jar (2.5 oz)	110	—	7
Graduates Meat Sticks	1 jar (2.5 oz)	110	—	7
Graduates Turkey Sticks	1 jar (2.5 oz)	120	—	8
STRAINED DINNERS				
Chicken & Rice w/ Vegetables (Beech-Nut)	4.5 oz	80	—	3
Chicken Noodle w/ Vegetables (Beech-Nut)	4.5 oz	90	—	3
STRAINED MEATS AND EGG YOLKS				
Veal (Beech-Nut)	2.8 oz	100	—	7
VEGETABLE				
Beech-Nut				
Stage 1 Butternut Squash	1 jar (2.5 oz)	30	0	0
Stage 1 Butternut Squash	1 jar (4 oz)	50	0	0
Stage 1 Carrots Sweet Tender	1 jar (4 oz)	50	0	0
Stage 1 Carrots Tender Sweet	1 jar (2.5 oz)	30	0	0
Stage 1 Green Beans (Spanish label)	1 jar (2.5 oz)	20	0	0
Stage 1 Green Beans Tender Young	1 jar (4 oz)	35	0	0
Stage 1 Peas Tender Sweet	1 jar (2.5 oz)	40	0	0
Stage 1 Peas Tender Sweet	1 jar (4 oz)	60	0	0
Stage 1 Sweet Potatoes Tender Golden	1 jar (2.5 oz)	50	0	0
Stage 1 Sweet Potatoes Tender Golden	1 jar (4 oz)	80	0	0
Stage 2 Carrots & Peas	1 jar (4 oz)	50	0	0
Stage 2 Creamed Corn	1 jar (4 oz)	90	0	0
Stage 2 Garden Vegetables	1 jar (4 oz)	50	0	0
Stage 2 Mixed Vegetables	1 jar (4 oz)	45	0	0
Stage 3 Carrots	1 jar (6 oz)	70	0	0
Stage 3 Green Beans	1 jar (6 oz)	50	0	0
Stage 3 Sweet Potatoes	1 jar (6 oz)	110	0	0

FOOD	PORTION	CALS.	SAT. FAT	FAT
Earth's Best				
Carrots	1 jar (4.5 fl oz)	40	—	0
Carrots & Parsnips	1 jar (4.5 fl oz)	60	—	0
Corn & Butternut Squash	1 jar (4.5 fl oz)	90	—	2
Garden Vegetables	1 jar (4.5 fl oz)	70	—	0
Green Beans & Rice	1 jar (4.5 fl oz)	40	—	1
Peas & Brown Rice	1 jar (4.5 fl oz)	80	—	0
Spinach & Potatoes	1 jar (4.5 fl oz)	60	—	2
Sweet Potatoes	1 jar (4.5 fl oz)	60	—	1
Winter Squash	1 jar (4.5 fl oz)	50	—	0
Gerber				
1st Foods Carrots	1 jar (2.5 oz)	25	0	0
1st Foods Green Beans	1 jar (2.5 oz)	25	0	0
1st Foods Peas	1 jar (2.5 oz)	30	0	0
1st Foods Squash	1 jar (2.5 oz)	25	0	0
1st Foods Sweet Potatoes	1 jar (2.5 oz)	45	0	0
2nd Foods Beets	1 jar (4 oz)	45	0	0
2nd Foods Carrots	1 jar (4 oz)	30	0	0
2nd Foods Creamed Corn	1 jar (4 oz)	80	—	1
2nd Foods Creamed Spinach	1 jar (4 oz)	50	—	1
2nd Foods Garden Vegetables	1 jar (4 oz)	45	—	1
2nd Foods Green Beans	1 jar (4 oz)	35	—	0
2nd Foods Mixed Vegetables	1 jar (4 oz)	50	—	1
2nd Foods Peas	1 jar (4 oz)	60	—	1
2nd Foods Squash	1 jar (4 oz)	35	0	0
2nd Foods Sweet Potatoes	1 jar (4 oz)	70	0	0
3rd Foods Broccoli Carrots Cheese	1 jar (6 oz)	80	—	2
3rd Foods Carrots	1 jar (6 oz)	50	0	0
3rd Foods Creamed Green Beans	1 jar (6 oz)	80	—	1
3rd Foods Mixed Vegetables	1 jar (6 oz)	70	0	0
3rd Foods Peas	1 jar (6 oz)	80	—	1
3rd Foods Squash	1 jar (6 oz)	60	—	1
3rd Foods Sweet Potatoes	1 jar (6 oz)	100	0	0
Graduates Carrots	1 jar (4.5 oz)	30	0	0

FOOD	PORTION	CALS.	SAT. FAT	FAT
Graduates Green Beans	1 jar (4.5 oz)	30	0	0
Graduates Peas	1 jar (4.5 oz)	60	0	0
Graduates Potatoes	1 jar (4.5 oz)	50	0	0

BACON
(*see also* BACON SUBSTITUTES)

Armour Lower Salt, cooked	1 strip	38	—	3
Armour Star, cooked	1 strip	38	—	3
Black Label, cooked	2 slices (0.5 oz)	80	3	7
Black Label Center Cut, cooked	3 slices (0.5 oz)	70	3	6
Black Label Low Salt, cooked	2 slices (0.5 oz)	80	3	7
Hillshire	1 slice	120	—	12
Hormel Bacon Bits	1 tsp (7 g)	30	1	2
Hormel Bacon Pieces	1 tsp (7 g)	25	1	2
Hormel Microwave, cooked	2 slices (0.5 oz)	70	2	5
Jones Sliced	1 slice	130	—	13
Nathan's Beef, cooked	3 slices	100	—	7
Old Smokehouse, cooked	2 slices (0.5 oz)	80	3	7
Oscar Mayer Bacon Bits	1 tbsp (7 g)	25	1	2
Oscar Mayer Center Cut, cooked	3 slices (0.5 oz)	70	2	6
Oscar Mayer, cooked	2 slices (0.4 oz)	60	2	5
Oscar Mayer Lower Sodium, cooked	2 slices (0.5 oz)	60	2	5
Oscar Mayer Thick Cut, cooked	1 slice (0.4 oz)	50	2	4
Range Brand, cooked	2 slices (0.7 oz)	100	4	9
Red Label, cooked	2 slices (0.5 oz)	80	3	7
breakfast strips, beef, cooked	3 strips (34 g)	153	5	12
breakfast strips, cooked	3 strips (34 g)	156	—	12
cooked	3 strips	109	3	9
gammon, lean & fat, grilled	4.2 oz	274	—	15
grilled	2 slices (1.7 oz)	86	—	4

BACON SUBSTITUTES

Bac'n Pieces McCormick	2 tsp	20	—	tr
Bac-Os	2 tsp (5 g)	25	—	1
Harvest Direct Bacon Style Bits	3.5 oz	320	2	15
Lightlife Fakin' Bacon	3 strips (2 oz)	79	tr	3

FOOD	PORTION	CALS.	SAT. FAT	FAT
Louis Rich Turkey Bacon	1 slice (0.5 oz)	30	1	3
Morningstar Farms Breakfast Strips	3 (25 g)	80	—	6
Stripples Worthington	4 strips (33 g)	120	—	9
bacon substitute	1 strip	25	—	2

BAGEL
FRESH

FOOD	PORTION	CALS.	SAT. FAT	FAT
cinnamon raisin	1 (3½ in)	194	tr	1
cinnamon raisin, toasted	1 (3½ in)	194	tr	1
egg	1 (3½ in)	197	tr	2
egg, toasted	1 (3½ in)	197	tr	2
oat bran	1 (3½ in)	181	tr	1
oat bran, toasted	1 (3½ in)	181	tr	1
onion	1 (3½ in)	195	tr	1
plain	1 (3½ in)	195	tr	1
plain, toasted	1 (3½ in)	195	tr	1
poppy seed	1 (3½ in)	195	tr	1

FROZEN

FOOD	PORTION	CALS.	SAT. FAT	FAT
Bagel Sandwich Ham And Cheese (Weight Watchers)	1 (3 oz)	210	2	6
Cinnamon & Raisin (Sara Lee)	1 (3 oz)	240	—	2
Cinnamon Raisin (Sara Lee)	1 (2.5 oz)	200	—	2
Cinnamon 'N Raisin (Lender's)	1 (2.5 oz)	200	—	1
Egg (Lender's)	1 (2 oz)	150	—	1
Egg (Sara Lee)	1 (2.5 oz)	200	—	2
Egg (Sara Lee)	1 (3 oz)	250	—	2
Ham & Cheese On A Bagel (Great Starts)	3 oz	240	—	8
Oat Bran (Sara Lee)	1 (2.5 oz)	180	—	1
Oat Bran (Sara Lee)	1 (3 oz)	220	—	1
Onion (Lender's)	1 (2 oz)	160	—	1
Onion (Sara Lee)	1 (2.5 oz)	190	—	1
Onion (Sara Lee)	1 (3 oz)	230	—	1
Plain (Lender's)	1 (2 oz)	150	—	1
Plain (Sara Lee)	1 (2.5 oz)	190	—	1
Plain (Sara Lee)	1 (3 oz)	230	—	1
Poppy Seed (Sara Lee)	1 (2.5 oz)	190	—	1
Poppy Seed (Sara Lee)	1 (3 oz)	230	—	1
Sesame Seed (Sara Lee)	1 (2.5 oz)	190	—	1
Sesame Seed (Sara Lee)	1 (3 oz)	240	—	2

FOOD	PORTION	CALS.	SAT. FAT	FAT

BAKING POWDER
Calumet	1 tsp	3	—	tr
Clabber Girl	1 tsp	0	0	0
Davis	1 tsp	6	0	0
baking powder	1 tsp	5	0	0
low sodium	1 tsp	5	0	0

BAKING SODA
Arm & Hammer	1 tsp	0	0	0
baking soda	1 tsp	0	0	0

BALSAM PEAR
leafy tips, cooked	½ cup	10	—	tr
leafy tips, raw	½ cup	7	—	tr
pods, cooked	½ cup	12	—	tr

BAMBOO SHOOTS
CANNED
Empress Sliced	2 oz	14	0	0
La Choy	¼ cup	6	tr	tr
sliced	1 cup	25	tr	1

FRESH
cooked	½ cup	15	tr	tr
raw	½ cup	21	tr	tr

BANANA
DRIED
powder	1 tbsp	21	tr	tr

FRESH
Chiquita	1 (3.5 oz)	110	—	0
Dole	1	120	—	1
banana	1	105	tr	tr
mashed	1 cup	207	tr	1

JUICE
Libby's Nectar	6 oz	110	0	0

BARLEY
Arrowhead	¼ cup (1.7 oz)	170	0	1
Arrowhead Hulless	¼ cup (1.6 oz)	140	0	1
Quaker Medium Pearled	¼ cup	172	—	1
Quaker Quick Pearled	¼ cup	172	—	1
Scotch Medium Pearled	¼ cup	172	—	1
Scotch Quick Pearled	¼ cup	172	—	1
pearled, cooked	½ cup	97	tr	tr
pearled, uncooked	½ cup	352	tr	1

FOOD	PORTION	CALS.	SAT. FAT	FAT
BASIL				
fresh, chopped	2 tbsp	1	tr	tr
ground	1 tsp	4	—	tr
leaves, fresh	5	1	tr	tr
BASS				
FRESH				
freshwater, raw	3 oz	97	1	3
sea, cooked	3 oz	105	1	2
sea, raw	3 oz	82	tr	2
striped, baked	3 oz	105	1	3
BAY LEAF				
crumbled	1 tsp	2	tr	tr
BEAN SPROUTS				
(see also individual bean names)				
CANNED				
La Choy	⅔ cup	8	tr	tr
BEANS				
(see also individual names)				
CANNED				
Baked (Allen)	½ cup (4.5 oz)	150	1	1
Baked Beans (Brick Oven)	½ cup	160	—	2
Baked Beans Fat Free (Van Camp's)	½ cup	130	0	0
Baked Beans Premium (Van Camp's)	½ cup (4.6 oz)	140	0	1
Barbecue Beans (Campbell)	½ can (7.88 oz)	210	—	4
Barbecue Beans Texas Style (S&W)	½ cup	135	—	1
Barbeque Baked Beans (B&M)	⅞ cup	310	—	6
Beanee Weenee (Van Camp's)	1 cup (9 oz)	320	4	14
Beanee Weenee Baked Flavor (Van Camp's)	1 cup (9 oz)	410	4	14
Beanee Weenee Barbeque (Van Camp's)	1 cup (9 oz)	340	4	14
Beans & Wieners (Hormel)	1 can (7.5 oz)	290	4	13
Big John's Beans 'n Fixin's (Hunt's)	4 oz	170	1	6
Boston Baked (Health Valley)	7.5 oz	190	—	tr

FOOD	PORTION	CALS.	SAT. FAT	FAT
Boston Baked No Salt Added (Health Valley)	7.5 oz	190	—	tr
Brown Sugar Beans (Van Camp's)	½ cup (4.6 oz)	170	1	3
Chili (Gebhardt)	4 oz	115	tr	1
Cut Green & Shelled Beans Seasoned w/ Pork (Luck's)	7.25 oz	200	—	6
Fast Menu Honey Baked Organic Beans w/ Tofu Weiner (Health Valley)	7.5 oz	150	—	4
Four Bean Salad (Hanover)	½ cup	80	—	0
Home Style Beans (Campbell)	½ can (8 oz)	220	—	4
Honey Baked (B&M)	8 oz	4	—	4
Hot Chili Beans (Campbell)	½ can (7.75 oz)	180	—	4
Hot N Spicy Baked (B&M)	8 oz	240	1	3
Kid's Kitchen Beans & Weiners (Hormel)	1 cup (7.5 oz)	310	5	13
Maple Baked (B&M)	8 oz	240	1	2
Maple Baked (Friends)	8 oz	240	1	2
Maple Sugar Beans (S&W)	½ cup	150	—	1
Mexe-Beans (Old El Paso)	½ cup	163	0	1
Mexi-Beans With Jalapeno (Trappey)	½ cup (4.5 oz)	130	1	2
Mexican Beans With Jalapeno (Brown Beauty)	½ cup (4.5 oz)	120	0	1
Mexican Style Chili Beans (Van Camp's)	½ cup	110	1	2
Mixed Bean Salad Marinated (S&W)	½ cup	90	—	1
Mixed Beans Seasoned w/ Pork (Luck's)	7.25 oz	200	—	5
Old Fashioned Beans in Molasses & Brown Sugar Sauce (Campbell)	½ can (8 oz)	230	—	3
Pork & Beans in Tomato Sauce (Campbell)	½ can (8 oz)	200	—	3
Pork And Beans (Crest Top)	½ cup (4.5 oz)	130	1	1
Pork And Beans (Hunt's)	4 oz	135	tr	1
Pork And Beans (Trappey)	½ cup (4.5 oz)	110	1	1
Pork And Beans (Van Camp's)	½ cup	110	1	2
Pork And Beans (Wagon Master)	½ cup (4.5 oz)	110	1	1

FOOD	PORTION	CALS.	SAT. FAT	FAT
Pork And Beans in Tomato Sauce (Green Giant)	½ cup	90	—	1
Pork And Beans With Jalapeno (Trappey)	½ cup (4.5 oz)	130	1	2
Pork 'N Beans (S&W)	½ cup	130	—	2
Ranchero Beans (Chi-Chi's)	½ cup (4.3 oz)	100	0	1
Refried (Casa Fiesta)	3.5 oz	110	—	2
Refried (Chi-Chi's)	½ cup (4.2 oz)	130	1	6
Refried (Gebhardt)	4 oz	100	1	2
Refried (Old El Paso)	¼ cup	55	—	tr
Refried (Rosarita)	4 oz	100	1	2
Refried Potatoes (Allen)	½ cup (4.5 oz)	150	1	3
Refried Spicy (Old El Paso)	¼ cup	35	0	1
Refried Vegetarian (Old El Paso)	¼ cup	70	—	1
Refried Vegetarian (Rosarita)	4 oz	100	1	2
Refried With Cheese (Old El Paso)	¼ cup	36	1	1
Refried With Green Chilies (Old El Paso)	¼ cup	49	—	tr
Refried With Sausages (Old El Paso)	¼ cup	180	—	8
Refried & Green Chili (Little Pancho)	½ cup	80	0	0
Refried Jalapeno (Gebhardt)	4 oz	115	—	2
Refried Spicy (Rosarita)	4 oz	100	1	2
Refried With Bacon (Rosarita)	4 oz	110	1	2
Refried With Green Chilies (Rosarita)	4 oz	90	1	2
Refried With Nacho Cheese (Rosarita)	4 oz	110	1	2
Refried With Onions (Rosarita)	4 oz	110	1	2
Smokey Ranch (S&W)	½ cup	130	—	2
Spicy (McIlhenny)	1 oz	7	tr	tr
Three Bean Salad (Green Giant)	½ cup	70	0	tr
Tomato Baked Beans (B&M)	8 oz	230	1	3

FOOD	PORTION	CALS.	SAT. FAT	FAT
Vegetarian (Campbell)	½ cup (7.75 oz)	170	—	1
Vegetarian Baked Beans (B&M)	8 oz	230	—	3
Vegetarian in Tomato Sauce (Van Camp's)	½ cup (4.6 oz)	110	0	1
Vegetarian w/ Miso (Health Valley)	7.5 oz	180	—	1
baked beans, plain	½ cup	118	tr	1
baked beans, vegetarian	½ cup	118	tr	1
baked beans w/ beef	½ cup	161	2	5
baked beans w/ franks	½ cup	182	3	8
baked beans w/ pork	½ cup	133	1	2
baked beans w/ pork & sweet sauce	½ cup	140	1	2
baked beans w/ pork & tomato sauce	½ cup	123	1	1
refried beans	½ cup	134	1	1
DRIED				
Bean Cuisine Black Turtle	½ cup	115	—	1
FROZEN				
Romano Bean Medley (Hanover)	½ cup	25	—	0
MIX				
Florentine Beans With Bow Ties (Bean Cuisine)	½ cup	199	2	7
Pasta & Beans Country French With Gemelli (Bean Cuisine)	½ cup	214	1	8
TAKE-OUT				
baked beans	½ cup	190	2	6
barbecue beans	3.5 oz	120	tr	tr
four bean salad	3.5 oz	100	tr	tr
refried beans	½ cup	43	1	2
three bean salad	¾ cup	230	1	11
BEAR				
simmered	3 oz	220	—	11
BEAVER				
roasted	3 oz	140	—	6
simmered	3 oz	141	—	5
BEECHNUTS				
dried	1 oz	164	2	14

FOOD	PORTION	CALS.	SAT. FAT	FAT

BEEF

(*see also* BEEF DISHES, VEAL)

Beef is graded according to its marbling, the little flecks of fat in the muscle. Beef graded "Prime" has the highest percentage of fat, followed by "Choice" with less fat and "Select" with the least fat.

CANNED

FOOD	PORTION	CALS.	SAT. FAT	FAT
Corned Beef (Hormel)	2 oz	120	3	7
Corned Beef Hash (Hormel)	1 cup (8.3 oz)	390	10	24
Corned Beef Hash (Mary Kitchen)	1 can (7.5 oz)	350	9	22
Potted Meat (Hormel)	4 tbsp (2 oz)	60	3	7
Roast Beef (Underwood)	2.08 oz	140	5	11
Roast Beef Mesquite Smoked (Underwood)	2.08 oz	126	5	11
Roast Beef Hash (Hormel)	1 cup (8.3 oz)	390	10	24
Roast Beef Hash (Mary Kitchen)	1 can (7.5 oz)	348	9	21
Roast Beef Light (Underwood)	2.08 oz	90	2	6
corned beef	1 oz	71	—	4
corned beef	3 oz	85	4	5
corned beef hash	3 oz	155	5	10

DRIED

FOOD	PORTION	CALS.	SAT. FAT	FAT
Hormel Pillow Pack	10 slices (1 oz)	45	1	1
Hormel Sliced	10 slices (1 oz)	50	1	2

FRESH

Note that values for cooked beef may differ slightly from values for raw beef. When meat is cooked some moisture and fat are lost, changing the nutritional value slightly. As a rule of thumb it can be assumed that a 4-ounce raw portion will equal a 3-ounce cooked portion of meat.

FOOD	PORTION	CALS.	SAT. FAT	FAT
Chuck Roast, raw (Dakota Lean)	3 oz	80	—	2
Eye Round, raw (Dakota Lean)	3 oz	80	—	2
Filet (Double J)	3.5 oz	130	3	4
Flank Steak, raw (Dakota Lean)	3 oz	80	—	1
Ground, raw (Dakota Lean)	3 oz	88	—	2
NY Strip (Double J)	3.5 oz	133	3	4

FOOD	PORTION	CALS.	SAT. FAT	FAT
Outside Round, raw (Dakota Lean)	3 oz	80	—	1
Rib Eye (Double J)	3.5 oz	134	3	5
Ribeye, raw (Dakota Lean)	3 oz	90	—	2
Sirloin Tip, raw (Dakota Lean)	3 oz	90	—	3
Strip Loin, raw (Dakota Lean)	3 oz	90	—	2
Tenderloin, raw (Dakota Lean)	3 oz	70	—	1
Top Butt (Double J)	3.5 oz	136	3	5
Top Round, raw (Dakota Lean)	3 oz	80	—	1
bottom round, lean & fat				
trim 0″, Choice, roasted	3 oz	172	3	8
trim 0″, Select, braised	3 oz	171	2	6
trim 0″, Select, roasted	3 oz	150	2	24
trim 0″, braised	3 oz	193	3	26
trim ¼″, Choice, braised	3 oz	241	6	15
trim ¼″, Choice, roasted	3 oz	221	5	14
trim ¼″, Select, braised	3 oz	220	5	13
trim ¼″, Select, roasted	3 oz	199	4	11
brisket, lean & fat				
flat half, trim 0″, braised	3 oz	183	3	8
flat half, trim ¼″, braised	3 oz	309	9	24
point half, trim 0″, braised	3 oz	304	10	24
point half, trim ¼″, braised	3 oz	343	12	29
whole, trim 0″, braised	3 oz	247	6	17
whole, trim ¼″, braised	3 oz	327	11	27
chuck arm pot roast, lean & fat, trim 0″, braised	3 oz	238	6	14
chuck arm pot roast, lean & fat, trim ¼″, braised	3 oz	282	8	20
chuck blade roast, lean & fat, trim 0″, braised	3 oz	284	8	21
chuck blade roast, lean & fat, trim ¼″, braised	3 oz	293	9	22
corned beef brisket, cooked	3 oz	213	5	16

FOOD	PORTION	CALS.	SAT. FAT	FAT
eye of round, lean & fat				
trim 0″, Choice, roasted	3 oz	153	8	5
trim 0″, Select, roasted	3 oz	137	1	4
trim ¼″, Choice, roasted	3 oz	205	5	12
trim ¼″, Select, roasted	3 oz	184	4	10
flank, lean & fat, trim 0″, braised	3 oz	224	6	14
flank, lean & fat, trim 0″, broiled	3 oz	192	5	11
ground				
extra lean, broiled medium	3 oz	217	5	14
extra lean, broiled well done	3 oz	225	5	14
extra lean, fried medium	3 oz	216	5	14
extra lean, fried well done	3 oz	224	5	14
extra lean, raw	4 oz	265	8	19
lean, broiled medium	3 oz	231	6	16
lean, broiled well done	3 oz	238	6	15
low-fat w/ carrageenan, raw	4 oz	160	4	7
regular, broiled medium	3 oz	246	7	18
regular, broiled well done	3 oz	248	7	17
porterhouse steak, lean & fat, trim ¼″, Choice, broiled	3 oz	260	8	19
porterhouse steak, lean only, trim ¼″, Choice, broiled	3 oz	185	4	9
rib eye, small end, lean & fat, trim 0″, Choice, broiled	3 oz	261	8	19
rib, lean & fat				
large end, trim 0″, roasted	3 oz	300	10	24
large end, trim ¼″, broiled	3 oz	295	10	24
large end, trim ¼″, roasted	3 oz	310	10	25
small end, trim 0″, broiled	3 oz	252	7	18
small end, trim ¼″, broiled	3 oz	285	9	22

FOOD	PORTION	CALS.	SAT. FAT	FAT
small end, trim ¼", roasted	3 oz	295	10	24
whole, trim ¼", Choice, broiled	3 oz	306	10	25
whole, trim ¼", Choice, roasted	3 oz	320	11	27
whole, trim ¼", Prime, roasted	3 oz	348	12	30
whole, trim ¼", Select, broiled	3 oz	274	9	21
whole, trim ¼", Select, roasted	3 oz	286	9	23
shank crosscut, lean & fat, trim ¼", Choice, simmered	3 oz	224	5	12
short loin top loin				
lean & fat, trim 0", Choice, broiled	1 steak (5.4 oz)	353	7	19
lean & fat, trim 0", Choice, broiled	3 oz	193	4	10
lean & fat, trim 0", Select, broiled	1 steak (5.4 oz)	309	5	14
lean & fat, trim ¼", Choice, broiled	1 steak (6.3 oz)	536	15	38
lean & fat, trim ¼", Choice, broiled	3 oz	253	7	18
lean & fat, trim ¼", Prime, broiled	1 steak (6.3 oz)	582	17	43
lean & fat, trim ¼", Select, broiled	1 steak (6.3 oz)	473	12	31
lean only, trim 0", Choice, broiled	1 steak (5.2 oz)	311	5	14
lean only, trim ¼", Choice, broiled	1 steak (5.2 oz)	314	6	15
shortribs, lean & fat, Choice, braised	3 oz	400	15	36
t-bone steak, lean & fat, trim ¼", Choice, broiled	3 oz	253	7	18
t-bone steak, lean only, trim ¼", Choice, broiled	3 oz	182	4	9
tenderloin				
lean & fat, trim 0", Choice, broiled	3 oz	208	5	12
lean & fat, trim 0", Select, broiled	3 oz	194	4	11

FOOD	PORTION	CALS.	SAT. FAT	FAT
tenderloin *(cont.)*				
lean & fat, trim ¼", Choice, broiled	3 oz	259	7	19
lean & fat, trim ¼", Choice, roasted	3 oz	288	9	22
lean & fat, trim ¼", Prime, broiled	3 oz	270	8	20
lean & fat, trim ¼", Select, roasted	3 oz	275	8	21
lean only, trim 0", Select, broiled	3 oz	170	3	7
lean only, trim ¼", Choice, broiled	3 oz	188	4	10
lean only, trim ¼", Select, broiled	3 oz	169	3	7
tip round, lean & fat				
trim 0", Choice, roasted	3 oz	170	3	8
trim 0", Select, roasted	3 oz	158	2	6
trim ¼", Choice, roasted	3 oz	210	5	13
trim ¼", Prime, roasted	3 oz	233	6	15
trim ¼", Select, roasted	3 oz	191	4	10
top round, lean & fat				
trim 0", Choice, braised	3 oz	184	2	6
trim 0", Select, braised	3 oz	170	2	5
trim ¼", Choice, braised	3 oz	221	4	11
trim ¼", Choice, broiled	3 oz	190	3	9
trim ¼", Choice, fried	3 oz	235	5	13
trim ¼", Prime, broiled	3 oz	195	3	9
trim ¼", Select, braised	3 oz	199	3	8
trim ¼", Select, broiled	3 oz	175	3	7
top sirloin, lean & fat				
trim 0", Choice, broiled	3 oz	194	4	10
trim 0", Select, broiled	3 0z	166	3	6
trim ¼", Choice, broiled	3 oz	228	6	14
trim ¼", Choice, fried	3 oz	277	8	19
trim ¼", Select, broiled	3 oz	208	5	12
tripe, raw	4 oz	111	2	4
FROZEN				
patties, broiled medium	3 oz	240	7	17
READY-TO-USE				
Deli-Thin Roast Beef (Oscar Mayer)	4 slices (1.8 oz)	60	1	2
Roast Beef (Healthy Choice)	1.9 oz	60	1	2

FOOD	PORTION	CALS.	SAT. FAT	FAT
Weight Watchers Oven Roasted Cured Deli Thin	5 slices (⅓ oz)	10	—	tr

BEEF DISHES
CANNED

FOOD	PORTION	CALS.	SAT. FAT	FAT
Beef Stew (Wolf Brand)	1 cup	179	—	8
Dinty Moore				
American Classics Beef Stew	1 bowl (10 oz)	260	6	13
American Classics Meatloaf With Mashed Potatoes	1 bowl (10 oz)	300	5	13
American Classics Roast Beef With Mashed Potatoes	1 bowl (10 oz)	240	2	5
American Classics Salisbury Steak	1 bowl (10 oz)	310	6	14
Beef Stew	1 can (7.5 oz)	190	4	10
Beef Stew	1 cup (8.3 oz)	230	7	14
Meatball Stew	1 cup (8.4 oz)	260	7	16
Microwave Cup Beef Stew	1 cup (7.5 oz)	190	4	10
Microwave Cup Corned Beef Hash	1 cup (7.5 oz)	350	9	22
Microwave Cup Hearty Burger Stew	1 cup (7.5 oz)	240	5	13
Microwave Cup Meatball Stew	1 cup (7.5 oz)	240	7	15
Sliced Potatoes & Beef	1 can (7.5 oz)	230	4	9
Hormel				
Beef Goulash	1 can (7.5 oz)	230	5	11
Micro Cup Meals Beef Stew	1 cup (7.5 oz)	180	4	9
Roast Beef With Gravy	2 oz	60	1	2
Manwich Mexican, as prep	1 sandwich	310	5	13
Sloppy Joe, as prep Manwich	1 sandwich	310	5	13
FROZEN				
Chefwich Beef w/ Barbecue Sauce	1	340	—	10
Ovenstuffs Beef/Chedder Deli Melt	1 (4.75 oz)	390	—	22
Tyson Microwave BBQ Sandwich	1 sandwich	200	—	3

FOOD	PORTION	CALS.	SAT. FAT	FAT
MIX				
Hamburger Helper				
Beef Noodle, as prep	1 cup	330	—	15
Beef Romanoff, as prep	1 cup	350	—	16
Beef Taco, as prep	1 cup	330	—	14
Cheddar 'n Bacon, as prep	1 cup	380	—	19
Cheeseburger Macaroni, as prep	1 cup	370	—	19
Cheesy Italian, as prep	1 cup	370	—	18
Chili Macaroni, as prep	1 cup	330	—	14
Hamburger Hash, as prep	1 cup	320	—	15
Hamburger Pizza Dish, as prep	1 cup	360	—	14
Hamburger Stew, as prep	1 cup	300	—	14
Lasagne, as prep	1 cup	340	—	14
Meat Loaf, as prep	5 oz	360	—	22
Nacho Cheese, as prep	1 cup	360	—	15
Pizzabake, as prep	⅙ pkg (4.5 oz)	320	—	14
Potatoes Au Gratin, as prep	1 cup	350	—	18
Potatoes Stroganoff, as prep	1 cup	330	—	16
Rice Oriental, as prep	1 cup	340	—	14
Sloppy Joe Bake, as prep	5 oz	340	—	15
Spaghetti, as prep	1 cup	340	—	14
Stroganoff, as prep	1 cup	390	—	20
Tacobake, as prep	⅙ pkg (5.75 oz)	320	—	15
Zesty Italian, as prep	1 cup	340	—	13
Lipton Microeasy Hearty Beef Stew	¼ pkg	71	—	1
Lipton Microeasy Homestyle Meatloaf	¼ pkg	87	—	2
Manwich Seasoning Mix, as prep	1 sandwich	320	5	13
TAKE-OUT				
bubble & squeak	5 oz	186	—	13
cornish pasty	1 (8 oz)	847	—	52
irish stew	1 cup (7 oz)	280	9	16
kebab, indian	1 (5.4 oz)	553	—	40
kheena	6.7 oz	781	—	71

FOOD	PORTION	CALS.	SAT. FAT	FAT
koftas	5	280	—	22
roast beef sandwich, plain	1	346	4	14
roast beef sandwich w/ cheese	1	402	9	18
roast beef submarine sandwich w/ tomato, lettuce, mayonnaise	1	411	7	13
samosa	1 (4 oz)	652	—	62
shepherd's pie	6 oz	196	—	10
steak & kidney pie w/ top crust	1 slice (5 oz)	400	—	26
steak sandwich w/ tomato, lettuce, salt, mayonnaise	1	459	4	14
stew	6 oz	208	—	13
stew w/ vegetables	1 cup	220	4	11
stroganoff	¾ cup	260	11	19
swiss steak	4.6 oz	214	3	9
toad in the hole	1 (4.7 oz)	383	—	29

BEEFALO
roasted	3 oz	160	2	5

BEER AND ALE
(see also MALT)

Amstel Light	12 oz	95	—	0
Anheuser Busch Natural Light	12 oz	110	—	0
Bud Light	12 oz	108	—	0
Coors	12 oz	132	0	0
Coors Extra Gold	12 oz	147	0	0
Coors Light	12 oz	105	0	0
Hamm's	12 oz	137	0	0
Killian's	12 oz	212	0	0
Michelob Light	12 oz	134	0	0
Miller Lite	12 oz	96	0	0
Molson Light	12 oz	109	0	0
Old Milwaukee	12 oz	145	0	0
Old Milwaukee Light	12 oz	122	0	0
Olympia	12 oz	143	0	0
Pabst	12 oz	143	0	0
Piels Light	12 oz	136	0	0
Schaefer	12 oz	138	0	0
Schaefer Light	12 oz	111	0	0
Schlitz	12 oz	145	0	0

FOOD	PORTION	CALS.	SAT. FAT	FAT
Schlitz Light	12 oz	99	0	0
Schmidts Light	12 oz	96	0	0
Signature	12 oz	150	0	0
Stroh	12 oz	142	0	0
Stroh Light	12 oz	115	0	0
Winterfest	12 oz	167	0	0
ale brown	10 oz	77	0	0
ale pale	10 oz	88	0	0
beer light	12 oz	100	0	0
beer regular	12 oz	146	0	0
lager	10 oz	80	0	0
stout	10 oz	102	0	0
NONALCOHOLIC				
Guiness Kaliber	12 oz	43	0	0
Hamm's	12 oz	55	0	0
Kingsbury	12 fl oz	60	0	0
Pabst	12 oz	55	0	0
Spirit	12 oz	80	0	0

BEETS
CANNED

FOOD	PORTION	CALS.	SAT. FAT	FAT
Cut (Seneca)	½ cup	35	0	0
Diced (Seneca)	½ cup	35	0	0
Diced Tender (S&W)	½ cup	40	0	0
Harvard (Seneca)	½ cup	80	0	0
Julienne French Style (S&W)	½ cup	40	0	0
Pickled (Seneca)	½ cup	35	0	0
Pickled Whole Extra Small (S&W)	½ cup	70	0	0
Pickled w/ Onions (Seneca)	2 tbsp	20	0	0
Pickled w/ Red Wine Vinegar Sliced (S&W)	70	0	0
Sliced (Seneca)	½ cup	35	0	0
Sliced Small Premium (S&W)	½ cup	40	0	0
Sliced Water Pack (S&W)	½ cup	35	0	0
Whole (Seneca)	½ cup	35	0	0
Whole Small (S&W)	½ cup	40	0	0
harvard	½ cup	89	tr	tr
pickled	½ cup	75	tr	tr
sliced	½ cup	27	tr	tr

FOOD	PORTION	CALS.	SAT. FAT	FAT
FRESH				
greens, cooked	½ cup	20	tr	tr
greens, raw	½ cup	4	tr	tr
greens, raw, chopped	½ cup	4	tr	tr
raw, sliced	½ cup (2.4 oz)	29	tr	tr
sliced, cooked	½ cup (3 oz)	38	tr	tr
whole, cooked	2 (3.5 oz)	44	tr	tr
whole, raw	2 (5.7 oz)	70	tr	tr
JUICE				
beet juice	3.5 oz	36	0	0

BEVERAGES

(*see* BEER AND ALE, CHAMPAGNE, COFFEE, DRINK MIXERS, FRUIT DRINKS, MALT, MINERAL/BOTTLED WATER, LIQUOR/LIQUEUR, SODA, TEA/HERBAL TEA, WINE, WINE COOLERS)

BISCUIT

FOOD	PORTION	CALS.	SAT. FAT	FAT
FROZEN				
Egg, Canadian Bacon & Cheese (Great Starts)	5.2 oz	420	—	22
Sausage (Great Starts)	4.7 oz	410	—	22
Sausage Biscuit (Weight Watchers)	3 oz	220	2	11
HOME RECIPE				
buttermilk	1 (2 oz)	212	3	10
oatcakes	2 (4 oz)	115	—	5
plain	1 (2 oz)	212	3	10
MIX				
Biscuit Mix (Arrowhead)	¼ cup (1.2 oz)	120	0	1
Bisquick	½ cup (2 oz)	240	2	8
Bisquick Reduced Fat	½ cup (2 oz)	210	1	4
Buttermilk Biscuit Mix, not prep (Health Valley)	1 oz	100	—	1
Buttermilk, as prep (Jiffy)	1	170	2	4
Jiffy	¼ cup (1.1 oz)	130	1	5
Jiffy, as prep	1	150	3	7
buttermilk	1 (2 oz)	191	2	7
plain	1 (2 oz)	191	2	7
READY-TO-EAT				
Old Fashioned Arnold	1	60	—	3
REFRIGERATED				
1869 Brand Baking Powder	1	100	1	5
1869 Brand Butter Tastin'	1	100	1	5
1869 Brand Buttermilk	1	100	1	5
Ballard Ovenready	1	50	0	1

FOOD	PORTION	CALS.	SAT. FAT	FAT
Ballard Ovenready Buttermilk	1	50	0	1
Big Country Southern Style	1	100	tr	4
Hungry Jack				
Butter Tastin' Flaky	1	90	tr	4
Buttermilk Flaky	1	90	tr	4
Buttermilk Fluffy	1	90	1	4
Extra Rich Buttermilk	1	50	0	1
Flaky	1	80	tr	4
Honey Tastin' Flaky	1	90	tr	4
Pillsbury				
Big Country Butter Tastin'	1	100	tr	4
Big Country Buttermilk	1	100	tr	4
Heat N' Eat Big Premium	2	280	3	15
Butter	1	50	0	1
Buttermilk	1	50	0	1
Country	1	50	0	1
Deluxe Heat N' Eat Buttermilk	2	170	1	5
Good 'N Buttery Fluffy	1	90	1	5
Hearty Grains Multi-Grain	1	80	0	2
Hearty Grains Oatmeal Raisin	1	90	tr	2
Tender Layer Buttermilk	1	50	0	1
Roman Meal	2 (2.4 oz)	180	1	4
Roman Meal Honey Nut Oat Bran	1 (1.5 oz)	131	1	5
buttermilk	1 (1 oz)	98	1	4
plain	1 (1 oz)	98	1	4
TAKE-OUT				
plain	1	276	9	34
w/ egg	1	315	6	20
w/ egg & bacon	1	457	10	31
w/ egg & sausage	1	582	15	39
w/ egg & steak	1	474	9	28
w/ egg, cheese & bacon	1	477	11	31
w/ ham	1	387	11	18
w/ sausage	1	485	14	32
w/ steak	1	456	7	26

FOOD	PORTION	CALS.	SAT. FAT	FAT
BISON				
roasted	3 oz	122	1	2
BLACK BEANS				
CANNED				
Allen Seasoned	½ cup (4.5 oz)	120	1	2
Health Valley Fast Menu Organic Black Beans With Tofu Weiners	7.5 oz	150	—	1
Health Valley Fast Menu Western Black Beans With Garden Vegetable	7.5 oz	160	—	5
Progresso	½ cup	90	—	1
Trappey Seasoned	½ cup (4.5 oz)	120	1	2
DRIED				
cooked	1 cup	227	tr	1
MIX				
Mahatma Black Beans & Rice	1 cup	200	0	2
Pasta & Beans Black Beans With Fusilli (Bean Cuisine)	½ cup	174	1	4
BLACKBERRIES				
CANNED				
Allen-Wolco	½ cup (5.3 oz)	60	0	1
in heavy syrup	½ cup	118	—	tr
FRESH				
blackberries	½ cup	37	—	tr
FROZEN				
Big Valley	⅔ cup (4.9 oz)	70	0	0
unsweetened	1 cup	97	—	1
BLACKEYE PEAS				
CANNED				
Allen	½ cup (4.5 oz)	110	1	1
Allen Fresh Shell	½ cup (4.4 oz)	120	1	1
Allen With Bacon	½ cup (4.5 oz)	105	1	2
Allen With Snaps	½ cup (4.4 oz)	120	1	1
Dorman Fresh Shell	½ cup (4.4 oz)	120	1	1
East Texas Fair	½ cup (4.5 oz)	110	1	1
East Texas Fair Fresh Shell	½ cup (4.4 oz)	120	1	1
East Texas Fair With Snaps	½ cup (4.4 oz)	120	1	1
Homefolks Fresh Shell	½ cup (4.4 oz)	120	1	1

FOOD	PORTION	CALS.	SAT. FAT	FAT
Homefolks With Jalapeno	½ cup (4.4 oz)	120	1	1
Homefolks With Snaps	½ cup (4.4 oz)	120	1	1
Seasoned w/ Pork Luck's	7.25 oz	200	—	6
Sunshine With Bacon	½ cup (4.5 oz)	105	1	2
Trappey With Bacon	½ cup (4.5 oz)	120	1	2
Trappey With Bacon And Jalapeno	½ cup (4.4 oz)	110	1	2
w/ pork	½ cup	199	1	4
DRIED				
cooked	1 cup	198	tr	1
FROZEN				
Fresh Like	3.5 oz	138	—	1

BLINTZE

Apple (Empire)	2 (4.4 oz)	220	2	6
Apple Raisin (Golden)	1 (2.25 oz)	80	0	2
Blueberry (Empire)	2 (4.4 oz)	190	1	4
Blueberry (Golden)	1 (2.25 oz)	90	0	1
Cheese (Empire)	2 (4.4 oz)	200	2	6
Cheese (Golden)	1 (2.25 oz)	80	1	2
Cherry (Empire)	2 (4.4 oz)	200	1	4
Cherry (Golden)	1 (2.25 oz)	95	0	1
Potato (Empire)	2 (4.4 oz)	190	2	6
Potato (Golden)	1 (2.25 oz)	90	1	2
TAKE-OUT				
cheese	2	186	3	6

BLUEBERRIES

CANNED				
In Heavy Syrup (S&W)	½ cup	111	0	0
in heavy syrup	1 cup	225	—	1
FRESH				
blueberries	1 cup	82	—	1
FROZEN				
Big Valley	¾ cup (4.9 oz)	70	0	0
unsweetened	1 cup	78	—	1

BLUEFIN

fillet, baked	4.1 oz	186	1	6

BLUEFISH

fresh, baked	3 oz	135	1	5

BOAR

wild, roasted	3 oz	136	1	4

FOOD	PORTION	CALS.	SAT. FAT	FAT
BOK CHOY				
Dole, shredded	½ cup	5	—	tr
BORAGE				
FRESH				
cooked, chopped	3.5 oz	25	—	1
raw, chopped	½ cup	9	—	tr
BOYSENBERRIES				
canned, in heavy syrup	1 cup	226	—	tr
frozen, unsweetened	1 cup	66	—	tr
JUICE				
Smucker's	8 oz	120	0	0
Smucker's Juice Sparkler	10 oz	130	—	tr
BRAINS				
beef, pan-fried	3 oz	167	3	13
beef, simmered	3 oz	136	2	11
lamb, braised	3 oz	124	2	9
lamb, fried	3 oz	232	5	19
pork, braised	3 oz	117	2	8
veal, braised	3 oz	115	—	8
veal, fried	3 oz	181	—	14
BRAN				
Fast Menu Oat Pilaf w/ Garden Vegetables (Health Valley)	7.5 oz	210	—	7
Oat (Hodgson Mill)	¼ cup (1.3 oz)	120	1	3
Oat (Roman Meal)	1 oz	94	tr	3
Oat Bran (Arrowhead)	⅓ cup (1.4 oz)	150	0	3
Oat Bran (Mother's)	⅓ cup	92	tr	2
Quaker Unprocessed Bran	2 tbsp	8	0	tr
Super Bran (H-O)	⅓ cup	110	0	2
Toasted Wheat Bran (Kretschmer)	⅓ cup	57	tr	2
Wheat (Hodgson Mill)	¼ cup (0.5 oz)	30	0	1
Wheat Bran (Arrowhead)	¼ cup (0.6 oz)	30	0	1
Wheat Bran (Good Shepherd)	1 oz	80	—	1
corn	⅓ cup	56	tr	tr
oat, cooked	½ cup	44	tr	tr
oat, dry	½ cup	116	tr	3
rice, dry	⅓ cup	88	1	6
wheat, dry	½ cup	65	tr	1

FOOD	PORTION	CALS.	SAT. FAT	FAT
BRAZIL NUTS				
dried, unblanched	1 oz	186	5	19
BREAD				
(*see also* BAGEL, BISCUIT, BREADSTICK, CROISSANT, ENGLISH MUFFIN, MUFFIN, ROLL, SCONE)				
CANNED				
Brown Bread (B&M)	½ in slice (1.6 oz)	92	0	0
Brown Bread (Friends)	1 slice (1.6 oz)	92	0	0
Brown Bread Raisins (B&M)	½ in slice (1.6 oz)	94	0	0
Brown Bread w/ Raisin (Friends)	1 slice (1.6 oz)	94	0	0
Brown Bread New England Recipe (S&W)	2 slices	76	0	0
boston brown	1 slice (1.6 oz)	88	tr	1
HOME RECIPE				
banana	1 slice (2 oz)	195	1	6
cornbread, as prep w/ 2% milk	1 piece (2.3 oz)	173	1	5
cornbread, as prep w/ whole milk	1 piece (2.3 oz)	176	1	5
datenut	½ in slice	92	—	3
irish soda bread	1 slice (2 oz)	174	1	3
pita whole wheat	1–6 in	247	—	1
pumpkin	1 slice (1 oz)	94	1	4
white, as prep w/ 2% milk	1 slice	81	tr	2
white, as prep w/ nonfat dry milk	1 slice	78	tr	1
white, as prep w/ whole milk	1 slice	82	tr	2
whole wheat	1 slice	71	—	tr
whole wheat	1 slice	79	tr	2
MIX				
Corn Bread (Ballard)	⅛ bread	140	—	3
Corn Bread (Dromedary)	1 piece (2 in x 2 in)	130	—	3
Corn Bread Easy Mix (Aunt Jemima)	⅙ cake	210	—	7
Cornbread Blue Cornmeal (Zia Foods)	1 piece (1.2 oz)	110	—	6
Cracked Wheat (Natural Ovens)	2 slices (2.4 oz)	140	0	1
English Muffin Bread (Natural Ovens)	2 slices (2.4 oz)	140	0	1
Executive Fitness Sunny Millet (Natural Ovens)	2 slices (2.6 oz)	160	0	2

FOOD	PORTION	CALS.	SAT. FAT	FAT
Garden Bread (Natural Ovens)	1 oz	50	0	1
Glorious Cinnamon & Raisin Fat Free (Natural Ovens)	2 slices (2.1 oz)	110	0	1
Honey 'N Flax (Natural Ovens)	2 slices (2.5 oz)	140	0	1
Hunger Filler Bread (Natural Ovens)	2 slices (2.1 oz)	110	0	2
Light Wheat (Natural Ovens)	2 slices (2.2 oz)	84	0	1
Nutty Natural Wheat Bread (Natural Ovens)	2 slices (2.5 oz)	140	0	2
Seven Grain Herb (Natural Ovens)	2 slices (2.5 oz)	140	0	1
Soft Hearth Whole Wheat (Natural Ovens)	2 slices (2 oz)	100	0	2
Soft Sandwich Very Low Fat (Natural Ovens)	2 slices (2.3 oz)	110	0	1
Stay Slim (Natural Ovens)	2 slices (2 oz)	100	0	2
cornbread	1 piece (2 oz)	189	2	6
READY-TO-EAT				
100% Whole Wheat Wonder	1 slice (1 oz)	70	0	1
100% Whole Wheat Soft Wonder	2 slices (1.6 oz)	110	0	2
12 Grain Natural Arnold	1 slice (0.8 oz)	60	0	0
7 Grain Hearty Slice Pepperidge Farm	2 slices	180	0	2
9 Grain & Nut (Matthew's)	1 slice	80	—	3
Augusto Pan De Aqua (Arnold)	1 oz	80	—	1
Austrian Wheat (Bread Du Jour)	3 in slice (1 oz)	130	0	2
Bran'nola Country Oat (Arnold)	1 slice (1.3 oz)	90	0	3
Bran'nola Country Oat (Brownberry)	1 slice	90	0	2
Bran'nola Dark Wheat (Arnold)	1 slice (1.3 oz)	90	0	3
Bran'nola Hearty Wheat (Arnold)	1 slice (1.3 oz)	100	0	3
Bran'nola Nutty Grains (Arnold)	1 slice (1.3 oz)	90	0	3
Bran'nola Original (Arnold)	1 slice (1.3 oz)	90	0	2

FOOD	PORTION	CALS.	SAT. FAT	FAT
Bran'nola Original (Brownberry)	1 slice	85	—	1
Bran'nola Hearty Wheat (Brownberry)	1 slice	88	—	2
Bran'nola Nutty Grains (Brownberry)	1 slice	85	—	2
Brown & Serve Mini Loaf (Roman Meal)	½ loaf (2 oz)	136	tr	2
Butter Crust (Freihofer's)	1 slice	70	—	1
Canadian Oat (Freihofer's)	1 slice	80	—	1
Cinnamon (Matthew's)	1 slice	70	—	1
Cinnamon (Pepperidge Farm)	1 slice	90	—	3
Cinnamon Chip (Arnold)	1 slice	80	—	2
Cinnamon Raisin (Arnold)	1 slice (0.9 oz)	70	0	1
Cinnamon Raisin (Wonder)	1 slice (1 oz)	70	0	1
Club Pullman (Freihofer's)	1 slice	70	tr	1
Country Bran Bakery Light (Arnold)	1 slice (0.8 oz)	40	tr	0
Cracked Wheat (Pepperidge Farm)	1 slice	70	—	1
Cracked Wheat (Roman Meal)	1 slice (1.4 oz)	92	tr	1
Cracked Wheat (Wonder)	1 slice (1 oz)	70	0	1
Cranberry (Arnold)	1 slice (0.9 oz)	70	0	1
Crunchy Oat 1½ lb Loaf (Pepperidge Farm)	2 slices	190	1	4
Date Walnut (Pepperidge Farm)	1 slice	90	—	3
Focaccia (Dicarlo's)	⅛ bread (2 oz)	130	0	2
French (Bread Du Jour)	3 in slice (1 oz)	130	0	1
French (Wonder)	1 slice (1 oz)	80	0	2
French Fully Baked (Pepperidge Farm)	2 oz	150	—	2
French Light (Wonder)	2 slices (1.6 oz)	80	0	1
French Parisian (Dicarlo's)	2 slices (1 oz)	70	0	1
French Stick Extra Sour (Parisian)	2 oz	150	—	1
French Stick Francisco (Arnold)	1 slice (1 oz)	70	—	2
French Stick Savoni (Arnold)	1 oz	80	—	tr
French Stick Sweet (Parisian)	2 oz	154	—	2
French Twin (Pepperidge Farm)	1 oz	80	—	1

FOOD	PORTION	CALS.	SAT. FAT	FAT
French Twin Loaves Francisco (Arnold)	2 slices (2 oz)	150	—	2
Golden (Matthew's)	1 slice	70	—	1
Granola (Wonder)	1 slice (1.5 oz)	100	0	2
Health Nut (Brownberry)	1 slice	71	—	3
Hearty Buttermilk & Biscuit White (Home Pride)	1 slice (1.3 oz)	100	0	2
Hearty Deli Rye (Home Pride)	1 slice (2 oz)	140	0	2
Hearty Golden Honey Wheat (Home Pride)	1 slice (1.3 oz)	90	0	2
Hearty Honey Oats & Cracked Wheat (Home Pride)	1 slice (1.4 oz)	100	0	2
Hearty Seven Grain Multi Grain (Home Pride)	1 slice (1.3 oz)	100	0	2
Hearty Wheat Light (Roman Meal)	1 slice (0.8 oz)	42	tr	tr
Hi-Fibre (Monks' Bread)	1 slice	50	—	1
Honey Bran (Pepperidge Farm)	1 slice	90	—	1
Honey Bran Light (Wonder)	2 slices (1.6 oz)	80	0	1
Honey Nut Oat Bran (Roman Meal)	1 slice (1 oz)	72	tr	2
Honey Oat Bran (Roman Meal)	1 slice (1 oz)	70	—	1
Honey Wheat (Home Pride)	1 slice (1 oz)	70	—	1
Italian (Weight Watchers)	1 slice (0.8 oz)	38	tr	tr
Italian (Wonder)	1 slice (1.1 oz)	80	0	1
Italian Bakery Light (Arnold)	1 slice (0.7 oz)	40	0	tr
Italian Brown & Serve (Pepperidge Farm)	1 oz	80	1	1
Italian Family (Wonder)	1 slice (1 oz)	70	—	1
Italian Francisco (Arnold)	1 slice (1 oz)	70	—	1
Italian Light (Wonder)	2 slices (1.6 oz)	80	0	1
Italian No Seeds (Freihofer's)	1 slice	70	—	1
Italian Seeded (Freihofer's)	1 slice	70	—	1
Italian Sliced (Pepperidge Farm)	1 slice	70	—	1
Italian Stick Francisco (Arnold)	1 oz	90	—	1

FOOD	PORTION	CALS.	SAT. FAT	FAT
Kid (Wonder)	1 slice (0.9 oz)	70	0	1
Lite Diet (Freihofer's)	1 slice	40	—	0
Malsovit	1 slice	66	tr	1
Multi-Grain (Weight Watchers)	1 slice (0.8 oz)	41	tr	1
Nine Grain Light (Wonder)	2 slices (1.6 oz)	80	0	1
Oat (Roman Meal)	1 slice (1 oz)	69	tr	1
Oat (Weight Watchers)	1 slice (0.8 oz)	42	tr	1
Oat Bran (Matthew's)	1 slice	65	—	0
Oat Bran (Roman Meal)	1 slice (1 oz)	68	tr	1
Oat Bran Light (Roman Meal)	1 slice (0.8 oz)	42	tr	tr
Oatmeal (Pepperidge Farm)	1 slice	70	—	1
Oatmeal Light (Wonder)	2 slices (1.6 oz)	90	0	1
Oatmeal 1½ lb Loaf (Pepperidge Farm)	1 slice	90	—	1
Oatmeal Bakery (Arnold)	1 slice	60	0	1
Oatmeal Bakery Light (Arnold)	1 slice	40	0	tr
Oatmeal Light (Pepperidge Farm)	1 slice	45	0	0
Oatmeal Natural (Brownberry)	1 slice	63	—	1
Oatmeal Raisin (Arnold)	1 slice (0.9 oz)	60	0	tr
Oatmeal Soft (Brownberry)	1 slice	48	—	1
Oatmeal Very Thin Sliced (Pepperidge Farm)	1 slice	40	—	1
Old Fashion (Freihofer's)	1 slice	70	—	1
Onion Rye (August Bros)	1 slice	80	—	1
Pita Oat Bran (Sahara)	½ pocket (1 oz)	66	—	tr
Pita Wheat (Arnold)	½ pocket (1 oz)	71	—	0
Pita White (Arnold)	½ pocket (0.5 oz)	71	0	0
Pita White (Sahara)	½ pocket	78	—	1
Pita Whole Wheat (Matthew's)	1	210	—	2
Pumpernickel (Arnold)	1 slice (1.1 oz)	70	0	1
Pumpernickel (August Bros)	1 slice	80	—	1
Pumpernickel (August Bros)	1 slice (24 oz loaf)	90	—	1
Pumpernickel (Beefsteak)	1 slice (1 oz)	70	0	1
Pumpernickel Family (Pepperidge Farm)	1 slice	80	—	1
Pumpernickel Party (Pepperidge Farm)	4 slices	60	—	1

FOOD	PORTION	CALS.	SAT. FAT	FAT
Raisin (Malsovit)	1 slice	77	tr	1
Raisin (Monks' Bread)	1 slice	70	—	2
Raisin (Sunmaid)	1 slice	70	tr	tr
Raisin (Weight Watchers)	1 slice (0.9 oz)	55	tr	tr
Raisin Bran (Brownberry)	1 slice	61	—	1
Raisin Cinnamon (Brownberry)	1 slice	66	—	1
Raisin Walnut (Brownberry)	1 slice	68	—	3
Raisin With Cinnamon (Pepperidge Farm)	1 slice	90	—	2
Rite Diet (Freihofer's)	2 slices	90	—	1
Round Top (Roman Meal)	1 slice (1 oz)	67	tr	1
Rye (Weight Watchers)	1 slice (0.8 oz)	38	tr	tr
Rye (Wonder)	1 slice (1 oz)	70	0	1
Rye Bakery Soft Light (Arnold)	1 slice (1.1 oz)	40	0	tr
Rye Bakery Soft Seeded (Arnold)	1 slice (1.1 oz)	70	0	1
Rye Bakery Soft Unseeded (Arnold)	1 slice (1.1 oz)	70	0	1
Rye Hearty (Beefsteak)	1 slice (1 oz)	70	0	1
Rye Light (Beefsteak)	2 slices (1.6 oz)	70	0	1
Rye Light (Wonder)	2 slices (1.6 oz)	70	0	1
Rye Mild (Beefsteak)	2 slices (1.4 oz)	90	0	1
Rye Soft (Beefsteak)	1 slice (1 oz)	70	0	1
Rye With Seeds (Augusto Bros)	1 slice (1 lb loaf)	80	—	1
Rye Without Seeds (August Bros)	1 slice	80	—	1
Rye Dijon (Pepperidge Farm)	1 slice	50	—	1
Rye Dijon Real Jewish (Arnold)	1 slice	70	—	tr
Rye Dijon Thick Sliced (Pepperidge Farm)	1 slice	70	—	1
Rye Dill (Arnold)	1 slice (1.1 oz)	60	0	1
Rye Family (Pepperidge Farm)	1 slice (32 g)	80	—	1
Rye N' Pump (Augusto Bros)	1 slice	90	—	1
Rye Party (Pepperidge Farm)	4 slices	60	—	1
Rye Real Jewish Melba Thin (Arnold)	1 slice (0.7 oz)	40	0	tr

FOOD	PORTION	CALS.	SAT. FAT	FAT
Rye Real Jewish Unseeded (Arnold)	1 slice	80	—	tr
Rye Seedless Family (Pepperidge Farm)	1 slice	80	—	1
Rye Soft (Pepperidge Farm)	1 slice	70	—	1
Rye Soft Pumpernickel (Freihofer's)	1 slice	70	—	1
Rye Soft Dill & Onion (Freihofer's)	1 slice	70	—	1
Rye Soft No Seeds (Freihofer's)	1 slice	70	—	1
Rye Soft Seeded (Freihofer's)	1 slice	70	—	1
Rye Stub Pullman (Freihofer's)	1 slice	70	—	1
Rye With Caraway Real Jewish (Arnold)	1 slice	70	—	tr
Rye With Seeds (August Bros)	1 slice (24 oz loaf)	90	—	1
Rye Without Seeds Real Jewish (Arnold)	1 slice (1.1 oz)	70	0	tr
Sandwich (Roman Meal)	1 slice (0.8 oz)	55	tr	1
Sesame Wheat (Pepperidge Farm)	2 slices	190	1	3
Seven Grain (Home Pride)	1 slice (0.9 oz)	60	0	1
Seven Grain (Roman Meal)	1 slice (1 oz)	67	tr	1
Seven Grain Light (Roman Meal)	1 slice (0.8 oz)	42	tr	1
Sodium Free (Matthew's)	1 slice	70	—	2
Sourdough (Wonder)	1 slice (1.2 oz)	90	0	2
Sourdough Francisco (Arnold)	1 slice	90	—	1
Sourdough Light (Roman Meal)	1 slice (0.8 oz)	41	tr	tr
Sourdough Light (Wonder)	2 slices (1.6 oz)	80	0	1
Sourdough Whole Grain Light (Roman Meal)	1 slice (0.8 oz)	40	tr	tr
Sprouted Wheat (Pepperidge Farm)	1 slice	70	—	2
Sun Grain (Roman Meal)	1 slice (1 oz)	70	tr	2
Sunbeam King (Freihofer's)	1 slice	70	—	1
Sunflower & Bran (Monks' Bread)	1 slice	70	—	1

FOOD	PORTION	CALS.	SAT. FAT	FAT
Texas Toast (Wonder)	1 slice (1.4 oz)	100	0	1
The Original (Freihofer's)	1 slice	70	—	1
Twelve Grain (Roman Meal)	1 slice (1 oz)	70	tr	2
Twelve Grain Light (Roman Meal)	1 slice (0.8 oz)	42	tr	tr
Vienna (Wonder)	1 slice (1 oz)	70	0	1
Vienna Light (Pepperidge Farm)	1 slice	45	0	0
Vienna Thick Sliced (Pepperidge Farm)	1 slice	70	—	1
Wheat (Freihofer's)	1½ slices	70	—	1
Wheat (Home Pride)	1 slice (0.9 oz)	70	0	1
Wheat (Weight Watchers)	1 slice (0.8 oz)	40	tr	tr
Wheat Family (Wonder)	1 slice (0.9 oz)	70	0	1
Wheat Golden Country Style (Wonder)	2 slices (1.4 oz)	100	0	2
Wheat Hearty (Beefsteak)	1 slice (1 oz)	70	0	1
Wheat Light (Home Pride)	3 slices (2.1 oz)	110	0	2
Wheat Light (Roman Meal)	1 slice (0.8 oz)	41	tr	tr
Wheat Light (Wonder)	2 slices (1.6 oz)	80	0	1
Wheat Soft (Beefsteak)	1 slice (1 oz)	70	0	1
Wheat 1½ lb Loaf (Pepperidge Farm)	1 slice	90	—	2
Wheat Apple Honey (Brownberry)	1 slice	69	—	2
Wheat Berry Honey (Arnold)	1 slice (1.1 oz)	80	0	2
Wheat Brick Oven (Arnold)	1 slice (0.8 oz)	60	0	2
Wheat Calcium Light (Wonder)	2 slices (1.6 oz)	80	0	1
Wheat Cottage (America's Own)	1 slice	70	—	1
Wheat Family (Pepperidge Farm)	1 slice	70	—	1
Wheat Golden Light (Arnold)	1 slice (0.8 oz)	40	0	tr
Wheat Light (Pepperidge Farm)	1 slice	45	0	0
Wheat Natural (Arnold)	1 slice (1.3 oz)	80	0	1
Wheat Rite Diet (Freihofer's)	2 slices	90	—	1
Wheat Small (Freihofer's)	1½ slices	70	—	1
Wheat Soft (Brownberry)	1 slice	74	—	2

FOOD	PORTION	CALS.	SAT. FAT	FAT
Wheat Split Top (Freihofer's)	1 slice	70	—	1
Wheat Stub Pullman (Freihofer's)	1 slice	70	—	1
Wheat Very Thin Sliced (Pepperidge Farm)	1 slice	35	0	0
Wheatberry Honey (Roman Meal)	1 slice (1 oz)	67	tr	1
Wheatberry Light (Roman Meal)	1 slice (0.8 oz)	42	tr	tr
White (Freihofer's)	1 slice	70	—	1
White (Home Pride)	1 slice (0.9 oz)	70	0	1
White (Monks' Bread)	1 slice	60	—	1
White (Weight Watchers)	1 slice (0.8 oz)	40	tr	tr
White (Wonder)	1 slice (0.9 oz)	70	0	1
White Calcium (Wonder)	2 slices (1.6 oz)	100	0	1
White Light (Home Pride)	3 slices (0.9 oz)	110	0	2
White Light (Roman Meal)	1 slice (0.8 oz)	41	tr	tr
White Light (Wonder)	2 slices (1.6 oz)	80	0	1
White Light Brick Oven (Arnold)	1 slice (0.8 oz)	40	0	tr
White Premium Light (Arnold)	1 slice	40	0	tr
White Robust (Beefsteak)	1 slice (1 oz)	70	0	1
White Thin Sliced Brick Oven (Arnold)	1 slice	40	—	tr
White With Buttermilk (Wonder)	1 slice (1 oz)	80	0	1
White Brick Oven (Arnold)	1 slice (0.8 oz)	60	0	1
White Calcium Light (Wonder)	2 slices (1.6 oz)	80	0	1
White Cottage (America's Own)	1 slice	70	—	1
White Country (Arnold)	1 slice (1.3 oz)	100	tr	2
White Country (Pepperidge Farm)	2 slices	190	1	2
White Extra Fiber Brick Oven (Arnold)	1 slice (0.9 oz)	50	0	tr
White Grain (Home Pride)	1 slice (1 oz)	60	0	1
White Large Family Thin Slice (Pepperidge Farm)	1 slice	70	—	1
White Sandwich (Pepperidge Farm)	2 slices	130	—	2
White Split Top (Freihofer's)	1 slice	70	—	1

FOOD	PORTION	CALS.	SAT. FAT	FAT
White Thin Slice (Pepperidge Farm)	1 slice	80	—	2
White Toasting (Pepperidge Farm)	1 slice	90	—	1
White Very Thin Sliced (Pepperidge Farm)	1 slice	40	0	0
White Whole Special Recipe (Stroehmann)	1 slice	70	—	1
White Whole Special Recipe Kids (Stroehmann)	1 slice	60	—	tr
Whole Grain Sourdough (Roman Meal)	1 slice (1 oz)	66	tr	1
Whole Grain 100% (Roman Meal)	1 slice (1.4 oz)	91	tr	1
Whole Wheat (Matthew's)	1 slice	70	—	1
Whole Wheat 100% (Freihofer's)	1 slice	75	—	1
Whole Wheat 100% (Roman Meal)	1 slice (1 oz)	64	tr	1
Whole Wheat 100% Light (Roman Meal)	1 slice (0.8 oz)	42	tr	tr
Whole Wheat 100% Light Brick Oven (Arnold)	1 slice (0.8 oz)	40	—	tr
Whole Wheat 100% Stoneground (Arnold)	1 slice (0.8 oz)	50	0	1
Whole Wheat 100% Stoneground (Monks' Bread)	1 slice	70	—	1
Whole Wheat 100% Stoneground (Wonder)	1 slice (1.2 oz)	80	0	2
Whole Wheat Hearty 100% Stoneground (Home Pride)	1 slice (1.4 oz)	90	0	2
Whole Wheat Thin Slice (Pepperidge Farm)	1 slice	60	—	1
Wonder Calcium Enriched (Wonder)	1 slice (1 oz)	70	0	1
Wonder Light Calcium Enriched (Wonder)	2 slices (1.6 oz)	80	0	1
cracked wheat	1 slice	65	tr	1
egg	1 slice (1.4 oz)	115	1	2
french	1 loaf (1 lb)	1270	4	18
french	1 slice (1 oz)	78	tr	1
gluten	1 slice	47	tr	tr

FOOD	PORTION	CALS.	SAT. FAT	FAT
italian	1 loaf (1 lb)	1255	1	4
italian	1 slice (1 oz)	81	tr	1
navajo fry	1 (10.5 in diam)	527	3	15
navajo fry	1 (5 in diam)	296	2	9
oat bran	1 slice	71	tr	1
oat bran reduced calorie	1 slice	46	tr	1
oatmeal	1 slice	73	tr	1
oatmeal reduced calorie	1 slice	48	tr	1
pita	1 reg (2 oz)	165	tr	1
pita	1 sm (1 oz)	78	tr	tr
pita whole wheat	1 reg (2 oz)	170	tr	2
pita whole wheat	1 sm (1 oz)	76	tr	1
protein	1 slice	47	tr	tr
pumpernickel	1 slice	80	tr	1
raisin	1 slice	71	tr	1
rice bran	1 slice	66	tr	1
rye	1 slice	83	tr	1
rye reduced calorie	1 slice	47	tr	1
seven grain	1 slice	65	tr	1
sourdough	1 slice (1 oz)	78	tr	1
vienna	1 slice (1 oz)	78	tr	1
wheat berry	1 slice	65	tr	1
wheat bran	1 slice	89	tr	1
wheat germ	1 slice	74	tr	1
wheat reduced calorie	1 slice	46	tr	1
white	1 slice	67	tr	1
white, cubed	1 cup	80	tr	1
white reduced calorie	1 slice	48	tr	1
white, toasted	1 slice	67	tr	1
whole wheat	1 slice	70	tr	1
REFRIGERATED				
Crusty French Loaf (Pillsbury)	1	60	0	tr
Hearty Grains Country Oatmeal Twists (Pillsbury)	1	80	tr	2
Hearty Grains Cracked Wheat Twists (Pillsbury)	1	80	0	2
Pipin' Hot Wheat Loaf (Pillsbury)	1	70	0	2
Pipin' Hot White Loaf (Pillsbury)	1	70	0	2
Roman Meal Loaf (Roman Meal)	1 slice (1 oz)	85	1	3

FOOD	PORTION	CALS.	SAT. FAT	FAT
TAKE-OUT				
chapatis, as prep w/ fat	1 (2.5 oz)	230	—	9
chapatis, as prep w/o fat	1 (2.5 oz)	141	—	1
cornbread	2" x 2" (1.4 oz)	107	1	2
cornstick	1 (1.3 oz)	101	1	4
naan	1 (6 oz)	571	—	21
papadums, fried	2 (1.5 oz)	81	—	4
paratha	1 (4.4 oz)	403	—	18

BREAD COATING

FOOD	PORTION	CALS.	SAT. FAT	FAT
Don's Chuck Wagon Batter All Purpose Mix (Hodgson Mill)	¼ cup (1 oz)	100	0	0
Don's Chuck Wagon Batter Chicken Frying Mix (Hodgson Mill)	¼ cup (1 oz)	95	0	0
Don's Chuck Wagon Batter Fish & Chips Mix (Hodgson Mill)	¼ cup (1 oz)	100	0	0
Don's Chuck Wagon Batter Fish Mix (Hodgson Mill)	¼ cup (1 oz)	95	0	0
Don's Chuck Wagon Batter Mushroom Mix (Hodgson Mill)	¼ cup (1 oz)	95	0	0
Don's Chuck Wagon Batter Onion Ring Mix (Hodgson Mill)	¼ cup (1 oz)	100	0	0
Don's Chuck Wagon Batter Seafood Seasoned Frying Mix (Hodgson Mill)	¼ cup (1 oz)	95	0	1
Fryin' Magic (Little Crow)	0.5 oz	43	—	tr
Golden Dipt Breading Frying Mix	1 oz	90	0	0
Golden Dipt Chicken Frying Mix	1 oz	90	0	0
Golden Dipt Onion Ring Mix	1 oz	100	0	0
Mrs. Dash Crispy Coating Mix	0.5 oz	63	—	1
Oven Fry Homestyle Flour Recipe for Chicken	¼ pkg	85	—	2

FOOD	PORTION	CALS.	SAT. FAT	FAT
Shake 'N Bake				
Extra Crispy Oven Fry for Pork	¼ pkg (1 oz)	120	—	3
Italian Herb Recipe	¼ pkg (½ oz)	77	—	1
Original Barbecue Recipe for Chicken	¼ pkg (½ oz)	93	—	2
Original Barbecue Recipe for Pork	¼ pkg (½ oz)	38	—	1
Original Country Mild Recipe	¼ pkg (½ oz)	76	—	4
Original Recipe for Chicken	¼ pkg (½ oz)	75	—	2
Original Recipe for Fish	¼ pkg (½ oz)	73	—	1
Original Recipe for Pork	¼ pkg (½ oz)	41	—	1

BREAD MACHINE

FOOD	PORTION	CALS.	SAT. FAT	FAT
MIX				
Dromedary Country White	½ in slice (2 oz)	140	1	1
Dromedary Italian Herb	½ in slice (1.8 oz)	140	2	3
Dromedary Stoneground Wheat	½ slice (1.8 oz)	140	1	2
Pillsbury Cracked Wheat	1/12 pkg (1.3 oz)	130	0	2

BREADCRUMBS

FOOD	PORTION	CALS.	SAT. FAT	FAT
4C Salt Free	1 tbsp (0o.5 oz)	50	—	1
4C Seasoned	1 tbsp (0o.5 oz)	50	—	1
4C Toasted	1 tbsp (0.5 oz)	50	—	1
4C Toasted Salt Free	1 tbsp (0.5 oz)	50	—	1
Arnold Italian	½ oz	50	0	tr
Arnold Plain	½ oz	50	0	tr
Contadina	⅓ cup	100	—	2
Devonsheer Italian Style	1 oz	104	—	1
Devonsheer Plain	1 oz	108	—	1
Friday's Seasoned	1 oz	56	—	tr
Jaclyn's Organic Whole Wheat Italian Style	½ oz	28	—	1
Jaclyn's Organic Whole Wheat Plain	½ oz	28	—	1
Progresso Italian Style	2 tbsp	60	—	tr
Progresso Plain	2 tbsp	60	—	tr
dry	1 cup	426	1	6
dry seasoned	1 cup (4 oz)	441	1	3
fresh	⅔ cup	76	tr	1

BREADFRUIT

FOOD	PORTION	CALS.	SAT. FAT	FAT
breadfruit	3.5 oz	109	—	tr

FOOD	PORTION	CALS.	SAT. FAT	FAT
fresh	¼ small	99	—	tr
seeds, cooked	1 oz	48	tr	1
seeds, raw	1 oz	54	tr	2
seeds, roasted	1 oz	59	tr	tr

BREADNUTTREE SEEDS
dried	1 oz	104	tr	tr

BREADSTICKS
FOOD	PORTION	CALS.	SAT. FAT	FAT
Brown & Serve Soft (Roman Meal)	1 (2.7 oz)	181	tr	3
Cheese (Angonoa)	5 (1 oz)	120	1	3
Cheese (Lance)	2	20	0	0
Cheese Mini (Angonoa)	16 (1 oz)	120	1	3
Deli Garlic Fat Free (Stella D'Oro)	5	60	0	0
Deli Original Fat Free (Stella D'Oro)	5	60	0	0
Garlic (Angonoa)	6 (1 oz)	120	0	2
Garlic (J. J. Cassone)	1 (1.6 oz)	150	0	3
Garlic (Keebler)	2	30	tr	tr
Garlic (Lance)	2	30	0	0
Garlic (Stella D'Oro)	1	35	—	1
Grissini Garlic Fat Free (Stella D'Oro)	3	60	—	0
Grissini Original Fat Free (Stella D'Oro)	3	60	—	0
Italian (Bread Du Jour)	1 (1.9 oz)	130	0	2
Italian Style Plain (Angonoa)	5 (1 oz)	120	1	3
Low Sodium With Sesame Seed (Angonoa)	6 (1 oz)	130	1	4
Onion (Angonoa)	6 (1 oz)	120	1	2
Onion (Keebler)	2	30	tr	tr
Onion (Stella D'Oro)	1	40	—	1
Pizza Mini (Angonoa)	26 (1 oz)	120	0	2
Plain (Keebler)	2	30	tr	tr
Plain (Lance)	2	30	0	0
Regular (Stella D'Oro)	1	40	—	1
Regular Sodium Free (Stella D'Oro)	2	80	—	2
Roman Meal, refrigerated	1 (1.4 oz)	117	1	4
Sesame (Keebler)	2	30	tr	1
Sesame (Lance)	2	30	0	0
Sesame Low Fat (Stella D'Oro)	2	70	—	1

FOOD	PORTION	CALS.	SAT. FAT	FAT
Sesame Mini (Angonoa)	16 (1 oz)	130	1	4
Sesame Sodium Free (Stella D'Oro)	1	50	—	3
Sesame Royale (Angonoa)	6 (1 oz)	130	1	4
Soft Bread Sticks (Pillsbury)	1	100	tr	2
Sourdough (Bread Du Jour)	1 (1.9 oz)	130	0	1
Traditional Garlic Fat Free (Stella D'Oro)	2	70	0	0
Traditional Original Fat Free (Stella D'Oro)	2	70	0	0
Wheat (Stella D'Oro)	1	40	—	1
Whole Wheat Mini (Angonoa)	14 (1 oz)	130	1	4
onion poppyseed home recipe	1	64	—	1
plain	1	41	tr	1
plain	1 sm	25	tr	1

BREAKFAST BAR
(see also BREAKFAST DRINKS, NUTRITIONAL SUPPLEMENTS)

FOOD	PORTION	CALS.	SAT. FAT	FAT
Carnation				
Chewy Chocolate Chip	1 (1.26 oz)	150	3	6
Chewy Peanut Butter Chocolate Chip	1 (1.26 oz)	140	2	5
Chocolate Chunk Granola	1 (1.26 oz)	140	2	5
Honey & Oats Granola	1 (1.26 oz)	130	2	4
Nutri-Grain				
Apple	1 (1.3 oz)	150	1	5
Blueberry Kellogg's	1 bar (1.3 oz)	140	1	4
Raspberry	1 (1.3 oz)	150	1	5
Strawberry	1 (1.3 oz)	150	1	5

BREAKFAST DRINKS
(see also BREAKFAST BAR, NUTRITIONAL SUPPLEMENTS)

FOOD	PORTION	CALS.	SAT. FAT	FAT
Carnation				
Instant Breakfast Cafe Mocha	1 can (10 fl oz)	220	1	3
Instant Breakfast Cafe Mocha	1 pkg	130	0	1
Instant Breakfast Cafe Mocha	1 pkg + skim milk (9 fl oz)	220	tr	1
Instant Breakfast Classic Chocolate Malt	1 pkg	130	1	2

FOOD	PORTION	CALS.	SAT. FAT	FAT
Instant Breakfast Classic Chocolate Malt	1 pkg + skim milk (9 fl oz)	220	1	1
Instant Breakfast Creamy Milk Chocolate	1 can (10 fl oz)	220	1	3
Instant Breakfast Creamy Milk Chocolate	1 pkg	130	1	1
Instant Breakfast Creamy Milk Chocolate	1 pkg + skim milk (9 fl oz)	220	1	1
Instant Breakfast Creamy Milk Chocolate	8 fl oz	220	2	3
Instant Breakfast French Vanilla	1 pkg	130	0	0
Instant Breakfast French Vanilla	1 pkg + skim milk	220	tr	1
Instant Breakfast Strawberry Creme	1 pkg	130	0	0
Instant Breakfast Strawberry Creme	1 pkg + skim milk	220	tr	1
Instant Breakfast No Sugar Added Classic Chocolate	1 pkg	70	1	2
Instant Breakfast No Sugar Added Classic Chocolate	1 pkg + skim milk (9 fl oz)	160	1	2
Instant Breakfast No Sugar Added Creamy Milk Chocolate	1 pkg	70	1	1
Instant Breakfast No Sugar Added Creamy Milk Chocolate	1 pkg + skim milk (9 fl oz)	160	1	1
Instant Breakfast No Sugar Added French Vanilla	1 pkg	70	0	0
Instant Breakfast No Sugar Added French Vanilla	1 pkg + skim milk (9 fl oz)	150	tr	1
Instant Breakfast No Sugar Added Strawberry Creme	1 pkg	70	0	0
Instant Breakfast No Sugar Added Strawberry Creme	1 pkg + skim milk (9 fl oz)	150	tr	1

FOOD	PORTION	CALS.	SAT. FAT	FAT
Instant Breakfast Chocolate Malt, as prep w/ whole milk (Pillsbury)	1 serving	290	—	9
Instant Breakfast Chocolate, as prep w/ whole milk (Pillsbury)	1 serving	290	—	9
Instant Breakfast Strawberry, as prep w/ whole milk (Pillsbury)	1 serving	290	—	9
Instant Breakfast Vanilla, as prep w/ whole milk (Pillsbury)	1 serving	300	—	9
orange drink, powder	3 rounded tsp	93	0	0
orange drink powder, as prep w/ water	6 oz	86	0	0

BROAD BEANS
CANNED
broad beans	1 cup	183	tr	1

DRIED
cooked	1 cup	186	tr	1

FRESH
cooked	3.5 oz	56	tr	tr

BROCCOLI
FRESH
Dole	1 med spear	40	—	1
chopped, cooked	½ cup	22	tr	tr
raw, chopped	½ cup	12	tr	tr

FROZEN
Baby Spears (Birds Eye)	⅔ cup	29	0	tr
Broccoli w/ Cheese in Pastry (Pepperidge Farm)	1	230	—	16
Chopped (Big Valley)	¾ cup	5	0	0
Chopped (Birds Eye)	⅔ cup	25	0	0
Cut (Hanover)	½ cup	25	—	0
Cuts (Big Valley)	¾ cup (3 oz)	25	0	0
Cuts (Green Giant)	½ cup	12	0	0
Farm Fresh Spears (Birds Eye)	¾ cup	30	0	0
Florets (Hanover)	½ cup	30	—	0
Florets Deluxe (Birds Eye)	½ cup	25	0	0
Fresh Like	3.5 oz	26	—	tr

FOOD	PORTION	CALS.	SAT. FAT	FAT
Harvest Fresh Cut (Green Giant)	½ cup	16	0	0
Harvest Fresh Spears (Green Giant)	½ cup	20	0	0
In Butter Sauce (Green Giant)	½ cup	40	tr	2
In Cheese Sauce (Green Giant)	½ cup	60	tr	2
Mini Spears Select (Green Giant)	4–5 spears	18	0	0
One Serve Cuts in Butter Sauce (Green Giant)	1 pkg	45	tr	2
One Serve Cuts in Cheese Sauce (Green Giant)	1 pkg	70	tr	3
Polybag Cuts (Birds Eye)	½ cup	25	0	0
Polybag Deluxe Florets (Birds Eye)	⅔ cup	25	0	0
Spears (Birds Eye)	⅔ cup	25	0	0
Valley Combinations Broccoli Fanfare (Green Giant)	½ cup	80	—	2
With Cheese Sauce (Birds Eye)	½ pkg	110	2	5
chopped, cooked	½ cup	25	tr	tr
spears, cooked	10 oz pkg	69	tr	tr
spears, cooked	½ cup	25	tr	tr

BROWNIE

FROZEN

FOOD	PORTION	CALS.	SAT. FAT	FAT
Brownie Ala Mode (Weight Watchers)	1	180	tr	4
Chocolate Brownie (Weight Watchers)	1 (1.25 oz)	100	tr	3
Mint Frosted (Weight Watchers)	1 (1.23 oz)	100	tr	5
Monterey Hot Fudge Chocolate Chunk Brownie (Pepperidge Farm)	1	480	14	26
Newport Hot Fudge Brownie (Pepperidge Farm)	1	400	10	20

HOME RECIPE

FOOD	PORTION	CALS.	SAT. FAT	FAT
plain	1 (0.8 oz)	112	2	7
w/ nuts	1 (0.8 oz)	95	—	6

FOOD	PORTION	CALS.	SAT. FAT	FAT
MIX				
Brownie With Hot Fudge MicroRave Single (Betty Crocker)	1	350	3	12
Deluxe Family-Size Fudge Brownie (Pillsbury)	2	150	—	7
Deluxe Fudge Brownie (Pillsbury)	2	150	—	6
Deluxe Fudge Brownie w/ Walnuts (Pillsbury)	2	150	—	8
Estee Lite	2	100	2	4
Frosted MicroRave (Betty Crocker)	1	180	2	7
Fudge, as prep (Jiffy)	1	160	1	4
Fudge Family Size (Betty Crocker)	1	150	1	5
Fudge Light (Betty Crocker)	1	100	—	1
Fudge MicroRave (Betty Crocker)	1	150	2	6
Fudge Microrave (Pillsbury)	1	190	—	9
Fudge Regular Size (Betty Crocker)	1	150	1	6
Supreme Caramel (Betty Crocker)	1	120	1	4
Supreme Frosted (Betty Crocker)	1	160	2	6
Supreme German Chocolate (Betty Crocker)	1	160	2	7
Supreme Original (Betty Crocker)	1	140	1	6
Supreme Party (Betty Crocker)	1	160	2	6
Supreme Walnut (Betty Crocker)	1	140	1	7
The Ultimate Caramel Fudge Chunk Brownie (Pillsbury)	2	170	—	7
The Ultimate Chunky Triple Fudge Brownie (Pillsbury)	2	170	—	7
The Ultimate Double Fudge Brownie (Pillsbury)	2	160	—	6

FOOD	PORTION	CALS.	SAT. FAT	FAT
The Ultimate Rockey Road Fudge Brownie (Pillsbury)	2	170	—	8
Walnut MicroRave (Betty Crocker)	1	160	2	7
plain	1 (1.2 oz)	139	1	7
plain low calorie	1 (0.8 oz)	84	1	2
READY-TO-EAT				
Brownie (Tastykake)	1 (85 g)	340	3	14
Brownie Bites (Hostess)	5 (2 oz)	260	4	14
Brownie Bites Walnut (Hostess)	5 (2 oz)	270	4	15
Charlotte Fudgey Brownie (Pepperidge Farm)	1	220	4	11
Fudge (Little Debbie)	1 pkg (2.1 oz)	270	3	13
Fudge (Little Debbie)	1 pkg (2.5 oz)	310	3	15
Fudge (Little Debbie)	1 pkg (2.9 oz)	360	3	17
Fudge (Little Debbie)	1 pkg (3.6 oz)	450	4	21
Fudge Nut (Frito Lay)	3 oz	360	—	14
Lance	1 pkg (78 g)	320	3	12
Tahoe Milk Chocolate Pecan (Pepperidge Farm)	1	210	3	10
Westport Fudgey Brownies w/ Walnuts (Pepperidge Farm)	1	220	4	11
w/ nuts	1 (1 oz)	100	2	4
w/o nuts	1 (2 oz)	243	3	10

BRUSSELS SPROUTS
FRESH

FOOD	PORTION	CALS.	SAT. FAT	FAT
Dole	½ cup	19	—	tr
cooked	½ cup	30	tr	tr
cooked	1 sprout	8	tr	tr
raw	½ cup	19	tr	tr
raw	1 sprout	8	tr	tr
FROZEN				
Birds Eye	½ cup	35	0	tr
Fresh Like	3.5 oz	37	—	tr
Green Giant	½ cup	7	0	0
Hanover	½ cup	40	—	0
In Butter Sauce (Green Giant)	½ cup	40	tr	1
Whole (Big Valley)	5–8 pieces (3 oz)	35	0	0
cooked	½ cup	33	tr	tr

FOOD	PORTION	CALS.	SAT. FAT	FAT
BUCKWHEAT				
Brown Groats Roasted (Wolff's)	1 cup (8 oz)	900	—	4
Flour (Wolff's)	1 cup (8 oz)	860	—	5
Kasha Coarse, cooked (Wolff's)	¼ cup (1.6 oz)	170	0	2
Kasha Fine, cooked (Wolff's)	¼ cup (1.6 oz)	170	0	2
Kasha Medium, cooked (Wolff's)	¼ cup (1.6 oz)	170	0	2
Kasha Whole, cooked (Wolff's)	¼ cup (1.6 oz)	170	0	2
White Grits (Wolff's)	1 cup (8 oz)	840	—	3
flour, whole groat	1 cup	402	tr	4
groats, roasted, cooked	½ cup	91	tr	tr
groats, roasted, uncooked	½ cup	283	tr	2
BUFFALO				
water, roasted	3 oz	111	1	2
BULGAR				
Good Shepherd	¼ cup (43 g)	150	—	1
Hodgson Mill	¼ cup (1.4 oz)	120	0	1
cooked	½ cup	76	tr	tr
uncooked	½ cup	239	—	tr
BURBOT (FISH)				
fresh, baked	3 oz	98	tr	1
BURDOCK ROOT				
cooked	1 cup	110	—	tr
raw	1 cup	85	—	tr
BUTTER				
(*see also* BUTTER BLENDS, BUTTER SUBSTITUTES, MARGARINE)				
REGULAR				
Cabot	1 tsp	35	3	4
Cabot Unsalted	1 tsp	35	3	4
Crystal Salted	1 tbsp (0.5 oz)	102	7	11
Crystal Unsalted	1 tbsp (0.5 oz)	102	7	11
Hotel Bar	1 tsp	35	—	4
Keller's	1 tsp	35	—	4
Land O'Lakes	1 tbsp (0.5 oz)	100	7	11
Land O'Lakes Light	1 tbsp	50	4	6
Land O'Lakes Unsalted	1 tsp	35	4	7
butter	1 pat	36	3	4

FOOD	PORTION	CALS.	SAT. FAT	FAT
butter	1 stick (4 oz)	813	57	92
butter oil	1 cup	1795	127	204
butter oil	1 tbsp	112	8	13
clarified butter	3.5 oz	876	62	99
WHIPPED				
Land O'Lakes	1 tbsp (0.3 oz)	70	5	7
Land O'Lakes Unsalted	1 tbsp	60	5	7
butter	4 oz	542	38	61
butter	1 pat	27	2	3

BUTTER BEANS
CANNED

FOOD	PORTION	CALS.	SAT. FAT	FAT
Allen Baby	½ cup (4.5 oz)	120	1	1
Allen Large	½ cup (4.5 oz)	120	0	1
Hanover	½ cup	80	—	0
Hanover in Sauce	½ cup	100	—	0
Luck's Speckled Seasoned w/ Pork	7.5 oz	230	—	8
S&W Tender Cooked	½ cup	100	0	0
Sunshine	½ cup (4.5 oz)	120	0	1
Trappey Large White With Bacon	½ cup (4.5 oz)	110	0	1
Trappey's Baby White With Bacon (Trappey)	½ cup (4.5 oz)	130	1	2
Van Camp's	½ cup	110	0	1

BUTTER BLENDS
(see also BUTTER, BUTTER SUBSTITUTES, MARGARINE)
REGULAR

FOOD	PORTION	CALS.	SAT. FAT	FAT
Blue Bonnet Better Blend	1 tbsp	90	2	11
Blue Bonnet Better Blend Unsalted	1 tbsp	90	1	11
Country Morning Blend (Land O'Lakes)	1 tbsp	100	3	11
Country Morning Blend Light (Land O'Lakes)	1 tbsp (0.5 oz)	50	3	6
Country Morning Blend Unsalted (Land O'Lakes)	1 tbsp	100	3	11
butter blend	1 stick	811	32	91
SOFT				
Blue Bonnet Better Blend	1 tbsp	90	2	11
Country Morning Blend Light Tub (Land O'Lakes)	1 tbsp (0.5 oz)	50	3	6

FOOD	PORTION	CALS.	SAT. FAT	FAT
Country Morning Blend Tub (Land O'Lakes)	1 tbsp	100	2	11
Downey's Cinnamon Honey-Butter	1 tbsp	52	—	1
Downey's Original Honey-Butter	1 tbsp	52	—	1
Le Slim Cow	1 tbsp	40	2	4
Touch of Butter Stick	1 tbsp	90	2	10
Touch of Butter Tub	1 tbsp	50	1	6

BUTTER SUBSTITUTES
(see also BUTTER BLENDS, MARGARINE)

Butter Buds Mix	1 tsp (2 g)	5	0	0
Butter Buds Sprinkles	1 tsp (2 g)	5	0	0
Molly McButter	½ tsp (1 g)	3	—	tr
Molly McButter w/ Bacon	½ tsp (1 g)	4	—	tr
Molly McButter w/ Cheese	½ tsp (0.9 g)	4	—	tr
Molly McButter w/ Sour Cream	½ tsp (1.1 g)	4	—	tr

BUTTERBUR

canned fuki, chopped	1 cup	3	—	tr
fresh fuki, raw	1 cup	13	—	tr

BUTTERFISH

baked	3 oz	159	—	9
fillet, baked	1 oz	47	—	3

BUTTERNUTS

dried	1 oz	174	tr	16

BUTTERSCOTCH
(see also CANDY)

CABBAGE
FRESH

Dole	½ med head	18	—	0
Dole Napa, shredded	½ cup	6	—	tr
chinese pak-choi, raw, shredded	½ cup	5	tr	tr
chinese pak-poi, shredded, cooked	½ cup	10	tr	tr
chinese pe-tsai, raw, shredded	1 cup	12	tr	tr
chinese pe-tsai, shredded, cooked	1 cup	16	tr	tr

FOOD	PORTION	CALS.	SAT. FAT	FAT
danish raw	1 head (2 lbs)	228	tr	2
danish raw, shredded	½ cup (1.2 oz)	9	tr	tr
danish shredded, cooked	½ cup (2.6 oz)	17	tr	tr
green, raw	1 head (2 lbs)	228	tr	2
green, raw, shredded	½ cup (1.2 oz)	9	tr	tr
green, shredded, cooked	½ cup (2.6 oz)	17	tr	tr
red, raw, shredded	½ cup	10	tr	tr
red, shredded, cooked	½ cup	16	tr	tr
savoy, raw, shredded	½ cup	10	tr	tr
savoy, shredded, cooked	½ cup	18	tr	tr
HOME RECIPE				
coleslaw w/ dressing	¾ cup	147	2	11
TAKE-OUT				
coleslaw w/ dressing	½ cup	42	tr	2
stuffed cabbage	1 (6 oz)	373	12	22
sweet & sour red cabbage	4 oz	61	—	3
vinegar & oil coleslaw	3.5 oz	150	1	9

CAKE

(*see also* BROWNIE, COOKIES, DANISH PASTRY, DOUGHNUT, PIE)

FOOD	PORTION	CALS.	SAT. FAT	FAT
FROSTING/ICING				
Butter Pecan Ready-to-Spread (Betty Crocker)	½₂ tub	170	2	7
Cake & Cookie Decorator all colors except chocolate (Pillsbury)	1 tbsp	70	—	2
Cake & Cookie Decorator Chocolate (Pillsbury)	1 tbsp	60	—	2
Cherry Ready-to-Spread (Betty Crocker)	½₂ tub	160	2	6
Chocolate Creamy Homestyle (Duncan Hines)	1 oz	130	2	5
Chocolate Ready-to-Spread (Betty Crocker)	½₂ tub	160	2	7
Chocolate Chip Ready-to-Spread (Betty Crocker)	½₂ tub	170	3	7
Chocolate Fudge (Pillsbury)	for ⅙ cake	110	—	5
Chocolate Fudge, as prep (Betty Crocker)	½₂ mix	180	2	6
Chocolate Light Ready-to-Spread (Betty Crocker)	½₂ tub	130	1	2

FOOD	PORTION	CALS.	SAT. FAT	FAT
Chocolate With Candy Coated Chocolate Chips Ready-to-Spread (Betty Crocker)	1/12 tub	160	2	7
Chocolate With Dinosaurs Ready-to-Spread (Betty Crocker)	1/12 tub	160	2	7
Chocolate With Turbo Racers Ready-to-Spread (Betty Crocker)	1/12 tub	160	2	7
Coconut Almond Frosting Mix (Pillsbury)	for 1/12 cake	160	—	10
Coconut Pecan Frosting Mix (Pillsbury)	for 1/12 cake	150	—	7
Coconut Pecan Ready-to-Spread (Betty Crocker)	1/12 tub	160	3	9
Coconut Pecan, as prep (Betty Crocker)	1/12 mix	180	2	8
Cream Cheese Ready-to-Spread (Betty Crocker)	1/12 tub	170	2	7
Creamy Milk Chocolate, as prep (Betty Crocker)	1/12 mix	170	1	5
Creamy Vanilla, as prep (Betty Crocker)	1/12 mix	170	1	5
Dark Dutch Fudge Ready-to-Spread (Betty Crocker)	1/12 tub	160	2	7
Fluffy White Frosting Mix (Pillsbury)	for 1/12 cake	60	0	0
Frost It Hot Chocolate (Pillsbury)	for 1/8 cake	50	0	0
Frost It Hot Fluffy White (Pillsbury)	for 1/8 cake	50	0	0
Frosting Supreme Caramel Pecan (Pillsbury)	for 1/12 cake	160	—	8
Frosting Supreme Chocolate Chip (Pillsbury)	for 1/12 cake	150	—	5
Frosting Supreme Chocolate Fudge (Pillsbury)	for 1/12 cake	150	—	6
Frosting Supreme Chocolate Mint (Pillsbury)	for 1/12 cake	150	—	7
Frosting Supreme Coconut Almond (Pillsbury)	for 1/12 cake	150	—	9

FOOD	PORTION	CALS.	SAT. FAT	FAT
Frosting Supreme Coconut Pecan (Pillsbury)	for ½ cake	160	—	10
Frosting Supreme Cream Cheese (Pillsbury)	for ½ cake	160	—	6
Frosting Supreme Double Dutch (Pillsbury)	for ½ cake	140	—	6
Frosting Supreme Lemon (Pillsbury)	for ½ cake	160	—	6
Frosting Supreme Milk Chocolate (Pillsbury)	for ½ cake	150	—	6
Frosting Supreme Mocha (Pillsbury)	for ½ cake	150	—	6
Frosting Supreme Sour Cream Vanilla (Pillsbury)	for ½ cake	160	—	6
Frosting Supreme Strawberry (Pillsbury)	for ½ cake	160	—	6
Frosting Supreme Vanilla (Pillsbury)	for ½ cake	160	—	6
Fudge (Jiffy)	¼ cup (1.2 oz)	150	2	4
Funetti Chocolate Fudge (Pillsbury)	½ can	140	—	6
Funfetti Vanilla Pink (Pillsbury)	½ can	150	—	6
Funfetti Vanilla White (Pillsbury)	½ can	150	—	6
Lemon Ready-to-Spread (Betty Crocker)	½ tub	170	2	6
Lite Frosting, as prep (Estee)	3 tbsp (0.7 oz)	100	0	3
Milk Chocolate Creamy Homestyle (Duncan Hines)	1 oz	130	2	5
Milk Chocolate Light Ready-to-Spread (Betty Crocker)	½ tub	140	1	2
Milk Chocolate Ready-to-Spread (Betty Crocker)	½ tub	160	2	6
Rainbow Chip Ready-to-Spread (Betty Crocker)	½ tub	170	3	7
Sour Cream Chocolate Ready-to-Spread (Betty Crocker)	½ tub	160	2	7
Sour Cream White Ready-to-Spread (Betty Crocker)	½ tub	160	2	6

FOOD	PORTION	CALS.	SAT. FAT	FAT
Vanilla (Pillsbury)	for ⅙ cake	120	—	5
Vanilla Creamy Homestyle (Duncan Hines)	1 oz	140	2	5
Vanilla Ready-to-Spread (Betty Crocker)	½ tub	160	2	6
Vanilla Light Ready-to-Spread (Betty Crocker)	½ tub	140	1	2
Vanilla With Teddy Bears Ready-to-Spread (Betty Crocker)	½ tub	160	2	6
White (Jiffy)	¼ cup (1.2 oz)	150	1	5
White Fluffy, as prep (Betty Crocker)	½ mix	70	0	0
FROZEN				
Amhurst Apple Crumb Coffee Cake (Pepperidge Farm)	1	220	7	11
Apple Crisp (Weight Watchers)	1 (3.5 oz)	190	tr	5
Apple Crisp Cake Light (Sara Lee)	1 (3 oz)	150	—	2
Apple 'N Spice Bake Dessert Lights (Pepperidge Farm)	1 piece (4.25 oz)	170	0	2
Banana Single Layer Iced Cake (Sara Lee)	1 slice (1.7 oz)	170	—	6
Berkshire Apple Crisp (Pepperidge Farm)	1	250	4	8
Black Forest Cake Light (Sara Lee)	1 (3.6 oz)	170	—	5
Black Forest Two Layer Cake (Sara Lee)	1 slice (2.5 oz)	190	—	8
Blueberry Turnovers (Pepperidge Farm)	1	310	—	19
Boston Cream Supreme (Pepperidge Farm)	1 (2⅞ oz)	290	6	14
Brownie Cheesecake (Weight Watchers)	1 (3.5 oz)	200	1	5
Butter Pound (Pepperidge Farm)	1 slice (1 oz)	130	3	7
Carrot Classic (Pepperidge Farm)	1 cake	260	6	16
Carrot Light (Sara Lee)	1 (2.5 oz)	170	—	4
Carrot Single Layer Iced Cake (Sara Lee)	1 slice (2.4 oz)	250	—	13

FOOD	PORTION	CALS.	SAT. FAT	FAT
Carrot w/ Cream Cheese Icing (Pepperidge Farm)	1 slice (1.5 oz)	150	3	9
Charleston Peach Melba Shortcake (Pepperidge Farm)	1	220	3	5
Cheese Sweet Roll (Weight Watchers)	1 (2.25 oz)	180	—	4
Cheesecake Original Cherry (Sara Lee)	1 slice (3.2 oz)	243	—	8
Cheesecake Original Plain (Sara Lee)	1 slice (2.8 oz)	230	—	11
Cheesecake Original Strawberry (Sara Lee)	1 slice (3.2 oz)	222	—	8
Cherries & Cream Cake (Weight Watchers)	1 (3 oz)	150	tr	2
Cherries Supreme Dessert Lights (Pepperidge Farm)	1 piece (3.25 oz)	170	0	11
Cherry Turnover (Pepperidge Farm)	1	310	—	19
Chocolate Cake (Weight Watchers)	1 (2.5 oz)	180	tr	5
Chocolate Cake Free & Light (Sara Lee)	1 slice (1.7 oz)	110	—	0
Chocolate Eclair (Weight Watchers)	1 (2.1 oz)	120	tr	4
Chocolate Fudge Large Layer (Pepperidge Farm)	1 slice (1⅝ oz)	180	3	10
Chocolate Fudge Strip Large Layer (Pepperidge Farm)	1 piece (1⅝ oz)	170	3	9
Chocolate Mousse Cake Dessert Lights (Pepperidge Farm)	1 piece (2.5 oz)	190	3	9
Cholesterol Free Pound (Pepperidge Farm)	1 slice (1 oz)	110	—	6
Cobbler Apple (Pet-Ritz)	⅙ cake (4.33 oz)	290	—	9
Cobbler Blackberry (Pet-Ritz)	⅙ cake (4.33 oz)	250	—	10
Cobbler Blueberry (Pet-Ritz)	⅙ cake (4.33 oz)	270	—	12
Cobbler Cherry (Pet-Ritz)	⅙ cake (4.33 oz)	280	—	10
Cobbler Peach (Pet-Ritz)	⅙ cake (4.33 oz)	260	—	10
Cobbler Strawberry (Pet-Ritz)	⅙ cake (4.33 oz)	290	—	9

FOOD	PORTION	CALS.	SAT. FAT	FAT
Coconut Classic (Pepperidge Farm)	1 cake	230	4	11
Coconut Large Layer (Pepperidge Farm)	1 slice (1⅝ oz)	180	3	8
Coffee Cake All Butter Butter Streusel (Sara Lee)	1 slice (1.4 oz)	160	—	7
Coffee Cake All Butter Cheese (Sara Lee)	1 slice (2 oz)	210	—	11
Coffee Cake All Butter Pecan (Sara Lee)	1 slice (1.4 oz)	160	—	8
Coffee Cake w/ Cinnamon Streusel (Weight Watchers)	2.25 oz	160	—	4
Devil's Food Large Layer (Pepperidge Farm)	1 slice (1⅝ oz)	180	3	9
Double Chocolate Cake Light (Sara Lee)	1 (2.5 oz)	150	—	5
Double Chocolate Classic (Pepperidge Farm)	1 cake	250	4	13
Double Chocolate Three Layer Cake (Sara Lee)	1 slice (2.2 oz)	220	—	11
Double Fudge (Weight Watchers)	1 piece (2.75 oz)	190	tr	4
Elfin Loaves Apple Cinnamon	1	180	1	4
Elfin Loaves Banana	1	190	1	7
Elfin Loaves Blueberry	1	170	1	4
Elfin Loaves Carrot	1	210	1	10
French Cheesecake (Sara Lee)	1 slice (2.9 oz)	250	—	16
French Cheesecake Light (Sara Lee)	1 (3.2 oz)	150	—	4
Fruit Squares Apple (Pepperidge Farm)	1	220	—	12
Fruit Squares Cherry (Pepperidge Farm)	1	230	—	12
Fudge Golden Classic (Pepperidge Farm)	1 cake	260	4	14
German Chocolate Classic (Pepperidge Farm)	1 cake	250	4	13
German Chocolate Large Layer (Pepperidge Farm)	1 slice (1⅝ oz)	180	4	10
Golden Large Layer (Pepperidge Farm)	1 slice (1⅝ oz)	180	3	9

FOOD	PORTION	CALS.	SAT. FAT	FAT
Lemon Cake Supreme Dessert Lights (Pepperidge Farm)	1 piece (2.75 oz)	170	1	5
Lemon Coconut Classic Cake (Pepperidge Farm)	3 oz	280	—	13
Lemon Coconut Supreme (Pepperidge Farm)	1 piece (3 oz)	280	6	13
Lemon Cream Cake Light (Sara Lee)	1 (3.2 oz)	180	—	6
Lemon Cream Supreme (Pepperidge Farm)	1 piece (1⅝ oz)	170	3	9
Manhattan Strawberry Cheesecake (Pepperidge Farm)	1	300	5	9
Peach Melba Supreme (Pepperidge Farm)	1 (3⅛ oz)	270	3	7
Peach Parfait Dessert Lights (Pepperidge Farm)	1 piece (4.25 oz)	150	1	5
Peach Turnover (Pepperidge Farm)	1	310	—	18
Pineapple Cream Supreme (Pepperidge Farm)	1 piece (2 oz)	190	2	7
Pound Cake All Butter Family Size (Sara Lee)	1 slice (1 oz)	130	—	7
Pound Cake All Butter Original (Sara Lee)	1 slice (1 oz)	130	—	7
Pound Cake Free & Light (Sara Lee)	1 slice (1 oz)	70	—	0
Raspberry Turnovers (Pepperidge Farm)	1	310	—	17
Raspberry Vanilla Swirl Dessert Lights (Pepperidge Farm)	1 piece (3.25 oz)	160	1	5
Strawberry Cheesecake (Weight Watchers)	1 piece (3.9 oz)	180	2	4
Strawberry French Cheesecake Light (Sara Lee)	1 (3.5 oz)	150	—	2
Strawberry Shortcake Dessert Lights (Pepperidge Farm)	1 piece (3 oz)	170	1	5
Strawberry Shortcake Two Layer Cake (Sara Lee)	1 slice (2.5 oz)	190	—	8

FOOD	PORTION	CALS.	SAT. FAT	FAT
Strawberry Strip Large Layer (Pepperidge Farm)	1 piece (1.5 oz)	160	3	8
Strawberry Yogurt Dessert Free & Light (Sara Lee)	1 slice (2.2 oz)	120	—	1
Vanilla Fudge Swirl Classic (Pepperidge Farm)	1 cake	250	4	11
Vanilla Large Layer (Pepperidge Farm)	1 slice (1⅝ oz)	190	3	8
boston cream pie	⅙ cake (3.2 oz)	232	2	8
eclair w/ chocolate icing & custard filling, frzn	1	205	—	10
HOME RECIPE				
angelfood	1⁄12 cake (1.9 oz)	142	tr	tr
boston cream pie	⅙ cake (3.3 oz)	293	4	12
carrot w/ cream cheese icing	1 cake (10 in diam tube)	6175	66	328
carrot w/ cream cheese icing	1⁄12 cake (3.9 oz)	484	5	29
cheesecake	1⁄12 cake (4.5 oz)	456	18	9
cheesecake w/ cherry topping	1⁄12 cake (5 oz)	359	13	23
chocolate w/o frosting	1⁄12 cake (3.3 oz)	340	5	14
chocolate w/o frosting	2 layers (39.9 oz)	4067	62	172
chocolate cupcake creme filled w/ frosting	1 (1.8 oz)	188	2	7
coffeecake creme-filled chocolate frosting	⅙ cake (3.2 oz)	298	3	10
coffeecake crumb topped cinnamon	1⁄12 cake (2.1 oz)	240	2	12
cream puff w/ custard filling	1 (4.6 oz)	336	5	20
cream puff shell	1 (2.3 oz)	239	4	17
eclair	1 (3 oz)	262	4	16
fruitcake	1⁄36 cake (2.9 oz)	302	1	10
fruitcake dark	1 cake (7½ in x 2¼ in)	5185	48	228
gingerbread	⅛ cake (2.6 oz)	264	3	12
pineapple upside down	⅛ cake (4 oz)	367	3	14
pound	1 loaf (8½″ × 3½″)	1935	21	94
pound cake	1 slice (1 oz)	120	1	5
sheet cake w/ white frosting	1 cake (9 in sq)	4020	42	129
sheet cake w/ white frosting	⅑ cake	445	5	14

FOOD	PORTION	CALS.	SAT. FAT	FAT
sheet cake w/o frosting	⅑ cake	315	3	12
sheet cake w/o frosting	1 cake (9 in sq)	2830	30	108
shortcake	1 (2.3 oz)	225	2	9
sponge	1/12 cake (2.2 oz)	140	1	2
white w/ coconut frosting	1/12 cake (3.9 oz)	399	4	12
white w/o frosting	1/12 cake (2.6 oz)	264	2	9
yellow w/o frosting	1/12 cake (2.4 oz)	245	3	10
yellow w/o frosting	2 layers (28.7 oz)	2947	32	119
MIX				
Angel Food (Duncan Hines)	1/12 pkg (1.3 oz)	140	0	0
Angel Food Confetti (Betty Crocker)	1/12 cake	150	0	0
Angel Food Traditional (Betty Crocker)	1/12 cake	130	0	0
Angel Food Lemon Custard (Betty Crocker)	1/12 cake	150	0	0
Angel Food White (Betty Crocker)	1/12 cake	150	0	0
Apple Cinnamon Coffee Cake (Pillsbury)	⅛ cake	240	—	7
Apple Streusel MicroRave (Betty Crocker)	⅙ cake	240	3	11
Apple Streusel MicroRave No Cholesterol Recipe (Betty Crocker)	⅙ cake	210	2	8
Banana Quick Bread (Pillsbury)	1/12 loaf	170	—	6
Bisquick	½ cup (2 oz)	240	2	8
Bisquick Reduced Fat	½ cup (2 oz)	210	1	4
Blueberry Nut Quick Bread (Pillsbury)	1/12 loaf	150	—	4
Butter Chocolate (Betty Crocker)	1/12 cake	280	7	14
Butter Pecan SuperMoist (Betty Crocker)	1/12 cake	250	1	11
Butter Pecan No Cholesterol Recipe (Betty Crocker)	1/12 cake	220	2	7
Butter Recipe (Pillsbury)	1/12 cake	260	—	12
Butter Yellow (Betty Crocker)	1/12 cake	260	6	11
Carrot (Betty Crocker)	1/12 cake	250	2	10
Carrot (Dromedary)	1/12 cake	232	—	15

FOOD	PORTION	CALS.	SAT. FAT	FAT
Carrot No Cholesterol Recipe (Betty Crocker)	1/12 cake	210	2	6
Cheese Cake Lite No-Bake (Royal)	1/8 pie	130	0	3
Cheese Cake Real No-Bake (Royal)	1/8 pie	160	—	3
Cheesecake (Jell-O)	1/8 cake	277	—	13
Cheesecake New York Style (Jell-O)	1/8 cake	283	—	12
Cherry Chip (Betty Crocker)	1/12 cake	190	1	3
Cherry Nut Quick Bread (Pillsbury)	1/12 loaf	180	—	5
Chocolate Chip (Betty Crocker)	1/12 cake	290	3	15
Chocolate Chip (Pillsbury)	1/12 cake	270	—	14
Chocolate Chip No Cholesterol Recipe (Betty Crocker)	1/12 cake	220	2	8
Chocolate Chocolate Chip (Betty Crocker)	1/12 cake	260	3	12
Chocolate Fudge (Betty Crocker)	1/12 cake	260	3	12
Chocolate Lite Cake & Frosting Mix (Batter Lite)	1/6 of cake	110	—	2
Chocolate Microwave (Pillsbury)	1/8 cake	210	—	12
Chocolate Pudding Classic Dessert (Betty Crocker)	1/6 cake	230	—	5
Chocolate With Chocolate Frosting (Pillsbury)	1/8 cake	300	—	17
Chocolate With Vanilla Frosting (Pillsbury)	1/8 cake	300	—	17
Cinnamon Pecan Streusel Microwave (Betty Crocker)	1/6 cake	280	3	12
Cinnamon Pecan Streusel Microwave No Cholesterol (Betty Crocker)	1/6 cake	230	2	7
Cobbler Apple Crumb (Dromedary)	1/8 cake	237	—	6
Cobbler Cherry Crumb (Dromedary)	1/8 cake	231	—	6

FOOD	PORTION	CALS.	SAT. FAT	FAT
Coffee Cake Easy Mix (Aunt Jemima)	⅛ cake	160	—	5
Cranberry Quick Bread (Pillsbury)	1/12 loaf	160	—	4
Cupcake Yellow With Chocolate Frosting (Duncan Hines)	1	180	2	0
Date Nut (Dromedary)	½ cake	183	—	8
Date Nut Roll (Dromedary)	½ in slice	80	—	2
Date Quick Bread (Pillsbury)	1/12 loaf	160	—	2
Devil's Food (Betty Crocker)	1/12 cake	260	3	12
Devil's Food (Pillsbury)	1/12 cake	270	—	14
Devil's Food, as prep (Jiffy)	⅛ cake	220	2	6
Devil's Food Chocolate Frosting MicroRave (Betty Crocker)	⅙ cake	310	5	17
Devil's Food Moist Deluxe (Duncan Hines)	1/12 cake (1.5 oz)	290	3	15
Devil's Food No Cholesterol Recipe (Betty Crocker)	1/12 cake	220	2	7
Devil's Food SuperMoist Light (Betty Crocker)	1/12 cake	200	2	4
Devil's Food SuperMoist Light No Cholesterol Recipe (Betty Crocker)	1/12 cake	180	1	3
Devil's Food With Chocolate Frosting MicroRave Single (Betty Crocker)	1	440	6	18
Double Chocolate Supreme Microwave (Pillsbury)	⅛ cake	330	—	19
Double Lemon Supreme Microwave (Pillsbury)	⅛ cake	300	—	15
French Vanilla Moist Deluxe (Duncan Hines)	1/12 cake (1.5 oz)	250	2	11
Fudge Marble (Pillsbury)	1/12 cake	270	—	12
Fudge Marble Moist Deluxe (Duncan Hines)	1/12 cake (1.5 oz)	250	2	11
German Chocolate (Betty Crocker)	1/12 cake	260	3	12

FOOD	PORTION	CALS.	SAT. FAT	FAT
German Chocolate (Pillsbury)	1/12 cake	250	—	11
German Chocolate Chocolate Frosting MicroRave (Betty Crocker)	1/6 cake	320	5	18
German Chocolate No Cholesterol Recipe (Betty Crocker)	1/12 cake	220	2	8
Gingerbread (Dromedary)	1 piece (2 in x 2 in)	100	—	2
Gingerbread (Pillsbury)	3 in sq	190	—	4
Gingerbread Classic Dessert (Betty Crocker)	1/9 cake	22	2	7
Gingerbread Classic Dessert No Cholesterol Recipe (Betty Crocker)	1/9 cake	210	2	6
Golden Pound Classic Dessert (Betty Crocker)	1/12 cake	200	3	9
Golden Vanilla (Betty Crocker)	1/12 cake	280	3	14
Golden Vanilla No Cholesterol Recipe (Betty Crocker)	1/12 cake	220	2	7
Golden Vanilla Rainbow Chip Frosting MicroRave (Betty Crocker)	1/6 cake	320	5	18
Golden Yellow, as prep (Jiffy)	1/5 cake	220	1	5
Lemon (Betty Crocker)	1/12 cake	260	3	11
Lemon (Pillsbury)	1/12 cake	250	—	11
Lemon Chiffon Classic Dessert (Betty Crocker)	1/12 cake	200	—	5
Lemon Microwave (Pillsbury)	1/8 cake	220	—	13
Lemon No Cholesterol Recipe (Betty Crocker)	1/12 cake	220	2	7
Lemon Pudding Classic Dessert (Betty Crocker)	1/6 cake	230	—	5
Lemon Supreme Moist Deluxe (Duncan Hines)	1/12 cake (1.5 oz)	250	2	11
Lemon With Lemon Frosting (Pillsbury)	1/8 cake	300	—	17
Lite Chocolate (Estee)	1/5 cake (1.7 oz)	190	2	4

FOOD	PORTION	CALS.	SAT. FAT	FAT
Lite Pound, as prep (Estee)	⅕ cake (1.7 oz)	200	2	4
Lite White, as prep (Estee)	⅕ cake (1.7 oz)	200	2	4
Marble (Betty Crocker)	1/12 cake	260	3	11
Marble No Cholesterol Recipe (Betty Crocker)	1/12 cake	220	2	7
Milk Chocolate (Betty Crocker)	1/12 cake	260	3	12
Milk Chocolate No Cholesterol Recipe (Betty Crocker)	1/12 cake	210	2	7
Nut Quick Bread (Pillsbury)	1/12 loaf	170	—	6
Pineapple Upsidedown Classic Dessert (Betty Crocker)	⅑ cake	250	4	10
Pound (Dromedary)	½ in slice	150	—	6
Rainbow Chip (Betty Crocker)	1/12 cake	250	3	11
Sour Cream Chocolate (Betty Crocker)	1/12 cake	260	3	12
Sour Cream Chocolate No Cholesterol Recipe (Betty Crocker)	1/12 cake	220	2	8
Sour Cream White (Betty Crocker)	1/12 cake	180	1	3
Spice (Betty Crocker)	1/12 cake	260	2	11
Spice No Cholesterol Recipe (Betty Crocker)	1/12 cake	220	2	7
Strawberry (Pillsbury)	1/12 cake	260	—	11
Streusel Swirl Cinnamon (Pillsbury)	1/16 cake	260	—	11
Streusel Swirl Cinnamon Microwave (Pillsbury)	⅛ cake	240	—	11
Streusel Swirl Lemon (Pillsbury)	1/16 cake	270	—	11
Tunnel of Fudge Bundt (Pillsbury)	1/16 cake	270	—	12
Tunnel of Fudge Bundt Microwave (Pillsbury)	⅛ cake	290	—	17
White (Betty Crocker)	1/12 cake	240	2	9
White (Pillsbury)	1/12 cake	240	—	10
White, as prep (Jiffy)	⅕ cake	210	1	5

FOOD	PORTION	CALS.	SAT. FAT	FAT
White Lite Cake & Frosting Mix (Batter Lite)	1/6 of cake	110	—	2
White No Cholesterol Recipe (Betty Crocker)	1/12 cake	220	2	7
White SuperMoist Light (Betty Crocker)	1/12 cake	180	1	3
Whole Wheat Baking Mix (Hain)	1½ oz	150	—	1
Yellow (Betty Crocker)	1/12 cake	260	3	11
Yellow (Pillsbury)	1/12 cake	260	—	12
Yellow Moist Deluxe (Duncan Hines)	1/12 cake (1.5 oz)	250	2	11
Yellow SuperMoist Light (Betty Crocker)	1/12 cake	200	2	4
Yellow SuperMoist Light No Cholesterol Recipe (Betty Crocker)	1/12 cake	190	1	3
Yellow Chocolate Frosting MicroRave (Betty Crocker)	1/6 cake	300	4	17
Yellow Microwave (Pillsbury)	1/8 cake	220	—	13
Yellow No Cholesterol Recipe (Betty Crocker)	1/12 cake	220	3	7
Yellow With Chocolate Frosting (Pillsbury)	1/8 cake	300	—	17
Yellow With Chocolate Frosting MicroRave Single (Betty Crocker)	1	440	6	19
angelfood	1/12 cake (1.8 oz)	129	tr	tr
angelfood	10 in cake (20.9 oz)	1535	tr	2
carrot w/o frosting	1/12 cake (2.5 oz)	239	2	11
carrot w/o frosting	2 layers (29.6 oz)	2886	22	133
cheesecake no-bake	1/8 cake (3.5 oz)	271	7	13
chocolate pudding type w/o frosting	1/12 cake (2.7 oz)	270	3	14
chocolate pudding type w/o frosting	2 layers (32.4 oz)	3234	35	172
chocolate w/o frosting	1/12 cake (2.3 oz)	198	2	8
chocolate w/o frosting	2 layers (26.8 oz)	2393	21	92
chocolate w/o frosting low sodium	1/10 cake (1.3 oz)	116	1	3
coffeecake crumb topped cinnamon	1/8 cake (2 oz)	178	1	5

FOOD	PORTION	CALS.	SAT. FAT	FAT
devil's food w/o frosting	½ cake (2.3 oz)	198	2	8
devil's food w/ chocolate frosting	1 cake (9 in diam)	3755	56	136
devil's food w/ chocolate frosting	⅟₁₆ cake	235	4	8
fudge w/o frosting	½ cake (2.3 oz)	198	2	8
german chocolate pudding type w/ coconut nut frosting	½ cake (3.9 oz)	404	5	21
gingerbread	1 cake (8 in sq)	1575	10	39
gingerbread	⅛ cake (2.4 oz)	207	2	7
lemon w/o frosting no sugar low sodium	⅟₁₀ cake (1.3 oz)	118	tr	3
marble pudding type w/o frosting	½ cake (2.6 oz)	253	2	12
marble pudding type w/o frosting	2 layers (30.6 oz)	3021	27	148
white pudding type w/o frosting	½ cake (2.4 oz)	244	2	10
white pudding type w/o frosting	2 layers (29 oz)	2915	23	123
white w/o frosting	½ cake (2.2 oz)	190	1	5
white w/o frosting	2 layer cake (26 oz)	2265	9	57
white w/o frosting no sugar low sodium	⅟₁₀ cake (1.3 oz)	118	tr	3
yellow pudding-type w/o frosting	½ cake (2.6 oz)	257	2	12
yellow pudding-type w/o frosting	2 layers (31 oz)	3084	28	139
yellow w/ chocolate frosting	⅟₁₆ cake	235	3	8
yellow w/o frosting	½ cake (2.2 oz)	202	1	6
yellow w/o frosting	2 layers (26.5 oz)	2415	12	71
yellow w/ chocolate frosting	1 cake (9 in diam)	3895	92	175
READY-TO-EAT				
Angel Food Ring (Hostess)	⅙ cake (1.6 oz)	150	2	3
Apple Puffs (Entenmann's)	1 (3 oz)	280	—	13
Apple Strudel Old Fashioned (Entenmann's)	1 serving (1.5 oz)	120	—	5
Cheese Topped Buns (Entenmann's)	1 (2.3 oz)	240	—	12

FOOD	PORTION	CALS.	SAT. FAT	FAT
Cinnamon Buns (Entenmann's)	1 (2.1 oz)	230	—	10
Cinnamon Filbert Ring (Entenmann's)	1 serving (1.5 oz)	190	—	12
Coffee Cake Cheese (Entenmann's)	1 serving (1.6 oz)	150	—	7
Coffee Cake Cheese Filled Crumb (Entenmann's)	1 serving (1.4 oz)	130	—	6
Coffee Cake Crumb (Entenmann's)	1 serving (1.3 oz)	160	—	7
Danish Ring (Entenmann's)	1 serving (1.5 oz)	180	—	10
Danish Ring Pecan (Entenmann's)	1 serving (1.5 oz)	190	—	12
Danish Ring Walnut (Entenmann's)	1 serving (1.5 oz)	190	—	12
Danish Twist Lemon (Entenmann's)	1 serving (1.2 oz)	140	—	7
Danish Twist Raspberry (Entenmann's)	1 serving (1.2 oz)	140	—	7
Date Nut Loaf (Thomas')	1 oz	90	—	2
Dessert Shells Chocolate Covered (Dutch Mill)	1 (0.5 oz)	80	2	5
Devil's Food Cake Fudge Iced (Entenmann's)	1 serving (1.2 oz)	130	—	5
French Crumb Cake All Butter (Entenmann's)	1 serving (1.6 oz)	180	—	8
Fruit Cake Holiday (Hostess)	⅙ cake (5.3 oz)	490	2	14
Louisiana Crunch Cake (Entenmann's)	1 serving (1.7 oz)	180	—	8
Pound Cake (Hostess)	⅙ cake (3.2 oz)	350	4	16
Pound Loaf All Butter (Entenmann's)	1 serving (1 oz)	110	—	5
Pound Loaf Sour Cream (Entenmann's)	1 serving (1 oz)	120	—	7
Thick Fudge Golden Cake (Entenmann's)	1 serving (1.2 oz)	130	—	6
angelfood	1 cake (11.9 oz)	876	tr	3
angelfood	¹⁄₁₂ cake (1 oz)	73	tr	tr
bakewell tart	1 slice (3 oz)	410	—	27
battenburg cake	1 slice (2 oz)	204	—	10
cheesecake	1 cake (9 in diam)	3350	120	213
cheesecake	⅙ cake (2.8 oz)	256	9	18

FOOD	PORTION	CALS.	SAT. FAT	FAT
cherry fudge w/ chocolate frosting	⅛ cake (2.5 oz)	187	3	9
chocolate w/ chocolate frosting	⅛ cake (2.2 oz)	235	3	11
coffeecake cheese	⅙ cake (2.7 oz)	258	4	12
coffeecake crumb topped cheese	⅙ cake (2.7 oz)	258	4	12
coffeecake crumb topped cinnamon	⅛ cake (2.2 oz)	263	4	15
coffeecake fruit	⅛ cake (1.8 oz)	156	1	5
crumpets toasted	2 (4 oz)	119	—	1
eccles cake	1 slice (2 oz)	285	—	16
eclair	1 (1.4 oz)	149	—	10
fruitcake	1 piece (1.5 oz)	139	tr	4
madeira cake	1 slice (1 oz)	98	—	4
pound	¹⁄₁₀ cake (1 oz)	117	3	6
pound cake	1 cake (8½ x 3½ x 3 in)	1935	52	94
pound cake	1 slice (1 oz)	110	3	12
sour cream pound	¹⁄₁₀ cake (1 oz)	117	1	5
sponge	¹⁄₁₂ cake (1.3 oz)	110	tr	1
strudel apple	1 piece (2½ oz)	195	2	8
treacle tart	1 slice (2.5 oz)	258	—	10
vanilla slice	1 slice (2½ oz)	248	—	13
white w/ white frosting	1 cake (9 in diam)	4170	33	148
white w/ white frosting	¹⁄₁₆ cake	260	2	9
yellow w/ vanilla frosting	⅛ cake (2.2 oz)	239	2	9
yellow w/ chocolate frosting	1 cake (9" diam)	3895	92	175
yellow w/ chocolate frosting	⅛ cake (2.2 oz)	242	3	11
REFRIGERATED				
Apple Turnovers (Pillsbury)	1	170	2	8
Cheesecake (Baby Watson)	1 slice (3.8 oz)	390	18	30
Cheesecake Light (Baby Watson)	¹⁄₁₆ cake (3.9 oz)	280	9	16
Cherry Turnovers (Pillsbury)	1	170	2	8
Coffee Cake Cinnamon Swirl (Pillsbury)	⅛ cake	180	2	9
Coffee Cake Pecan Streusel (Pillsbury)	⅛ cake	180	2	9
Pastry Pockets (Pillsbury)	1	240	3	13

FOOD	PORTION	CALS.	SAT. FAT	FAT
SNACK				
All Butter Pound Cake (Sara Lee)	1	200	—	11
Apple Delights (Little Debbie)	1 pkg (1.2 oz)	140	2	5
Apple Light & Fruity (Drake's)	1 (1.2 oz)	90	—	1
Apple Oatmeal (Lance)	1 pkg (51 g)	200	3	9
Apple Twist (Hostess)	1 (2.5 oz)	220	2	4
Apple-Roos (Little Debbie)	1 pkg (1.5 oz)	150	0	3
Banana Nut Muffin Loaves (Little Debbie)	1 pkg (1.9 oz)	210	2	9
Banana Twins (Little Debbie)	1 pkg (2.2 oz)	250	2	10
Baseball Yellow Cakes (Hostess)	1 (1.6 oz)	160	1	3
Be My Valentine (Little Debbie)	1 pkg (2.2 oz)	280	3	14
Blueberry Light & Fruity (Drake's)	1 (1.2 oz)	90	—	1
Butter Cream Cream Filled Cupcake (Tastykake)	1 (32 g)	120	1	4
Cherry Cordials (Little Debbie)	1 pkg (1.3 oz)	160	2	8
Choc-O-Jel (Little Debbie)	1 pkg (1.2 oz)	150	2	7
Choco-Cakes (Little Debbie)	1 pkg (2.1 oz)	250	3	13
Choco-Cakes (Little Debbie)	1 pkg (2.2 oz)	240	3	12
Choco-Diles (Hostess)	1 (1.8 oz)	210	7	10
Choco-Licious (Hostess)	1 (1.5 oz)	170	3	6
Chocolate (Little Debbie)	1 pkg (3 oz)	360	4	17
Chocolate Cream Filled Cupcake (Tastykake)	1 (34 g)	130	1	5
Chocolate Cupcake (Tastykake)	1 (30 g)	100	1	3
Chocolate Chip (Little Debbie)	1 pkg (2.4 oz)	290	3	15
Chocolate Fudge Cake (Sara Lee)	1	190	—	10
Chocolate Twins (Little Debbie)	1 pkg (2.4 oz)	240	2	9
Christmas Tree Cakes (Little Debbie)	1 pkg (1.5 oz)	190	2	9

FOOD	PORTION	CALS.	SAT. FAT	FAT
Cinnaminis Original (Hostess)	5 (2.4 oz)	300	4	17
Cinnamon Raisin Light & Fruity (Drake's)	1 (1.2 oz)	90	—	1
Cinnamon Roll (Hostess)	1 (2.3 g)	220	3	6
Classic Cheesecake (Sara Lee)	1	200	—	14
Coconut (Little Debbie)	1 pkg (2.1 oz)	270	3	13
Coconut (Little Debbie)	1 pkg (2.4 oz)	300	4	14
Coconut Rounds (Little Debbie)	1 pkg (1.2 oz)	140	3	7
Coffee Cake				
(Drake's)	1 (1.1 oz)	140	—	6
(Little Debbie)	1 pkg (1.9 oz)	220	1	7
Apple Cinnamon (Sara Lee)	1	290	—	13
Apple Streusel (Little Debbie)	1 pkg (2 oz)	220	1	7
Butter Streusel (Sara Lee)	1	230	—	12
Chocolate Crumb (Drake's)	1 (2.5 oz)	245	—	9
Cinnamon Crumb (Drake's)	½ cake (1.3 oz)	150	—	6
Pecan (Sara Lee)	1	280	—	16
Small (Drake's)	1 (2 oz)	220	—	9
Creamies Banana Treat (Tastykake)	1	138	—	3
Creamies Chocolate (Tastykake)	1	174	—	7
Creamies Vanilla (Tastykake)	1	182	—	8
Crumb Cake (Hostess)	1 (1.9 oz)	210	3	8
Crumb Cake Light (Hostess)	1 (1.8 oz)	150	0	1
Cup Cakes Chocolate (Hostess)	1 (1.6 oz)	170	3	5
Cup Cakes Chocolate Light (Hostess)	1 (1.4 oz)	120	0	2
Cup Cakes Orange (Hostess)	1 (1.5 oz)	160	2	5
Deluxe Carrot Cake (Sara Lee)	1	180	—	7
Dessert Cups (Hostess)	1 (1 oz)	90	0	2

FOOD	PORTION	CALS.	SAT. FAT	FAT
Devil Cremes (Little Debbie)	1 pkg (1.6 oz)	190	2	8
Devil Cremes (Little Debbie)	1 pkg (3.2 oz)	380	3	17
Devil Dog (Drake's)	1 (1.5 oz)	160	—	6
Devil Squares (Little Debbie)	1 pkg (2.2 oz)	260	3	13
Ding Dongs (Hostess)	1 (1.3 oz)	160	6	9
Dunking Sticks (Lance)	1 (39 g)	190	3	10
Easter Basket Cakes (Little Debbie)	1 pkg (2.5 oz)	310	3	15
Fancy Cakes (Little Debbie)	1 pkg (2.4 oz)	300	3	15
Fig Cake (Lance)	1 pkg (60 g)	210	1	3
Fruit Loaf (Hostess)	1 (3.8 oz)	350	1	10
Fudge Crispy (Little Debbie)	1 pkg (1.1 oz)	170	3	10
Fudge Round (Little Debbie)	1 pkg (2.5 oz)	290	3	12
Fudge Round (Little Debbie)	1 pkg (3 oz)	350	4	14
Fudge Rounds (Little Debbie)	1 pkg (1.2 oz)	140	1	5
Funny Bones (Drake's)	1 (1.25 oz)	150	—	8
Golden Cremes (Little Debbie)	1 pkg (1.5 oz)	170	2	7
Golden Cremes (Little Debbie)	1 pkg (3 oz)	330	3	15
Ho Ho's (Hostess)	1 (1 oz)	130	4	6
Holiday Cakes Chocolate (Little Debbie)	1 pkg (2.4 oz)	290	3	14
Holiday Cakes Vanilla (Little Debbie)	1 pkg (2.5 oz)	310	3	15
Holiday Cakes (Hostess)	1 (1.6 oz)	160	1	3
Honey Bun (Little Debbie)	1 pkg (3 oz)	380	6	23
Honey Bun (Little Debbie)	1 pkg (4 oz)	510	8	31
Honey Bun Glazed (Hostess)	1 (2.7 oz)	320	9	19
Honey Bun Iced (Hostess)	1 (3.4 oz)	390	9	20
Honey Buns (Lance)	1 (85 g)	330	4	14
Honeybun Glazed (Tastykake)	1 pkg (92 g)	360	4	20
Honeybun Iced (Tastykake)	1 pkg (92 g)	350	3	15
Hopper Cakes (Hostess)	1 (1.6 oz)	160	1	3
Jelly Rolls (Little Debbie)	1 pkg (2.1 oz)	230	2	7
Junior Chocolate (Tastykake)	1 pkg (94 g)	340	3	12
Junior Coconut (Tastykake)	1 pkg (94 g)	300	3	6
Junior Lemon (Tastykake)	1 pkg (94 g)	310	3	7
Junior Orange (Tastykake)	1 pkg (94 g)	340	3	9
Kandy Kake Chocolate (Tastykake)	1 (19 g)	80	2	3

FOOD	PORTION	CALS.	SAT. FAT	FAT
Kandy Kake Coconut (Tastykake)	1 (19 g)	80	3	4
Kandy Kake Peanut Butter (Tastykake)	1 (19 g)	90	2	4
Koffe Kake Cream Filled (Tastykake)	1 (29 g)	110	1	4
Koffee Kake Junior (Tastykake)	1 pkg (71 g)	260	2	8
Kreme Kup (Tastykake)	1 (25 g)	90	1	3
Krimpet Butterscotch (Tastykake)	1 (28 g)	100	1	3
Krimpet Jelly (Tastykake)	1 (28 g)	90	1	1
Krimpet Strawberry (Tastykake)	1 (28 g)	100	1	2
Lemon Stix (Little Debbie)	1 pkg (1.5 oz)	210	3	10
Lil Angels (Hostess)	1 (1 oz)	90	1	2
Marshmallow Supremes (Little Debbie)	1 pkg (1.1 oz)	130	1	5
Mint Sprints (Little Debbie)	1 pkg (1.5 oz)	230	3	13
Nutty Bar (Little Debbie)	1 pkg (2 oz)	290	3	17
Oatmeal Cake (Lance)	1 (57 g)	240	3	11
Pastry Pocket Apple (Tastykake)	1 (85 g)	320	4	18
Pastry Pocket Cheese (Tastykake)	1 (85 g)	330	5	19
Pastry Pocket Cherry (Tastykake)	1 (85 g)	330	4	17
Pecan Spinners (Hostess)	1 (1 oz)	110	1	5
Pecan Twins (Little Debbie)	1 pkg (2 oz)	220	1	9
Pecan Twirls (Lance)	1 pkg (57 g)	220	—	8
Pecan Twirls (Tastykake)	1 (28 g)	110	—	1
Pop-Tarts				
Apple Cinnamon	1	210	1	6
Blueberry	1	210	1	6
Brown Sugar Cinnamon	1	210	2	8
Cherry	1	210	1	6
Chocolate Graham	1	210	2	6
Frosted Brown Sugar Cinnamon	1	210	1	7
Frosted Cherry	1	210	1	5
Frosted Chocolate Fudge	1	200	1	5
Frosted Chocolate Vanilla Creme	1	200	1	5

FOOD	PORTION	CALS.	SAT. FAT	FAT
Pop-Tarts *(cont.)*				
Frosted Grape	1	200	1	5
Frosted Raspberry	1	220	1	5
Frosted Strawberry	1	200	1	5
Strawberry	1	210	1	6
Pound Cake (Drake's)	1	110	—	5
Pumpkin Delights (Little Debbie)	1 pkg (1.1 oz)	130	1	5
Raisin Cake (Lance)	1 (57 g)	230	3	10
Ring Ding (Drake's)	1 (1.5 oz)	180	—	10
Ring Ding Mint (Drake's)	1 (1.5 oz)	190	—	11
Royale Chocolate Cupcake (Tastykake)	1 (46 g)	170	2	7
Smiley Faces Cherry (Little Debbie)	1 pkg (1.2 oz)	140	1	5
Smiley Faces Pumpkin (Little Debbie)	1 pkg (1 oz)	130	1	5
Snack Cake Chocolate (Little Debbie)	1 pkg (2.5 oz)	300	3	15
Snack Cake Vanilla (Little Debbie)	1 pkg (2.6 oz)	320	3	16
Sno Balls (Hostess)	1 (1.6 oz)	160	3	5
Spice (Little Debbie)	1 pkg (2.5 oz)	300	3	15
Star Crunch (Little Debbie)	1 pkg (1.1 oz)	140	1	6
Star Crunch (Little Debbie)	1 pkg (2.6 oz)	330	3	14
Sunny Doodle (Drake's)	1 (1 oz)	100	—	3
Suzy Q's (Hostess)	1 (2 oz)	220	4	9
Suzy Q's Banana (Hostess)	1 (2 oz)	220	1	10
Swirls Caramel Pecan (Hostess)	1 (2 oz)	140	6	15
Swiss Rolls (Little Debbie)	1 pkg (2.1 oz)	250	3	12
Swiss Rolls (Little Debbie)	1 pkg (2.7 oz)	320	4	15
Swiss Rolls (Little Debbie)	1 pkg (3.2 oz)	380	4	18
Tasty Too Chocolate Cream Filled Cupcake (Tastykake)	1 (32 g)	100	1	1
Tasty Too Vanilla Cream Filled Cupcake (Tastykake)	1 (32 g)	100	1	1
Tasty Twists (Tastykake)	1 (4 g)	18	—	1
Teddy Berries (Little Debbie)	1 pkg (1.2 oz)	130	1	4
Tiger Tails (Hostess)	1 (1.5 oz)	160	3	6
Toast-R-Cakes BlueBerry	1	110	—	3
Toast-R-Cakes Bran	1	103	—	3
Toast-R-Cakes Corn	1	120	—	4

FOOD	PORTION	CALS.	SAT. FAT	FAT
Toaster Tart				
(Pepperidge Farm)				
Apple Cinnamon	1	170	3	7
Blueberry	1	190	1	5
Cheese	1	190	3	10
Strawberry	1	190	2	7
Toastettes (Nabisco)				
Apple	1	190	1	5
Blueberry	1	190	1	5
Cherry	1	190	1	5
Frosted Apple	1	190	1	5
Frosted Blueberry	1	190	—	0
Frosted Brown Sugar Cinnamon	1	190	1	5
Frosted Cherry	1	190	1	5
Frosted Fruit Punch	1	190	1	5
Frosted Fudge	1	200	1	5
Frosted Strawberry	1	190	1	5
Strawberry	1	190	1	5
Twinkies (Hostess)	1 (1.4 oz)	140	2	4
Twinkies Banana (Hostess)	2 (2.7 oz)	300	2	13
Twinkies Devil Food (Hostess)	2 (2.7 oz)	300	5	12
Twinkies Lights (Hostess)	1 (1.4 oz)	120	0	2
Twinkies Strawberry Fruit 'n Creme (Hostess)	1 (1.6 oz)	150	1	3
Vanilla (Little Debbie)	1 pkg (3 oz)	370	4	18
Vanilla Cremes (Little Debbie)	1 pkg (1.4 oz)	170	2	7
Yankee Doodle (Drake's)	1 (1 oz)	100	—	4
Yodel's (Drake's)	1 (1 oz)	150	—	9
Zebra Cakes (Little Debbie)	1 pkg (2.6 oz)	150	3	16
devil's food cupcake w/ chocolate frosting	1	120	4	4
devil's food w/ creme filling	1 (1 oz)	105	4	4
sponge w/ creme filling	1 (1.5 oz)	155	1	5
toaster pastry apple	1 (1.75 oz)	204	1	5
toaster pastry blueberry	1 (1.75 oz)	204	1	5
toaster pastry brown sugar cinnamon	1 (1.75 oz)	206	2	7
toaster pastry cherry	1 (1.75 oz)	204	1	5
toaster pastry strawberry	1 (1.75 oz)	204	1	5
TAKE-OUT				
baklava	1 oz	126	4	9

FOOD	PORTION	CALS.	SAT. FAT	FAT
strudel	1 piece (4.1 oz)	272	4	8
trifle w/ cream	6 oz	291	—	16

CALZONE
cheese	1 (12 oz)	1020	24	54

CANADIAN BACON
Hormel	2 oz	70	2	3
Jones	1 slice	30	—	1
Oscar Mayer	2 slices (1.6 oz)	50	1	2
unheated	2 slices (1.9 oz)	89	1	4

CANDY
(*see also* MARSHMALLOW)

FOOD	PORTION	CALS.	SAT. FAT	FAT
100 Grand (Nestle)	1 bar (1.5 oz)	200	5	8
3 Musketeers	1 (2.1 oz)	260	5	8
3 Musketeers	2 bars fun size (1.1 oz)	140	3	5
5th Avenue	1 (2.1 oz)	290	—	13
After Eight Dark Chocolate Wafer Thin Mints (Rowntree)	1	35	—	1
Almond Butter Dome (Godiva)	3 pieces (1.5 oz)	240	6	17
Almond Joy	1 (1.76 oz)	250	—	14
Areo Bar (Nestle)	1 bar (1.45 oz)	210	7	13
Baby Ruth (Nestle)	1 bar (2.1 oz)	280	7	12
Baby Ruth Fun Size (Nestle)	2 pieces	200	5	9
Bar None	1 (1.5 oz)	240	—	14
Bit-O-Honey	1.7 oz	200	—	4
Bits O Brickle	1 tbsp (0.5 oz)	80	2	5
Bonus Bar	1 bar (2.1 oz)	290	7	16
Bouchee Au Chocolat (Godiva)	1 piece (1.5 oz)	210	6	11
Bouchee Ivory Raspberry (Godiva)	1 piece (1 oz)	160	3	9
Breath Savers Sugar Free Cinnamon	1 candy	2	0	0
Breath Savers Sugar Free Peppermint	1 candy	2	0	0
Breath Savers Sugar Free Spearmint	1 candy	2	0	0
Breath Savers Sugar Free Wintergreen	1 candy	2	0	0

FOOD	PORTION	CALS.	SAT. FAT	FAT
Buncha Crunch (Nestle)	1 pkg (1.4 oz)	90	5	10
Butter Mints (Kraft)	1	8	0	0
Butterfinger (Nestle)	1 bar (2.1 oz)	280	6	11
Butterfinger BB's (Nestle)	1 pkg (1.7 oz)	230	7	10
Butterfinger Fun Size (Nestle)	2 bars (1.6 oz)	200	4	8
Butternut Bar	1 bar (1.8 oz)	250	5	14
Butterscotch Discs (Brock)	3 pieces (0.6 oz)	70	0	0
Candy Corn (Brock)	21 pieces (1.4 oz)	150	0	0
Candy Rolls (Brock)	2 rolls (0.5 oz)	50	0	0
Caramel Dots (Brock)	3 pieces (1.3 oz)	140	1	3
Caramello	1 (1.6 oz)	220	—	11
Caramels (Kraft)	1	30	0	1
Caramels Chocolate & Vanilla No Sugar Added (Estee)	5 (1.3 oz)	150	1	5
Caroby Almond Bar (Natural Touch)	4 sections (28 g)	150	—	10
Caroby Milk Bar (Natural Touch)	4 sections (28 g)	150	—	9
Caroby Milk Free Bar (Natural Touch)	4 sections (28 g)	160	—	11
Caroby Mint Bar (Natural Touch)	4 sections (28 g)	150	—	9
Certs	1 piece (1.67 g)	6	0	0
Certs Sugar Free	1 piece (1.67 g)	7	0	0
Certs Mini Sugar Free (Certs)	1 piece (0.365 g)	1	0	0
Charleston Chew (Cambridge)	1 pkg (1.9 oz)	230	6	7
Charleston Chew! Chocolate (Pearson's)	½ bar	120	—	3
Charleston Chew! Strawberry (Pearson's)	½ bar	120	—	3
Charleston Chew! Vanilla (Pearson's)	½ bar	120	—	3
Charms Blow Pop	1 (0.7 oz)	80	0	0
Charms Pop	1 (0.6 oz)	70	0	0
Chocolate Covered Cherries Dark Chocolate (Cellas)	2 pieces (1 oz)	100	3	4
Chocolate Covered Cherries Milk Chocolate (Cellas)	2 pieces (1 oz)	110	3	4

FOOD	PORTION	CALS.	SAT. FAT	FAT
Chocolate Fudgies (Kraft)	1	35	0	1
Chocolaty Peanut Bar (Lance)	1 (57 g)	320	6	18
Chuckles	4 pieces (1.4 oz)	140	0	0
Chunky (Nestle)	1 bar (1.4 oz)	200	6	11
Cinnamon Discs (Brock)	3 pieces (0.6 oz)	70	0	0
Circus Peanuts (Brock)	11 pieces (2.5 oz)	260	0	0
Clorets Mints (Clorets)	1 piece (1.67 g)	6	0	0
Coconut Mountains (Brock)	4 pieces (1.4 oz)	170	1	6
Crunch Fun Size (Nestle)	4 bars (1.5 oz)	200	6	10
Crunch 'N Munch Candied (Franklin)	1.25 oz	170	—	7
Crunch 'N Munch Caramel (Franklin)	1.25 oz	160	—	5
Crunch 'N Munch Maple Walnut (Franklin)	1.25 oz	160	—	6
Crunch 'N Munch Toffee (Franklin)	1.25 oz	160	—	5
Dark Chocolate (Estee)	½ bar (1.4 oz)	200	8	14
Dark Chocolate (Whitman's)	3 pieces (1.4 oz)	200	6	10
Dove				
Dark Chocolate	1 bar (1.3 oz)	200	5	12
Dark Chocolate	¼ bar (1.5 oz)	230	5	14
Dark Chocolate Miniatures	7 (1.5 oz)	230	5	14
Milk Chocolate	¼ bar (1.5 oz)	230	8	13
Milk Chocolate	1 bar (1.3 oz)	200	7	7
Milk Chocolate Miniatures	7 (1.5 oz)	230	8	13
Fruit Basket (Brock)	3 pieces (0.6 oz)	60	0	0
Fruit Kisses (Brock)	3 pieces (0.6 oz)	70	0	0
Glitters (Brock)	2 pieces (0.5 oz)	50	0	0
Gold Ballotin (Godiva)	3 pieces (1.5 oz)	210	4	10
Golden Almond	½ bar	260	—	17
Golden III	½ bar	250	1	15
Goobers (Nestle)	1 pkg (1.38 oz)	210	5	13
Good & Fruity	1 box (1.8 oz)	140	—	1
Good & Plenty Snacksize	3 boxes (1.5 oz)	140	0	0
Gum Drops Assorted Fruit Sugar Free (Estee)	23 (1.4 oz)	140	0	0
Gum Drops Licorice (Estee)	23 (1.4 oz)	140	0	0

FOOD	PORTION	CALS.	SAT. FAT	FAT
Gummy Bears (Brock)	5 pieces (1.4 oz)	130	0	0
Gummy Bears Sugar Free (Estee)	16 (1.4 oz)	140	0	0
Gummy Squirms (Brock)	5 pieces (1.3 oz)	120	0	0
Hard Candies Assorted Fruit Sugar Free (Estee)	5 (0.5 oz)	60	0	0
Hard Candies Assorted Mint Sugar Free (Estee)	5 (0.5 oz)	60	0	0
Hard Candies Butterscotch Sugar Free (Estee)	2 (0.4 oz)	50	0	0
Hard Candies Peppermint Swirls Sugar Free (Estee)	3 (0.5 oz)	60	0	0
Hard Candies Tropical Fruit Sugar Free (Estee)	5 (0.5 oz)	60	0	0
Heath	1 bar (1.4 oz)	210	7	13
Hershey Bar	1 (1.55 oz)	240	—	14
Hershey Bar with Almonds	1 (1.45 oz)	230	—	14
Hershey's Kisses	9 pieces (1.46 oz)	220	—	13
Jelly Beans (Brock)	12 pieces (1.4 oz)	140	0	0
Jelly Beans (Just Born)	1 oz	108	—	tr
Jolly Rancher	3 pieces (0.6 oz)	60	0	0
Junior Mints	12 pieces	120	—	3
Junior Mints (Cambridge)	1 pkg (1.6 oz)	190	3	4
Just Born Sugar Coated	1½ oz	148	—	tr
Just Born Toasted Coconut	1⅜ oz	140	—	2
Kit Kat Wafer	1 (1.63 oz)	250	—	13
Krackel	1 (1.55 oz)	230	—	13
Laffy Taffy (Beich's)				
Apple Chews	1 oz	110	—	1
Banana Chews	1 oz	110	—	1
Grape Chews	1 oz	110	—	1
Passion Punch Chews	1 oz	110	—	1
Strawberry Chews	1 oz	110	—	1
Sweet & Sour Cherry Chews	1 oz	110	—	1
Watermelon Chews	1 oz	110	—	1
Lemon Drops (Brock)	3 pieces (0.5 oz)	60	0	0
Lifesaver Holes Sunshine Fruits	1 candy	2	0	0
Lifesafer Holes Tangerine	1 candy	2	0	0
Lifesaver Lollipops All Flavors	1	45	—	0
Lifesaver Sugar Free	1 piece	8	—	0

FOOD	PORTION	CALS.	SAT. FAT	FAT
Lifesavers				
Christmas Lollipops	1	40	0	0
Easter Pops	1	40	0	0
Fancy Fruits	1 candy	8	0	0
Fruit Juicers Citrus Fruits	1 candy	8	0	0
Fruit Juicers Easter Egg-Sortments	1 candy	10	0	0
Fruit Juicers Fruit Punch	1 candy	8	0	0
Fruit Juicers Grape	1 candy	8	0	0
Fruit Juicers Lollipops	1	40	0	0
Fruit Juicers Mixed Berries	1 candy	8	0	0
Fruit Juicers Strawberry	1 candy	8	0	0
Gummi Savers Grape	1 candy	12	0	0
Gummi Savers Mixed Berry	1 candy	12	0	0
Sunshine Fruits	1 candy	8	0	0
Tropical Fruits	1 candy	8	0	0
Valentine Pops	1	40	0	0
Wild Cherry	1 candy	8	0	0
Lollipops Assorted Fruit Sugar Free (Estee)	2 (0.5 oz)	60	0	0
M&M's				
Almond	1 pkg (1.5 oz)	220	4	12
Mint	1 pkg (1.7 oz)	230	6	10
Mint	1.5 oz	200	5	9
Peanut	1 fun size (0.7 oz)	110	2	5
Peanut	1 pkg (1.7 oz)	250	5	13
Peanut	1.5 oz	220	5	11
Peanut	½ bag king size (1.6 oz)	240	5	12
Peanut Butter	1 fun size (0.7 oz)	110	3	6
Peanut Butter	1 pkg (1.6 oz)	240	6	13
Peanut Butter	1.5 oz	220	5	11
Plain	1 pkg (1.7 oz)	230	10	10
Plain	1 pkg fun size (0.7 oz)	100	3	5
Plain	1.5 oz	200	5	9
Plain	½ pkg king size (1.6 oz)	220	6	9
Semisweet	0.5 oz	70	2	4

FOOD	PORTION	CALS.	SAT. FAT	FAT
Mars	1 bar (1.8 oz)	240	5	13
Mars Almond Bar	2 fun size (1.3 oz)	190	4	10
Milk Chocolate (Estee)	½ bar (1.4 oz)	230	10	17
Milk Chocolate With Almonds (Estee)	½ bar (1.4 oz)	230	9	17
Milk Chocolate With Crisp Rice (Estee)	1 bar (2.3 oz)	370	15	26
Milk Chocolate With Fruit & Nuts (Estee)	½ bar (1.4 oz)	220	9	16
Milk Duds	1 box (1.8 oz)	230	6	8
Milk Duds (Snack Size)	4 boxes (1.3 oz)	160	4	5
Milkshake Bar	1 bar (1.8 oz)	220	4	7
Milky Way	1 bar (2.1 oz)	280	5	11
Milky Way	2 fun size (1.4 oz)	180	4	7
Milky Way Miniature	5 (1.5 oz)	190	4	7
Milky Way Dark	1 bar (1.8 oz)	220	5	8
Milky Way Dark	1 fun size (0.7 oz)	90	2	3
Mint Chocolate (Estee)	½ bar (1.4 oz)	200	8	14
Mounds	1 (1.9 oz)	260	—	14
Mr. Goodbar	1 (1.75 oz)	290	—	19
Munch Bar	1.4 oz	220	4	14
NECCO Mint Lozenges	1 piece	12	—	tr
Nestle Crunch Bar	1.5 oz	230	7	12
Nestle Milk Chocolate Bar	1.45 oz	220	7	13
Nestle Crunch (Nestle)	1 bar (1.55 oz)	230	7	12
Nips Butter Rum (Pearson)	2 pieces (0.5 oz)	60	2	2
Nips Caramel (Pearson)	2 pieces (0.5 oz)	60	2	2
Nips Chocolate Mint (Pearson)	2 pieces (0.5 oz)	60	2	2
Nips Chocolate Parfait (Pearson)	2 pieces (0.5 oz)	60	2	2
Nips Licorice (Pearson)	2 pieces (0.5 oz)	60	2	2
Nips Peanut Butter Parfait (Pearson)	2 pieces (0.5 oz)	60	2	2
Oh Henry! (Nestle)	1 bar (1.8 oz)	230	4	9
Orange Slices (Brock)	4 pieces (1.5 oz)	140	0	0
PB Max	2 (1.6 oz)	240	5	15
PB Max	2 fun size (1.2 oz)	180	4	12
Party Mints (Brock)	9 pieces (0.5 oz)	60	0	0
Party Mints (Kraft)	1	8	0	0
PayDay	1 bar (1.85 oz)	240	2	12

FOOD	PORTION	CALS.	SAT. FAT	FAT
Peanut Bar (Lance)	1 pkg (50 g)	260	3	14
Peanut Brittle (Kraft)	1 oz	130	1	5
Peanut Brittle No Sugar Added (Estee)	⅓ box (1.5 oz)	210	2	9
Peanut Butter Crunch (Brock)	3 pieces (0.6 oz)	80	—	2
Peanut Butter Cups (Estee)	1 (0.3 oz)	40	4	3
Peanut Butter Cups (Estee)	5 (1.3 oz)	200	7	12
Peanut Chews (Goldenberg's)	4 pieces (1.7 oz)	215	—	7
Pez	1 roll (0.3 oz)	30	0	0
Pom Pom (Cambridge)	1 pkg (1.6 oz)	200	5	6
Pops Assorted (Brock)	2 (0.5 oz)	60	0	0
Popscotch (Lance)	1 pkg (35 g)	160	1	6
Raisinets (Nestle)	1 pkg (1.58 oz)	200	4	8
Reese's Peanut Butter Cups	1 (1.8 oz)	280	—	17
Reese's Pieces	1.85 oz	260	—	11
Rolo Carmels in Milk Chocolate	8 pieces (1.93 oz)	270	—	12
Skittles	1 pkg (2.2 oz)	250	1	3
Skittles	1.5 oz	170	0	2
Skittles				
Original	2 pkg fun size (1.4 oz)	160	0	2
Tart-N-Tangy	1 bag (2.2 oz)	250	1	3
Tart-N-Tangy	1.5 oz	170	0	2
Tart-N-Tangy	2 bags fun size (1.4 oz)	160	0	2
Tropical	1 bag (2.2 oz)	250	1	3
Tropical	1.5 oz	170	0	2
Tropical	2 bags fun size (1.4 oz)	160	0	2
Wild Berry	1 bag (2.2 oz)	250	1	3
Wild Berry	1.5 oz	170	0	2
Wild Berry	2 bags fun size (1.4 oz)	160	0	2
Skor Toffee Bar	1 (1.4 oz)	220	—	14
Snickers	1 bar (2.1 oz)	280	5	14
Snickers	2 bars fun size (1.4 oz)	190	4	9
Snickers Miniatures	4 (1.3 oz)	170	3	8
Snickers Peanut Butter	1 bar (2 oz)	310	7	20
Sno Caps (Nestle)	1 pkg (2.3 oz)	300	8	13

FOOD	PORTION	CALS.	SAT. FAT	FAT
Solitaires With Almonds	½ bag	260	—	17
Sour Balls (Brock)	3 pieces (0.6 oz)	70	0	0
Sour Sharks (Brock)	23 pieces (2.5 oz)	30	2	3
Spearmint Starlights (Brock)	3 pieces (0.6 oz)	60	0	0
Special Dark Sweet Chocolate Bar (Hershey)	1 (1.45)	220	—	12
Spice Drops (Brock)	12 pieces (1.4 oz)	130	0	0
Spice Stix And Drops	14 pieces (1.6 oz)	140	0	0
Starburst				
California Fruits	1 stick (2.1 oz)	240	1	5
California Fruits	8 pieces (1.4 oz)	160	1	4
Strawberry Fruits	1 stick (2.1 oz)	240	1	5
Strawberry Fruits	8 pieces (1.4 oz)	160	1	3
Tropical Fruits	1 stick (2.1 oz)	240	1	5
Tropical Fruits	8 pieces (1.4 oz)	160	1	3
Starlight Mints (Brock)	3 pieces (0.6 oz)	60	0	0
Sugar Babies (Cambridge)	1 pkg (1.7 oz)	190	2	2
Sugar Babies Tidbits	1 pkg	180	—	2
Sugar Daddy	1 pop	150	—	1
Sugar Daddy (Cambridge)	1 pkg (1.7 oz)	200	3	3
Swedish Fish Red	19 pieces (1.4 oz)	150	—	1
Switzer Cherry Bites	12 pieces (1.6 oz)	50	0	0
Switzer Licorice Bites	12 pieces (1.6 oz)	46	0	0
Symphony Almond/ Butterchips	1 (1.4 oz)	220	—	14
Symphony Milk Chocolate	1 (1.4 oz)	220	—	13
Toffee (Brock)	6 pieces (1.5 oz)	170	2	5
Toffee Sugar Free (Estee)	5 (0.5 oz)	60	0	0
Tootsie Roll	1 (1 oz)	110	0	2
Tootsie Roll Dots	12 (1.5 oz)	160	0	0
Tootsie Roll Midgees	6 (1.4 oz)	160	1	3
Tootsie Roll Pop	1 (0.6 oz)	60	0	0
Truffle Amaretto Di Saronno (Godiva)	2 pieces (1.5 oz)	210	6	12
Truffle Deluxe Liqueur (Godiva)	2 pieces (1.5 oz)	210	6	13
Turtles Pecan Caramel Candy (Nestle)	2 pieces (1.2 oz)	160	3	9
Twix				
Caramel	1 (1 oz)	140	3	7
Caramel	1 fun size (0.6 oz)	80	2	4
Caramel	2 (1 pkg (2 oz)	280	5	14

FOOD	PORTION	CALS.	SAT. FAT	FAT
Twix *(cont.)*				
Cookies-N-Creme	1 (0.8 oz)	130	3	8
Fudge N Crunchy	1 (0.7 oz)	110	2	6
Peanut Butter	1 (0.9 oz)	130	3	8
Twizzlers (Y&S Candies)	4 pieces (1.4 oz)	130	—	1
Velamints	1 mint	9	—	0
Velamints Cocoamint	1 mint	8	—	0
Whatchamacallit	1 (1.8 oz)	260	—	13
Whoppers	1 pkg (1.8 oz)	230	8	10
Y&S Bites Cherry	1 oz	100	—	1
York Peppermint Patty	1 (1.5 oz)	180	—	4
Zagnut Bar	1 bar (1.8 oz)	230	4	9
Zero Bar	2 pieces (1.4 oz)	170	3	6
candied cherries	1 cherry	12	—	tr
candied citron	1 oz	89	—	tr
candied lemon peel	1 oz	90	—	tr
candied orange peel	1 oz	90	—	tr
candied pineapple slice	1 slice (2 oz)	179	—	tr
candy corn	1 oz	105	0	0
caramels chocolate	1 oz	115	3	3
caramels plain	1 oz	115	3	3
chocolate	1 oz	145	5	9
chocolate crisp	1 oz	140	4	7
chocolate w/ almonds	1 oz	150	5	10
chocolate w/ peanuts	1 oz	155	4	11
dark chocolate	1 oz	150	6	10
fruit pastilles	1 tube (1.4 oz)	101	—	0
fudge, chocolate	1 oz	115	2	3
fudge, vanilla	1 oz	115	2	3
gum drops	1 oz	100	tr	tr
hard candy	1 oz	110	0	0
jelly beans	1 oz	105	tr	tr
marzipan	3.5 oz	497	—	25
mint fondant	1 oz	105	0	0
nougat nut cream	3.5 oz	342	—	31

CANTALOUPE

FRESH

FOOD	PORTION	CALS.	SAT. FAT	FAT
Chiquita	1 cup	70	—	0
Dole	¼ melon	50	—	0
cubed	1 cup	57	—	tr
fresh	½ melon	94	—	1
FROZEN				
Balls (Big Valley)	¾ cup (4.9 oz)	40	0	0

FOOD	PORTION	CALS.	SAT. FAT	FAT
CAPERS				
Reese	1 tsp (5 g)	0	0	0
CARAMBOLA				
fresh	1	42	—	tr
CARAWAY				
seed	1 tsp	7	tr	tr
CARDAMOM				
ground	1 tsp	6	tr	tr
CARDOON				
FRESH				
cardoon, cooked	3.5 oz	22	tr	tr
raw, shredded	½ cup	36	tr	tr
CARIBOU				
roasted	3 oz	142	1	4
CARISSA				
fresh	1	12	—	tr
CAROB				
carob mix	3 tsp	45	0	0
carob mix, as prep w/ whole milk	9 oz	195	5	8
flour	1 cup	185	tr	1
flour	1 tbsp	14	tr	tr
CARP				
FRESH				
cooked	3 oz	138	1	6
cooked	1 fillet (6 oz)	276	2	12
roe, raw	3½ oz	130	—	2
CARROTS				
CANNED				
Diced (Seneca)	½ cup	20	0	0
Diced Fancy (S&W)	½ cup	30	0	0
Julienne French Style Fancy (S&W)	½ cup	30	0	0
Sliced (Allen)	½ cup (4.5 oz)	35	0	1
Sliced (Crest Top)	½ cup (4.5 oz)	35	0	1
Sliced (Seneca)	½ cup	30	0	0
Sliced Fancy (S&W)	½ cup	30	0	0

FOOD	PORTION	CALS.	SAT. FAT	FAT
Sliced Water Pack (S&W)	½ cup	30	0	0
Whole Tiny Fancy (S&W)	½ cup	30	0	0
slices	½ cup	17	tr	tr
slices, low sodium	½ cup	17	tr	tr
FRESH				
Dole	1 med	40	—	1
baby, raw	1 (½ oz)	6	tr	tr
raw	1 (2.5 oz)	31	tr	tr
raw, shredded	½ cup	24	tr	tr
slices, cooked	½ cup	35	tr	tr
FROZEN				
Baby Whole Deluxe (Birds Eye)	½ cup	40	0	0
Carrots (Big Valley)	½ cup (3 oz)	35	0	0
Crinkle Sliced (Hanover)	½ cup	35	—	0
Fresh Like	3.5 oz	42	—	tr
Harvest Fresh Baby (Green Giant)	½ cup	18	0	0
Polybag Sliced (Birds Eye)	¾ cup	35	0	0
slices, cooked	½ cup	26	tr	tr
JUICE				
Hain	6 fl oz	80	0	0
Hollywood	6 fl oz	80	0	0
Odwalla	8 fl oz	70	0	0
canned	6 oz	73	tr	tr
CASABA				
cubed	1 cup	45	—	tr
fresh	⅒ melon	43	—	tr
CASHEWS				
Cashew Butter Raw (Hain)	2 tbsp	190	3	15
Cashew Butter Raw Unsalted (Hain)	2 tbsp	210	3	19
Cashew Butter Toasted (Hain)	2 tbsp	210	3	17
Cashews (Beer Nuts)	1 pkg (1 oz)	170	—	13
Fancy (Planters)	1 oz	170	2	14
Frito Lay	1 oz	170	—	14
Honey Roasted (Eagle)	1 oz	170	—	12
Honey Roasted (Planters)	1 oz	170	2	12
Honey Roasted Halves (Fisher)	1 oz	150	3	13
Honey Roasted Whole (Fisher)	1 oz	150	3	13

FOOD	PORTION	CALS.	SAT. FAT	FAT
Lance	1 pkg (32 g)	190	3	15
Low Salt (Eagle)	1 oz	170	—	14
Oil Roasted Halves (Fisher)	1 oz	170	3	15
Oil Roasted Whole (Fisher)	1 oz	170	3	15
Unsalted Halves (Planters)	1 oz	170	2	14
Whole Salted (Guy's)	1 oz	170	—	14
cashew butter w/o salt	1 tbsp	94	2	8
dry roasted	1 oz	163	3	13
dry roasted, salted	1 oz	163	3	13
oil roasted	1 oz	163	3	14
oil roasted, salted	1 oz	163	3	14

CASSAVA
fresh, raw	3.5 oz	120	tr	tr

CATFISH
channel, breaded & fried	3 oz	194	3	11

CATSUP
Estee Imitation Sodium Free	1 pkg (0.5 oz)	15	—	0
Hain Natural	1 tbsp	16	0	0
Hain Natural No Salt Added	1 tbsp	16	0	0
Healthy Choice	1 tbsp (0.5 oz)	10	0	0
Heinz	1 tbsp	16	0	0
Heinz Hot	1 tbsp	14	0	0
Heinz Lite	1 tbsp	8	0	0
Hunt's	1 tbsp	15	0	tr
Hunt's No Salt Added	1 tbsp	20	—	tr
McIlhenny	1 tbsp (0.6 oz)	23	tr	tr
McIlhenny Spicy Ketchup	1 tbsp (0.6 oz)	23	tr	tr
Smucker's	1 tsp	8	0	0
Weight Watchers	2 tsp	8	0	0
catsup	1 tbsp	16	tr	tr
catsup	1 pkg (.2 oz)	6	tr	tr
low sodium	1 tbsp	16	tr	tr

CAULIFLOWER
FRESH
Dole	⅙ med head	18	—	0
Dole Green	⅙ head	35	0	0
cooked	½ cup (2.2 oz)	14	tr	tr
flowerets, cooked	3 (2 oz)	12	tr	tr
flowerets raw	3 (2 oz)	14	tr	tr

FOOD	PORTION	CALS.	SAT. FAT	FAT
FROZEN				
Cauliflower (Birds Eye)	⅔ cup	23	—	tr
Cauliflower (Hanover)	½ cup	20	—	0
Cuts (Green Giant)	½ cup	12	0	0
Florets (Big Valley)	¾ cup (3 oz)	25	0	0
Florets (Hanover)	½ cup	20	—	0
Fresh Like	3.5 oz	26	—	tr
In Cheese Sauce (Green Giant)	½ cup	60	tr	2
One Serve in Cheese Sauce (Green Giant)	1 pkg	80	3	3
Polybag (Birds Eye)	½ cup	20	0	0
With Cheese Sauce (Birds Eye)	½ pkg	90	2	5
cooked	½ cup	17	tr	tr
JARRED				
Hot & Spicy (Vlasic)	1 oz	4	0	0
Sweet (Vlasic)	1 oz	35	0	0
CAVIAR				
black granular	1 oz	71	—	5
black granular	1 tbsp	40	—	3
red granular	1 oz	71	—	5
red granular	1 tbsp	40	—	3
CELERIAC				
fresh, cooked	3.5 oz	25	—	tr
fresh, raw	½ cup	31	—	tr
CELERY				
DRIED				
seed	1 tsp	8	tr	tr
FRESH				
Dole	2 med stalks	20	—	0
diced, cooked	½ cup	13	tr	tr
raw	1 stalk (1.3 oz)	6	tr	tr
raw, diced	½ cup	10	tr	tr
FROZEN				
Fresh Like	3.5 oz	14	—	tr
CELTUCE				
raw	3.5 oz	22	—	tr
CEREAL				
COOKED				
4 Grain + Flax (Arrowhead)	¼ cup (1.6 oz)	150	0	2

FOOD	PORTION	CALS.	SAT. FAT	FAT
5-Bran Kashi (Kashi)	2.5 oz	281	—	6
7 Grain (Arrowhead)	⅓ cup (1.4 oz)	140	0	2
Apple Cinnamon (Roman Meal)	1.2 oz	105	tr	2
Barley Plus (Erewhon)	1 oz	110	—	1
Bear Mush (Arrowhead)	1 oz	100	0	0
Brown Rice Cream (Erewhon)	1 oz	110	—	1
Coco Wheat (Little Crow)	3 tbsp (36 g)	130	—	1
Corn Flakes (Ralston)	1¼ cup (1.1 oz)	120	0	0
Cream of Rice (Nabisco)	1 oz	100	0	0
Cream of Rye (Roman Meal)	1.3 oz	111	tr	1
Cream of Wheat Instant (Nabisco)	1 oz	100	tr	tr
Cream of Wheat Quick (Nabisco)	1 oz	100	tr	tr
Cream of Wheat Regular (Nabisco)	1 oz	100	0	0
Enriched White Hominy Grits Quick (Aunt Jemima)	3 tbsp	101	—	tr
Enriched White Hominy Grits Quick (Quaker)	3 tbsp	101	—	tr
Enriched White Hominy Grits Regular (Aunt Jemima)	3 tbsp	101	—	tr
Enriched White Hominy Grits Regular (Quaker)	3 tbsp	101	—	tr
Enriched Yellow Hominy Quick Grits (Quaker)	3 tbsp	101	—	tr
Farina not prep (H-O)	3 tbsp	120	0	0
Farina Instant (H-O)	1 pkg	110	0	0
Farina (Pillsbury)	⅔ cup	80	—	tr
Hominy Quick Grits, uncooked (Albers)	¼ cup	150	—	0
Instant Grits White Hominy (Quaker)	1 pkg	79	tr	tr
Instant Grits w/ Imitation Bacon Bits (Quaker)	1 pkg	101	—	tr
Instant Grits w/ Imitation Ham Bits (Quaker)	1 pkg	99	—	tr
Instant Grits w/ Real Cheddar Cheese (Quaker)	1 pkg	104	1	1

FOOD	PORTION	CALS.	SAT. FAT	FAT
Irish Oatmeal (McCann's)	1 oz	110	—	2
Kashi (Kashi)	2 oz	177	—	1
Maltex	1 oz	105	tr	1
Maypo 30 Second	1 oz	100	tr	1
Maypo Vermont Style	1 oz	105	tr	1
Maypo With Oat Bran	1 oz	130	tr	2
Mix'n Eat Cream of Wheat (Nabisco)				
Brown Sugar Cinnamon	1 pkg (1.25 oz)	130	0	0
Apple & Cinnamon	1 pkg (1.25 oz)	130	0	0
Maple Brown Sugar	1 pkg (1.25 oz)	130	0	0
Our Original	1 pkg (1.25 oz)	100	0	0
Oat Bran (Quaker)	⅓ cup	92	tr	2
Oat Bran Natural Apples & Cinnamon (Health Valley)	¼ cup	100	—	tr
Oat Bran Natural Raisins & Spice (Health Valley)	¼ cup	100	—	tr
Oat Bran w/ Toasted Wheat Germ (Erewhon)	1 oz	115	—	2
Oat Flakes Rolled (Arrowhead)	⅓ cup (1.2 oz)	130	1	3
Oat Groats (Arrowhead)	¼ cup (1.5 oz)	160	1	3
Oatmeal Cinnamon Graham Cookie (Quaker)	1 pkg (1.4 oz)	140	—	2
Oatmeal Radical Raspberry (Quaker)	1 pkg (1.4 oz)	150	—	3
Oatmeal Strawberries 'N Stuff (Quaker)	1 pkg (1.4 oz)	140	—	2
Oatmeal Instant				
(H-O)	½ cup	130	0	2
(H-O)	1 pkg	110	0	2
Apple Cinnamon (Erewhon)	1.25 oz	145	—	3
Apple Cinnamon (H-O)	1 pkg	130	0	2
Apple Raisin (Erewhon)	1.3 oz	150	—	2
Apples & Cinnamon, cooked (Quaker)	1 pkg	118	tr	2
Cinnamon & Spice, cooked (Quaker)	1 pkg	164	tr	2
Dates & Walnuts (Erewhon)	1.2 oz	130	—	3
Extra Fortified Apples & Spice, cooked (Quaker)	1 pkg	133	tr	2

FOOD	PORTION	CALS.	SAT. FAT	FAT
Extra Fortified Raisins & Cinnamon, cooked (Quaker)	1 pkg	129	tr	2
Extra Fortified Regular, cooked (Quaker)	1 pkg	95	tr	2
Maple & Brown Sugar, cooked (Quaker)	1 pkg	152	tr	2
Maple Brown Sugar (H-O)	1 pkg	160	0	2
Maple Spice (Erewhon)	1.2 oz	140	—	3
Original (Arrowhead)	1 oz	100	—	0
Peaches & Cream Flavors, cooked (Quaker)	1 pkg	129	1	2
Raisin & Spice (H-O)	1 pkg	150	0	2
Raisin & Spice, cooked (Quaker)	1 pkg	149	tr	2
Raisin, Dates & Walnuts, cooked (Quaker)	1 pkg	141	tr	4
Regular, cooked (Quaker)	1 pkg	94	tr	2
Strawberries & Cream Flavors, cooked (Quaker)	1 pkg	129	1	2
Sweet 'n Mellow (H-O)	1 pkg	150	0	2
With Added Oat Bran (Erewhon)	1.25 oz	125	—	3
Oats Gourmet (H-O)	⅓ cup	100	0	2
Oats 'n Fiber (H-O)	1 pkg	110	0	2
Oats 'n Fiber (H-O)	⅓ cup	100	0	2
Oats 'n Fiber Apple & Bran (H-O)	1 pkg	130	0	2
Oats 'n Fiber Raisin & Bran (H-O)	1 pkg	150	0	2
Oats, Old Fashion, cooked (Quaker)	⅔ cup	99	tr	2
Oats, Quick (H-O)	½ cup	130	0	2
Oats, Quick, cooked (Quaker)	⅔ cup	99	tr	2
Oats, Wheat, Dates, Raisins, Almonds Cereal, not prep (Roman Meal)	⅓ cup (1.3 oz)	129	tr	2

FOOD	PORTION	CALS.	SAT. FAT	FAT
Oats, Wheat, Honey, Coconut, Almonds Cereal, not prep (Roman Meal)	⅓ cup (1.3 oz)	155	3	5
Original (Roman Meal)	1 oz	83	tr	1
Original With Oats (Roman Meal)	1.2 oz	108	tr	1
Rice & Shine (Arrowhead)	¼ oz (1.5 oz)	150	0	1
Spelt (Good Shepherd)	1 oz	90	—	tr
Wheat Flakes Rolled (Arrowhead)	⅓ cup (1.2 oz)	110	0	1
Wheatena	⅓ cup (1.4 oz)	150	0	1
Whole Wheat Hot Natural Cereal, cooked (Quaker)	⅔ cup	92	tr	1
corn grits, instant, as prep	1 pkg (.8 oz)	82	—	tr
corn grits, quick	1 cup	579	tr	2
corn grits, quick	1 tbsp	36	tr	tr
corn grits, quick, cooked	1 cup	146	tr	1
corn grits, regular	1 cup	579	tr	2
corn grits, regular, cooked	1 cup	146	tr	1
farina, cooked	¾ cup	87	tr	tr
farina, dry	1 tbsp	40	0	0
oatmeal, cooked	1 cup	145	tr	2
oatmeal, dry	1 cup	311	tr	5
oatmeal instant, cooked w/o salt	1 cup	145	tr	2
oatmeal quick, cooked w/o salt	1 cup	145	tr	2
oatmeal regular, cooked w/o salt	1 cup	145	tr	2
READY-TO-EAT				
100% Bran (Nabisco)	⅓ cup	70	0	2
100% Natural Bran w/ Apples & Cinnamon (Health Valley)	¼ cup	100	—	1
All-Bran (Kellogg's)	⅓ cup (1 oz)	70	0	1
All-Bran w/ Extra Fiber (Kellogg's)	½ cup (1 oz)	50	0	0
Almond Delight (Ralston)	1 cup	210	0	3
Alpha-Bits (Post)	1 cup (1 oz)	111	—	1
Alpha-Bits Marshmallow Sweetened Letter Shaped Oats (Post)	1 cup	110	—	1
Amaranth Flakes (Arrowhead)	1 cup (1.2 oz)	130	0	2

FOOD	PORTION	CALS.	SAT. FAT	FAT
Apple Cinnamon Natural (Grist Mill)	½ cup (1.9 oz)	260	2	10
Apple Cinnamon Squares (Kellogg's)	½ cup (1 oz)	90	0	1
Apple Corns (Arrowhead)	1 cup (1.5 oz)	150	0	2
Apple Jacks (Kellogg's)	1 cup (1 oz)	110	0	0
Apple Raisin Crisp (Kellogg's)	⅔ cup (1 oz)	130	0	0
Aztec (Erewhon)	1 oz	100	—	0
Basic 4 (General Mills)	¾ cup	130	—	2
Blue Corn Flakes 100% Organic (Health Valley)	½ cup	90	—	tr
Blueberry Squares (Kellogg's)	½ cup (1 oz)	90	0	0
Booberry (General Mills)	1 cup	110	—	1
Bran (Grist Mill)	½ cup	250	6	8
Bran Buds (Kellogg's)	⅓ cup (1 oz)	70	0	1
Bran Cereal w/ Dates 100% Organic (Health Valley)	¼ cup	100	—	1
Bran Cereal w/ Raisins 100% Organic (Health Valley)	¼ cup	100	—	1
Bran Flakes (Arrowhead)	1 oz	100	0	1
Bran Flakes (Kellogg's)	⅔ cup (1 oz)	90	0	0
Bran Flakes (Ralston)	¾ cup (1.1 oz)	110	0	1
Cap'n Crunch (Quaker)	¾ cup	113	1	2
Cap'n Crunch's Crunchberries (Quaker)	¾ cup	113	1	2
Cap'n Crunch's Peanut Butter Crunch (Quaker)	¾ cup	119	1	3
Cheerios (General Mills)	1¼ cup	110	—	2
Cheerios Apple Cinnamon (General Mills)	¾ cup (1 oz)	110	—	2
Cheerios Honey Nut (General Mills)	¾ cup (1 oz)	110	—	1
Cheerios-to-Go (General Mills)	1 pkg (0.75 oz)	80	—	2
Cheerios-to-Go Apple Cinnamon (General Mills)	1 pkg (1 oz)	110	—	2
Cheerios-to-Go Honey Nut (General Mills)	1 pkg (1 oz)	110	—	1
Chex Corn (Ralston)	1¼ cup (1 oz)	110	0	0
Chex Double (Ralston)	1¼ cup (1 oz)	120	0	0

FOOD	PORTION	CALS.	SAT. FAT	FAT
Chex Graham (Ralston)	1 cup (1.8 oz)	210	0	2
Chex Multi-Bran (Ralston)	1¼ cup	220	0	2
Chex Rice (Ralston)	1 cup (1.1 oz)	120	0	0
Chex Wheat (Ralston)	¾ cup (1.8 oz)	190	0	1
Cinnamon Mini Buns (Kellogg's)	¾ cup (1 oz)	110	0	1
Cinnamon Toast Crunch (General Mills)	¾ cup (1 oz)	120	—	3
Clusters (General Mills)	½ cup (1 oz)	110	—	2
Cocoa Crispy Rice (Ralston)	1 cup (1.8 oz)	200	0	1
Cocoa Crunchies (Ralston)	¾ cup (1.1 oz)	120	0	1
Cocoa Krispies (Kellogg's)	¾ cup (1 oz)	110	0	0
Cocoa Pebbles (Post)	⅞ cup	113	—	1
Cocoa Puffs (General Mills)	1 cup (1 oz)	110	—	1
Coconut (Heartland)	1 oz	130	—	5
Common Sense Oat Bran (Kellogg's)	¾ cup (1 oz)	100	0	1
Common Sense Oat Bran w/ Raisins (Kellogg's)	¾ cup (1.3 oz)	130	0	1
Cookie-Crisp (Ralston)	1 cup (1 oz)	120	0	2
Corn Flakes (Estee)	1 pkg (1 oz)	90	0	0
Corn Flakes (Kellogg's)	1 cup (1 oz)	100	0	0
Corn Pops (Kellogg's)	1 cup (1 oz)	110	0	0
Count Chocula (General Mills)	1 cup (1 oz)	110	—	1
Country Corn Flakes (General Mills)	1 cup	110	—	tr
Cracklin' Oat Bran (Kellogg')	½ cup (1 oz)	110	1	3
Crisp Crunch (Ralston)	¾ cup (1.1 oz)	120	0	1
Crisp Rice (Ralston)	1¼ cup (1.2 oz)	130	0	0
Crispix (Kellogg's)	1 cup (1 oz)	110	0	0
Crispy Brown Rice (Erewhon)	1 oz	110	—	1
Crispy Critters (Post)	1 cup (1 oz)	110	0	0
Crispy Wheats 'n Raisins (General Mills)	¾ cup (1 oz)	100	—	1
Crunchy Nut Ohls (Quaker)	1 cup	127	2	4
Double Dip Crunch (Kellogg's)	⅔ cup (1 oz)	110	0	0
Fiber 7 Flakes 100% Organic (Health Valley)	½ cup	90	—	tr

FOOD	PORTION	CALS.	SAT. FAT	FAT
Fiber 7 Flakes w/ Raisins 100% Organic (Health Valley)	½ cup	90	—	tr
Fiber One (General Mills)	½ cup (1 oz)	60	—	1
Frankenberry (General Mills)	1 cup	110	—	1
Froot Loops (Kellogg's)	1 cup (1 oz)	110	0	1
Frosted Mini-Wheats (Kellogg's)	4 biscuits (1 oz)	100	0	0
Frosted Mini-Wheats Bite Size (Kellogg's)	½ cup (1 oz)	100	0	0
Frosted Bran (Kellogg's)	⅔ cup (1 oz)	100	0	0
Frosted Flakes (Kellogg's)	¾ cup (1 oz)	110	0	0
Frosted Flakes (Ralston)	¾ cup (1.1 oz)	120	0	0
Frosted Krispies (Kellogg's)	¾ cup (1 oz)	110	0	0
Fruit & Fiber Dates, Raisins & Walnuts (Post)	⅔ cup	120	—	2
Fruit & Fiber Tropical Fruit (Post)	⅔ cup	125	—	3
Fruit & Fitness (Health Valley)	1 cup (2 oz)	220	—	4
Fruit Lites Corn (Health Valley)	½ cup	45	0	0
Fruit Lites Rice (Health Valley)	½ cup (0.5 oz)	45	—	1
Fruit Lites Wheat (Health Valley)	½ cup	45	—	1
Fruit 'n Wheat (Erewhon)	1 oz	100	—	1
Fruit Rings (Ralston)	¾ cup (0.9 oz)	100	0	1
Fruit Wheats Apple (Nabisco)	1 oz	90	0	0
Fruitful Bran (Kellogg's)	⅔ cup (1.4 oz)	120	0	0
Fruity Marshmallow Krispies (Kellogg's)	1¼ cups (1.3 oz)	140	0	0
Fruity Pebbles (Post)	⅞ cup	113	—	1
Fruity Yummy Mummy (General Mills)	1 cup (1 oz)	110	—	1
Golden Grahams (General Mills)	¾ cup	110	—	1
Grape-Nuts (Post)	¼ cup	105	0	0
Grape-Nuts Raisin (Post)	¼ cup (1 oz)	102	0	0
Healthy Crunch Almond Date (Health Valley)	¼ cup (1 oz)	110	—	3

FOOD	PORTION	CALS.	SAT. FAT	FAT
Healthy Crunch Apple Cinnamon (Health Valley)	¼ cup	110	—	3
Healthy O's 100% Organic (Health Valley)	¾ cup	90	—	1
Honey Bunches Of Oats Honey Roasted (Post)	⅔ cup (1 oz)	111	—	2
Honey Bunches Of Oats With Almonds (Post)	⅔ cup (1 oz)	115	—	3
Honey Graham Oh!s (Quaker)	1 cup	122	2	3
Honeycomb (Post)	1⅓ cup	110	0	0
Just Right with Crunchy Nuggets (Kellogg's)	⅔ cup (1 oz)	110	0	1
Just Right w/ Raisins, Dates & Nuts (Kellogg's)	¾ cup (1.3 oz)	140	0	1
Kaboom (General Mills)	1 cup	110	—	1
Kamut Flakes (Arrowhead)	1 cup (1.1 oz)	120	0	1
Kashi Brittles Sesame/ Maple (Kashi)	3½ oz	473	—	19
Kashi Puffed (Kashi)	¾ oz	74	—	1
Kenmei (Kellogg's)	¾ cup (1 oz)	110	0	1
King Vitamin (Quaker)	1½ cup	110	—	1
Kix (General Mills)	1½ cup (1 oz)	110	—	1
Life (Quaker)	⅔ cup	101	—	2
Life Cinnamon (Quaker)	⅔ cup	101	—	2
Lites Puffed Corn (Health Valley)	½ (1 oz)	50	0	0
Lites Puffed Rice (Health Valley)	½ cup (1 oz)	50	0	0
Lites Puffed Wheat (Health Valley)	½ cup (1 oz)	50	0	0
Lucky Charms (General Mills)	1 cup (1 oz)	110	—	1
Magic Stair (Ralston)	¾ cup (1.1 oz)	120	0	1
Maple Corns (Arrowhead)	1 cup (1.9 oz)	190	1	3
Muesli Blueberry (Ralston)	1 cup (1.9 oz)	200	2	3
Muesli Cranberry (Ralston)	¾ cup (1.9 oz)	200	0	3
Muesli Peach (Ralston)	¾ cup (1.9 oz)	200	0	3
Muesli Raspberry (Ralston)	¾ cup (2 oz)	220	0	3
Muesli Strawberry (Ralston)	1 cup (1.9 oz)	210	2	3

FOOD	PORTION	CALS.	SAT. FAT	FAT
Mueslix Crispy Blend (Kellogg's)	⅔ cup (1.5 oz)	150	0	2
Mueslix Golden Crunch (Kellogg's)	½ cup (1.2 oz)	120	0	2
Multi Grain Flakes (Arrowhead)	1 cup (1.2 oz)	140	0	2
Multi Vitamin Whole Grain Flakes (Ralston)	1 cup (1.1 oz)	120	0	1
Natural Bran Flakes (Post)	⅔ cup	88	0	0
Nature O's (Arrowhead)	1 cup (1.1 oz)	130	1	2
Nut & Honey Crunch (Kellogg's)	⅔ cup (1 oz)	120	0	1
Nut & Honey Crunch O's (Kellogg's)	¾ cup (1 oz)	110	0	2
Nutri-Grain Almond Raisin (Kellogg's)	⅔ cup (1.4 oz)	140	0	2
Nutri-Grain Nuggets (Kellogg's)	¼ cup (1 oz)	90	0	0
Nutri-Grain Raisin Bran (Kellogg's)	1 cup (1.4 oz)	130	0	1
Nutri-Grain Wheat (Kellogg's)	⅔ cup (1 oz)	90	0	0
Oat & Honey Natural (Grist Mill)	½ cup (1.9 oz)	270	3	12
Oat Bran Flakes (Arrowhead)	1 cup (1.2 oz)	110	1	2
Oat Bran Flakes 100% Organic (Health Valley)	½ cup (1 oz)	100	—	tr
Oat Bran Flakes w/ Almonds & Dates 100% Organic (Health Valley)	½ cup (1 oz)	100	—	tr
Oat Bran Flakes w/ Raisins 100% Organic (Health Valley)	½ cup (1 oz)	100	—	tr
Oat Bran O'S 100% Organic (Health Valley)	½ cup (1 oz)	110	—	tr
Oat Bran O'S Fruit & Nuts (Health Valley)	½ cup (1 oz)	110	—	3
Oat Flakes (Post)	⅔ cup (1 oz)	107	—	1
Oat Squares (Quaker)	½ cup	105	—	2
Oat, Honey & Raisin Natural (Grist Mill)	½ cup (1.9 oz)	260	2	10
Oatbake Honey Bran (Kellogg's)	⅓ cup (1 oz)	110	1	3

FOOD	PORTION	CALS.	SAT. FAT	FAT
Oatbake Raisin Nut (Kellogg's)	⅓ cup (1 oz)	110	1	3
Oatmeal Crisp (General Mills)	½ cup (1 oz)	110	—	2
Oatmeal Raisin Crisp (General Mills)	½ cup (1.2 oz)	130	—	2
Orangeola Almonds & Dates (Health Valley)	¼ cup	110	—	3
Orangeola Bananas & Hawaiian Fruit (Health Valley)	¼ cup	120	—	4
Popeye Sweet Crunch (Quaker)	1 cup	113	1	2
Poppets (US Mills)	1 oz	110	—	1
Post Toasties Corn Flakes (Post)	1¼ cup	108	0	tr
Product 19 (Kellogg's)	1 cup (1 oz)	100	0	0
Puffed Corn (Arrowhead)	½ oz	50	0	0
Puffed Kamut	1 cup (0.6 oz)	50	0	0
Puffed Millet (Arrowhead)	½ oz	50	0	0
Puffed Rice (Arrowhead)	½ oz	50	0	0
Puffed Rice (Quaker)	1 cup	54	—	tr
Puffed Wheat (Arrowhead)	½ oz	50	0	0
Puffed Wheat (Quaker)	1 cup	50	0	tr
Quaker 100% Natural	¼ cup	127	3	6
Quaker 100% Natural Apples & Cinnamon	¼ cup	126	3	5
Quaker 100% Natural Raisins & Date	¼ cup	123	3	5
Raisin (Heartland)	1 oz	100	—	0
Raisin Bran (Erewhon)	1 oz	100	—	0
Raisin Bran (Estee)	1 pkg (1 oz)	90	0	1
Raisin Bran (Kellogg's)	¾ cup (1.4 oz)	120	0	1
Raisin Bran (Post)	⅔ cup (4 oz)	122	—	1
Raisin Bran (Ralston)	¾ cup (1.9 oz)	190	0	1
Raisin Bran Flakes 100% Organic (Health Valley)	½ cup	100	—	tr
Raisin Nut Bran	½ cup (1 oz)	110	—	3
Raisin Square (Kellogg's)	½ cup (1 oz)	90	0	tr
Real Oat Bran Almond Crunch (Health Valley)	¼ cup (1 oz)	110	—	3
Real Oat Bran Hawaiian Fruit (Health Valley)	¼ cup (1 oz)	130	—	3
Real Oat Bran Raisin Nut (Health Valley)	¼ (1 oz)	130	—	3

FOOD	PORTION	CALS.	SAT. FAT	FAT
Rice Bran O's (Health Valley)	½ cup	110	—	1
Rice Bran w/ Almonds & Dates (Health Valley)	½ cup (1 oz)	110	—	3
Rice Krispies Treats (Kellogg's)	¾ cup (1 oz)	110	0	1
Ruskets Biscuits (LaLoma)	2 biscuits (30 g)	110	0	0
S'Mores Grahams (General Mills)	¾ cup (1 oz)	120	—	2
Shredded Wheat (Quaker)	2 biscuits	132	—	1
Shredded Wheat 'n Bran (Nabisco)	⅔ cup (1 oz)	90	—	1
Shredded Wheat Spoon Size (Nabisco)	⅔ cup (1 oz)	90	0	1
Shredded Wheat w/ Oat Bran (Nabisco)	⅔ cup (1 oz)	100	0	1
Smacks (Kellogg's)	¾ cup (1 oz)	110	0	1
Special K (Kellogg's)	1 cup (1 oz)	100	0	1
Spelt Flakes (Arrowhead)	1 cup (1.1 oz)	100	0	1
Spelt Flakes (Good Shepherd)	1 oz	100	—	6
Sprouts 7 Bananas & Hawaiian Fruit (Health Valley)	¼ cup (1 oz)	90	—	1
Sprouts 7 Raisin (Health Valley)	¼ cup	90	—	1
Strawberry Squares (Kellogg's)	½ cup (1 oz)	90	0	tr
Super Golden Crisp (Post)	⅞ cup (1 oz)	104	0	0
Super-O's (Erewhon)	1 oz	110	—	0
Swiss Breakfast Raisin Nut (Health Valley)	¼ cup (1 oz)	100	—	3
Swiss Breakfast Tropical Fruit (Health Valley)	¼ cup (1 oz)	100	—	3
Tasteeos (Ralston)	1¼ cup (1.1 oz)	130	0	3
Tasteeos Apple Cinnamon (Ralston)	1 cup (1.2 oz)	130	0	2
Tasteeos Honey Nut (Ralston)	1 cup (1.2 oz)	130	0	2
Team (Nabisco)	1 cup	110	—	1
Total (General Mills)	1 cup (1 oz)	100	—	1
Total Corn Flakes (General Mills)	1 cup (1 oz)	110	—	tr
Total Raisin Bran (General Mills)	1 cup (1.5 oz)	140	—	1

FOOD	PORTION	CALS.	SAT. FAT	FAT
Triples (General Mills)	¾ cup (1 oz)	110	—	1
Trix (General Mills)	1 cup	110	—	1
Uncle Sam Cereal (US Mills)	1 oz	110	—	1
Weetabix	2 (1.3 oz)	142	—	1
Wheat Flakes (Erewhon)	1 oz	100	—	0
Wheaties (General Mills)	1 cup (1 oz)	100	—	1
all bran	½ cup (1 oz)	76	tr	1
bran flakes	¾ cup (1 oz)	90	tr	1
corn flakes	1¼ cup (1 oz)	110	tr	tr
corn flakes, low sodium	1 cup	100	—	tr
crispy rice	1 cup	111	—	tr
fortified oat flakes	1 cup	177	—	tr
puffed rice	1 cup	57	—	tr
puffed wheat	1 cup	44	—	tr
shredded wheat	1 biscuit	83	—	tr
sugar-coated corn flakes	¾ cup (1 oz)	110	tr	1

CHAMPAGNE

FOOD	PORTION	CALS.	SAT. FAT	FAT
Andre Blush	1 fl oz	22	0	0
Andre Brut	1 fl oz	21	0	0
Andre Cold Duck	1 fl oz	25	0	0
Andre Extra Dry	1 fl oz	23	0	0
Ballatore Gran Spumante Ballatore	1 fl oz	23	0	0
Eden Roc Brut	1 fl oz	21	0	0
Eden Roc Brut Rosé	1 fl oz	22	0	0
Eden Roc Extra Dry	1 fl oz	21	0	0
Tott's Blanc de Noir	1 fl oz	22	0	0
Tott's Brut	1 fl oz	20	0	0
Tott's Extra Dry	1 fl oz	21	0	0

CHAYOTE
FRESH

FOOD	PORTION	CALS.	SAT. FAT	FAT
cooked	1 cup	38	—	1
raw	1 (7 oz)	49	—	1
raw, cut up	1 cup	32	—	tr

CHEESE
(*See also* CHEESE DISHES, CHEESE SUBSTITUTES, COTTAGE CHEESE, CREAM CHEESE)
NATURAL

FOOD	PORTION	CALS.	SAT. FAT	FAT
Asiago (Frigo)	1 oz	110	—	9
Baby Swiss (Cracker Barrel)	1 oz	110	5	9

FOOD	PORTION	CALS.	SAT. FAT	FAT
Baby Swiss (Land O'Lakes)	1 oz	110	5	8
Baby Swiss Reduced Fat (Alpine Lace)	1 piece (1 oz)	90	4	20
Babybel (Laughing Cow)	1 oz	90	5	7
Babybel Mini (Laughing Cow)	1 (0.7 oz)	70	4	6
Babybel Mini Light (Laughing Cow)	1 (0.7 oz)	45	2	3
Blue (Frigo)	1 oz	100	—	8
Blue (Kraft)	1 oz	100	5	9
Blue (Sargento)	1 oz	100	—	8
Bonbel (Laughing Cow)	1 oz	100	5	8
Bonbel, Mini (Laughing Cow)	1 (0.7 oz)	70	4	6
Breakfast (Marin French Cheese)	1 oz	86	4	7
Brick (Kraft)	1 oz	110	5	9
Brick (Land O'Lakes)	1 oz	110	5	8
Brie (Bresse)	1 oz	110	5	9
Brie (Gerard)	1 oz	90	5	7
Brie (Marin French Cheese)	1 oz	86	4	7
Brie (Sargento)	1 oz	95	—	8
Brie Baby (Alouette)	1 oz	110	5	9
Brie Baby With Herbs (Alouette)	1 oz	110	5	9
Brie Light (Bresse)	1 oz	70	3	4
Brie With Herbs (Bresse)	1 oz	110	5	9
Burger Cheese (Sargento)	1 oz	106	—	9
Cajun (Sargento)	1 oz	110	—	9
Camembert (Marin French Cheese)	1 oz	86	4	7
Camembert (Sargento)	1 oz	85	—	7
Chavrie (Bongrain)	2 tbsp (0.8 oz)	40	2	3
Cheda-Jack Reduced Fat Low Sodium (Dorman)	1 oz	80	3	5
Chederella (Land O'Lakes)	1 oz	100	5	8
Cheddar				
(Armour)	1 oz	110	—	9
(Cabot)	1 oz	110	6	9
(Dorman)	1 oz	110	—	9
(Frigo)	1 oz	110	6	9
(Kraft)	1 oz	110	5	9
(Sargento)	1 oz	114	—	9

FOOD	PORTION	CALS.	SAT. FAT	FAT
Cheddar Curds Snack (Heluva Good Cheese)	1 oz	113	5	9
Cheddar Extra-Sharp (Heluva Good Cheese)	1 oz	110	5	9
Cheddar Extra-Sharp Premium (Father Time)	1 oz	110	5	9
Cheddar Fancy Shreds Fat Free (Healthy Choice)	1 oz	45	0	0
Cheddar Light (Land O'Lakes)	1 oz	70	3	4
Cheddar Mild (Heluva Good Cheese)	1 oz	110	5	9
Cheddar Mild Reduced Fat (Heluva Good Cheese)	1 oz	80	4	6
Cheddar Reduced Fat (Alpine Lace)	1 piece (1 oz)	80	3	5
Cheddar Sharp (Heluva Good Cheese)	1 oz	110	5	9
Cheddar Shredded (Heluva Good Cheese)	¼ cup (1 oz)	110	5	9
Cheddar Shreds Fat Free (Healthy Choice)	1 oz	45	0	0
Cheddar Very Low Sodium (Heluva Good Cheese)	1 oz	110	6	9
Cheddar Light (Bristol Gold)	1 oz	70	—	4
Cheddar Light With Simplesse (White Clover)	1 oz	80	—	4
Cheddar Lite (Frigo)	1 oz	80	3	5
Cheddar Lower Salt (Armour)	1 oz	110	—	9
Cheddar Mild MooTown Snackers Light (Sargento)	1 stick	70	—	5
Cheddar Mild Preferred Light (Sargento)	1 oz	90	—	5
Cheddar Mild Reduced Fat Light (Kraft)	1 oz	80	3	5
Cheddar Mild Shredded (Weight Watchers)	1 oz	80	3	5
Cheddar Mild Shredded Preferred Light (Sargento)	1 oz	90	—	5

FOOD	PORTION	CALS.	SAT. FAT	FAT
Cheddar Mild White (Weight Watchers)	1 oz	80	3	5
Cheddar Mild Yellow (Weight Watchers)	1 oz	80	3	5
Cheddar Mild Low Sodium White (Weight Watchers)	1 oz	80	3	5
Cheddar Mild Low Sodium Yellow (Weight Watchers)	1 oz	80	3	5
Cheddar New York (Sargento)	1 oz	114	—	9
Cheddar Reduced Fat Low Sodium (Dorman)	1 oz	80	3	5
Cheddar Sharp Light Reduced Fat White (Cracker Barrel)	1 oz	80	3	5
Cheddar Sharp Nut Log (Sargento)	1 oz	97	—	7
Cheddar Sharp Reduced Fat Light (Kraft)	1 oz	80	3	5
Cheddar Sharp White (Weight Watchers)	1 oz	80	3	5
Cheddar Sharp Yellow (Weight Watchers)	1 oz	80	3	5
Cheddar White Extra-Sharp (Heluva Good Cheese)	1 oz	110	5	9
Cheddar White Mild (Heluva Good Cheese)	1 oz	110	5	9
Cheddar White Sharp (Heluva Good Cheese	1 oz	110	5	9
Cheddar White Shredded (Heluva Good Cheese)	¼ cup (1 oz)	110	5	9
Cheddar White Very Low Sodium (Heluva Good Cheese)	1 oz	110	6	9
Chevre (Brier Run)	1 oz	61	—	5
Chub (Keller's)	2 tbsp (1 oz)	100	6	10
Chub (Quaker)	2 tbsp (1 oz)	100	6	10
Colby				
(Dorman)	1 oz	110	—	9
(Kraft)	1 oz	110	5	9
(Heluva Good Cheese)	1 oz	117	6	9
(Sargento)	1 oz	112	—	9

FOOD	PORTION	CALS.	SAT. FAT	FAT
Colby *(cont.)*				
(Weight Watchers)	1 oz	80	3	5
And Monterey Jack Reduced Fat Light (Kraft)	1 oz	80	3	5
Lower Salt (Armour)	1 oz	110	—	9
Light w/ Simplesse (White Clover)	1 oz	80	—	4
Reduced Fat Light (Kraft)	1 oz	80	3	5
Colby-Jack (Heluva Good Cheese)	1 oz	110	6	9
Colby-Jack (Sargento)	1 oz	109	—	9
Creme De Brie (Bresse)	2 tbsp (1 oz)	90	5	8
Creme De Brie Herb (Bresse)	2 tbsp (1 oz)	90	5	8
Delice De France	1 oz	110	5	9
Delice De France With Herbs	1 oz	110	5	9
Edam				
(Dorman)	1 oz	100	—	8
(Holland Farm)	1 oz	97	—	8
(Kraft)	1 oz	90	4	7
(May-Bud)	1 oz	100	6	8
(Sargento)	1 oz	101	—	8
Farmer (Friendship)	2 tbsp (1 oz)	50	2	3
Farmer (Holland Farm)	1 oz	102	—	8
Farmer No Salt Added (Friendship)	2 tbsp (1 oz)	50	2	3
Farmer's MooTown Snackers Light (Sargento)	1 stick	70	—	4
Farmer's Preferred Light (Sargento)	1 oz	80	—	5
Farmer's Shredded Preferred Light (Sargento)	1 oz	80	—	5
Feta (Churney)	1 oz	80	4	6
Feta (Frigo)	1 oz	100	—	8
Feta (Sargento)	1 oz	75	—	6
Finland Swiss (Sargento)	1 oz	107	—	8
Fontina (Sargento)	1 oz	110	—	9
French Onion Light (Bristol Gold)	1 oz	70	—	4

FOOD	PORTION	CALS.	SAT. FAT	FAT
Fruit Moos Apricot (Dannon)	3.5 oz	150	—	8
Fruit Moos Banana (Dannon)	3.5 oz	150	—	8
Fruit Moos Raspberry (Dannon)	3.5 oz	150	—	8
Fruit Moos Strawberry (Dannon)	3.5 oz	150	—	8
Garlic & Herb Light (Bristol Gold)	1 oz	70	—	4
Gjetost (Sargento)	1 oz	132	—	8
Gouda				
(Dorman)	1 oz	100	—	8
(Holland Farm)	1 oz	103	—	8
(Kraft)	1 oz	110	5	9
(Land O'Lakes)	1 oz	110	5	8
(May-Bud)	1 oz	100	6	8
(Sargento)	1 oz	101	—	8
Mini (Laughing Cow)	1 (0.7 oz)	80	4	6
Round (MayBud)	1 oz	100	6	8
Gourmet Parm (Sargento)	1 tbsp	20	—	1
Havarti (Casino)	1 oz	120	7	11
Havarti (Sargento)	1 oz	118	—	11
Havarti Lower Fat Garden Vegetable (New Holland)	1 oz	80	4	6
Havarti Reduced Fat (Alpine Lace)	1 piece (1 oz)	90	5	25
Hoop (Friendship)	4 oz	84	0	tr
Horseradish Light (Bristol Gold)	1 oz	70	—	4
Impastata (Frigo)	1 oz	60	—	5
Italian Style Grated Cheese (Sargento)	1 oz	108	—	8
Jarlsberg (Sargento)	1 oz	100	—	7
Limburger (Sargento)	1 oz	93	—	8
Limburger Little Gem Size (Mohawk Valley)	1 oz	90	5	8
Mexican Shreds Fat Free (Healthy Choice)	1 oz	45	0	0
Monterey Jack				
(Armour)	1 oz	110	—	9
(Cabot)	1 oz	80	5	5
(Dorman)	1 oz	100	—	8
(Heluva Good Cheese)	1 oz	100	6	8

FOOD	PORTION	CALS.	SAT. FAT	FAT
Monterey Jack *(cont.)*				
(Holland Farm)	1 oz	102	—	9
(Kraft)	1 oz	110	5	9
(Land O'Lakes)	1 oz	110	5	9
(Sargento)	1 oz	106	—	9
(Weight Watchers)	1 oz	80	3	5
Light w/ Simplesse (White Clover)	1 oz	70	—	4
Lower Salt (Armour)	1 oz	110	—	9
Reduced Fat (Alpine Lace)	1 oz	70	3	5
Reduced Fat Light (Kraft)	1 oz	80	3	5
Reduced Fat Low Sodium (Dorman)	1 oz	80	3	5
Shredded (Heluva Good Cheese)	1 oz	100	5	8
With Caraway Seeds (Kraft)	1 oz	100	5	8
With Jalapeno Peppers (Kraft)	1 oz	110	5	9
With Jalapenos (Heluva Good Cheese)	1 oz	100	6	8
With Peppers Reduced Fat Light (Kraft)	1 oz	80	3	5
Montrachet				
(Bongrain)	1 oz	70	4	6
Chive (Bongrain)	1 oz	70	4	6
Classic (Bongrain)	1 oz	70	4	6
Classic Herb (Bongrain)	1 oz	70	4	6
Herbs & Garlic (Bongrain)	1 oz	70	4	6
In Oil, drained (Bongrain)	1 oz	70	4	6
With Ash (Bongrain)	1 oz	70	4	6
Mozzarella				
(Land O'Lakes)	1 oz	80	4	6
(Weight Watchers)	1 oz	70	3	4
Fancy Shreds Fat Free (Healthy Choice)	1 oz	45	0	0
Free (Polly-O)	1 oz	35	0	0
Lite (Polly-O)	1 oz	60	2	3
Low Moisture (Kraft)	1 oz	90	4	7
Part Skim (Dorman)	1 oz	90	—	7
Part Skim (Polly-O)	1 oz	70	3	5

FOOD	PORTION	CALS.	SAT. FAT	FAT
Part Skim Low Moisture (Frigo)	1 oz	80	3	5
Part Skim Low Moisture (Kraft)	1 oz	80	3	5
Part Skim Low Moisture (Sargento)	1 oz	79	—	5
Part Skim Low Moisture Shredded (Heluva Good Cheese)	¼ cup (1 oz)	80	3	5
Part Skim Shredded (Polly-O)	¼ cup	80	4	5
Preferred Light (Sargento)	1 oz	60	—	3
Reduced Fat Light (Kraft)	1 oz	80	3	4
Reduced Fat Low Sodium (Dorman)	1 oz	80	3	4
Reduced Sodium Part Skim Low Moisture (Alpine Lace)	1 piece (1 oz)	70	3	5
Shredded (Weight Watchers)	1 oz	80	3	5
Shredded Free (Polly-O)	¼ cup	45	0	0
Shredded Lite (Polly-O)	¼ cup	60	2	3
Shredded Preferred Light (Sargento)	1 oz	60	—	3
Shreds Fat Free (Healthy Choice)	1 oz	45	0	0
Snack Stick Fat Free (Healthy Choice)	1 (1 oz)	45	0	0
Whole Milk (Heluva Good Cheese)	1 oz	80	4	6
Whole Milk (Polly-O)	1 oz	80	4	6
Whole Milk (Sargento)	1 oz	90	—	7
Whole Milk Low Moisture (Frigo)	1 oz	90	4	7
Whole Milk Shredded (Polly-O)	¼ cup	90	5	7
Mozzarella Ball Fat Free (Healthy Choice)	1 oz	45	0	0
Mozzarella Lite Whole Milk Low Moisture (Frigo)	1 oz	60	2	2
Muenster				
(Dorman)	1 oz	110	—	9
(Heluva Good Cheese)	1 oz	100	6	8

FOOD	PORTION	CALS.	SAT. FAT	FAT
Muenster *(cont.)*				
(Holland Farm)	1 oz	102	—	9
(Land O'Lakes)	1 oz	100	5	8
Light w/ Simplesse (White Clover)	1 oz	70	—	4
Low Sodium (Dorman)	1 oz	110	—	9
Red Rind (Sargento)	1 oz	104	—	9
Reduced Fat Low Sodium (Dorman)	1 oz	80	3	5
Reduced sodium (Alpine Lace)	1 oz	100	5	9
Naturally Slender (Northfield)	1 oz	90	—	7
New Holland	1 oz	90	5	7
New Holland Garlic	1 oz	90	5	7
New Holland Jalapeno	1 oz	80	4	6
New Holland Natural Vegetable	1 oz	80	4	6
Parmazest (Frigo)	1 oz	120	—	7
Parmesan				
(Dorman)	1 oz	110	—	7
And Romano Dry Grated (Frigo)	1 oz	130	—	9
And Romano Grated (Frigo)	1 oz	110	—	7
And Romano Grated (Sargento)	1 oz	111	—	7
Dry Grated (Frigo)	1 oz	130	—	9
Grated (Frigo)	1 oz	110	—	7
Grated (Kraft)	1 oz	130	5	9
Grated (Progresso)	1 tbsp	23	1	2
Grated (Sargento)	1 oz	129	—	9
Natural (Kraft)	1 oz	100	4	7
Shreds (Di Giorno)	2 tsp (5 g)	20	1	2
Whole (Frigo)	1 oz	110	—	7
Pizza Fancy Shreds Fat Free (Healthy Choice)	1 oz	45	0	0
Pizza Snack Stick Fat Free (Healthy Choice)	1 (1 oz)	45	0	0
Pizza Shredded (Frigo)	1 oz	65	—	3
Port Wine Nut Log (Sargento)	1 oz	97	—	7
Provolone				
(Dorman)	1 oz	90	—	7
(Frigo)	1 oz	100	5	7

FOOD	PORTION	CALS.	SAT. FAT	FAT
(Kraft)	1 oz	100	4	7
(Land O'Lakes)	1 oz	100	5	8
(Sargento)	1 oz	100	—	8
Lite (Frigo)	1 oz	70	2	4
Reduced Fat (Alpine Lace)	1 oz	70	3	5
Reduced Fat Low Sodium (Dorman)	1 oz	80	3	4
Quark (Brier Run)	1 oz	34	—	3
Queso Blanco (Sargento)	1 oz	104	—	9
Queso de Papa (Sargento)	1 oz	114	—	9
Ricotta				
Free (Polly-O)	¼ cup	50	0	0
Lite (Polly-O)	¼ cup	70	3	2
Lite (Sargento)	1 oz	24	—	1
Low Fat Low Salt (Frigo)	1 oz	30	—	1
Part Skim (Frigo)	1 oz	40	—	3
Part Skim (Polly-O)	¼ cup	90	4	6
Part Skim (Sargento)	1 oz	32	—	2
Whole Milk (Frigo)	1 oz	60	—	5
Whole Milk (Polly-O)	¼ cup	110	5	8
Romano				
(Dorman)	1 oz	100	—	7
(Sargento)	1 oz	110	—	8
Dry Grated (Frigo)	1 oz	130	—	9
Grated (Casino)	1 oz	130	6	9
Grated (Frigo)	1 oz	110	—	8
Grated (Progresso)	1 tbsp	23	1	2
Natural (Casino)	1 oz	100	4	7
Whole (Frigo)	1 oz	110	—	8
Sargento Brick	1 oz	95	—	9
Schloss (Marin French Cheese)	1 oz	86	4	7
Sheep's Milk (Hallow Road Farms)	1 oz	45	—	3
Smoke Light (Bristol Gold)	1 oz	70	—	4
Smokestick (Sargento)	1 oz	103	—	7
String (Frigo)	1 oz	80	—	5
String (Polly-O)	1 oz	90	—	6
String (Sargento)	1 oz	79	—	5
String Lite (Frigo)	1 oz	60	—	2
String Moo Town Snackers Light (Sargento)	1 stick	40	—	2
String Smoked (Sargento)	1 oz	79	—	5

FOOD	PORTION	CALS.	SAT. FAT	FAT
String w/ Jalapeno Peppers (Kraft)	1 oz	80	3	5
Swiss				
(Casino)	1 oz	110	5	8
(Dorman)	1 oz	100	—	8
(Frigo)	1 oz	110	—	8
(Heluva Good Cheese)	1 oz	112	5	8
(Kraft)	1 oz	110	5	8
(Land O'Lakes)	1 oz	110	6	8
(Sargento)	1 oz	107	—	8
Aged (Kraft)	1 oz	110	5	8
Almond Nut Log (Sargento)	1 oz	94	—	7
Light (Land O'Lakes)	1 oz	80	3	4
No Salt Added (Dorman)	1 oz	100	—	8
Reduced Fat (Alpine Lace)	1 oz	90	4	6
Reduced Fat (Kraft Light)	1 oz	90	3	5
Reduce Fat Low Sodium (Dorman)	1 oz	90	3	5
Very Low (Kraft)	1 oz	110	5	8
Wafer Thin Preferred Light (Sargento)	1 oz	80	—	4
Taco (Sargento)	1 oz	109	—	9
Taco Shredded (Frigo)	1 oz	110	—	9
Taco Shredded (Kraft)	1 oz	110	5	9
Tilsiter (Sargento)	1 oz	96	—	7
Tybo Red Wax (Sargento)	1 oz	98	—	7
Vitalait (Cabot)	1 oz	70	2	4
Vitalait Japapeno (Cabot)	1 oz	70	2	4
Washed Curd Cheese (Heluva Good Cheese)	1 oz	110	5	9
Weight Watchers Sharp Cheddar Cup	1½ cup (1 oz)	70	2	3
Wine Light (Bristol Gold)	1 oz	70	—	4
bel paese	3.5 oz	391	—	30
blue	1 oz	100	6	8
blue, crumbled	1 cup	477	25	39
brick	1 oz	105	5	8
brie	1 oz	95	—	8
caerphilly	1.4 oz	150	—	13
camembert	1 oz	85	4	7
camembert	1 wedge (1⅓ oz)	114	6	9

FOOD	PORTION	CALS.	SAT. FAT	FAT
caraway	1 oz	107	—	8
cheddar	1 oz	114	6	9
cheddar, reduced fat	1.4 oz	104	—	6
cheddar, shredded	1 cup	455	24	37
cheshire	1 oz	110	—	9
cheshire, reduced fat	1.4 oz	108	—	6
colby	1 oz	112	6	9
derby	1.4 oz	161	—	14
double gloucester	1.4 oz	162	—	14
edam	1 oz	101	5	8
edam, reduced fat	1.4 oz	92	—	4
emmentaler	3.5 oz	403	—	30
feta	1 oz	75	4	6
fontina	1 oz	110	5	9
fromage frais	1.6 oz	51	—	3
gjetost	1 oz	132	5	8
goat, hard	1 oz	128	7	10
goat-semi-soft	1 oz	103	6	8
goat, soft	1 oz	76	4	6
gorgonzola	3.5 oz	376	—	31
gouda	1 oz	101	5	8
gruyere	1 oz	117	5	9
lancashire	1.4 oz	149	—	12
leicester	1.4 oz	160	—	14
limburger	1 oz	93	5	8
lymeswold	1.4 oz	170	—	16
monterey	1 oz	106	—	9
mozzarella	1 oz	80	4	6
mozzarella	1 lb	1276	60	98
mozzarella, low moisture	1 oz	90	4	7
mozzarella, part skim	1 oz	72	3	5
mozzarella, part skim, low moisture	1 oz	79	3	5
muenster	1 oz	104	5	9
parmesan, grated	1 tbsp	23	1	2
parmesan, grated	1 oz	129	5	9
parmesan, hard	1 oz	111	5	7
port du salut	1 oz	100	5	8
provolone	1 oz	100	5	8
quark, 20% fat	3.5 oz	116	—	5
quark, 40% fat	3.5 oz	167	—	11
quark, made w/ skim milk	3.5 oz	78	—	tr
ricotta	½ cup	216	10	16
ricotta	1 cup	428	20	32
ricotta, part skim	½ cup	171	6	10

FOOD	PORTION	CALS.	SAT. FAT	FAT
ricotta, part skim	1 cup	340	12	19
romadur, 40% fat	3.5 oz	289	—	20
romano	1 oz	110	—	8
roquefort	1 oz	105	5	9
stilton, blue	1.4 oz	164	—	14
stilton, white	1.4 oz	145	—	13
swiss	1 oz	107	5	8
tilsit	1 oz	96	5	7
wensleydale	1.4 oz	151	—	13
yogurt cheese	1 oz	20	—	0
PROCESSED				
Alouette				
French Onion	2 tbsp (0.8 oz)	70	5	7
Garlic	2 tbsp (0.8 oz)	70	5	7
Salmon	2 tbsp (0.8 oz)	60	3	5
Scallions	2 tbsp (0.8 oz)	70	5	7
Spinach	2 tbsp (0.8 oz)	60	4	6
Alouette Light				
Dill Alouette	2 tbsp (0.8 oz)	50	3	4
Garlic Alouette	2 tbsp (0.8 oz)	50	3	4
Herb Alouette	2 tbsp (0.8 oz)	50	3	4
Herbs and Garlic Alouette	2 tbsp (0.8 oz)	50	3	4
Spring Vegetable Alouette	2 tbsp (0.8 oz)	50	3	4
Alpine Lace				
American	1 oz	80	4	6
American	1 slice (0.66 oz)	50	2	3
American Fat Free	1 piece (1 oz)	45	tr	tr
Cheddar Fat Free	1 piece (1 oz)	45	tr	tr
For Parmesan Lovers Fat Free	2 tsp (5 g)	10	0	0
Hot Pepper	1 piece (1 oz)	80	4	20
Mexican Macho Fat Free	2 tbsp (1 oz)	30	tr	tr
Mozzarella Fat Free	1 piece (1 oz)	45	tr	tr
Singles Fat Free	1 slice (0.66 oz)	25	0	0
Borden				
American Slices	1 oz	110	7	9
American Very Sharp	1 oz	110	—	9
Lite Line Mozzarella	1 oz	50	—	2
Lite Line Sharp Cheddar	1 oz	50	—	2
Lite Line Swiss	1 oz	50	—	2
Swiss Slices	1 oz	100	4	8
Cheez Whiz	1 oz	80	3	6

FOOD	PORTION	CALS.	SAT. FAT	FAT
Cheez Whiz Mild Mexican	1 oz	80	4	6
Cheez Whiz w/ Jalapeno Peppers	1 oz	80	4	6
Churney				
Diet Snack Cheddar Flavored	1 oz	70	—	3
Diet Snack Port Wine Flavored	1 oz	70	—	3
Cracker Barrel				
Cheese Ball Sharp Cheddar w/ Almonds	1 oz	100	3	7
Cheese Log Port Wine w/ Almonds	1 oz	90	3	6
Cheese Log Sharp Cheddar w/ Almonds	1 oz	90	3	6
Cheese Log Smokey Cheddar w/ Almonds	1 oz	90	3	6
Extra Sharp Cheddar	1 oz	90	4	7
Port Wine Cheddar	1 oz	100	4	7
Sharp Cheddar	1 oz	100	4	7
With Bacon	1 oz	90	4	7
Delico				
Alouette Cajun (Alouette)	2 tbsp (0.8 oz)	70	5	7
Alouette French Onion (Alouette)	2 tbsp (0.8 oz)	70	5	7
Alouette Garden Vegetable (Alouette)	2 tbsp (0.8 oz)	60	4	6
Alouette Garlic (Alouette)	2 tbsp (0.8 oz)	70	5	7
Alouette Horseradish and Chive (Alouette)	2 tbsp (0.8 oz)	60	4	7
Alouette Spinach (Alouette)	2 tbsp (0.8 oz)	60	4	6
Dorman's Lo-Chol Cheddar	1 oz	100	1	7
Dorman's Lo-Chol Colby	1 oz	100	1	7
Dorman's Lo-Chol Mozzarella	1 oz	90	1	6
Dorman's Lo-Chol Muenster	1 oz	100	1	7
Dorman's Lo-Chol Swiss	1 oz	100	1	7
Easy Cheese Sharp Cheddar Spread	1 oz	80	4	6
Formagg Shredded Provolone	1 oz	70	—	5

FOOD	PORTION	CALS.	SAT. FAT	FAT
Formaggio D'Oro				
Formagg	1 oz	70	3	5
Frigo Imitation Cheddar	1 oz	90	1	7
Frigo Imitation Mozzarella	1 oz	90	1	7
Harvest Moon American	1 oz	70	2	4
Healthy Choice				
Fat Free	1 oz	35	0	0
White Singles Fat Free	1 slice (0.75 oz)	30	0	0
Yellow Singles Fat Free	1 slice (0.67 oz)	25	0	0
Yellow Singles Fat Free	1 slice (0.75 oz)	30	0	0
Heluva Good Cheese				
American	1 slice (0.7)	45	3	5
Cheddar Sharp Cold Pack	2 tbsp (1 oz)	90	3	7
Cheddar Sharp With Bacon Cold Pack	2 tbsp (1 oz)	90	3	7
Cheddar Sharp With Horseradish Cold Pack	2 tbsp (1 oz)	90	3	7
Cheddar Sharp With Jalapenos Cold Pack	2 tbsp (1 oz)	90	3	7
Cheddar Sharp With Port Wine Cold Pack	2 tbsp (1 oz)	90	3	7
Hoffman American Yellow	1 oz	110	6	9
Hoffman Hot Pepper	1 oz	90	5	7
Hoffman Super Sharp	1 oz	110	6	9
Kraft				
American Cheese Spread	1 oz	80	3	6
American Grated	1 oz	130	4	7
American Singles	1 oz	90	4	7
American Singles White	1 oz	90	4	7
Cheese Food w/ Garlic	1 oz	90	4	7
Cheese Food w/ Jalapeno Peppers	1 oz	90	4	7
Cheese Spread w/ Bacon	1 oz	80	4	7
Cheez 'N Bacon Singles	1 oz	90	4	7
Deluxe American Cheese	1 oz	110	5	9
Deluxe Pimento Cheese	1 oz	100	5	8
Deluxe Swiss Cheese	1 oz	90	4	7
Free Singles	1 oz	45	0	0
Jalapeno Pepper Spread	1 oz	70	3	5
Jalapeno Spread	1 oz	80	4	6
Jalapeno Singles	1 oz	90	4	7

FOOD	PORTION	CALS.	SAT. FAT	FAT
Light Singles	1 oz	70	2	4
Light Singles American	1 oz	70	3	4
Light Singles Sharp Cheddar	1 oz	70	2	4
Light Singles Swiss	1 oz	70	2	3
Monterey Jack Singles	1 oz	90	4	7
Olives & Pimento Spread	1 oz	60	3	5
Pimento Singles	1 oz	90	4	7
Pimento Spread	1 oz	70	3	5
Pineapple Spread	1 oz	70	3	5
Sharp Singles	1 oz	100	5	8
Swiss Singles	1 oz	90	4	7
Lactaid American	3.5 oz	328	15	25
Land O'Lakes				
American	1 oz	110	6	9
American	1 slice (0.75 oz)	80	5	6
American	2 slices (1 oz)	100	6	9
American Less Salt	1 oz	110	6	9
American Light	1 oz	70	3	5
American Sharp	1 oz	110	6	9
American & Swiss	1 oz	100	6	8
Jalapeno Light	1 oz	70	3	4
Laughing Cow				
Assorted Wedge	1 (1 oz)	70	4	6
Cheesbits	6 pieces (1 oz)	70	4	6
Original Wedge	1 (1 oz)	70	4	6
Wedge Light	1 (1 oz)	50	2	3
Light N' Lively Singles American	1 oz	70	3	4
Light N' Lively Singles American White	1 oz	70	2	4
Light N' Lively Singles Sharp Cheddar	1 oz	70	2	4
Light N' Lively Singles Swiss	1 oz	70	2	3
Lunch Wagon Sandwich Slices	1 oz	90	1	7
Michael's Country Gourmet Spread				
French Onion	1 oz	48	—	5
Garden Vegetable	1 oz	48	—	5
Garlic & Herbs	1 oz	48	—	5
Mohawk Valley Limburger Cheese Spread	1 oz	70	3	6

FOOD	PORTION	CALS.	SAT. FAT	FAT
Nippy Cheese Food	1 oz	90	4	7
Old English Sharp American	1 oz	110	5	9
Old English Sharp Cheese Spread	1 oz	90	4	7
Price's				
Cheese & Bacon Spread	2 tbsp (1.1 oz)	90	3	7
Jalapeno Nacho Dip Hot	2 tbsp (1.1 oz)	80	3	7
Jalapeno Nacho Dip Mild	2 tbsp (1.1 oz)	80	3	7
Pimiento Cheese Spread	2 tbsp (1.1 oz)	80	3	7
Pimiento Cheese Spread Light	2 tbsp (1.1 oz)	60	1	4
Vegetable Garden	2 tbsp (1.1 oz)	70	2	5
Roka Blue Spread	1 oz	70	4	6
Rondele Soft Spreadable Garlic & Herbs	2 tbsp (1 oz)	100	6	9
Rondele Light Soft Spreadable Garlic & Herb Rondele	2 tbsp (0.9 oz)	60	3	4
Sargento				
American Hot Pepper	1 oz	106	—	9
American Sharp Spread	1 oz	106	—	9
American w/ Pimento	1 oz	106	—	9
Swiss	1 oz	95	—	7
Smart Beat American	1 slice (0.6 oz)	35	1	2
Smart Beat Low Sodium	1 slice (0.6 oz)	35	1	2
Smart Beat Sharp	1 slice (0.6 oz)	35	1	2
Spreadery				
Medium Cheddar	1 oz	70	2	4
Mild Mexican w/ Jalapeno Peppers	1 oz	70	3	4
Nacho	1 oz	70	2	4
Port Wine	1 oz	70	2	4
Sharp Cheddar	1 oz	70	2	4
Vermont White Cheddar	1 oz	70	2	4
Squeez-A-Snak Garlic	1 oz	80	4	7
Squeez-A-Snak Hickory Smoke	1 oz	80	4	7
Squeez-A-Snak Sharp	1 oz	80	4	7
Squeez-A-Snak w/Bacon	1 oz	90	4	7
Squeez-A-Snak w/ Jalapeno Pepper	1 oz	80	4	6
Velveeta				
Cheese Spread	1 oz	80	4	6

FOOD	PORTION	CALS.	SAT. FAT	FAT
Light Singles	1 oz	70	2	4
Mexican Hot	1 oz	80	3	6
Mexican Mild	1 oz	80	3	6
Pimento	1 oz	80	3	6
Shredded	1 oz	100	4	7
Shredded Hot Mexican w/ Jalapeno Peppers	1 oz	100	4	7
Shredded Mild Mexican w/ Jalapeno Peppers	1 oz	100	4	7
Slices	1 oz	90	4	6
Weight Watchers				
American Slices Low Sodium White	2 slices (0.66 oz)	35	1	1
American Slices Low Sodium Yellow	2 slices (0.66 oz)	35	1	1
American Slices White	2 slices (0.66 oz)	35	1	1
American Slices Yellow	2 slices (0.66 oz)	35	1	1
Port Wine Cup	1½ tbsp (1 oz)	70	2	3
Sharp Cheddar Slices	2 slices (0.66 oz)	35	1	1
Swiss Slices	2 slices (0.66 oz)	35	1	1
WisPride				
Chunk	1 oz	110	3	8
Garlic & Herb Cup	2 tbsp (1.1 oz)	100	4	7
Hickory Smoked Cup	2 tbsp (1.1 oz)	100	4	7
Port Wine Ball	2 tbsp (1.1 oz)	100	4	8
Port Wine Cup	2 tbsp (1.1 oz)	100	4	7
Port Wine Light Cup	2 tbsp (1.1 oz)	80	2	3
Sharp Ball	2 tbsp (1.1 oz)	100	4	8
Sharp Cup	2 tbsp (1.1 oz)	100	4	7
Sharp Light Cup	2 tbsp (1.1 oz)	80	2	3
Swiss Ball	2 tbsp (1.1 oz)	110	3	8
Sharp Cheddar Ball WisPride	2 tbsp (1.1 oz)	100	4	8
american	1 oz	93	4	7
american, cheese food	1 pkg (8 oz)	745	35	56
american, cheese food, cold pack	1 pkg (8 oz)	752	35	56
american, cheese spread	1 oz	82	4	6
american, cheese spread	1 jar (5 oz)	412	19	30
pimento	1 oz	106	6	9
swiss	1 oz	95	5	7
swiss, cheese food	1 pkg (8 oz)	734	—	55

FOOD	PORTION	CALS.	SAT. FAT	FAT

CHEESE DISHES

FROZEN

Mozzarella Cheese Nuggets (Banquet)	2.5 oz	230	—	12
Welsh Rarebit (Stouffer's)	¼ cup (1.1 oz)	120	4	9

HOME RECIPE

welsh rarebit, as prep w/ 1 white toast	1 slice	228	—	16

TAKE OUT

cheese omelette, as prep w/ 2 eggs	1 (6.8 oz)	519	—	44
fondue	½ cup	303	11	18
macaroni & cheese	6.3 oz	320	—	19

CHEESE SUBSTITUTES

Borden Taco-Mate	1 oz	100	2	7
Cheese Two	1 oz	90	1	7
Formagg				
American White	1 slice (0.66 oz)	60	1	4
American Yellow	1 slice (0.66 oz)	60	1	4
Caesar's Italian Garden American	1 oz	60	0	3
Cheddar	1 slice (0.66 oz)	60	tr	4
Cheddar Shredded	1 oz	60	0	3
Classic American	1 oz	60	0	3
Macaroni And Cheese Sauce	⅔ cup (5 oz)	190	0	2
Mozzarella Shredded	1 oz	60	0	3
Old World Mozzarella	1 oz	60	0	3
Parmesan Grated	2 tsp (5 g)	15	0	1
Swiss	1 oz	60	0	3
Swiss White	1 slice (0.66 oz)	60	1	4
Vintage Provolone Fromagg	1 oz	60	0	3
Zesty Jalapeno American	1 oz	60	0	3
Georgio's Imitation Cheddar Shredded	¼ cup (1 oz)	90	1	7
Georgio's Imitation Mozzarella Shredded	¼ cup (1 oz)	90	1	7
Golden Image American	1 oz	90	2	6
Golden Image Colby	1 oz	110	2	9
Golden Image Mild Cheddar	1 oz	100	2	9

FOOD	PORTION	CALS.	SAT. FAT	FAT
Sargento Imitation Cheddar	1 oz	85	—	6
Sargento Imitation Mozzarella	1 oz	80	—	6
White Wave				
Soy A Melt American Singles	1 slice (.75 oz)	60	1	4
Soy A Melt Cheddar	1 oz	80	1	5
Soy A Melt Cheddar Fat Free	1 oz	40	—	tr
Soy A Melt Garlic Herb	1 oz	80	1	5
Soy A Melt Jalapeno Jack	1 oz	80	1	5
Soy A Melt Monterey Jack	1 oz	80	1	5
Soy A Melt Mozzarella	1 oz	80	1	5
Soy A Melt Mozzarella Fat Free	1 oz	40	—	tr
Soy A Melt Mozzarella Singles	1 slice (.75 oz)	60	1	4
mozzarella	1 oz	70	1	3

CHERIMOYA

fresh	1	515	—	2

CHERRIES

CANNED

sour in heavy syrup	½ cup	232	tr	tr
sour in light syrup	½ cup	189	tr	tr
sour water packed	1 cup	87	tr	tr
sweet in heavy syrup	½ cup	107	tr	tr
sweet in light syrup	½ cup	85	tr	tr
sweet juice pack	½ cup	68	tr	tr
sweet water pack	½ cup	57	tr	tr

DRIED

Bing (Chukar)	2 oz	160	—	1
Rainer (Chukar)	2 oz	160	—	1
Tart (Chukar)	2 oz	170	0	0
Tart 'N Sweet (Chukar)	2 oz	180	0	0

FRESH

Dole	1 cup	90	—	1
sour	1 cup	51	tr	tr
sweet	10	49	tr	1

FOOD	PORTION	CALS.	SAT. FAT	FAT
FROZEN				
Dark Sweet (Big Valley)	¾ cup (4.9 oz)	90	0	0
sour unsweetened	1 cup	72	tr	1
sweet sweetened	1 cup	232	tr	tr
JUICE				
Hi-C	8 fl oz	130	0	0
Hi-C Box	8.45 fl oz	140	0	0
Juicy Juice Cherry	1 bottle (6 fl oz)	90	0	0
Juice Works Cherry	6 oz	100	—	0
Kool-Aid	8 oz	98	0	0
Kool-Aid Black Cherry	8 oz	98	0	0
Kool-Aid Sugar Free	8 oz	3	0	0
Kool-Aid Koolers	1 (8.45 oz)	142	0	0
Sipps Wild Cherry	8.45 oz	130	—	0
Smucker's Black Cherry Sparkler	10 oz	120	—	tr
Sucker's Black Cherry	8 oz	130	0	0
Tang Fruit Box	8.45 oz	121	0	0
Wylers Drink Mix Unsweetened Cherry	8 oz	2	—	0
Wylers Drink Mix Wild Cherry	8 oz	81	0	0
CHERVIL				
seed	1 tsp	1	—	tr
CHESTNUTS				
chinese, cooked	1 oz	44	tr	tr
chinese, dried	1 oz	103	tr	tr
chinese, raw	1 oz	64	tr	tr
chinese, roasted	1 oz	68	tr	tr
cooked	1 oz	37	tr	tr
dried, peeled	1 oz	105	tr	1
japanese, cooked	1 oz	16	tr	tr
japanese, dried	1 oz	102	tr	tr
japanese, raw	1 oz	44	tr	tr
japanese, roasted	1 oz	57	tr	tr
raw, peeled	1 oz	56	tr	tr
roasted	1 cup	350	1	3
roasted	1 oz	70	tr	1
CHEWING GUM				
Beech-Nut Cinnamon	1 piece	10	0	0
Beech-Nut Fruit	1 piece	10	0	0
Beech-Nut Peppermint	1 piece	10	0	0

FOOD	PORTION	CALS.	SAT. FAT	FAT
Beech-Nut Spearmint	1 piece	10	0	0
Big Red	1 stick	10	0	tr
Brock Bubble Gum	1 piece (0.2 oz)	20	0	0
Bubblicious Bubblicious	1 piece (7.9 g)	25	0	0
Bubble Yum Fruit Juice Variety	1 piece	20	0	0
Bubble Yum Luscious Lime	1 piece	25	0	0
Care*Free Sugarless All Flavors	1 piece	8	0	0
Care*Free Sugarless Bubble Gum All Flavors	1 piece	10	—	0
Chiclets	1 piece (1.59 g)	6	0	0
Chicklets Tiny Size	8 pieces (0.13 g)	tr	0	0
Clorets	1 piece (1.59 g)	6	0	0
Dentyne	1 piece (1.88 g)	6	0	0
Dentyne Cinn-A-Burst	1 piece (3.2 g)	9	0	0
Dentyne Sugar Free	1 piece (1.88 g)	5	0	0
Extra Sugar Free Cinnamon	1 piece	8	—	tr
Extra Sugar Free Spearmint & Peppermint	1 stick	8	—	tr
Extra Sugar Free Winter Fresh	1 piece	8	—	tr
Freedent Spearmint, Peppermint, & Cinnamon	1 stick	10	—	tr
Fresh-Up	1 piece (4.2 g)	13	0	0
Fruit Stripe	1 piece	8	0	0
Fruit Stripe Bubble Gum	1 piece	8	0	0
Fruit Stripe Variety Pack	1 piece	8	0	0
Hubba Bubba Bubble Gum Cola	1 piece	23	—	tr
Hubba Bubba Bubble Gum Sugarfree Original	1 piece	14	—	tr
Hubba Bubba Bubble Gum Sugarfree Grape	1 piece	13	—	tr
Hubba Bubba Original	1 piece	23	—	tr
Hubba Bubba Strawberry, Grape, Raspberry	1 piece	23	—	tr
Swell Bubble Gum	1 piece (3 g)	10	0	0
Trident	1 piece (1.88 g)	5	0	0
Trident Soft Bubble Gum	1 piece (3.3 g)	9	0	0
Wrigley's Doublemint	1 piece	10	—	tr

FOOD	PORTION	CALS.	SAT. FAT	FAT
Wrigley's Juicy Fruit	1 stick	10	—	tr
Wrigley's Spearmint	1 stick	10	—	tr

CHIA SEEDS

dried	1 oz	134	3	7

CHICKEN

(see also CHICKEN DISHES, CHICKEN SUBSTITUTES, DINNER, HOT DOG)

CANNED

FOOD	PORTION	CALS.	SAT. FAT	FAT
Chunk (Hormel)	2 oz	70	1	3
Chunk Breast (Hormel)	2 oz	60	1	2
Chunk Breast No Salt (Hormel)	2 oz	60	1	2
Chunk Style Mixin' Chicken (Swanson)	2.5 oz	130	—	8
Chunky (Underwood)	2.08 oz	150	3	9
Chunky Light Underwood	2.08 oz	80	1	2
Smoky Underwood	2.08 oz	150	2	8
White (Swanson)	2.5 oz	100	—	4
White & Dark (Swanson)	2.5 oz	100	—	4
chicken spread	1 tbsp	25	—	2
chicken spread	1 oz	55	—	3
chicken spread, barbeque flavored	1 oz	55	—	3
w/ broth	1 can (5 oz)	234	3	11
w/ broth	½ can (2.5 oz)	117	2	6

FRESH

FOOD	PORTION	CALS.	SAT. FAT	FAT
Breast (Tyson)	3 oz	116	—	2
Breast Oven Stuffer Roaster w/ skin, cooked (Perdue)	1 oz	42	1	2
Breast Quarters Fresh Young w/ skin, cooked (Perdue)	1 oz	48	1	3
Breast Skinless & Boneless Oven Stuffer Roaster, cooked (Perdue)	1 oz	31	tr	tr
Breast Skinless & Boneless, cooked (Perdue)	1 oz	30	tr	tr
Breast Split Fresh Young w/ skin, cooked (Perdue)	1 oz	45	1	3

FOOD	PORTION	CALS.	SAT. FAT	FAT
Breast Tender Skinless & Boneless, cooked (Perdue)	1 oz	29	tr	tr
Breast Thin-Sliced Skinless & Boneless Oven Stuffer, cooked (Perdue)	1 oz	31	tr	tr
Breast Whole Fresh Young w/ skin, cooked (Perdue)	1 oz	45	1	3
Cornish Hen (Tyson)	3.5 oz	250	—	15
Cornish Hen Dark Meat w/ skin, cooked (Perdue)	1 oz	43	1	3
Cornish Hen White Meat w/skin, cooked (Perdue)	1 oz	42	1	3
Drumstick (Tyson)	3 oz	131	—	4
Drumsticks Fresh Young w/ skin, cooked (Perdue)	1 oz	42	tr	2
Drumsticks Oven Stuffer, Roaster w/ skin, cooked (Perdue)	1 oz	41	tr	2
Ground Fresh Young, cooked (Perdue)	1 oz	49	1	3
Leg Quarters Fresh Young w/ skin, cooked (Perdue)	1 oz	49	1	4
Legs Fresh Young w/ skin, cooked (Perdue)	1 oz	51	2	4
Soup & Stew Baking Hen Dark Meat w/ skin, cooked (Perdue)	1 oz	41	1	3
Soup & Stew Baking Hen White Meat w/ skin, cooked (Perdue)	1 oz	41	1	2
Thigh (Tyson)	3 oz	152	—	7
Thighs Fresh Young w/ skin, cooked (Perdue)	1 oz	57	1	4
Thighs Skinless & Boneless, cooked (Perdue)	1 oz	30	tr	2
Thighs Skinless & Boneless Oven Stuffer Roaster, cooked (Perdue)	1 oz	34	1	2
Whole (Tyson)	3 oz	134	—	4

FOOD	PORTION	CALS.	SAT. FAT	FAT
Whole Fresh Young Dark Meat w/ skin, cooked (Perdue)	1 oz	47	1	3
Whole Fresh Young White Meat w/ skin, cooked (Perdue)	1 oz	43	tr	2
Whole Oven Stuffer Roaster Dark Meat w/ skin, cooked (Perdue)	1 oz	49	1	3
Whole Oven Stuffer Roaster White Meat w/ skin, cooked (Perdue	1 oz	44	tr	2
Wing (Tyson)	3 oz	147	—	6
Wing Drumettes Fresh Young w/ skin, cooked (Perdue)	1 oz	50	1	3
Wingettes Oven Stuffer Roaster w/ skin, cooked (Perdue)	1 oz	52	1	3
Wings Fresh Young w/ skin, cooked (Perdue)	1 oz	54	1	4
broiler/fryer				
back w/ skin, batter dipped, fried	½ back (2.5 oz)	238	4	16
back w/ skin, floured, fried	1.5 oz	146	2	9
back w/ skin, roasted	1 oz	96	2	7
back w/ skin, stewed	½ back (2.1 oz)	158	3	11
back w/o skin, fried	½ back (2 oz)	167	2	9
breast w/ skin, batter dipped, fried	½ breast (4.9 oz)	364	5	18
breast w/ skin, batter dipped, fried	2.9 oz	218	3	11
breast w/ skin, roasted	2 oz	115	1	5
breast w/ skin, roasted	½ breast (3.4 oz)	193	2	8
breast w/ skin, stewed	½ breast (3.9 oz)	202	2	8
breast w/o skin, fried	½ breast (3 oz)	161	1	4
breast w/o skin, roasted	½ breast (3 oz)	142	1	3
breast w/o skin, stewed	2 oz	86	tr	2
dark meat w/ skin, batter dipped, fried	5.9 oz	497	8	31
dark meat w/ skin, floured, fried	3.9 oz	313	5	19
dark meat w/ skin, roasted	3.5 oz	256	4	16

FOOD	PORTION	CALS.	SAT. FAT	FAT
dark meat w/ skin, stewed	3.9 oz	256	4	16
dark meat w/o skin, fried	1 cup (5 oz)	334	4	16
dark meat w/o skin, roasted	1 cup (5 oz)	286	4	14
dark meat w/o skin, stewed	3 oz	165	2	8
dark meat w/o skin, stewed	1 cup (5 oz)	269	3	13
drumstick w/ skin, batter dipped, fried	1 (2.6 oz)	193	3	11
drumstick w/ skin, floured, fried	1 (1.7 oz)	120	2	7
drumstick w/ skin, roasted	1 (1.8 oz)	112	2	6
drumstick w/ skin, stewed	1 (2 oz)	116	2	6
drumstick w/o skin, fried	1 (1.5 oz)	82	1	3
drumstick w/o skin, roasted	1 (1.5 oz)	76	1	2
drumstick w/o skin, stewed	1 (1.6oz)	78	1	3
leg w/ skin, batter dipped, fried	1 (5.5 oz)	431	7	26
leg w/ skin, floured, fried	1 (3.9 oz)	285	4	16
leg w/ skin, roasted	1 (4 oz)	265	4	15
leg w/ skin, stewed	1 (4.4 oz)	275	4	16
leg w/o skin, fried	1 (3.3 oz)	195	2	9
leg w/o skin, roasted	1 (3.3 oz)	182	2	8
leg w/o skin, stewed	1 (3.5 oz)	187	2	8
light meat w/ skin, batter dipped, fried	4 oz	312	5	17
light meat w/ skin, floured, fried	2.7 oz	192	3	9
light meat w/ skin, roasted	2.8 oz	175	2	9
light meat w/ skin, stewed	3.2 oz	181	3	9
light meat w/o skin, fried	1 cup (5 oz)	268	2	8
light meat w/o skin, roasted	1 oup (5 oz)	242	2	6

FOOD	PORTION	CALS.	SAT. FAT	FAT
broiler/fryer *(cont.)*				
light meat w/o skin, stewed	1 cup (5 oz)	223	2	6
neck w/ skin, stewed	1 (1.3 oz)	94	2	7
neck w/o skin, stewed	1 (.6 oz)	32	tr	1
skin, batter dipped, fried	4 oz	449	9	33
skin, batter dipped & fried	from ½ chicken (6.7 oz)	748	14	55
skin, floured, fried	from ½ chicken (2 oz)	281	7	24
skin, floured, fried	1 oz	166	4	14
skin, roasted	from ½ chicken (2 oz)	254	6	23
skin, stewed	2.5 oz	261	7	24
thigh w/ skin, batter dipped, fried	1 (3 oz)	238	4	14
thigh w/ skin, floured, fried	1 (2.2 oz)	162	3	9
thigh w/ skin, roasted	1 (2.2 oz)	153	3	10
thigh w/ skin, stewed	1 (2.4 oz)	158	3	10
thigh w/o skin, fried	1 (1.8 oz)	113	1	5
thigh w/o skin, roasted	1 (1.8 oz)	109	2	6
thigh w/o skin, stewed	1 (1.9 oz)	107	1	5
w/ skin, floured & fried	½ breast (3.4 oz)	218	2	9
w/ skin, floured fried	½ chicken (11 oz)	844	13	47
w/ skin, fried	½ chicken (16.4)	1347	22	81
w/ skin, neck & giblets, batter dipped & fried	1 chicken (2.3 lbs)	2987	48	180
w/ skin, neck & giblets, roasted	1 chicken (1.5 lbs)	1598	25	90
w/ skin, neck & giblets, stewed	1 chicken (1.6 lbs)	1625	26	93
w/ skin, roasted	½ chicken (10.5 oz)	715	11	41
w/ skin, stewed	½ chicken (11. 7 oz)	730	12	42
w/o skin, roasted	1 cup (5 oz)	266	3	10
w/o skin, fried	1 cup	307	3	13
w/o skin, stewed	1 cup (5 oz)	248	3	9
w/o skin, stewed	1 oz	54	1	3
wing w/ skin, batter dipped, fried	1 (1.7 oz)	159	3	11
wing w/ skin, floured, fried	1 (1.1 oz)	103	2	7

FOOD	PORTION	CALS.	SAT. FAT	FAT
wing w/ skin, roasted	1 (1.2 oz)	99	2	7
wing w/ skin, stewed	1 (1.4 oz)	100	2	7
capon w/ skin, neck & giblets, roasted	1 chicken (3.1 lbs)	3211	46	165
roaster dark meat w/o skin, roasted	1 cup (5 oz)	250	3	12
roaster light meat w/o skin, roasted	1 cup (5 oz)	214	2	6
roaster w/ skin, roasted	½ chicken (1.1 lbs)	1071	18	64
roaster w/ skin, neck & giblets, roasted	1 chicken (2.4 lbs)	2363	39	140
roaster w/o skin, roasted	1 cup (5 oz)	469	3	28
stewing dark meat w/o skin, stewed	1 cup (5 oz)	361	6	21
stewing w/ skin, stewed	½ chicken (9.2 oz)	744	13	49
stewing w/ skin, stewed	6.2 oz	507	9	34
stewing w/ skin, neck & giblets, stewed	1 chicken (1.3 lbs)	1636	29	107
FROZEN				
Tyson				
Breast Tenders Skinless	3.5 oz	120	—	1
Breasts Boneless	3.5 oz	210	—	12
Breasts Boneless Skinless	3.5 oz	130	—	2
Drums & Thighs	3.5 oz	270	—	17
Thighs Boneless Skinless	3.5 oz	200	—	10
FROZEN PREPARED				
Banquet				
Fried Chicken Breast Portions	5.75 oz	220	—	11
Fried Chicken Thighs & Drumsticks	6.25 oz	250	—	14
Hot'n Spicy Fried Chicken	6.4 oz	330	—	19
Hot'n Spicy Snack'n Chicken	3.75 oz	140	—	9
Original Fried Chicken	5.6 oz	290	—	17
Southern Fried Chicken	5.6 oz	290	—	17
Boneless Breast Tenders	2.25 oz	150	—	6
Boneless Chicken Nuggets	2.5 oz	200	—	13

FOOD	PORTION	CALS.	SAT. FAT	FAT
Banquet *(cont.)*				
Boneless Chicken Nuggets w/ Cheddar	2.5 oz	240	—	17
Boneless Chicken Patties	2.5 oz	190	—	12
Boneless Chicken Sticks	2.5 oz	210	—	14
Boneless Drum-Snackers	2.5 oz	210	—	14
Boneless Fried Breast Tenders	2.25 oz	160	—	7
Boneless Southern Fried Chicken Nuggets	2.5 oz	210	—	14
Boneless Southern Fried Chicken Patties	2.5 oz	200	—	12
Hot'n Spicy Chicken Nuggets	2.5 oz	240	—	18
Country Skillet				
Chicken Chunks	3 oz	260	—	16
Chicken Nuggets	3 oz	250	—	15
Chicken Patties	3 oz	230	—	15
Southern Fried Chicken Chunks	3 oz	270	—	18
Southern Fried Chicken Patties	3 oz	240	—	15
Empire Nuggets	5 (3 oz)	180	2	9
Empire Stix	4 (3.1 oz)	180	2	9
Healthy Balance				
Baked Boneless Breast Nuggets	2.25 oz	120	—	4
Baked Boneless Breast Patties	2.25 oz	120	—	4
Baked Boneless Breast Tenders	2.25 oz	120	—	4
Swanson				
Chicken Nibbles	3.25 oz	300	—	19
Chicken Nuggets	3 oz	230	—	14
Fried Chicken Breast Portion	4.5 oz	360	—	20
Pre-fried Chicken Parts	3.25 oz	270	—	16
Thighs & Drumsticks	3.25 oz	290	—	18
Tyson				
BBQ Breast Fillets	3 oz	110	—	2
Breaded Patties	3 oz	300	—	20
Breast Chunks	3 oz	240	—	17
Breast Fillets	3 oz	190	—	9

FOOD	PORTION	CALS.	SAT. FAT	FAT
Breast Patties	2.6 oz	220	—	15
Breast Tenders	3 oz	220	—	12
Chick'n Cheddar	2.6 oz	220	—	15
Chick'n Chunks	2.6 oz	220	—	15
Cordon Bleu Mini	1	90	—	4
Diced	3 oz	130	—	3
Grilled Sandwich	3.5 oz	200	—	5
Hors D'Oeuvres Mesquite Chunks	3.5 oz	100	—	1
Hot BBQ Breast Tenders	2.75 oz	110	—	3
Mesquite Breast Fillets	2.75 oz	100	—	2
Mesquite Breast Strips	2.75 oz	100	—	2
Mesquite Breast Tenders	2.75 oz	110	—	2
Microwave Breast Sandwich	4.25 oz	328	—	14
Microwave Chunks	3.5 oz	220	—	15
Microwave Tenders	3.5 oz	230	—	11
Microwave Chunks BBQ Sandwich	4 oz	230	—	6
Roasted Breasts	1 oz	50	—	3
Roasted Breast Fillets	1 oz	50	—	2
Roasted Half Chicken	1 oz	60	—	4
Roasted Thighs	1 oz	70	—	5
Roasted Whole Chicken	1 oz	60	—	4
Southern Fried Breast Fillets	3 oz	220	—	11
Southern Fried Breast Patties	2.6 oz	220	—	15
Southern Fried Chick'n Chunks	2.6 oz	220	—	15
Thick & Crispy Patties	2.6 oz	220	—	14
Weaver				
Batter Dipped Breast	4.4 oz	310	—	20
Batter Dipped Thighs/ Drums	3 oz	210	—	14
Batter Dipped Wings	4 oz	400	—	28
Breast Fillets	4.5 oz	270	—	13
Breast Fillets Strips	3.3 oz	200	—	10
Breast Patties	3 oz	205	—	11
Chicken Nuggets	2.6 oz	190	—	12
Crispy Dutch Frye Assorted	3.6 oz	290	—	18
Crispy Dutch Frye Breasts	4.5 oz	350	—	22

FOOD	PORTION	CALS.	SAT. FAT	FAT
Weaver *(cont.)*				
Crispy Dutch Frye Thighs/Drums	3.5 oz	290	—	19
Crispy Dutch Frye Wings	4 oz	400	—	28
Crispy Light Skinless	2.9 oz	170	—	9
Croquettes	2 pieces	280	—	16
Croquettes With Gravy	2 pieces + ½ cup gravy	282	—	18
Honey Batter Tenders	3 oz	220	—	12
Hot Wings	2.7 oz	170	—	11
Mini Drums Crispy	3 oz	210	—	12
Mini Drums Herbs & Spice	3 oz	200	—	11
Premium Tenders	3 oz	170	—	9
Roasted Drumsticks	1 oz	50	—	3
Rondelets Cheese	1 (2.6 oz)	190	—	11
Rondelets Italian	1 (2.6 oz)	190	—	11
Rondelets Original	1 (3 oz)	190	—	10
Weight Watchers Chicken Nuggets	5.9 oz	220	2	7
READY-TO-USE				
Carl Buddig	1 oz	50	2	3
Chicken By George				
Cajun	1 breast (4 oz)	120	1	4
Caribbean Grill	1 breast (4 oz)	150	1	4
Garlic & Herb	1 breast (4 oz)	120	1	3
Italian Bleu Cheese	1 breast (4 oz)	130	1	5
Lemon Herb	1 breast (4 oz)	120	1	3
Lemon Oregano	1 breast (4 oz)	130	1	4
Mesquite Barbecue	1 breast (4 oz)	120	5	2
Mustard Dill	1 breast (4 oz)	140	1	5
Roasted	1 breast (4 oz)	110	1	3
Teriyaki	1 breast (4 oz)	130	1	3
Tomato Herb With Basil	1 breast (4 oz)	140	1	5
Dutch Family Roll	1 oz	61	—	15
Empire				
Bologna	3 slices (1.8 oz)	200	2	7
Breast Battered & Breaded Fried	3 oz	170	2	8
Cutlets Battered & Breaded	1 (3.3 oz)	200	2	9
Drum & Thigh Fried	3 oz	240	4	16
Nuggets Battered & Breaded	5 (3 oz)	200	3	13

FOOD	PORTION	CALS.	SAT. FAT	FAT
Whole Barbecue	5 oz	280	5	17
Falls BBQ	3 oz	150	—	8
Healthy Choice Breast Oven Roasted	1.9 oz	60	1	2
Hebrew National Deli Thin Oven Roasted	1.8 oz	45	—	1
Hillshire				
Deli Select Breast Oven Roasted	1 slice	10	—	tr
Deli Select Breast Smoked	1 slice	10	—	tr
Flavor Pack 90–99% Fat Free Breast Smoked	1 slice (0.75 oz)	20	—	tr
Lunch 'N Munch Smoked Chicken/ Monterey Jack	1 pkg (4.5 oz)	350	—	20
Lunch 'N Munch Smoked Chicken/ Monterey Snickers	1 pkg (4.25 oz)	400	—	23
Longacre Roll	1 oz	65	—	17
Louis Rich				
Deluxe Oven Roasted Breast	1 slice (1 oz)	40	0	1
Hickory Smoked Breast	1 slice (1 oz)	30	0	1
Oven Roasted Breast	4 slices (1.8 oz)	60	1	2
White Oven Roasted	1 slice (1 oz)	40	1	3
Mr. Turkey Breast	1 slice (1 oz)	32	—	1
Oscar Mayer				
Deli-Thin Breast Honey Glazed	4 slices (1.8 oz)	60	0	1
Healthy Favorites Breast Oven Roasted	4 slices (1.8 oz)	40	0	0
Lunchables Chicken/ Monterey Jack	1 pkg (4.5 oz)	350	10	21
Lunchables Deluxe Chicken/Turkey	1 pkg (5.1 oz)	380	11	22
Lunchables Dessert Choc. Pudding/ Chicken/Jack	1 pkg (6.2 oz)	370	9	18
Smoked Breast	1 slice (1 oz)	25	tr	tr
Perdue Done It!				
BBQ Breast Half	1 oz	46	1	2
BBQ Drumsticks	1 oz	53	tr	2
BBQ Half Dark Meat	1 oz	57	1	4
BBQ Half White Meat	1 oz	40	tr	1

FOOD	PORTION	CALS.	SAT. FAT	FAT
Perdue Done It! *(cont.)*				
BBQ Thighs	1 oz	59	1	3
BBQ Wings	1 oz	62	3	4
Breast Roasted	1 oz	45	1	2
Cornish Hen Roasted Dark Meat	1 oz	45	1	3
Cornish Hen Roasted White Meat	1 oz	39	tr	1
Cutlets	3.5 oz	250	3	14
Drumsticks Roasted	1 oz	40	tr	1
Nuggets Cheese	1 (.67 oz)	54	1	4
Nuggets Fun Shaped	1 (.73 oz)	54	1	3
Nuggets Original	1 (.67 oz)	48	1	3
Tenders	1 oz	62	1	3
Thighs Roasted	1 oz	46	tr	2
Whole or Half Roasted Dark Meat	1 oz	51	1	3
Whole or Half Roasted White Meat	1 oz	37	tr	1
Wings Garlic & Herb	1 oz	61	1	4
Wings Hot & Spicy	1 oz	60	1	4
Tyson				
Bologna	1 slice	44	—	1
Breast Hickory Smoked	1 slice	25	—	1
Breast Honey Flavored	1 slice	25	—	1
Breast Oven Roasted	1 slice	25	—	1
Breast Oven Roasted Mesquite	1 slice	25	—	1
Roll	1 slice	26	—	1
Tyson Wings				
Barbecue	6–7 (3.5 oz)	218	—	14
Hot & Spicy	6–7 (3.5 oz)	218	—	14
Roasted	6–7 (3.5 oz)	218	—	14
Teriyaki	6–7 (3.5 oz)	218	—	14
Wampler Longacre				
Breast Deli Sliced Browned Roasted	1 oz	49	—	11
Breast Meat	1 oz	38	—	2
Breast Stuffed w/ Breading	8 oz	472	—	94
Breast Stuffed w/ Cordon Blue	6.5 oz	429	—	39
Diced Breast	1 oz	38	—	2
Roll Diced Breast	1 oz	49	—	11
Roll Sliced	1 oz	63	—	16

FOOD	PORTION	CALS.	SAT. FAT	FAT
Weaver Roasted Wings	1 oz	70	—	5
Weight Watchers				
Roasted & Smoked Breast	2 slices (.75 oz)	25	—	1
chicken roll light meat	1 pkg (6 oz)	271	3	13
chicken roll light meat	2 oz	90	1	4
poultry salad sandwich spread	1 tbsp	109	tr	2
poultry salad sandwich spread	1 oz	238	1	4
TAKE-OUT				
boneless, breaded & fried w/ barbecue sauce	6 pieces (4.6 oz)	330	6	18
boneless, breaded & fried w/ honey	6 pieces (4 oz)	339	5	18
boneless, breaded & fried w/ mustard sauce	6 pieces (4.6 oz)	323	6	17
boneless, breaded & fried w/ sweet & sour sauce	6 pieces (4.6 oz)	346	6	18
breast & wing, breaded & fried	2 pieces (5.7 oz)	494	8	30
drumstick, breaded & fried	2 pieces (5.2 oz)	430	7	27
thigh, breaded & fried	2 pieces (5.2 oz)	430	7	27

CHICKEN DISHES
(see also CHICKEN SUBSTITUTES, DINNER)

FOOD	PORTION	CALS.	SAT. FAT	FAT
CANNED				
American Classics Chicken & Noodles (Dinty Moore)	1 bowl (10 oz)	260	4	8
American Classics Chicken With Mashed Potatoes (Dinty Moore)	1 bowl (10 oz)	220	2	4
Chicken Cacciatore (Top Shelf)	1 bowl (10 oz)	210	1	3
Chicken & Dumplings (Swanson)	7½ oz	220	—	11
Chicken Acapulco Fiesta Chicken (Top Shelf)	1 bowl (10 oz)	420	8	16
Chicken Ala King (Swanson)	5¼ oz	190	—	12
Chicken Ala King (Top Shelf)	1 bowl (10 oz)	380	5	12
Chicken Stew (Swanson)	7⅝ oz	160	—	7

FOOD	PORTION	CALS.	SAT. FAT	FAT
Glazed Breast of Chicken (Top Shelf)	1 bowl (10 oz)	200	2	5
Microwave Cup Chicken & Dumpling (Dinty Moore)	1 cup (7.5 oz)	190	2	6
Microwave Cup Chicken Stew (Dinty Moore)	1 cup (7.5 oz)	180	2	8
Stew (Dinty Moore)	1 cup (8.5 oz)	220	3	11
FROZEN				
Kibun Chicken Pasta Salad w/ dressing	½ pkg	220	—	9
Kibun Chicken Pasta Salad w/o dressing	½ pkg	150	—	2
MicroMagic Chicken Sandwich	1 pkg (4.5 oz)	390	—	16
Ovenstuffs Chicken Turnover	1 (4.75 oz)	350	—	16
Weight Watchers Chicken & Broccoli Pita	1 (5.4 oz)	190	1	5
Weight Watchers Grilled Chicken Sandwich	1 (4 oz)	210	2	6
HOME RECIPE				
chicken & noodles	1 cup	365	5	18
chicken a la king	1 cup	470	13	34
MIX				
Lipton Microeasy Barbeque Chicken	¼ pkg	108	—	1
Lipton Microeasy Country Chicken	¼ pkg	78	—	1
Skillet Chicken Helper				
Cheesy Broccoli, as prep	⅕ pkg (7.5 oz)	270	—	6
Creamy Chicken, as prep	⅕ pkg (8.25 oz)	290	—	10
Creamy Mushroom, as prep	⅕ pkg (8 oz)	280	—	8
Fettucine Alfredo, as prep	⅕ pkg (7.5 oz)	270	—	8
Stir-Fried Chicken, as prep	⅕ pkg (7 oz)	330	—	11
READY-TO-USE				
Salad (Wampler Longacre)	1 oz	65	—	16
The Spreadables Chicken Salad	¼ can	100	—	6

FOOD	PORTION	CALS.	SAT. FAT	FAT
TAKE-OUT				
chicken & dumplings	¾ cup	256	4	12
chicken cacciatore	¾ cup	394	6	24
chicken paprikash	1½ cup	296	—	10
chicken pie w/ top crust	1 slice (5.6 oz)	472	—	31
fillet sandwich plain	1	515	9	29
fillet sandwich w/ cheese, mayonnaise, tomato, lettuce	1	632	12	39

CHICKEN SUBSTITUTES

FOOD	PORTION	CALS.	SAT. FAT	FAT
Harvest Direct TVP Poultry Chunks	3.5 oz	280	tr	1
Harvest Direct TVP Poultry Ground	3.5 oz	280	tr	1
Jaclyn's Salsa Chicken Style Dinner	11.5 oz	325	—	9
Jaclyn's Sesame Chicken Style Dinner	11.5 oz	345	—	8
Knox Mountain Farm Chick'N Wheat Mix	1 serv (⅛ pkg)	110	—	1
LaLoma				
Chicken Supreme, not prep	¼ cup (16 g)	50	0	0
Chik Nuggets	5 nuggets (85 g)	270	—	20
Fried Chicken	1 piece (57 g)	180	—	14
Fried Chicken w/ Gravy	2 pieces (85 g)	140	—	10
White Wave Meatless Sandwich Slices	2 slices (1.6 oz)	80	0	0
Worthington				
Chick-ketts	½ cup (84 g)	160	—	7
ChickStiks	1 (47 g)	110	—	7
Chicken Sliced	2 slices (57 g)	130	—	9
CrispyChik	1 patty (71 g)	220	—	15
CrispyChik	6 nuggets (85 g)	280	—	19
Cutlets	1.5 slices (92 g)	100	—	2
Diced Chik	¼ cup (60 g)	90	—	8
FriChik	2 pieces (90 g)	180	—	13
Golden Croquettes	5 pieces (106 g)	280	—	14
Savory Slices	2 slices (60 g)	90	—	8
Vegetarian Chicken Pie	1 (227 g)	380	—	20

CHICKPEAS
CANNED

FOOD	PORTION	CALS.	SAT. FAT	FAT
Allen Garbanzo	½ cup (4.4 oz)	120	1	3

FOOD	PORTION	CALS.	SAT. FAT	FAT
East Texas Fair Garbanzo	½ cup (4.4 oz)	120	1	3
Goya Spanish Style	7.5 oz	150	—	2
Green Giant Garbanzo	½ cup	90	—	2
Hanover	½ cup	100	—	1
Old El Paso Garbanzo	½ cup	190	—	tr
Progresso	½ cup	110	—	1
S&W Garbanzo Lite 50% Less Salt	½ cup	110	0	0
S&W Garbanzo Premium Large	½ cup	110	—	1
S&W Garbanzo Water Pack	½ cup	105	—	1
chickpeas	1 cup	285	tr	3
DRIED				
Bean Cuisine. Garbanzo	½ cup	115	—	1
cooked	1 cup	269	tr	4
REFRIGERATED				
Cedar's Hommus Tahini No Salt Added	2 tbsp (1 oz)	50	0	2

CHICORY
FRESH

FOOD	PORTION	CALS.	SAT. FAT	FAT
greens, raw, chopped	½ cup	21	tr	tr
roots, raw	1 (2.1 oz)	44	tr	tr
roots, raw, cut up	½ cup (1.6 oz)	33	tr	tr
witloof head, raw	1 (1.9 oz)	9	tr	tr
witloof, raw	½ cup	7	tr	tr

CHILI
CANNED

FOOD	PORTION	CALS.	SAT. FAT	FAT
Allen Mexican Chili Beans	½ cup (4.5 oz)	120	0	1
Brown Beauty Mexican Chili Beans	½ cup (4.5 oz)	120	0	1
Chi-Chi's San Antonio	1 cup (8.5 oz)	240	1	19
Dennison's				
Chili Beans in Chili Gravy	7.5 oz	180	—	1
Chili Con Carne w/ Beans	7.5 oz	310	—	15
Chili Con Carne w/o Beans	7.5 oz	300	—	19
Cook-Off Chili w/ Beans	7.5 oz	340	—	19
Chunky Chili w/ Beans	7.5 oz	310	—	14
Hot Chili Con Carne w/ Beans	7.5 oz	310	—	16
Gebhardt Hot w/ Beans	1 cup	470	10	27

FOOD	PORTION	CALS.	SAT. FAT	FAT
Gebhardt Plain	1 cup	530	16	43
Gebhardt w/ Beans	1 cup	495	10	28
Hain				
Spicy Tempeh	7.5 oz	160	—	4
Spicy Vegetarian	7.5 oz	160	—	1
Spicy Vegetarian Reduced Sodium	7.5 oz	170	—	1
Spicy With Chicken	7.5 oz	130	—	2
Health Valley				
Mild Vegetarian w/ Beans	5 oz	160	—	3
Mild Vegetarian w/ Beans No Salt Added	5 oz	160	—	3
Mild Vegetarian w/ Lentils	5 oz	140	—	4
Mild Vegetarian w/ Lentils No Salt Added	5 oz	140	—	4
Spicy Vegetarian w/ Beans	5 oz	160	—	4
Hormel				
Chili Mac	1 can (7.5 oz)	200	4	9
Chili No Beans	1 cup (8.3 oz)	410	13	30
Chili With Beans	1 cup (8.7 oz)	340	7	17
Chunky Chili With Beans	1 cup (8.7 oz)	330	6	16
Hot Chili No Beans	1 cup (8.3 oz)	410	13	30
Hot Chili With Beans	1 cup (8.7 oz)	340	7	17
Hot With Beans	1 can (7.5 oz)	250	5	11
Micro Cup Meals Chili Mac	1 cup (7.5 oz)	200	4	9
Micro Cup Meals Chili No Beans	1 cup (7.5 oz)	290	8	17
Micro Cup Meals Chili With Beans	1 cup (10.4 oz)	410	7	17
Micro Cup Meals Chili With Beans	1 cup (7.5 oz)	250	5	11
Micro Cup Meals Hot Chili With Beans	1 cup (7.5 oz)	250	5	11
No Beans	1 can (7.5 oz)	390	14	30
Turkey Chili With Beans	1 cup (8.7 oz)	220	1	3
Turkey Chili No Beans	1 cup (8.3 oz)	190	1	3
With Beans	1 can (7.5 oz)	250	5	11
Hunt's Chili Beans	4 oz	100	—	tr
Just Rite Hot w/ Beans	4 oz	195	4	10
Just Rite w/ Beans	4 oz	200	4	11

FOOD	PORTION	CALS.	SAT. FAT	FAT
Just Rite w/o Beans	4 oz	180	4	11
Luck's Hot Chili Beans	7.5 oz	200	—	2
Manwich Chili Fixin's, as prep	8 oz	290	5	14
Natural Touch Vegetarian	⅔ cup (190 g)	230	—	12
Old El Paso Chili Con Carne	1 cup	162	—	7
Old El Paso Chili With Beans	1 cup	217	—	10
S&W Chili Beans	½ cup	130	—	1
S&W Chili Makin's Original	½ cup	100	—	1
Van Camp's Chili Beanee Weenee	1 can (8 oz)	240	3	12
Van Camp's Chili w/ Beans	1 cup (8.9 oz)	350	8	21
Wolf Brand Chili-Mac	7.5 oz	317	—	20
Wolf Brand Extra Spicy w/ Beans	7.5 oz	324	—	21
Wolf Brand Extra Spicy w/o Beans	7.5 oz	363	—	25
Wolf Brand Plain	7.5 oz	330	—	22
Wolf Brand w/ Beans	7.5 oz	345	—	22
Wolf Brand w/o Beans	1 cup	387	—	27
Worthington	⅔ cup (141 g)	190	—	10
chili w/ beans	1 cup	286	6	14
DRIED				
powder	1 tsp	8	—	tr
DRY MIX				
Gebhardt Chili Powder	1 tsp	15	—	tr
Gebhardt Chili Quik Seasoning	1 tsp	10	—	tr
Hain Hot	¼ pkg	30	—	1
Hain Medium	¼ pkg	30	—	1
Hain Mild	¼ pkg	30	—	1
Nile Spice Chili'n Beans Original	1 pkg	150	0	2
Nile Spice Chili'n Beans Spicy	1 pkg	150	0	2
Old El Paso Seasoning Mix	⅛ pkg	21	—	1
FROZEN				
Lean Cuisine Three Bean	1 pkg (9 oz)	210	2	6
Lightlife	4.3 oz	110	tr	3
Stouffer's With Beans	1 pkg (8.75 oz)	270	4	10
Swanson Homestyle Chili Con Carne	8¼ oz	270	—	10

FOOD	PORTION	CALS.	SAT. FAT	FAT
Tyson Chicken Chili	3.5 oz	105	—	3
TAKE-OUT				
con carne w/ beans	8.9 oz	254	3	8

CHINESE CABBAGE
(see CABBAGE)

CHINESE FOOD
(see ORIENTAL FOOD)

CHINESE PRESERVING MELON
cooked	½ cup	11	tr	tr

CHIPS
(see also POPCORN, PRETZELS, SNACKS)

FOOD	PORTION	CALS.	SAT. FAT	FAT
CORN				
Fritos	34 pieces (1 oz)	150	—	10
Chili Cheese	34 pieces (1 oz)	160	—	10
Crisp 'N Thin	18 pieces (1 oz)	160	—	10
Dip Size	13 pieces (1 oz)	150	—	10
Non-Stop Nacho Cheese	34 pieces (1 oz)	150	—	9
Rowdy Rustlers Bar-B-Q	34 pieces (1 oz)	150	—	9
Wild 'N Mild	32 pieces (1 oz)	160	—	9
Health Valley	1 oz	160	—	11
Health Valley No Salt Added	1 oz	160	—	11
Health Valley w/ Cheddar Cheese	1 oz	160	—	10
Lance	1 pkg (50 g)	270	4	17
Lance BBQ	1 pkg (50 g)	260	3	16
Snyder's	1 oz	160	—	11
Snyder's BBQ	1 oz	160	—	11
Weight Watchers Corn Snacker	½ oz	60	—	2
Weight Watchers Corn Snackers Nacho Cheese	½ oz	60	—	2
Wise				
Corn Crunchies	1 oz	160	—	10
Crispy Corn Chips	1 oz	160	—	10
Crispy Corn Chips Nacho Cheese	1 oz	160	—	10
MULTIGRAIN				
Sunchips	12 pieces (1 oz)	150	—	8
Sunchips French Onion	12 pieces (1 oz)	140	—	7

FOOD	PORTION	CALS.	SAT. FAT	FAT
POTATO				
Barrel O' Fun	1 oz	150	2	9
Barrel O' Fun Barbeque	1 oz	145	2	9
Barrel O' Fun Sour Cream & Onion	1 oz	150	2	9
Butterfield Sticks	1 pkg (1.7 oz)	250	5	15
Butterfield Sticks	⅔ cup (1 oz)	150	3	9
Cape Cod	19 chips (1 oz)	150	2	8
Cottage Fries No Salt Added	1 oz	160	—	11
Eagle				
BBQ Thins	1 oz	150	—	10
Ranch Ridged	1 oz	160	—	10
Ridged	1 oz	150	—	10
Sour Cream & Onion	1 oz	150	—	10
Thins	1 oz	150	—	10
Eagle Kettle Fry				
BBQ Crunchy	1 oz	150	—	8
Cape Cod	1 oz	150	—	8
Cape Cod No Salt	1 oz	150	—	8
Cape Cod Waves	1 oz	150	—	8
Cape Cod Waves No Salt	1 oz	150	—	8
Dill & Sour Cream	1 oz	150	—	8
Dill & Sour Cream No Salt	1 oz	150	—	8
Extra Crunchy	1 oz	150	—	8
Idaho Russet	1 oz	150	—	8
Louisiana BBQ	1 oz	150	—	8
Health Valley				
Country Ripple	1 oz	160	—	10
Country Ripple No Salt Added	1 oz	160	—	10
Dip Chips	1 oz	160	—	10
Dip Chips No Salt Added	1 oz	160	—	10
Natural	1 oz	160	—	10
Natural No Salt Added	1 oz	160	—	10
Kelly's				
Bar-B-Q	1 oz	150	1	9
Crunchy	1 oz	150	1	9
Rippled	1 oz	150	1	9
Sour Cream n' Onion	1 oz	150	1	9
Unsalted	1 oz	150	1	10

FOOD	PORTION	CALS.	SAT. FAT	FAT
Lance				
BBQ	1 pkg (1⅛ oz)	190	3	12
Cajun Style	1 pkg (1 oz)	160	2	10
Hot Fries	1 pk (28 g)	160	2	10
Ripple	1 pkg (32 g)	190	4	15
Sour Cream & Onion	1 pkg (1⅛ oz)	190	3	12
Lay's	17 pieces (1 oz)	150	—	10
Bar-B-Q	17 pieces (1 oz)	150	—	9
Cheddar Cheese	17 pieces (1 oz)	150	—	10
Crunch Tators	16 pieces (1 oz)	150	—	8
Crunch Tators Amazin' Cajun	16 pieces (1 oz)	150	—	8
Crunch Tators Hoppin' Jalapeno	16 pieces (1 oz)	140	—	7
Crunch Tators Mighty Mesquite	16 pieces (1 oz)	150	—	8
Crunch Tators Supreme Sour Cream	16 pieces (1 oz)	150	—	8
Flamin' Hot	17 pieces (1 oz)	150	—	9
Kansas City Style Bar-B-Q	17 pieces (1 oz)	150	—	9
Salt & Vinegar	17 pieces (1 oz)	150	—	10
Sour Cream & Onion	17 pieces (1 oz)	160	—	10
Tangy Ranch	17 pieces (1 oz)	160	—	10
Unsalted	17 pieces (1 oz)	150	—	10
Louise's				
Fat-Free	30 chips (1 oz)	110	0	0
Fat-Free BBQ	30 chips (1 oz)	110	0	0
Fat-Free Maui Onion	30 chips (1 oz)	110	0	0
Fat-Free No-Salt	30 chips (1 oz)	110	0	0
Fat-Free Vinegar & Salt	30 chips (1 oz)	100	0	0
Low-Fat	30 chips (1 oz)	110	0	3
Mr. Phipps Tater Crisps Bar-B-Que	11 (0.5 oz)	60	tr	2
Mr. Phipps Tater Crisps Original	11 (0.05 oz)	60	tr	2
Mr. Phipps Tater Crisps Sour Cream 'n Onion	11 (0.5 oz)	60	tr	2
New York Deli	1 oz	160	—	11
Old Dutch Foods	1 oz	150	—	9
Augratin	1 oz	150	—	8
BBQ	1 oz	140	—	8
Dill Flavored	1 oz	150	—	8
Onion & Garlic	1 oz	150	—	9

FOOD	PORTION	CALS.	SAT. FAT	FAT
Old Dutch Foods *(cont.)*				
Ripple	1 oz	150	—	9
Sour Cream & Onion	1 oz	150	—	10
Pringle's				
BBQ	14 chips (1 oz)	150	3	10
Cheez-ums	14 chips (1 oz)	170	3	13
Original	14 chips (1 oz)	160	2	11
Ranch	14 chips (1 oz)	150	3	10
Rippled	10 chips (1 oz)	160	3	11
Sour Cream N'Onion	14 chips (1 oz)	160	3	10
Pringles Light				
BBQ Pringles	14 chips (0.9 oz)	130	1	6
Original Pringles	14 chips (0.9 oz)	130	1	6
Ranch Pringles	14 chips (0.9 oz)	130	1	6
Sour Cream 'N Onion Pringles	14 chips (0.9 oz)	130	1	6
Pringles Right				
BBQ Pringles	16 chips (1 oz)	140	2	7
Original Pringles	16 chips (1 oz)	140	2	7
Ranch Pringles	16 chips (1 oz)	140	2	7
Sour Cream 'N Onion Pringles	16 chips (1 oz)	140	2	7
Ruffles	18 chips (1 oz)	150	—	10
Cheddar Cheese & Sour Cream	18 chips (1 oz)	160	—	10
Light	18 chips (1 oz)	130	—	6
Mesquite Grille B-B-Q	18 chips (1 oz)	160	—	10
Monterey Jack Cheese Flavor Cheese Attack	18 chips (1 oz)	160	—	10
Ranch	18 chips (1 oz)	160	—	10
Sour Cream & Onion	18 chips (1 oz)	160	—	10
Sour Cream & Onion Light	18 chips (1 oz)	130	—	6
Snyder's	1 oz	150	—	10
BBQ	1 oz	150	—	10
Cheddar Bacon	1 oz	150	—	10
Coney Island	1 oz	150	—	10
Grilled Steak & Onion	1 oz	150	—	10
Hot Buffalo Wings	1 oz	150	—	10
Kosher Dill	1 oz	150	—	10
No Salt	1 oz	150	—	10
Salt & Vinegar	1 oz	150	—	10
Sausage Pizza	1 oz	150	—	10
Sour Cream & Onion	1 oz	150	—	10

FOOD	PORTION	CALS.	SAT. FAT	FAT
Sour Cream & Onion Unsalted	1 oz	150	—	10
Suprimos Cheddar & Jack	1 oz	140	—	6
Suprimos Cool Onion	1 oz	140	—	6
Weight Watchers				
Great Snackers Barbecue	½ oz	70	1	3
Great Snackers Cheddar Cheese	½ oz	70	1	3
Great Snackers Sour Cream & Onion	½ oz	70	1	3
Wise Natural	1 oz	160	—	11
Wise Ridgies Barbecue	1 oz	150	—	10
potato	1 pkg	1217	25	79
potato	1 oz	152	3	10
sticks	1 oz pkg	148	3	10
sticks	½ cup	94	2	6
TORTILLA				
Barrel O' Fun				
Nacho	1 oz	140	2	6
Tostado Yellow	1 oz	140	2	6
White	1 oz	140	2	6
Doritos				
Lightly Salted	16 (1 oz)	150	—	7
Salsa 'N Cheese	16 (1 oz)	150	—	8
Eagle				
Nacho	1 oz	150	—	8
Ranch	1 oz	150	—	8
Restaurant Style	1 oz	150	—	7
Strips	1 oz	150	—	8
Eagle	1 oz	150	—	8
Guiltless Gourmet Baked	22–26 (1 oz)	110	—	1
Hain				
Sesame	1 oz	140	—	7
Sesame Cheese	1 oz	160	—	8
Sesame No Salt Added	1 oz	140	—	7
Taco Style	1 oz	160	—	11
La FAMOUS	1 oz	140	—	7
La FAMOUS No Salt Added	1 oz	140	—	7
Lance Jalapeno Cheese	1 pkg (1⅛ oz)	160	—	8
Lance Nacho	1 pkg (32 g)	160	2	8
Louise's				
Low-Fat Nacho Cheese	30 chips (1 oz)	130	1	3
Low-Fat Ranch	30 chips (1 oz)	130	1	3

FOOD	PORTION	CALS.	SAT. FAT	FAT
Louise's *(cont.)*				
Low-Fat White Corn	30 chips (1 oz)	120	0	3
Old El Paso Crispy Corn	16 chips (1 oz)	150	—	8
Old El Paso NACHIPS	9 chips (1 oz)	150	—	7
Santitas	1 oz	140	—	7
Cantina Style	1 oz	140	—	6
Cantina Style Fajita Flavored	1 oz	140	—	7
Strips	1 oz	140	—	7
Snyder's	1 oz	140	—	7
Enchilada	1 oz	140	—	7
Nacho Cheese	1 oz	140	—	7
No Salt	1 oz	140	—	7
Ranch	1 oz	140	—	7
Tostitos	11 pieces (1 oz)	140	—	8
Bite Size	16 pieces (1 oz)	150	—	8
Restaurant Style Lime 'N Chili	7 pieces (1 oz)	150	—	7
Restaurant Style White Corn	7 pieces (1 oz)	150	—	6
Tostitos Baked	1 oz	110	—	1
Cool Ranch	1 oz	130	—	3
Unsalted	1 oz	110	—	1
Tyson				
Nacho Cheese	1 oz	140	—	7
Ranch Flavor	1 oz	140	—	2
Traditional	1 oz	140	—	7
Unsalted	1 oz	140	—	7
Wise BRAVOS	1 oz	150	—	8

CHITTERLINGS

FOOD	PORTION	CALS.	SAT. FAT	FAT
pork, simmered	3 oz	258	9	24

CHIVES

FOOD	PORTION	CALS.	SAT. FAT	FAT
fresh, chopped	1 tbsp	1	tr	tr
fresh, chopped	1 tsp	0	tr	tr
freeze-dried	1 tbsp	1	tr	tr

CHOCOLATE

(see also CANDY, CAROB, COCOA, ICE CREAM TOPPINGS, MILK DRINKS)

BAKING

FOOD	PORTION	CALS.	SAT. FAT	FAT
Baker's				
German Sweet	1 oz	143	—	10
German Sweet	¼ cup	200	—	12
Semi-Sweet	1 oz	135	—	9
Unsweetened	1 oz	141	—	15

FOOD	PORTION	CALS.	SAT. FAT	FAT
Hershey Premium Semi-Sweet	1 oz	140	—	8
Hershey Premium Unsweetened	1 oz	190	—	16
Nestle				
Choco Bake	.5 oz	80	5	8
Premier White	.5 oz	80	3	5
Semi-Sweet	.5 oz	70	3	4
Unsweetened	.5 oz	80	2	7
baking	1 oz	145	9	15
CHIPS				
Baker's	1 oz	143	—	8
Big Milk Chocolate	¼ cup	239	—	14
Big Semi-Sweet	¼ cup	220	—	13
Real Semi-Sweet	¼ cup	198	—	12
Semi-Sweet	¼ cup	197	—	9
Hershey				
Chunks Milk Chocolate	1 oz	160	—	9
Chunks Semi-Sweet	1 oz	140	—	8
Milk Chocolate	1 oz	150	—	12
Miniature Semi-Sweet	¼ cup (1.5 oz)	220	—	12
Mint Chocolate	¼ cup	230	—	12
Semi-Sweet	¼ cup (1.5 oz)	220	—	12
Nestle Morsels				
Milk Chocolate	1 tbsp	70	—	4
Mint Chocolate	1 tbsp	70	2	4
Rainbow	1 tbsp	70	2	3
Semi-Sweet	1 tbsp	40	—	4
Semi-Sweet Mini	1 tbsp	70	—	4
MIX				
Hershey Chocolate Milk Mix	3 tbsp	90	—	4
powder	2–3 heaping tsp	75	tr	1
powder, as prep w/ whole milk	9 oz	226	9	9
SYRUP				
Estee Choco-Syp	2 tbsp (1.2 oz)	50	0	0
Hershey's	2 tbsp	80	—	1
Quick Syrup Chocolate (Nestle)	1⅔ tbsp	110	—	1
chocolate	1 cup	653	2	3
chocolate	2 tbsp	82	tr	tr
chocolate, as prep w/ whole milk	9 oz	232	5	9

FOOD	PORTION	CALS.	SAT. FAT	FAT

CHOCOLATE MILK
(see CHOCOLATE, COCOA, MILK DRINKS)

CHUTNEY

FOOD	PORTION	CALS.	SAT. FAT	FAT
apple	1.2 oz	68	—	0
apple cranberry	1 tbsp	16	—	0
tomato	1.2 oz	54	—	0

CILANTRO

FOOD	PORTION	CALS.	SAT. FAT	FAT
fresh	¼ cup	1	—	tr

CINNAMON

FOOD	PORTION	CALS.	SAT. FAT	FAT
ground	1 tsp	6	tr	tr

CISCO

FOOD	PORTION	CALS.	SAT. FAT	FAT
raw	3 oz	84	2	2
smoked	3 oz	151	1	10
smoked	1 oz	50	tr	3

CLAMS
CANNED

FOOD	PORTION	CALS.	SAT. FAT	FAT
American Original Foods Quahogs	4 oz	66	1	tr
Doxsee Chopped	6.5 oz	90	—	tr
Doxsee Clam Juice	3 fl oz	4	0	0
Empress Whole Baby	4 oz	60	—	1
Gorton's Minced & Chopped	½ can	70	—	1
Progresso	½ cup	70	—	tr
Progresso Red Clam Sauce	½ cup	70	—	3
Progresso White Clam Sauce	½ cup	110	—	8
S&W Fancy Chopped	2 oz	28	—	0
S&W Fancy Minced	2 oz	28	—	0
S&W Whole Baby Chowder Clams	2 oz	33	—	0
Snow's Minced	6.5 oz	90	—	tr
liquid only	3 oz	2	—	tr
liquid only	1 cup	6	—	tr
meat only	3 oz	126	tr	2
meat only	1 cup	236	tr	3
FRESH				
cooked	3 oz	126	tr	2
cooked	20 sm	133	tr	2

FOOD	PORTION	CALS.	SAT. FAT	FAT
raw	20 sm	133	tr	2
raw	9 lg	133	tr	2
raw	3 oz	63	tr	1
FROZEN				
Fried (Mrs. Paul's)	2.5 oz	200	—	9
Microwave Chrunchy Clam Strips (Gorton's)	3.5 oz	330	6	22
Microwave Fried Clams (Mrs. Paul's)	2.5 oz	260	—	15
HOME RECIPE				
breaded & fried	20 sm	379	5	21
breaded & fried	3 oz	171	2	9
TAKE-OUT				
breaded & fried	¾ cup	451	7	26

CLOVES

FOOD	PORTION	CALS.	SAT. FAT	FAT
ground	1 tsp	7	tr	tr

COCOA
(*see also* CHOCOLATE)

FOOD	PORTION	CALS.	SAT. FAT	FAT
Carnation Hot Cocoa 70 Calorie	3 tsp (21 g)	70	—	tr
Carnation Hot Cocoa Milk Chocolate	1 pkg or 4 heaping tsp (1 oz)	110	—	1
Carnation Hot Cocoa Natural Mint	1 pkg or 4 heaping tsp	110	—	1
Carnation Hot Cocoa Rich Chocolate	1 pkg or 4 heaping tsp	110	—	1
Carnation Hot Cocoa Rich Chocolate w/ Marshmallows	1 pkg or 4 heaping tsp	110	—	1
Carnation Hot Cocoa Sugar Free Mint	1 pkg or 4 heaping tsp	50	—	tr
Carnation Hot Cocoa Sugar Free Rich Chocolate	1 pkg or 4 heaping tsp	50	—	tr
Hershey's Cocoa	⅓ cup	120	—	4
Hershey's European Cocoa	1 oz	90	—	3
Hills Bros. Hot Cocoa Sugar Free, as prep w/ water	6 oz	60	—	2
Hills Bros. Hot Cocoa, as prep w/ water	6 oz	110	—	2
Nestle	1 tbsp	15	0	1
Nestle Hot Cocoa Mix	1 oz	110	—	1

FOOD	PORTION	CALS.	SAT. FAT	FAT
Nestle Hot Cocoa Mix, as prep w/ 2% milk	6 oz	210	—	5
Nestle Hot Cocoa Mix, as prep w/ skim milk	6 oz	180	—	1
Nestle Hot Cocoa Mix, as prep w/ whole milk	6 oz	230	—	8
Nestle Hot Cocoa Mix w/ Marshmallows	1 oz	120	—	1
Nestle Hot Cocoa Mix w/ Marshmallows, as prep w/ 2% milk	6 oz	220	—	5
Nestle Hot Cocoa Mix w/ Marshmallows, as prep w/ skim milk	6 oz	190	—	1
Nestle Hot Cocoa Mix w/ Marshmallows, as prep w/ whole milk	6 oz	240	—	8
Swiss Miss Cocoa Diet	6 oz	20	—	tr
Swiss Miss Cocoa Lite, as prep	6 oz	70	—	tr
Swiss Miss Cocoa Sugar Free, as prep	6 oz	60	—	tr
Swiss Miss Cocoa Sugar Free w/ Sugar Free Marshmallows, as prep	6 oz	50	—	tr
Swiss Miss Hot Cocoa Bavarian Chocolate, as prep	6 oz	110	1	3
Swiss Miss Hot Cocoa Double Rich, as prep	4 oz	110	1	1
Swiss Miss Hot Cocoa Milk Chocolate, as prep	6 oz	110	tr	1
Swiss Miss Hot Cocoa w/ Mini Marshmallows, as prep	4 oz	110	tr	1
Ultra Slim-Fast Hot Cocoa as prep w/ water	8 oz	190	—	tr
Weight Watchers	1 pkg	60	0	0
hot cocoa	1 cup	218	6	9
mix, as prep w/ water	7 oz	103	1	1
mix w/ Nutrasweet, as prep w/ water	7 oz	48	tr	tr
powder	1 oz	102	1	1

FOOD	PORTION	CALS.	SAT. FAT	FAT
COCONUT				
Angel Flake Toasted (Bakers)	⅓ cup	212	—	17
Cream of Coconut (Coco Lopez)	2 tbsp	120	—	5
Premium Shred (Bakers)	⅓ cup	135	—	9
coconut water	1 cup	46	tr	tr
coconut water	1 tbsp	3	tr	tr
cream, canned	1 cup	568	47	52
cream, canned	1 tbsp	36	3	3
dried, sweetened, flaked	7 oz pkg	944	21	64
dried, sweetened, flaked	1 cup	351	57	24
dried, sweetened, flaked, canned	1 cup	341	22	24
dried, sweetened, shredded	1 cup	466	29	33
dried, sweetened, shredded	7 oz pkg	997	63	71
dried, toasted	1 oz	168	12	13
dried, unsweetened	1 oz	187	16	18
fresh	1 piece (1.5 oz)	159	13	15
fresh, shredded	1 cup	283	24	27
milk, canned	1 cup	445	43	48
milk, canned	1 tbsp	30	3	3
milk, frozen	1 cup	486	44	50
milk, frozen	1 tbsp	30	3	3
COD				
CANNED				
atlantic	3 oz	89	tr	1
atlantic	1 can (11 oz)	327	1	3
roe	3.5 oz	118	tr	3
DRIED				
atlantic	3 oz	246	tr	2
FRESH				
atlantic, raw	3 oz	70	tr	1
atlantic, cooked	1 fillet (6.3 oz)	189	tr	2
atlantic, cooked	3 oz	89	tr	1
pacific, baked	3 oz	95	tr	1
roe baked w/ butter & lemon juice	3.5 oz	126	—	3
roe, raw	3.5 oz	130		2
FROZEN				
Fishmarket Fresh (Gorton's)	5 oz	110		1

FOOD	PORTION	CALS.	SAT. FAT	FAT
Light Fillets (Mrs. Paul's)	1 fillet	240	—	11
Light Fillets (Van De Kamp's)	1 piece	250	2	11
Natural Fillets (Van De Kamp's)	4 oz	90	0	1

COFFEE
(*see also* COFFEE BEVERAGES, COFFEE SUBSTITUTES)

INSTANT

FOOD	PORTION	CALS.	SAT. FAT	FAT
Kava	1 tsp	2	0	0
cappuccino mix, as prep	7 oz	62	2	2
decaffeinated	1 rounded tsp	4	0	0
decaffeinated, as prep	6 oz	4	0	0
fresh mix, as prep	7 oz	57	3	3
mocha mix, as prep	7 oz	51	2	2
regular	1 rounded tsp	4	0	0
regular, as prep w/ water	6 oz	4	0	0
regular w/ chicory	1 rounded tsp	6	0	0
regular w/ chicory, as prep	6 oz	6	0	0

REGULAR

FOOD	PORTION	CALS.	SAT. FAT	FAT
brewed	6 oz	4	0	0

TAKE-OUT

FOOD	PORTION	CALS.	SAT. FAT	FAT
cafe au lait	1 cup (8 fl oz)	77	3	4
cafe brulot	1 cup (4.8 fl oz)	48	0	0
capuccino	1 cup (8 fl oz)	77	3	4
coffee con leche	1 cup (8 fl oz)	77	3	4
espresso	1 cup (3 fl oz)	2	0	0
irish coffee	1 serving (9 fl oz)	107	2	3
mocha	1 mug (9.6 fl oz)	202	9	15

COFFEE BEVERAGES
(*see also* COFFEE SUBSTITUTES)

FOOD	PORTION	CALS.	SAT. FAT	FAT
Chock O'ccino Cinnamon	8 oz	120	—	2
Chock O'ccino Coffee	8 oz	120	—	2
Chock O'ccino Mocha	8 oz	120	—	2
International Coffee (General Foods)				
Cafe Amaretto	6 oz	51	—	3
Cafe Francais	6 oz	55	—	3
Cafe Irish Creme	6 oz	55	—	3
Cafe Vienna	6 oz	59	—	2
Irish Mocha Mint	6 oz	51	—	2
Orange Cappuccino	6 oz	59	—	10
Sugar Free Cafe Francais	6 oz	35	—	2

FOOD	PORTION	CALS.	SAT. FAT	FAT
Sugar Free Cafe Irish Creme	6 oz	31	—	3
Sugar Free Cafe Vienna	6 oz	29	—	3
Sugar Free Irish Mocha Mint	6 oz	28	—	2
Sugar Free Orange Cappuccino	6 oz	29	—	2
Sugar Free Suisse Mocha	6 oz	29	—	2
Suisse Mocha	6 oz	53	—	3

COFFEE SUBSTITUTES

FOOD	PORTION	CALS.	SAT. FAT	FAT
Kaffree Roma (Natural Touch)	1 tsp	6	0	0
Postum Instant	6 oz	11	0	0
Postum Instant Coffee Flavored	6 oz	11	0	0
powder	1 tsp	9	tr	tr
powder, as prep w/ milk	6 oz	121	4	6
powder, as prep	6 oz	9	tr	tr

COFFEE WHITENERS
(see also MILK SUBSTITUTES)
LIQUID

FOOD	PORTION	CALS.	SAT. FAT	FAT
Coffee Rich	1 tbsp	20	—	2
Coffee-Mate	1 tbsp (0.5 fl oz)	16	tr	1
Grand Union	1 tbsp	24	—	2
International Delight				
Amaretto Naturally Yours	1 tbsp (0.6 fl oz)	45	0	2
Cinnamon Hazelnut Naturally Yours	1 tbsp (0.6 fl oz)	45	0	2
Irish Creme Naturally Yours	1 tbsp (0.6 fl oz)	45	0	2
Suisse Chocolate Mocha Naturally Yours	1 tbsp (0.6 fl oz)	45	0	2
International Delight No Fat				
Amaretto Naturally Yours	1 tbsp (0.5 fl oz)	30	0	0
French Vanilla Royale Naturally Yours	1 tbsp (0.5 fl oz)	30	0	0
Hawaiian Macadamia Naturally Yours	1 tbsp (0.5 fl oz)	30	0	0
Irish Creme Naturally Yours	1 tbsp (0.5 fl oz)	30	0	0

FOOD	PORTION	CALS.	SAT. FAT	FAT
Mocha Mix				
Fat-Free	1 tbsp (0.5 fl oz)	10	0	0
Lite	1 tbsp (0.5 fl oz)	10	0	tr
Lite	4 fl oz	80	2	7
Original	1 tbsp (0.5 fl oz)	20	0	2
Signature Flavors French Vanilla	1 tbsp (0.5 fl oz)	35	0	0
Signature Flavors Irish Creme	1 tbsp (0.5 fl oz)	35	0	0
Signature Flavors Kahlua	1 tbsp (0.5 fl oz)	35	0	0
Signature Flavors Mauna Loa Macadamia Nut	1 tbsp (0.5 fl oz)	35	0	0
nondairy, frzn	1 tbsp	20	tr	2
POWDER				
Coffee-Mate	1 tsp	10	1	1
Cremora	1 tsp	12	—	1
N-Rich Creamer	1 tsp	10	—	tr
Weight Watchers Dairy Creamer Instant Non-fat Dry Milk	1 pkg	10	0	0
nondairy	1 tsp	11	1	tr

COLESLAW
(see SALAD)

COLLARDS

fresh, cooked	½ cup	17	—	tr
fresh, raw, chopped	½ cup	6	—	tr
frozen, chopped, cooked	½ cup	31	—	tr

COOKIES
(see also BROWNIE, CAKE, DOUGHNUT, PIE)

HOME RECIPE				
chocolate chip as prep w/ butter	1 (0.42 oz)	78	2	5
chocolate chip as prep w/ margarine	1 (0.56 oz)	78	1	5
macaroons	1 (0.8 oz)	97	3	3
oatmeal	1 (0.5 oz)	67	1	3
oatmeal w/ raisins	1 (0.52 oz)	65	tr	2
peanut butter	1 (0.7 oz)	95	1	5
shortbread as prep w/ butter	1 (0.38 oz)	60	2	4

FOOD	PORTION	CALS.	SAT. FAT	FAT
shortbread as prep w/ margarine	1 (0.38 oz)	60	1	4
sugar as prep w/ butter	1 (0.49 oz)	66	2	3
sugar as prep w/ margarine	1 (0.49 oz)	66	1	3
MIX				
Chocolate Chip (Estee)	3	130	2	7
Chocolate Chip Big Batch (Betty Crocker)	2	120	—	6
Date Bar Classic Dessert (Betty Crocker)	1	60	1	2
chocolate chip	1 (0.56 oz)	79	1	4
oatmeal	1 (0.6 oz)	74	1	3
oatmeal raisin	1 (0.6 oz)	74	1	3
READY-TO-EAT				
7-Grain Oatmeal (Frookie)	1	45	1	2
Almond Crescents (Archway)	2 (0.8 oz)	100	1	4
Almond Shortbread (Mothers)	3	180	4	11
Almond Toast Mandel (Stella D'Oro)	1	60	—	1
Amaranth (Health Valley)	1	70	—	3
Angel Bars (Stella D'Oro)	1	80	—	5
Angel Wings (Stella D'Oro)	1	70	—	5
Angelica Goodies (Stella D'Oro)	1	110	—	4
Anginetti (Stella D'Oro)	1	30	—	1
Animal (Little Debbie)	1 pkg (1.5 oz)	190	2	5
Animal Cookies Candied (Grandma's)	5 (1 oz)	140	—	6
Animal Crackers (FFV)	9	110	—	3
Animal Crackers (Sunshine)	14 (1.1 oz)	140	1	4
Animal Crackers (Sunshine)	1 box (2 oz)	260	2	7
Animal Crackers Barnum's (Nabisco)	5 (0.5 oz)	60	tr	2
Animal Frackers (Frookie)	6	60	1	2
Anisette Sponge (Stella D'Oro)	1	50	—	1
Anisette Toast (Stella D'Oro)	1	50	—	1
Anisette Toast Jumbo (Stella D'Oro)	1	110	—	1

FOOD	PORTION	CALS.	SAT. FAT	FAT
Apple Cinnamon Oat Bran (Frookie)	1 lg	120	—	4
Apple Cinnamon Oat Bran (Frookie)	1	45	1	2
Apple Fruitins (Frookie)	1	60	tr	1
Apple N'Raisin (Archway)	1 (1.1 oz)	130	1	52
Apple Newtons (Nabisco)	1 (0.75 oz)	70	tr	2
Apple Newtons Fat Free (Nabisco)	1 (0.75 oz)	70	0	0
Apple Pastry Low Sodium (Stella D'Oro)	1	80	—	3
Apple Raisin Bar (Weight Watchers)	1	100	—	3
Apple Walnut Raisin (Bakery Wagon)	1	100	1	4
Apricot Filled (Archway)	1 (1 oz)	110	1	4
Arrowroot Biscuit National (Nabisco)	1 (0.25 oz)	20	tr	1
Bakers Bonus Oatmeal (Nabisco)	1 (0.5 oz)	80	tr	3
Barre Chocolat (LU)	1	65	—	3
Beacon Hill Chocolate Chocolate Walnut (Pepperidge Farm)	1	120	2	7
Bells and Stars (Archway)	3 (1 oz)	150	2	7
Biscos Sugar Wafers (Nabisco)	4 (0.5 oz)	70	tr	3
Biscos Waffle Cremes (Nabisco)	1 (0.25 oz)	40	tr	2
Biscottini Cashews (Stella D'Oro)	1	110	—	6
Blueberry Filled (Archway)	1 (1 oz)	110	2	4
Bordeaux (Pepperidge Farm)	2	70	1	3
Breakfast Treats (Stella D'Oro)	1	100	—	4
Brown Edge Wafers (Nabisco)	2½ (0.5 oz)	70	tr	2
Brownie Chocolate Nut (Pepperidge Farm)	2	110	2	7
Brownie Nut Large Cookie (Pepperidge Farm)	1	140	3	8
Brussels (Pepperidge Farm)	2	110	2	5

FOOD	PORTION	CALS.	SAT. FAT	FAT
Brussels Mint (Pepperidge Farm)	2	130	2	7
Bugs Bunny Graham (Nabisco)	5 (0.5 oz)	60	tr	2
Butter (Mother's)	5	140	3	6
Butter (Pally)	4 (0.88 oz)	100	2	3
Butter Chessman (Pepperidge Farm)	2	90	2	4
Buttercup (Keebler)	3	70	tr	3
Cameo (Nabisco)	1 (0.5 oz)	120	1	5
Cappucino (Pepperidge Farm)	1	50	1	3
Capri (Pepperidge Farm)	1	80	1	5
Caramel Patties (FFV)	2	150	—	7
Carrot Cake (Archway)	1 (1 oz)	120	1	5
Castelets Chocolate (Stella D'Oro)	1	60	—	3
Champagne (Pepperidge Farm)	2	110	—	6
Chantilly (Pepperidge Farm)	1	80	1	2
Chesapeake Chocolate Chunk Pecan (Pepperidge Farm)	1	120	2	7
Checkerboard Wafers (Mother's)	8	150	5	8
Cherry Filled (Archway)	1 (1 oz)	110	2	4
Cherry Nougat (Archway)	3 (1 oz)	150	2	9
Cheyenne Peanut Butter Milk Chocolate Chunk (Pepperidge Farm)	1	110	2	6
Chinese Dessert (Stella D'Oro)	1	170	—	9
Chip-A-Roos (Sunshine)	3 (1.3 oz)	190	4	10
Chips Ahoy! (Nabisco)				
Bite Size Chocolate Chip	6	70	1	3
Chewy	1 (0.5 oz)	60	1	3
Chocolate Chunk Pecan	1 (0.5 oz)	100	2	6
Chunky Chocolate Chip	1 (0.5 oz)	90	2	5
Oatmeal Chocolate Chip	1	90	2	5
Real Chocolate Chip	1 (0.5 oz)	50	tr	2
Rockers Chocolate Chip	1 (0.5 oz)	60	tr	3
Sprinkled Chocolate Chip	1	60	tr	3

FOOD	PORTION	CALS.	SAT. FAT	FAT
Chips Ahoy! *(cont.)*				
Striped Chocolate Chip	1	90	2	5
White Fudge Chunk	1 (0.5 oz)	90	2	5
Choc-O-Lunch (Lance)	1 pkg (37 g)	180	2	7
Choc-O-Mint (Lance)	1 pkg (35 g)	180	3	10
Chocolate (Weight Watchers)	3	80	—	3
Chocolate Chip (Archway)	1 (1 oz)	130	2	6
Chocolate Chip (Drake's)	2 (1 oz)	140	—	6
Chocolate Chip (Dutch Mill)	3 (1.1 oz)	160	3	10
Chocolate Chip (Entenmann's)	3 (0.9 oz)	140	—	7
Chocolate Chip (Famous Amos)	3 (1 oz)	140	—	6
Chocolate Chip (Frookie)	1	45	1	2
Chocolate Chip (Frookie)	1 lg	120	—	4
Chocolate Chip (Grandma's)	2 (2.75 oz)	370	—	17
Chocolate Chip (Mother's)	2	160	3	8
Chocolate Chip (Nutra/Balance)	1 (2 oz)	260	—	14
Chocolate Chip (Pepperidge Farm)	2	100	2	5
Chocolate Chip (Weight Watchers)	2	90	0	2
Chocolate Chip Angel (Mother's)	3	180	4	9
Chocolate Chip Bag (Archway)	3 (0.9 oz)	130	2	7
Chocolate Chip Bag (Mother's)	4	140	—	5
Chocolate Chip Bar (Tastykake)	1 (43 g)	190	2	8
Chocolate Chip Chewy (Little Debbie)	1 pkg (2 oz)	370	6	19
Chocolate Chip Crisp (Little Debbie)	1 pkg (1.5 oz)	210	4	12
Chocolate Chip Drop (Archway)	1 (1 oz)	140	3	10
Chocolate Chip Fudge (Lance)	1 (28 g)	130	2	5
Chocolate Chip Ice Box (Archway)	1 (1 oz)	140	3	7

FOOD	PORTION	CALS.	SAT. FAT	FAT
Chocolate Chip Large (Pepperidge Farm)	1	130	2	6
Chocolate Chip Mini (Archway)	12 (1.1 oz)	150	2	7
Chocolate Chip Mint (Frookie)	1	45	1	2
Chocolate Chip Parade (Mother's)	4	130	2	5
Chocolate Chip Pecan (Famous Amos)	3 (1 oz)	150	—	8
Chocolate Chip Rich'N Chewy (Grandma's)	3 (1 oz)	140	—	6
Chocolate Chip Snaps (Nabisco)	3 (0.5 oz)	70	tr	2
Chocolate Chip Soft (Lance)	1 (28 g)	130	2	5
Chocolate Chip & Toffee (Archway)	1 (1 oz)	140	2	7
Chocolate Chunk Macadamia Nut (Tastykake)	1 pkg (56 g)	310	5	14
Chocolate Chunk Pecan (Pepperidge Farm)	1	70	1	4
Chocolate Fudge Sandwich (Keebler)	1	80	1	4
Chocolate Snaps (Nabisco)	4 (0.5 oz)	70	1	2
Chocolate-Chocolate Chip (Drake's)	2 (1 oz)	130	—	5
Chocolatiers (LU)	4 (1.1 oz)	170	4	8
Chocolatiers Dipped (LU)	3 (1 oz)	170	9	11
Cinnamon Snaps (Archway)	12 (1.1 oz)	150	1	7
Circus Animals (Mother's)	6	140	5	6
Classics Chocolate Chip With Pecans (Sunshine)	1 (0.7 oz)	110	2	7
Classics Chocolate Chip With Walnuts (Sunshine)	1 (0.7 oz)	100	3	6
Classics Premier Chocolate Chip (Sunshine)	1 (0.7 oz)	100	3	5
Coated Graham (Lance)	1 pkg (50 g)	200	4	10
Cobbler Apple Cranberry Fat Free (Bakery Wagon)	1	70	0	0
Cobbler Mixed Fruit Fat Free (Bakery Wagon)	1	70	0	0

FOOD	PORTION	CALS.	SAT. FAT	FAT
Cobbler Raspberry Fat Free (Bakery Wagon)	1	70	0	0
Cobbler Apple Fat Free (Bakery Wagon)	1	70	0	0
Cocadas (Mother's)	5	150	3	7
Coconut (Drake's)	2 (1 oz)	130	—	5
Coconut (Estee)	4 (1 oz)	140	2	6
Coconut Macaroons (Dutch Mill)	3 (1 oz)	120	6	7
Coconut Macaroon (Archway)	1 (0.8 oz)	90	4	5
Coconut Macaroon (Drake's)	1 (1 oz)	135	—	7
Commodore (Keebler)	1	60	tr	2
Como Delight (Stella D'Oro)	1	150	—	7
Cookie Assortment (Delacre)	4 (1.1 oz)	130	6	<5
Cookie Jar Hermits (Archway)	1 (1 oz)	110	1	3
Cookie Parade (Mother's)	4	140	3	7
Cookie Wreaths (Little Debbie)	1 pkg (0.6 oz)	90	1	5
Cookies 'N Fudge Party Grahams (Nabisco)	1 (0.25 oz)	45	tr	2
Cookies 'N Fudge Striped (Nabisco)	1 (0.5 oz)	60	1	3
Cookies 'N Fudge Striped Wafers (Nabisco)	1 (0.5 oz)	70	tr	4
Cookies Mates (Keebler)	2	50	1	2
Creme Filled Chocolate (Little Debbie)	1 pkg (1.8 oz)	260	3	11
Creme Filled Chocolated (Little Debbie)	1 pkg (1.2 oz)	180	2	8
Creme Wafers Chocolate (Estee)	7 (1.1 oz)	160	2	8
Creme Wafers Lemon (Estee)	5 (1.2 oz)	170	2	8
Creme Wafers Peanut Butter (Estee)	5 (1.2 oz)	170	2	9
Creme Wafers Triple Decker Banana Split (Estee)	3 (0.9 oz)	140	2	7

FOOD	PORTION	CALS.	SAT. FAT	FAT
Creme Wafers Triple Decker Chocolate, Caramel & Peanut Butter (Estee)	3 (0.9 oz)	140	1	7
Creme Wafers Vanilla (Estee)	7 (1.1 oz)	160	1	7
Creme Wafers Vanilla & Strawberry (Estee)	5 (1.2 oz)	170	1	8
Dakota Milk Chocolate Oatmeal (Pepperidge Farm)	1	110	2	6
Danish Imported (Nabisco)	2 (0.5 oz)	70	tr	4
Dark Chocolate (Archway)	1 (1 oz)	110	1	4
Date Pecan (Pepperidge Farm)	2	110	2	5
Deep Night Fudge (Stella D'Oro)	1	65	—	4
Devil's Food Cakes (Nabisco)	1 (0.75 oz)	70	tr	1
Dinosaur Grrrahams (Mother's)	2	130	1	3
Dinosaur Grrrahams Chocolate (Salerno)	1 pkg (1.25 oz)	167	—	5
Dinosaur Grrrahams Cinnamon (Salerno)	1 pkg (1.25 oz)	165	—	5
Dinosaur Grrrahams Orignal (Salerno)	1 pkg (1.25 oz)	156	—	3
Dixie Vanilla (Sunshine)	2 (0.9 oz)	120	1	5
Double Fudge (Mother's)	3	170	4	8
Dunkaroos (General Mills)	1 pkg (1 oz)	130	1	5
Duplex Creme (Mother's)	3	170	4	8
Dutch Apple Bars (Stella D'Oro)	1	110	—	3
Dutch Chocolate (Archway)	1 (1 oz)	120	1	4
Easter Puffs (Little Debbie)	1 pkg (1.2 oz)	140	1	5
Egg Biscuits Low Sodium (Stella D'Oro)	3	120	—	3
Egg Biscuits Sugared (Stella D'Oro)	1	80	—	1
Egg Jumbo (Stella D'Oro)	1	50	—	1
English Tea (Mother's)	2	180	4	7
Famous Chocolate Wafers (Nabisco)	2½ (0.5 oz)	70	tr	2

FOOD	PORTION	CALS.	SAT. FAT	FAT
Fancy Fruit Chunks (Health Valley)				
Apricot Almond	2	90	—	4
Date Pecan	2	90	—	4
Raisin Oat Bran	2	70	—	2
Tropical Fruit	2	90	—	3
Fancy Peanut Chunks (Health Valley)	2	90	—	3
Fat Free (Health Valley)				
Apple Spice	3	75	—	tr
Apricot Delight	3	75	—	tr
Date Delight	3	75	—	tr
Hawaiian Fruit	3	75	—	tr
Jumbos Apple Raisin	1	70	—	tr
Jumbos Raisin	1	70	—	tr
Jumbos Raspberry	1	70	—	tr
Raisin Oatmeal	3	75	—	tr
Fiber Jumbos Blueberry Nut (Health Valley)	1	100	—	3
Fiber Jumbos Chunky Pecan (Health Valley)	1	100	—	3
Fiber Jumbos Raisin Nut (Health Valley)	1	100	—	3
Fig Bar (Lance)	1 pkg (42 g)	150	1	2
Fig Bar (Mother's)	2	130	1	4
Fig Bar Fat Free (Mother's)	1	70	0	0
Fig Bar Whole Wheat (Mother's)	2	130	2	5
Fig Bar Whole Wheat Fat Free (Mother's)	1	70	0	0
Fig Bars (Sunshine)	2 (1 oz)	110	1	3
Fig Bars Apple Low Fat (Estee)	2 (1 oz)	100	0	1
Fig Bars Cranberry Low Fat (Estee)	2 (1 oz)	100	0	1
Fig Bars Low Fat (Archway)	2 (1.1 oz)	100	0	1
Fig Bars Low Fat (Estee)	2 (1 oz)	100	0	0
Fig Bars Vanilla (FFV)	1	60	—	1
Fig Bars Whole Wheat (FFV)	1	60	—	1
Fig Fruitins (Frookie)	1	60	tr	1
Fig Newtons (Nabisco)	1 (0.5 oz)	60	tr	1
Fig Newtons Fat Free (Nabisco)	1 (0.75 oz)	70	0	0

FOOD	PORTION	CALS.	SAT. FAT	FAT
Figaroos (Little Debbie)	1 pkg (1.5 oz)	160	1	4
Figaroos (Little Debbie)	1 pkg (2 oz)	200	1	5
Flaky Flix Fudge (Mother's)	2	140	5	7
Flaky Flix Vanilla (Mother's)	2	140	5	8
Fortune (La Choy)	1	15	—	tr
French Vanilla Creme (Keebler)	1	80	tr	4
Frosted Holiday (Mother's)	4	130	5	6
Frosty Lemon (Archway)	1 (1 oz)	120	1	5
Frosty Orange (Archway)	1 (1 oz)	120	1	4
Fruit & Fitness (Health Valley)	5	200	—	6
Fruit And Honey Bar (Archway)	1 (1 oz)	110	1	4
Fruit Bar No Fat (Archway)	1 (1 oz)	90	0	0
Fruit Cake (Archway)	1 (1.1 oz)	140	2	7
Fruit Delight Apple Cinnamon Fat Free (Stella D'Oro)	1	70	0	0
Fruit Delight Peach Apricot Fat Free (Stella D'Oro)	1	70	0	0
Fruit Delight Raspberry Fat Free (Stella D'Oro)	1	70	0	0
Fruit Filled Apricot-Raspberry (Pepperidge Farm)	2	100	2	4
Fruit Filled Strawberry (Pepperidge Farm)	2	100	2	5
Fruit Filled Bar Apple (Weight Watchers)	1	80	0	tr
Fruit Filled Bar Raspberry (Weight Watchers)	1	80	0	tr
Fruit Jumbos Almond Date (Health Valley)	1	70	—	3
Fruit Jumbos Oat Bran (Health Valley)	1	70	—	2
Fruit Jumbos Raisin Nut (Health Valley)	1	70	—	3
Fruit Jumbos Tropical Fruit (Health Valley)	1	70	—	3
Fruit Slices (Stella D'Oro)	1	60	—	2
Fruit Slices Fat Free (Stella D'Oro)	1	50	0	0
Fudge (Estee)	4 (1 oz)	150	2	7

FOOD	PORTION	CALS.	SAT. FAT	FAT
Fudge Bar (Tastykake)	1 (50 g)	200	2	7
Fudge Bowl Crowns (Mother's)	2	140	4	6
Fudge Bowl Nuggets (Mother's)	2	140	4	6
Fudge Chocolate Chip (Grandma's)	2 (2.75 oz)	350		13
Fudge Family Bears Vanilla (Sunshine)	2 (1 oz)	140	2	6
Fudge Macaroons (Little Debbie)	1 pkg (1 oz)	140	4	8
Fudge Mint Patties (Sunshine)	2 (0.8 oz)	130	4	7
Fudge Nut Bar (Archway)	1 (1 oz.)	110	1	5
Fudge Striped Shortbread (Sunshine)	3 (1.1 oz)	160	5	8
Fun Chip Mini (Archway)	12 (1.1 oz)	140	1	6
FundaMiddles Vanilla Creme In Chocolate Graham Shells (General Mills)	1 pkg (0.8 oz)	110	1	4
Gaucho Peanut Butter (Mother's)	2	190	3	10
Geneva (Pepperidge Farm)	2	130	2	6
Ginger (Little Debbie)	1 pkg (0.7 oz)	90	1	3
Ginger Boys Calcium Enriched (FFV)	6	120	—	3
Ginger Snaps (Bakery Wagon)	5	160	2	7
Ginger Snaps (Sunshine)	7 (1 oz)	130	1	5
Ginger Snaps Old Fashioned (Nabisco)	2 (0.5 oz)	60	tr	1
Ginger Spice (Frookie)	1	45	1	2
Gingerbread Man (Mother's)	6	140	2	6
Gingerman (Pepperidge Farm)	2	70	0	3
Gingersnaps (Archway)	5 (1.1 oz)	130	1	5
Golden Bars (Stella D'Oro)	1	110	—	4
Golden Fruit Apple (Sunshine)	1 (0.7 oz)	80	0	1
Golden Fruit Cranberry Low Fat (Sunshine)	1 (0.7 oz)	70	0	1
Golden Fruit Raisin (Sunshine)	1 (0.7 oz)	80	0	2

FOOD	PORTION	CALS.	SAT. FAT	FAT
Grab Cookie Bits Chocolate (Grandma's)	8 (1 oz)	140	—	6
Grab Cookie Bits Peanut Butter (Grandma's)	8 (1 oz)	140	—	6
Grab Cookie Bits Vanilla (Grandma's)	8 (1 oz)	140	—	6
Graham (Nabisco)	2	60	tr	1
Graham Amaranth (Health Valley)	7	110	—	3
Graham Chocolate (Nabisco)	1 (0.5 oz)	50	1	3
Graham Honey (Health Valley)	7	100	—	4
Graham Honey Fiber Enriched (Keebler)	2	90	1	2
Graham Kitchen Rich (Keebler)	2	60	1	2
Graham Oat Bran (Health Valley)	7	120	—	3
Grahams Cinnamon (Sunshine)	2 (1.1 oz)	140	2	6
Grahams Fudge Dipped (Sunshine)	4 (1.2 oz)	170	6	9
Grahams Honey (Sunshine)	2 (1 oz)	120	1	4
Grahamy Bears (Sunshine)	1 pkg (2 oz)	260	2	10
Grahamy Bears (Sunshine)	10 (1.1 oz)	140	1	5
Granola No Fat (Archway)	1 (0.5 oz)	50	0	0
Hazelnut (Pepperidge Farm)	2	110	2	6
Hermit (Drake's)	1 (2 oz)	230	—	7
Heyday Caramel & Peanut (Nabisco)	1 (0.75 oz)	110	2	6
Heyday Fudge (Nabisco)	1	110	2	6
Holiday Pak (Archway)	3 (1.1 oz)	150	2	8
Holiday Rings & Stars (Stella D'Oro)	1	47	—	1
Holiday Trinkets (Stella D'Oro)	1	40	2	2
Homeplate (Keebler)	1	60	—	2
Honey Fruit Bars (Bakery Wagon)	1	100	1	3
Honey Jumbos Crisp Cinnamon (Health Valley)	1	70	—	4

FOOD	PORTION	CALS.	SAT. FAT	FAT
Honey Jumbos Crisp Peanut Butter (Health Valley)	1	70	—	2
Honey Jumbos Fancy Oat Bran (Health Valley)	2	130	—	4
Honey Maid Cinnamon (Nabisco)	2 (0.5 oz)	60	tr	1
Honey Maid Grahams (Nabisco)	2 (0.5 oz)	60	tr	1
Hostess Assortment (Stella D'Oro)	1	40	—	2
Hydrox (Sunshine)	3	150	2	7
Hydrox Reduced Fat (Sunshine)	3 (1.1 oz)	130	1	4
Iced Gingerbread (Archway)	3 (1.1 oz)	140	1	5
Iced Molasses (Archway)	1 (1 oz)	110	1	5
Iced Molasses (Bakery Wagon)	1	100	1	3
Iced Molasses Mini (Bakery Wagon)	3	130	1	3
Iced Oatmeal (Archway)	1 (1 oz)	120	1	5
Iced Oatmeal (Mother's)	2	120	2	4
Iced Oatmeal (Sunshine)	2 (0.9 oz)	120	1	5
Iced Oatmeal Bag (Mother's)	4	120	2	4
Iced Raisin (Mother's)	2	180	7	8
Ideal Bars (Nabisco)	1 (0.75 oz)	90	2	5
Irish Oatmeal (Pepperidge Farm)	2	90	1	5
Jelly Tarts (FFV)	2	110	—	4
Keebies (Keebler)	1	80	tr	3
Kichel Low Sodium (Stella D'Oro)	21	150	—	9
Krisp Kreem Wafers (Keebler)	2	50	—	3
Lady Stella Assortment (Stella D'Oro)	1	40	—	2
Lem-O-Lunch (Lance)	1 pkg (48 g)	240	2	11
Lemon (Estee)	4 (1 oz)	140	1	6
Lemon Coolers (Sunshine)	5 (1 oz)	140	2	6
Lemon Nekot (Lance)	1 pkg (42 g)	220	4	11
Lemon Nut Crunch (Pepperidge Farm)	1 pkg (42 g)	220	4	11

FOOD	PORTION	CALS.	SAT. FAT	FAT
Lido (Pepperidge Farm)	1	90	1	5
Linzer (Pepperidge Farm)	1	120	1	4
Little Schoolboy Dark Chocolate (LU)	2 (0.9 oz)	130	3	7
Lorna Doone	2	70	tr	4
MLB Double Header Duplex (Mother's)	3	170	4	8
Macaroon (Mother's)	2	150	4	8
Mallomars (Nabisco)	1 (0.5 oz)	60	1	3
Mallopuffs (Sunshine)	1 (0.6 oz)	70	2	2
Malt (Lance)	1 pkg (35 g)	190	2	11
Mandarin Chocolate Chip (Frookie)	1	45	1	2
Margherite Chocolate (Stella D'Oro)	1	70	—	3
Margherite Vanilla (Stella D'Oro)	1	70	—	3
Marias (Mother's)	3	170	2	6
Marie LU (LU)	3 (1.2 oz)	170	2	6
Marshmallow Puffs (Nabisco)	1 (0.75 oz)	90	1	4
Marshmallow Twirls (Nabisco)	1 (1 oz)	130	1	5
Milano (Pepperidge Farm)	2	120	2	6
Milk Chocolate Macadamia (Pepperidge Farm)	2	140	—	8
Mini Chocolate Chip (Sunshine)	5 (1.1 oz)	160	3	8
Mini Fudge Royale (Sunshine)	15 (1.1 oz)	160	5	8
Mint Milano (Pepperidge Farm)	2	150	2	7
Mint Sandwich (FFV)	2	160	—	7
Molasses Crisps (Pepperidge Farm)	2	70	0	3
Mystic Mint	1 (0.5 oz)	90	3	5
Nantucket Chocolate Chunk (Pepperidge Farm)	1	120	2	6
Nassau (Pepperidge Farm)	1	80	1	5
New Orleans Cake (Archway)	1 (1 oz)	110	1	4
Nilla Wafers (Nabisco)	3	60	tr	2
North Poles (Mother's)	2	140	6	7

FOOD	PORTION	CALS.	SAT. FAT	FAT
Nut-O-Lunch (Lance)	1 oz	140	—	5
Nutter Butter Bites (Nabisco)	4½ (0.5 oz)	70	tr	3
Nutter Butter Peanut Butter (Nabisco)	1 (0.5 oz)	70	tr	3
Nutter Butter Peanut Creme (Nabisco)	2 (0.5)	80	tr	4
Oat Bran Animal (Health Valley)	7	110	—	4
Oat Bran Fruit & Nut (Health Valley)	2	110	—	4
Oat Bran Muffin (Frookie)	1	45	1	2
Oat Bran Muffin (Frookie)	1 lg	120	—	4
Oatmeal (Archway)	1	110	—	4
Oatmeal (Drake's)	2 (1 oz)	120	—	5
Oatmeal (Lance)	1 (57 g)	130	1	5
Oatmeal (Mother's)	2	110	2	5
Oatmeal Apple Filled (Archway)	1 (1 oz)	110	1	3
Oatmeal Apple Filled (Bakery Wagon)	1	90	1	3
Oatmeal Apple Spice (Grandma's)	2 (2.75 oz)	330	—	12
Oatmeal Calcium Enriched (FFV)	5	130	—	5
Oatmeal Chocolate Chip (Mother's)	2	120	2	5
Oatmeal Chocolate Chip (Sunshine)	3 (1.3 oz)	170	3	8
Oatmeal Chocolate Chunk (Bakery Wagon)	1	100	1	3
Oatmeal Country Style (Sunshine)	3 (1.2 oz)	170	2	7
Oatmeal Creme (Drake's)	1 (2 oz)	240	—	9
Oatmeal Crisp (Little Debbie)	1 pkg (1.5 oz)	210	3	11
Oatmeal Date Filled (Archway)	1 (1 oz)	110	1	4
Oatmeal Date Filled (Bakery Wagon)	1	90	1	3
Oatmeal Large (Pepperidge Farm)	1	120	1	6
Oatmeal Lights (Little Debbie)	1 pkg (1.3 oz)	140	1	4

FOOD	PORTION	CALS.	SAT. FAT	FAT
Oatmeal Mini (Archway)	12 (1.1 oz)	150	2	8
Oatmeal Pecan (Archway)	1 (1 oz)	120	2	5
Oatmeal Raisin (Archway)	1 (1 oz)	110	1	4
Oatmeal Raisin (Dutch Mill)	3 (1 oz)	130	2	6
Oatmeal Raisin (Estee)	4 (1 oz)	130	1	5
Oatmeal Raisin (Famous Amos)	3 (1 oz)	134	—	6
Oatmeal Raisin (Frookie)	1	45	1	2
Oatmeal Raisin (Frookie)	1 lg	120	—	4
Oatmeal Raisin (Little Debbie)	1 pkg (2.7 oz)	320	3	13
Oatmeal Raisin (Mother's)	5	150	2	7
Oatmeal Raisin (Nutra/Balance)	1 (2 oz)	240	—	9
Oatmeal Raisin (Pepperidge Farm)	2	110	2	5
Oatmeal Raisin (Weight Watchers)	2	90	0	tr
Oatmeal Raisin Bar (Tastykake)	1 (50 g)	210	2	8
Oatmeal Raisin Bran (Archway)	1 (1 oz)	110	1	4
Oatmeal Raspberry Filled (Bakery Wagon)	1	100	1	3
Oatmeal Soft (Bakery Wagon)	1	100	1	4
Oatmeal Spice (Weight Watchers)	3	80	—	2
Oatmeal Walnut Chocolate Chip (Mother's)	2	130	2	6
Oatmeal Walnut Raisin (Bakery Wagon)	1	100	1	4
Old Fashion Chocolate Chip (Keebler)	1	80	1	4
Old Fashion Double Fudge (Keebler)	1	80	2	4
Old Fashion Oatmeal (Keebler)	1	80	1	4
Old Fashion Peanut Butter (Keebler)	1	80	1	4
Old Fashion Sugar (Keebler)	1	80	1	3
Old Fashioned Chocolate Chip (Pepperidge Farm)	2	100	2	5

FOOD	PORTION	CALS.	SAT. FAT	FAT
Old Fashioned Molasses (Archway)	1 (1 oz)	120	1	3
Old Fashioned Windmill (Archway)	1 (0.7 oz)	100	1	4
Old Time Molasses (Grandma's)	2 (2.75 oz)	320	—	9
Orange Milano (Pepperidge Farm)	2	150	2	7
Oreo	1 (0.5 oz)	50	tr	2
Oreo Double Stuf	1	70	1	4
Oreo Fudge Covered	1	110	2	6
Oreo Mini	5 (0.5 oz)	70	tr	3
Oreo White Fudge Covered	1	110	4	6
Orleans (Pepperidge Farm)	3	90	2	6
Orleans Sandwich (Pepperidge Farm)	2	120	2	8
Paris (Pepperidge Farm)	2	100	—	5
Party Treats (Archway)	3 (1.1 oz)	140	2	7
Peach-Apricot Pastry Sodium Free (Stella D'Oro)	1	80	—	3
Peanut Butter (Archway)	1 (1 oz)	140	—	7
Peanut Butter (Grandma's)	2 (2.75 oz)	410	—	30
Peanut Butter (Little Debbie)	1 pkg (1.5 oz)	210	3	10
Peanut Butter & Chip (Archway)	3 (0.9 oz)	130	2	7
Peanut Butter & Jelly Sandwiches (Little Debbie)	1 pkg (1.1 oz)	130	1	5
Peanut Butter Bar (Frito Lay)	1.75 oz	270	—	16
Peanut Butter Bars (Little Debbie)	1 pkg (1.9 oz)	270	3	15
Peanut Butter Creme Filled Wafer (Lance)	1 pkg (50 g)	240	3	10
Peanut Butter Nougat (Archway)	3 (1.1 oz)	160	2	9
Peanut Butter Sandwich (FFV)	2	170	—	8
Peanut Butter Wafers (Drake's)	1 (2.25 oz)	324	—	16
Peanut Clusters (Little Debbie)	1 pkg (1.4 oz)	190	2	11

FOOD	PORTION	CALS.	SAT. FAT	FAT
Pecan Crunch (Archway)	6 (1.1 oz)	150	2	8
Pecan Goldens (Mother's)	2	170	2	11
Pecan Ice Box (Archway)	1 (1 oz)	140	2	7
Pecan Malted Nougat (Archway)	3 (1.1 oz)	160	2	10
Pecan Shortbread (Little Debbie)	1 pkg (1.5 oz)	220	3	13
Pecan Shortbread (Pepperidge Farm)	1	70	2	5
Pecan Spinwheels (Little Debbie)	1 pkg (1 oz)	110	1	4
Pecan Supremes (Nabisco)	1 (0.5 oz)	80	1	5
Pfeffernusse (Archway)	2 (1.3 oz)	140	0	1
Pfeffernusse Spice Drops (Stella D'Oro)	1	40	—	1
Pims (LU)	1	50	0	1
Pineapple Filled (Archway)	1 (0.9 oz)	100	1	4
Pinwheels (Nabisco)	1 (1 oz)	130	2	5
Pirouettes Chocolate Laced (Pepperidge Farm)	2	70	1	4
Pirouettes Original (Pepperidge Farm)	2	70	1	4
Pitter Patter (Keebler)	1	90	tr	4
Prune Pastry Dietetic (Stella D'Oro)	1	90	—	3
Pure Chocolate Middles (Nabisco)	1 (0.5 oz)	80	2	5
Rainbow Wafers (Mother's)	8	150	5	8
Raisin Bran (Pepperidge Farm)	2	110	2	5
Raisin Oatmeal (Archway)	1 (1 oz)	130	1	5
Raisin Oatmeal Bag (Archway)	3 (1 oz)	130	2	6
Raisin Soft (Grandma's)	2 (2.75 oz)	320	—	10
Raspberry Newtons (Nabisco)	1 (0.75 oz)	70	tr	2
Raspberry Filled (Archway)	1 (1 oz)	110	1	4
Regal Grahams (FFV)	2	140	—	7
Rocky Road (Archway)	1 (1 oz)	130	2	6
Roman Egg Biscuits (Stella D'Oro)	1	140	—	5
Royal Dainty (FFV)	2	120	—	6
Royal Nuggets (Stella D'Oro)	1	2	—	tr

FOOD	PORTION	CALS.	SAT. FAT	FAT
Ruth's Golden Oatmeal (Archway)	1 (1 oz)	120	1	5
Sandwich Chocolate (Estee)	3 (1.2 oz)	160	2	6
Sandwich Original (Estee)	3 (1.2 oz)	160	2	6
Sandwich Peanut Butter (Estee)	3 (1.2 oz)	160	1	7
Sandwich Vanilla (Estee)	3 (1.2 oz)	160	1	5
Sante Fe Oatmeal Raisin (Pepperidge Farm)	1	100	1	4
Sausalito Milk Chocolate Macadamia (Pepperidge Farm)	1	120	2	7
School House Cookies (Sunshine)	20 (1.1 oz)	140	1	5
Select Assortment (Archway)	3 (0.9 oz)	130	2	6
Sesame Regina (Stella D'Oro)	1	50	—	2
Seville (Pepperidge Farm)	2	100	—	5
Shortbread (Pepperidge Farm)	2	150	2	8
Shortbread (Weight Watchers)	3	80	—	2
Shortbread Reduced Fat (Estee)	4 (1 oz)	130	1	4
Snackwell's				
Chocolate Chip	6 (0.5 oz)	60	tr	1
Cinnamon Graham Snacks	9 (0.5 oz)	50	0	0
Devil's Food Cakes	1 (0.5 oz)	60	0	0
Oatmeal Raisin	1 (0.5 oz)	60	tr	1
Social Tea (Nabisco)	3 (0.5 oz)	70	tr	2
Soft Molasses Drop (Archway)	1 (1 oz)	110	1	4
Soft Sugar (Archway)	1 (1 oz)	110	1	4
Soft'n Chewy Chocolate Chocolate Chip (Tastykake)	1 (32 g)	170	2	7
Soft'n Chewy Chocolate Chip (Tastykake)	1 (39 g)	170	2	7
Soft'n Chewy Oatmeal Raisin (Tastykake)	1 (39 g)	160	1	5
Southport (Pepperidge Farm)	2	170	—	10

FOOD	PORTION	CALS.	SAT. FAT	FAT
Strawberry Filled (Archway)	1 (1 oz)	110	1	4
Strawberry Newtons (Nabisco)	1 (0.75 oz)	70	tr	2
Striped Shortbread (Mother's)	3	170	5	8
Sugar (Archway)	1 (1 oz)	120	1	4
Sugar (Mother's)	2	140	2	6
Sugar (Pepperidge Farm)	2	100	2	5
Sugar Wafers Chocolate (Sunshine)	3 (0.9 oz)	130	2	7
Sugar Wafers Peanut Butter (Sunshine)	4 (1.1 oz)	170	2	9
Sugar Wafers Vanilla (Sunshine)	3 (0.9 oz)	130	2	6
Sunshine Almond Crescents (Sunshine)	4 (1.1 oz)	150	2	6
Sunshine Iced Gingerbread (Sunshine)	5 (1 oz)	130	2	6
Sunshine Jingles (Sunshine)	6 (1.1 oz)	150	1	5
Swiss Fudge (Stella D'Oro)	1	70	—	3
T. C. Rounds (FFV)	2	160	—	8
Tahiti (Pepperidge Farm)	1	90	2	6
Tango (FFV)	2	160	—	5
Teddy Grahams (Nabisco)				
Bearwich Chocolate & Vanilla Creme	4	70	tr	3
Bearwich Chocolate Creme w/ Peanut Butter	4 (0.5 oz)	70	tr	3
Bearwich Cinnamon w/ Vanilla Creme	4	70	tr	3
Bearwich Vanilla & Chocolate Creme	4	70	tr	3
Chocolate Graham	11	60	tr	2
Cinnamon Graham	11	60	tr	2
Honey Graham	11	60	tr	2
Vanilla And Beach Bears	11 (0.5 oz)	60	tr	2
Vanilla And Holiday Bears	11 (0.5 oz)	60	tr	2
Vanilla And Rockin' Bears	11 (0.5 oz)	60	tr	2
Vanilla Graham	11	60	tr	2
The Great Tofu (Health Valley)	2	90	—	3

FOOD	PORTION	CALS.	SAT. FAT	FAT
The Great Wheat Free (Health Valley)	2	80	—	3
Tryslet Assortment (Mother's)	2	140	3	7
Trolley Cakes Devilsfood (FFV)	2	120	—	2
Tru Blu Chocolate (Sunshine)	2	160	1	7
Tru Blu Lemon (Sunshine)	1	70	1	3
Tru Blu Vanilla (Sunshine)	1	8	1	3
Truffle Lu (LU)	4 (1.2 oz)	180	7	11
Van-O-Lunch (Lance)	1 pkg (37 g)	180	2	7
Vanilla (Estee)	4 (1 oz)	140	1	6
Vanilla Sugar Wafer (Tastykake)	1 (6 g)	36	0	2
Vanilla Wafer (Archway)	5 (1.1 oz)	130	1	4
Vanilla Wafers (FFV)	8	120	—	5
Vanilla Wafers (Keebler)	4	80	—	4
Vanilla Wafers (Mother's)	6	150	2	6
Vanilla Wafers (Sunshine)	7 (1.1 oz)	150	2	7
Vanilla Wafers Cholesterol Free (Bakery Wagon)	6	130	2	4
Vienna Fingers (Sunshine)	2 (1 oz)	140	2	6
Vienna Fingers Low Fat (Sunshine)	2 (1 oz)	130	1	4
Walnut Fudge (Mother's)	2	130	3	7
Wedding Cakes (Archway)	3 (1.1 oz)	160	2	8
Zoo Pals (Mother's)	14	140	2	5
Zurich (Pepperidge Farm)	1	60	1	2
animal crackers	11 (1 oz)	126	1	4
animal crackers	1 (2.5 g)	11	tr	tr
animal crackers	1 box (2.4 oz)	299	4	9
butter	1 (5 g)	23	1	1
chocolate chip	1 (0.4 oz)	48	1	2
chocolate chip	1 box (1.9 oz)	233	5	12
chocolate chip low fat	1 (0.25 oz)	45	tr	1
chocolate chip low sugar low sodium	1 (0.24 oz)	31	1	1
chocolate chip soft-type	1 (0.5 oz)	69	1	4
chocolate w/ creme filling	1 (0.35 oz)	47	tr	2
chocolate w/ creme filling chocolate coated	1 (0.60 oz)	82	1	5
chocolate w/ creme filling sugar free low sodium	1 (0.35 oz)	46	1	2

FOOD	PORTION	CALS.	SAT. FAT	FAT
chocolate w/ extra creme filling	1 (0.46 oz)	65	1	3
chocolate wafer	1 (0.2 oz)	26	tr	1
chocolate wafer cookie crumbs	½ cup (5.9 oz)	728	6	25
digestive biscuits plain	2	141	—	7
fig bars	1 (0.56 oz)	56	tr	1
fortune	1 (0.28 oz)	30	tr	tr
fudge	1 (0.73 oz)	73	tr	1
gingersnaps	1 (0.24 oz)	29	tr	1
graham	1 square (0.24 oz)	30	tr	1
graham chocolate covered	1 (0.49 oz)	68	2	3
graham cracker crumbs	½ cup (4.4 oz)	540	3	13
graham honey	1 (0.24 oz)	30	tr	1
ladyfingers	1 (0.38 oz)	40	tr	1
marshmallow chocolate coated	1 (0.46 oz)	55	1	2
marshmallow pie chocolate coated	1 (1.4 oz)	165	2	7
molasses	1 (0.5 oz)	65	tr	2
oatmeal	1 (0.52 oz)	71	1	4
oatmeal	1 (0.6 oz)	81	1	3
oatmeal soft-type	1 (0.5 oz)	61	tr	2
oatmeal raisin	1 (0.6 oz)	81	1	3
oatmeal raisin low sugar no sodium	1 (0.24 oz)	31	1	1
oatmeal raisin soft-type	1 (0.5 oz)	61	tr	2
peanut butter soft-type	1 (0.5 oz)	69	1	4
shortbread	1 (0.28 oz)	40	tr	2
sugar	1 (0.52 oz)	72	1	3
sugar low sugar sodium free	1 (0.24 oz)	30	tr	1
sugar wafers w/ creme filling	1 (0.12 oz)	18	tr	1
sugar wafers w/ creme filling sugar free sodium free	1 (0.14 oz)	20	tr	1
vanilla sandwich	1 (0.35 oz)	48	tr	2
vanilla wafers	1 (0.21 oz)	28	tr	1
REFRIGERATED				
Chocolate Chip (Pillsbury)	1	70	tr	3
Oatmeal Raisin (Pillsbury)	1	60	tr	2
Peanut Butter (Pillsbury)	1	70	tr	3

FOOD	PORTION	CALS.	SAT. FAT	FAT
Sugar (Pillsbury)	1	70	tr	3
chocolate chip	1 (0.42 oz)	59	1	3
chocolate chip unbaked	1 oz	126	2	6
oatmeal	1 (0.4 oz)	56	1	3
oatmeal raisin	1 (0.4 oz)	56	1	3
peanut butter	1 (0.4 oz)	60	1	3
peanut butter dough	1 oz	130	2	7
sugar	1 (0.42 oz)	58	1	3
sugar dough	1 oz	124	2	6

CORIANDER

leaf, dried	1 tsp	2	—	tr
leaf, fresh	¼ cup	1	—	tr
seed	1 tsp	5	tr	tr

CORN

(see also BRAN, CEREAL, CORNMEAL, FLOUR)

CANNED

50% Less Salt No Sugar Added (Green Giant)	½ cup	50	—	1
Corn (Green Giant)	½ cup	70	0	0
Cream Style (Green Giant)	½ cup	100	—	tr
Cream Style (Owatonna)	½ cup	100	0	1
Cream Style, Diet (S&W)	½ cup	100	—	1
Cream Style Premium Homestyle (S&W)	½ cup	105	—	1
Deli Corn (Green Giant)	½ cup	80	—	tr
Golden Kernel 50% Less Salt (Green Giant)	½ cup	70	—	tr
Golden Vacuum Packed (Green Giant)	½ cup	80	0	0
Mexi Corn (Green Giant)	½ cup	80	—	tr
No Salt No Sugar (Green Giant)	½ cup	80	—	tr
Sweet 'N Natural (S&W)	½ cup	90	—	1
Sweet Select (Green Giant)	½ cup	60	—	1
White Vacuum Packed (Green Giant)	½ cup	80	0	0
Whole Kernel (Seneca)	½ cup	80	0	1
Whole Kernel in Brine (Owatonna)	½ cup	90	—	1
Whole Kernel Natural Pack (Seneca)	½ cup	80	0	1
Whole Kernel Tender Young (S&W)	½ cup	90	—	1

FOOD	PORTION	CALS.	SAT. FAT	FAT
Whole Kernel Vacuum Pack (Owatonna)	½ cup	100	—	1
Whole Kernel Water Pack (S&W)	½ cup	80	—	1
cream style	½ cup	93	—	1
w/ red & green peppers	½ cup	86	—	1
white	½ cup	66	—	1
yellow	½ cup	66	—	1
FRESH				
on the cob, cooked, w/ butter	1 ear	155	2	3
white, cooked	½ cup	89	tr	1
white, raw	½ cup	66	tr	1
yellow, cooked	1 ear (2.7 oz)	83	tr	1
yellow, cooked	½ cup	89	tr	1
yellow, raw	1 ear (3 oz)	77	tr	1
yellow, raw	½ cup	66	tr	1
FROZEN				
Big Ears (Birds Eye)	1 ear	160	tr	1
Cob Corn (Fresh Like)	1 ear (3 in)	96	—	1
Cob Corn (Fresh Like)	1 ear (5 in)	96	—	1
Cob Corn (Ore Ida)	1 ear (6.1 oz)	180	0	3
Cob Corn Mini-Gold (Ore Ida)	1 (2.65 oz)	90	tr	tr
Cob Corn Mini-Gold (Ore Ida)	1 ear (3.1 oz)	90	0	1
Cream Style (Green Giant)	½ cup	110	0	1
Fritters (Mrs. Paul's)	2	240	—	9
Harvest Fresh Niblets (Green Giant)	½ cup	80	—	1
Harvest Fresh White Shoepeg (Green Giant)	½ cup	90	—	1
In Butter Sauce (Birds Eye)	½ cup	90	1	2
In Butter Sauce (Green Giant)	½ cup	100	1	2
Little Ears (Birds Eye)	2 ears	130	tr	1
Nibblers Corn on the Cob (Green Giant)	2 ears	120	—	1
Niblet Ears (Green Giant)	1 ear	120	—	1
Niblets (Green Giant)	½ cup	90	tr	—
On the Cob (Birds Eye)	1 ear	120	tr	1
One Serve Corn on the Cob (Green Giant)	1 pkg	120	tr	1

FOOD	PORTION	CALS.	SAT. FAT	FAT
One Serve Niblets in Butter Sauce (Green Giant)	1 pkg	120	tr	2
Polybag Cut (Birds Eye)	½ cup	80	tr	1
Polybag Deluxe Tender Sweet (Birds Eye)	½ cup	80	tr	1
Souffle (Stouffer's)	½ cup (2.4 oz)	170	2	7
Super Sweet Nibblers Corn on the Cob (Green Giant)	2 ears	90	—	2
Super Sweet Niblet (Green Giant Select)	½ cup	60	—	1
Super Sweet Niblet Ears (Green Giant)	1 ear	90	—	2
Sweet (Birds Eye)	½ cup	80	tr	1
White (Green Giant Select)	½ cup	90	—	1
White in Butter Sauce (Green Giant)	½ cup	100	tr	2
White Shoepeg (Hanover)	½ cup	80	—	0
White Sweet (Hanover)	½ cup	80	—	0
Yellow Sweet (Hanover)	½ cup	80	—	0
cooked	½ cup	67	tr	tr
on the cob, cooked	1 ear (2.2 oz)	59	tr	tr
SHELF STABLE				
Golden Whole Kernel (Pantry Express)	½ cup	60	0	tr
TAKE-OUT				
fritters	1 (1 oz)	62	tr	2
scalloped	½ cup	258	1	7

CORN CHIPS
(see CHIPS)

CORNISH HENS
(see CHICKEN)

CORNMEAL

FOOD	PORTION	CALS.	SAT. FAT	FAT
Albers White	1 oz	100	0	0
Albers Yellow	1 oz	100	0	0
White (Aunt Jemima)	3 tbsp	102	—	1
White (Quaker)	3 tbsp	102	—	1
Yellow (Arrowhead)	¼ cup (1.2 oz)	120	0	1
Enriched Yellow (Quaker)	3 tbsp	102	—	1
corn grits, cooked	1 cup	146	tr	tr
corn grits, uncooked	1 cup	579	tr	2
degermed	1 cup	506	tr	2

FOOD	PORTION	CALS.	SAT. FAT	FAT
self-rising, degermed	1 cup	489	tr	2
whole grain	1 cup	442	tr	4
HOME RECIPE				
hush puppies	1 (.75 oz)	74	tr	3
hush puppies	5 (2.7 oz)	256	3	12
MIX				
Arrowhead Corn Bread	¼ cup (1.2 oz)	120	—	1
Aunt Jemima				
Bolted White Mix	3 tbsp	99	—	1
Buttermilk Self-Rising White Mix	3 tbsp	101	—	1
Self Rising Yellow Mix	3 tbsp	100	—	1
Self-Rising White Mix	3 tbsp	98	—	1
Golden Dipt				
Corny Dog Batter Mix	1 oz	100	0	0
Hush Puppy Deluxe Mix	1.25 oz	120	0	0
Hush Puppy Jalapeno Mix	1.25 oz	120	0	0
Hush Puppy With Onion	1.25 oz	120	0	0
Hodgson Mill Yellow	¼ cup (1 oz)	100	0	1
Hodgson Mill Yellow Self Rising	¼ cup (1 oz)	90	0	1
Kentucky Kernal White Corn Meal Mix	¼ cup (1 oz)	100	0	1
Miracle Maize Complete as prep	1 piece (1.5 oz)	193	—	3
Miracle Maize Country Style as prep	1 piece 2 in x 2 in (1.8 oz)	230	—	5
Miracle Maize Sweet as prep	1 piece 2 in x 2 in (1.8 oz)	236	—	5

CORNSALAD

FOOD	PORTION	CALS.	SAT. FAT	FAT
raw	1 cup	12	—	tr

CORNSTARCH

FOOD	PORTION	CALS.	SAT. FAT	FAT
Argo	1 cup	460	0	tr
Argo	1 tbsp	30	0	0
Hodgson Mill	2 tsp (0.4 oz)	35	0	0
Kingsford's	1 cup	460	—	tr
Kingsford's	1 tbsp	30	—	tr
cornstarch	⅛ cup	164	tr	tr

COTTAGE CHEESE

FOOD	PORTION	CALS.	SAT. FAT	FAT
Axelrod Nonfat	½ cup (4.4 oz)	90	0	0
Borden 4%	½ cup	120	—	5

FOOD	PORTION	CALS.	SAT. FAT	FAT
Borden 5% Dry Curd	½ cup	80	—	1
Borden Unsalted 4%	½ cup	120	—	5
Breakstone 2%	4 oz	100	1	2
Breakstone 4% Small Curd	4 oz	110	3	5
Breakstone 4% w/ Pineapple	4 oz	140	3	5
Breakstone Dry Curd No Salt Added	4 oz	90	0	0
Cabot	4 oz	120	3	5
Cabot Light	4 oz	90	1	1
Friendship California Style	½ cup	115	3	5
Friendship Lowfat No Salt Added	½ cup	90	1	1
Friendship Lowfat Pineapple	½ cup (4 oz)	120	1	1
Friendship Lowfat 1%	½ cup (4 oz)	90	1	1
Friendship Nonfat	½ cup (4 oz)	80	0	0
Friendship Nonfat Plus Peach	½ cup (4 oz)	110	0	0
Friendship Pot Style	½ cup (4 oz)	90	2	3
Friendship w/ Pineapple	½ cup (4 oz)	140	3	4
Knudsen 2%	4 oz	100	1	2
Knudsen 2% w/ Fruit Cocktail	4 oz	130	2	2
Knudsen 2% w/ Mandarin Orange	4 oz	110	2	2
Knudsen 2% w/ Peach	6 oz	170	2	2
Knudsen 2% w/ Pear	4 oz	110	2	2
Knudsen 2% w/ Pineapple	4 oz	170	2	2
Knudsen 2% w/ Spiced Apple	4 oz	180	2	2
Knudsen 2% w/ Strawberry	4 oz	170	2	2
Knudsen 4% Large Curd	4 oz	120	3	5
Knudsen 4% Small Curd	4 oz	120	3	5
Knudsen Nonfat	4 oz	90	0	0
Lactaid 1%	4 oz	72	1	1
Light N'Lively 1%	4 oz	80	1	2
Light N'Lively 1% Garden Salad	4 oz	80	1	2
Light N'Lively 1% Peach & Pineapple	4 oz	100	1	1
Lite-Line Lowfat 1½%	½ cup	90	—	2
Sargento Pot Cheese	1 oz	26	—	tr

FOOD	PORTION	CALS.	SAT. FAT	FAT
Sealtest 2%	4 oz	100	1	2
Viva Nonfat	½ cup	70	0	0
Weight Watchers 1%	½ cup	90	—	1
Weight Watchers 2%	½ cup	100	—	2
creamed	4 oz	117	3	5
creamed	1 cup	217	6	9
creamed w/ fruit	4 oz	140	2	4
dry curd	4 oz	96	tr	tr
dry curd	1 cup	123	tr	1
lowfat 1%	4 oz	82	1	1
lowfat 1%	1 cup	164	1	2
lowfat 2%	4 oz	101	1	2
lowfat 2%	1 cup	203	3	4

COTTONSEED

FOOD	PORTION	CALS.	SAT. FAT	FAT
kernels, roasted	1 tbsp	51	1	4

COUGH DROPS

FOOD	PORTION	CALS.	SAT. FAT	FAT
Halls	1 (3.8 g)	15	0	0
Halls Plus	1 (4.7 g)	18	0	0
Halls With Vitamin C	1 (3.8 g)	14	0	0

COWPEAS

CANNED

FOOD	PORTION	CALS.	SAT. FAT	FAT
common	1 cup	184	tr	1

DRIED

| catjang, cooked | 1 cup | 200 | tr | 1 |

FRESH

| leafy tips, chopped, cooked | 1 cup | 12 | tr | tr |
| leafy tips, raw, chopped | 1 cup | 10 | tr | tr |

FROZEN

| cooked | ½ cup | 112 | tr | tr |

CRAB

CANNED

FOOD	PORTION	CALS.	SAT. FAT	FAT
Dungeness Crab (S&W)	3.25 oz	81	—	2
blue	3 oz	84	tr	1
blue	1 cup	133	tr	2

FRESH

alaska king, cooked	1 leg (4.7 oz)	129	tr	2
alaska king, cooked	3 oz	82	tr	1
alaska king, raw	1 leg (6 oz)	144	tr	1
alaska king, raw	3 oz	71	tr	1
blue, cooked	1 cup	138	tr	2

FOOD	PORTION	CALS.	SAT. FAT	FAT
blue, cooked	3 oz	87	tr	2
blue raw	1 crab (.7 oz)	18	tr	tr
blue raw	3 oz	74	tr	1
dungeness, raw	1 crab (5.7 oz)	140	tr	2
dungeness, raw	3 oz	73	tr	1
queen, steamed	3 oz	98	tr	1
FROZEN				
Crab Crisp (King & Prince)	4 oz	310	—	19
Crab Del Rey (King & Prince)	4 oz	205	—	12
Deviled Crab (Mrs. Paul's)	1 cake	180	—	9
Deviled Crab Miniatures (Mrs. Paul's)	3.5 oz	240	—	12
READY-TO-USE				
crab cakes	1 cake (2.1 oz)	93	1	5
TAKE-OUT				
baked	1 (3.8 oz)	160	tr	2
cake	1 (2 oz)	160	2	10
soft-shell, fried	1 (4.4 oz)	334	4	18

CRACKER CRUMBS

Corn Flake Crumbs (Kellogg's)	¼ cup (1 oz)	100	0	0
Cracker Meal (Golden Dipt)	1 oz	100	0	0
Cracker Meal (Keebler)	1 cup	100	tr	3
Cracker Meal (Lance)	1 oz	100	—	1
Cracker Meal (Nabisco)	2 tbsp	50	tr	0
Graham Crumbs (Keebler)	1 cup	520	tr	14
Zesty Meal (Keebler)	1 cup	85	2	10

CRACKERS

(*see also* CRACKER CRUMBS)

American Classic (Nabisco)				
Cracked Wheat	4	70	tr	4
Dairy Butter	4	70	tr	3
Golden Sesame	4	70	tr	3
Toasted Poppy	4	70	tr	3
American Heritage Sesame (Sunshine)	9 (1.1 oz)	160	2	9
American Heritage Wheat & Bran (Sunshine)	9 (1 oz)	140	2	7
Armenian Thin Bread (Venus)	2 (0.9 oz)	100	tr	1

FOOD	PORTION	CALS.	SAT. FAT	FAT
Bacon Cheese (Eagle)	1 oz	140	—	6
Bacon Flavored (Nabisco)	7 (0.5 oz)	70	tr	4
Better Chedders (Nabisco)	10 (0.5 oz)	70	tr	4
Better Chedders Low Salt (Nabisco)	10 (0.5 oz)	70	tr	4
Bonnie (Lance)	1 pkg (349)	160	2	7
Bran Wafers Salt Free (Venus)	5 (0.5 oz)	60	—	1
Breadflats (J. J. Flats)				
Caraway	1	52	—	1
Caraway And Salt	1	51	—	1
Cinnamon	1	53	—	1
Flavorall	1	52	—	1
Garlic	1	52	—	1
Oat Bran	1	49	—	1
Onion	1	53	—	1
Plain	1	53	—	1
Poppy	1	53	—	1
Sesame	1	55	—	2
Brown Rice (Sesmark)	15 (1 oz)	120	0	2
Butter Crackers (Goya)	1	40	—	1
Butter Thins (Pepperidge Farm)	4	70	1	3
Captain Wafers (Lance)	2	30	0	1
Captain Wafers Very Low Sodium (Lance)	2	30	0	1
Captain Wafers w/ Cream Cheese & Chives (Lance)	1.3 oz	170	2	9
Cheddar Thins (FFV)	7	70	—	2
Cheddar Wedges (Nabisco)	3	70	tr	3
Cheese (Eagle)	1 oz	130	—	6
Cheese (Hain)	1 oz	130	—	6
Cheese Crackers With Peanut Butter (Little Debbie)	1 pkg (0.9 oz)	140	2	7
Cheese Crackers w/ Peanut Butter (Little Debbie)	1 pkg (1.4 oz)	210	3	11
Cheese Filled (Frito Lay)	6 (1.5 oz)	210	—	10
Cheese Thins (Sesmark)	15 (1 oz)	130	0	3
Cheese-on-Wheat (Lance)	1.3 oz	180	2	9
Cheez-It (Sunshine)	1 pkg (1.5 oz)	220	3	12
Cheez-It (Sunshine)	1 pkg (2 oz)	290	4	16
Cheez-It (Sunshine)	27 (1 oz)	160	2	8

FOOD	PORTION	CALS.	SAT. FAT	FAT
Cheez-It Hot & Spicy (Sunshine)	1 pkg (1.5 oz)	220	2	12
Cheez-It Hot & Spicy (Sunshine)	26 (1 oz)	160	2	8
Cheez-It Low Sodium (Sunshine)	27 (1 oz)	160	2	8
Cheez-It Party Mix (Sunshine)	½ cup (1 oz)	140	1	5
Cheez-It Reduced Fat (Sunshine)	30 (1 oz) (1.9 oz)	130	1	5
Cheez-It White Cheddar (Sunshine)	1 pkg (1.5 oz)	220	3	12
Cheez-It White Cheddar (Sunshine)	26 (1 oz)	160	2	9
Cheez 'n Crackers (Handi-Snacks)	1 pkg	120	5	9
Cheez 'n Crackers Bacon (Handi-Snacks)	1 pkg	130	4	9
Chicken in a Biskit (Nabisco)	7	80	1	5
Club (Keebler)	2	30	tr	2
Corn Crackers Salt Free (Venus)	5 (0.5 oz)	60	tr	1
Cracked Wheat (Pepperidge Farm)	3	100	1	4
Cracked Wheat Wafers Salt Free (Venus)	5 (0.5 oz)	60	tr	1
Cracker Bread (Venus)	5 (0.5 oz)	60	tr	1
Cracker Crisp Country Butter (McCrackens)	1 oz	140	—	8
Cracker Crisp Sour Cream & Chives (McCrackens)	1 oz	140	—	8
Cracker Crisp Tangy Cheddar (McCrackens)	1 oz	140	—	8
Cracker Crisp Toasted Wheat (McCrackens)	1 oz	140	—	8
Cracker Snacks Cheddar (Frito Lay)	13–16 (1 oz)	70	—	4
Cracker Snacks Zesty Italian (Frito Lay)	13–16 (1 oz)	70	—	3
Crackups (Nabisco)	15 (0.5 oz)	70	tr	3
Crisp Bread Dark Finn Crisp (Ryvita)	2	38	—	tr
Crisp Bread Dark Rye (Ryvita)	1	26	—	tr

FOOD	PORTION	CALS.	SAT. FAT	FAT
Crisp Bread Dark w/ Caraway Seeds Finn Crisp (Ryvita)	2	38	—	tr
Crisp Bread Light Rye (Ryvita)	1	26	—	tr
Crisp Bread Toasted Sesame Rye (Ryvita)	1	31	—	tr
Crispbread Garlic (Weight Watchers)	2	30	0	0
Crispy Graham (Pepperidge Farm)	4	70	0	2
Crown Pilot (Nabisco)	1	70	tr	2
Double Cheddar (FFV)	7	70	—	2
English Water Biscuits (Pepperidge Farm)	4	70	0	1
Escort (Nabisco)	3	70	tr	4
Flutters Garden Herb (Pepperidge Farm)	0.75 oz	100	1	4
Flutters Golden Sesame (Pepperidge Farm)	0.75 oz	100	1	5
Flutters Original Butter (Pepperidge Farm)	0.75 oz	100	1	4
Flutters Toasted Wheat (Pepperidge Farm)	0.75 oz	100	1	5
Garden Vegetable (Pepperidge Farm)	5	60	0	2
Goldfish (Pepperidge Farm)				
Cheddar Cheese	1 pkg (1.5 oz)	190	2	6
Cheese Thins	4	50	0	2
Original	1 oz	130	1	5
Parmesan Cheese	1 oz	120	1	4
Pizza Flavored	1 oz	130	1	5
Pretzel	1 oz	110	—	3
Gourmet Flatbread Caraway & Rye (Adrienne's)	2	20	—	tr
Gourmet Flatbread Classic Island (Adrienne's)	2	20	—	tr
Gourmet Flatbread Slightly Onion (Adrienne's)	2	20	—	tr
Gourmet Flatbread Ten Grain (Adrienne's)	2	20	0	tr
Goya Crackers	1	30	—	0
Ham & Cheese Crispy Wafers (FFV)	7	70	—	2

FOOD	PORTION	CALS.	SAT. FAT	FAT
Harvest Crisps 5 Grain (Nabisco)	6	60	—	2
Harvest Crisps Oat (Nabisco)	6	60	—	2
Hearty Wheat (Pepperidge Farm)	4	100	1	5
Herb Stoned Wheat (Health Valley)	13	55	—	2
Herb Stoned Wheat No Salt (Health Valley)	13	55	—	2
Hi Ho (Sunshine)	9 (1.1 oz)	160	2	9
Hi Ho Butter Flavored (Sunshine)	9 (1.1 oz)	160	2	9
Hi Ho Cracked Pepper (Sunshine)	9 (1.1 oz)	160	2	9
Hi Ho Low Salt (Sunshine)	9 (1.1 oz)	160	2	9
Hi Ho Multi Grain (Sunshine)	9 (1.1 oz)	160	2	9
Hi Ho Reduced Fat (Sunshine)	10 (1.1 oz)	140	1	5
Hi Ho Whole Wheat (Sunshine)	9 (1.1 oz)	150	2	8
Hors D'oeuvre (Venus)	3 (0.5 oz)	60	tr	2
Ideal Crispbread Extra Thin	3	48	0	0
Ideal Crispbread Fiber Thins	2	41	—	1
Ideal Crispbread Oatbran Thins	2	50	0	0
Kavli	1 piece	40	—	tr
Krispy Cracked Pepper (Sunshine)	5 (0.5 oz)	60	0	2
Krispy Fat Free (Sunshine)	5 (0.5 oz)	60	0	0
Krispy Mild Cheddar (Sunshine)	5 (0.5 oz)	60	1	2
Krispy Original (Sunshine)	5 (0.5 oz)	60	0	2
Krispy Soup & Oyster Crackers (Sunshine)	17 (0.5 oz)	60	0	2
Krispy Unsalted Tops (Sunshine)	5 (0.5 oz)	60	0	2
Krispy Whole Wheat (Sunshine)	5 (0.5 oz)	60	0	2
Lanchee (Lance)	1 pkg (35 g)	180	2	11
Lavash Wafer Bread Crisp Original (Venus)	2 (0.5 oz)	60	tr	1

FOOD	PORTION	CALS.	SAT. FAT	FAT
Lavash Wafer Bread Crisp Sesame (Venus)	2 (0.5 oz)	60	tr	1
Melba Rounds (Devonsheer)				
Garlic	0.5 oz	56	—	1
Honey Bran	0.5 oz	52	—	1
Onion	0.5 oz	51	—	1
Plain	0.5 oz	53	—	1
Plain Unsalted	0.5 oz	52	—	1
Rye	0.5 oz	53	—	1
Sesame	0.5 oz	57	—	2
Melba Toast Garlic (Keebler)	2	25	tr	tr
Melba Toast Long (Keebler)	2	30	tr	tr
Melba Toast Oblong (Lance)	2	30	0	0
Melba Toast Onion (Keebler)	2	25	tr	tr
Melba Toast Plain (Keebler)	2	25	tr	tr
Melba Toast Plain (Lance)	2	20	0	0
Melba Toast Pumpernickel (Old London)	0.5 oz	54	—	1
Melba Toast Round Garlic (Lance)	2	20	0	0
Melba Toast Round Onion (Lance)	2	20	0	0
Melba Toast Rye (Old London)	0.5 oz	52	—	1
Melba Toast Sesame (Keebler)	2	25	tr	tr
Melba Toast Sesame (Old London)	0.5 oz	55	—	2
Melba Toast Sesame Unsalted (Old London)	0.5 oz	55	—	2
Melba Toast Wheat (Old London)	0.5 oz	51	—	1
Melba Toast White (Old London)	0.5 oz	51	—	1
Melba Toast White Unsalted (Old London)	0.5 oz	51	—	1
Melba Toast Whole Grain (Old London)	0.5 oz	52	—	1

FOOD	PORTION	CALS.	SAT. FAT	FAT
Melba Toast Whole Grain Unsalted (Old London)	0.5 oz	53	—	1
Melba Toast Sesame (Lance)	2	25	0	0
Multi Grain (Pepperidge Farm)	4	70	0	2
NAB Cheese Peanut Butter Sandwich (Nabisco)	4 (1 oz)	130	1	7
NAB Peanut Butter Toast Sandwich (Nabisco)	4 (1 oz)	130	1	7
Nekot (Lance)	1.5 oz	210	2	10
Nip-Chee (Lance)	1.3 oz	180	2	8
Nips Cheese (Nabisco)	13	70	tr	3
Oat Bran Krisp (Ralston)	2	60	—	3
Oat Bran Wafers (Venus)	5 (0.5 oz)	60	—	1
Oat Bran Wafers Salt Free (Venus)	5 (0.5 oz)	60	tr	1
Oat Thins (Nabisco)	8 (0.5 oz)	70	tr	3
Ocean Crisp (FFV)	1	60	—	1
Old Brussels Cheddar Waferettes (Venus)	5 (0.5 oz)	80	1	5
Old Brussels Jalapeno Waferettes (Venus)	5 (0.5 oz)	80	1	5
Onion (Hain)	1 oz	130	—	6
Onion No Salt Added (Hain)	1 oz	130	—	6
Oyster Crackers (Lance)	1 pkg (14 g)	70	1	2
Oyster Crackers Large (Keebler)	26	80	tr	2
Oyster Crackers Small (Keebler)	50	80	tr	2
Oysterettes (Nabisco)	18	60	tr	1
Peanut Butter & Cheese (Eagle)	1 oz	280	—	16
Penut Butter Filled (Frito Lay)	6 (1.5 oz)	210	—	10
Peanut Butter 'n Cheez Crackers (Handi-Snacks)	1 pkg	190	4	14
Peanut Butter Wheat (Lance)	1 pkg (37 g)	190	2	11
Pita Crisps (Tuscany)	1 oz	90	—	1
Pita Crisps Sesame (Tuscany)	1 oz	96	—	2
Premium Bits (Nabisco)	16 (0.5 oz)	70	tr	3
Premium Saltine (Nabisco)	5 (0.5 oz)	60	tr	2

FOOD	PORTION	CALS.	SAT. FAT	FAT
Premium Saltine Fat Free (Nabisco)	5	50	0	0
Premium Saltine Low Salt (Nabisco)	5	60	tr	2
Premium Saltine Unsalted Tops (Nabisco)	5	60	tr	2
Premium Soup & Oyster (Nabisco)	20 (0.5 oz)	60	tr	1
Premium With Multi-Grain (Nabisco)	5	60	tr	2
Rice Bran (Health Valley)	7	130	—	4
Rice Thins Original (Sesmark)	15 (1 oz)	130	0	3
Rice Thins Teriyaki Flavored (Sesmark)	13 (1 oz)	130	0	3
Rich (Hain)	1 oz	130	—	5
Rich No Salt Added (Hain)	1 oz	130	—	5
Ritz (Nabisco)	4 (0.5 oz)	70	tr	4
Ritz Bits (Nabisco)	22 (0.5 oz)	70	tr	4
Ritz Bits Cheese (Nabisco)	22 (0.5 oz)	70	tr	4
Ritz Bits Cheese Pizza (Nabisco)	5 (0.5 oz)	80	1	5
Ritz Bits Cheese Sandwiches (Nabisco)	6 (0.5 oz)	80	1	5
Ritz Bits Low Salt (Nabisco)	22 (0.5 oz)	70	tr	4
Ritz Bits Nacho Cheese (Nabisco)	6 (0.5 oz)	80	1	5
Ritz Bits Peanut Butter Sandwiches (Nabisco)	6 (0.5 oz)	80	tr	4
Ritz Low Salt (Nabisco)	4 (0.5 oz)	70	tr	4
Rounds Bacon (Old London)	0.5 oz	53	—	1
Rounds Garlic (Old London)	0.5 oz	56	—	1
Rounds Onion (Old London)	0.5 oz	52	—	1
Rounds Rye (Old London)	0.5 oz	52	—	1
Rounds Sesame (Old London)	0.5 oz	56	—	2
Rounds White (Old London)	0.5 oz	48	—	1
Rounds Whole Grain (Old London)	0.5 oz	54	—	1
Royal Lunch (Nabisco)	1 (0.5 oz)	60	tr	2

FOOD	PORTION	CALS.	SAT. FAT	FAT
Rye (Hain)	1 oz	120	—	4
Rye No Salt Added (Hain)	1 oz	120	—	4
Rye-Chee (Lance)	1 pkg (41 g)	190	2	9
Rye Twins (Lance)	2	30	0	1
Rye Wafers Low Salt (Venus)	5 (0.5 oz)	60	tr	1
Rykrisp Natural	2	40	0	0
Rykrisp Seasoned	2	45	—	1
Rykrisp Seasoned Twindividuals	2	45	—	1
Rykrisp Sesame	2	50	—	2
Saltines (Lance)	2	25	0	1
Saltines Slug Pack (Lance)	4	50	0	1
Savory Thins Original (Sesmark)	15 (1 oz)	125	0	2
Sesame (Hain)	1 oz	140	—	7
Sesame (Pepperidge Farm)	4	80	1	4
Sesame Crisp (FFV)	2	120	—	3
Sesame No Salt Added (Hain)	1 oz	140	—	7
Sesame Stoned Wheat (Health Valley)	13	55	—	2
Sesame Stoned Wheat No Salt Added (Health Valley)	13	55	—	2
Sesame Thins Cheddar (Sesmark)	9 (1 oz)	150	1	8
Sesame Thins Garlic (Sesmark)	9 (1 oz)	150	1	8
Sesame Thins Original (Sesmark)	9 (1 oz)	150	1	8
Sesame Thins Unsalted (Sesmark)	11 (1 oz)	150	1	8
Sesame Twins (Lance)	2	40	0	1
Seven Grain Vegetable Stoned Wheat (Health Valley)	13	55	—	2
Seven Grain Vegetable Stoned Wheat No Salt Added (Health Valley)	13	55	—	2
Snack Crackers Toasted Rye (Keebler)	2	30	tr	2
Snack Crackers Toasted Sesame (Keebler)	2	30	tr	2

FOOD	PORTION	CALS.	SAT. FAT	FAT
Snack Crackers Toasted Wheat (Keebler)	2	30	tr	2
Snack Mix Classic (Pepperidge Farm)	1 oz	140	1	8
Snack Mix Lightly Smoked (Pepperidge Farm)	1 oz	150	1	9
Snack Sticks Cheese (Pepperidge Farm)	8	130	2	5
Snack Sticks Pretzel (Pepperidge Farm)	8	120	0	3
Snack Sticks Pumpernickel (Pepperidge Farm)	8	140	1	6
Snack Sticks Sesame (Pepperidge Farm)	8	140	1	5
Snackbread High Fiber (Ryvita)	1	14	—	tr
Snackbread Original Wheat (Ryvita)	1	20	—	tr
Snackwell's Cheese	18 (0.5 oz)	60	tr	1
Snackwell's Wheat	5 (0.5 oz)	50	0	0
Snorkles Fun Cheddar (Nabisco)	27 (0.5 oz)	60	tr	2
Snorkles Fun Pizza (Nabisco)	27 (0.5 oz)	60	tr	2
Snorkles Fun Ranch (Nabisco)	27 (0.5 oz)	60	tr	2
Sociables (Nabisco)	6 (0.5 oz)	70	tr	3
Sour Cream & Chive (Hain)	1 oz	130	—	6
Sour Cream & Chive No Salt Added (Hain)	1 oz	130	—	6
Sourdough (Hain)	0.5 oz	65	—	3
Sourdough Low Salt (Hain)	1 oz	130	—	5
Spicy Lightly Smoked (Pepperidge Farm)	1 oz	140	1	8
Stoned Wheat (FFV)	4	60	—	1
Stoned Wheat (Health Valley)	13	55	—	2
Stoned Wheat No Salt Added (Health Valley)	13	55	—	2
Stoned Wheat Wafers Bite Size (Venus)	7 (0.5 oz)	60	tr	1
Swiss Cheese (Nabisco)	7	70	tr	3

FOOD	PORTION	CALS.	SAT. FAT	FAT
Tam Tams (Manischewitz)	10	147	—	8
Tam Tams No Salt (Manischewitz)	10	138	—	7
Tams Garlic (Manischewitz)	10	153	—	8
Tams Onion (Manischewitz)	10	150	—	8
Tams Wheat (Manischewitz)	10	150	—	8
Tid Bits Cheese (Nabisco)	15	70	tr	4
Toastchee (Lance)	1 pkg (39 g)	190	2	11
Toasted Bacon Snack Crackers (Keebler)	2	30	tr	2
Toasted Onion Snack Crackers (Keebler)	2	30	tr	2
Toasted Pumpernickel Snack Crackers (Keebler)	2	30	tr	2
Toasted Rice (Pepperidge Farm)	4	60	0	2
Toasted Wheat w/ Onion (Pepperidge Farm)	4	80	1	3
Toasty (Lance)	1 pkg (35 g)	180	2	10
Toasty Crackers w/ Peanut Butter (Little Debbie)	1 pkg (0.9 oz)	140	2	7
Toasty Crackers w/ Peanut Butter (Little Debbie)	1 pkg (1.4 oz)	200	2	10
Town House (Keebler)	2	35	tr	2
Triscuit (Nabisco)	3 (0.5 oz)	60	tr	2
Triscuit Deli-Style Rye (Nabisco)	3 (0.5 oz)	60	tr	2
Triscuit Low Salt (Nabisco)	3 (0.5 oz)	60	tr	2
Triscuit Wheat 'n Bran (Nabisco)	3 (0.5 oz)	60	tr	2
Tuscany Toast	1 oz	95	—	2
Tuscany Toast Pepato	1 oz	93	—	2
Tuscany Toast Pesto	1 oz	96	—	2
Tuscany Toast Tomato	1 oz	95	—	2
Twigs Sesame & Cheese Sticks (Nabisco)	5 (0.5 oz)	70	tr	4
Uneeda Biscuit Unsalted Tops (Nabisco)	2 (0.5 oz)	60	tr	2
Unsalted (Estee)	1 (0.5 oz)	70	1	2
Vegetable (Hain)	1 oz	130	—	5

FOOD	PORTION	CALS.	SAT. FAT	FAT
Vegetable No Salt Added (Hain)	1 oz	130	—	5
Vegetable Thins (Nabisco)	6 (0.5 oz)	70	tr	4
Waldorf Sodium Free (Keebler)	2	30	tr	1
Wasa Crispbread Breakfast	1	50	—	1
Wasa Crispbread Extra Crisp	1	25	0	0
Wasa Crispbread Falu Rye	1	30	0	0
Wasa Crispbread Fiber Plus	1	35	—	1
Wasa Crispbread Golden Rye	1	30	0	0
Wasa Crispbread Hearty Rye	1	50	0	0
Wasa Crispbread Light Rye	1	25	0	0
Wasa Crispbread Royal	½	26	0	0
Wasa Crispbread Savory Sesame	1	30	—	1
Wasa Crispbread Sesame Rye	1	30	—	1
Wasa Crispbread Sesame Wheat	1	60	—	2
Wasa Crispbread Toasted Wheat	1	50	—	1
Water Crackers Fat Free (Venus)	5 (0.5 oz)	55	0	0
Waverly (Nabisco)	4 (0.5 oz)	70	tr	3
Waverly Low Salt (Nabisco)	4	70	tr	3
Wheat Crackers with Chedder Cheese (Little Debbie)	1 pkg (0.9 oz)	140	2	7
Wheat Crispy Wafers (FFV)	6	70	—	3
Wheat Twins (Lance)	2	30	0	1
Wheat Thins (Nabisco)	8 (0.5 oz)	70	tr	3
Wheat Thins Low Salt (Nabisco)	8 (0.5 oz)	70	tr	3
Wheat Thins Multi-Grain (Nabisco)	8 (0.5 oz)	60	tr	2
Wheat Thins Nutty (Nabisco)	7	70	tr	4
Wheat Wafers Low Salt (Venus)	5 (0.5 oz)	60	tr	2

FOOD	PORTION	CALS.	SAT. FAT	FAT
Wheatswafer (Lance)	2	30	0	1
Wheatsworth Stone Ground (Nabisco)	4 (0.5 oz)	70	tr	3
Wholegrain Wheat (Keebler)	2	30	tr	1
Zesta Saltine (Keebler)	2	25	tr	1
Zesta Saltine Unsalted Top (Keebler)	2	25	tr	1
Zings! Cheddar (Nabisco)	15 (0.5 oz)	70	tr	3
Zings! Original (Nabisco)	15 (0.5 oz)	70	tr	3
Zings! Ranch (Nabisco)	15 (0.5 oz)	70	tr	3
Zwieback (Nabisco)	2 (0.5 oz)	60	tr	1
cheese	1 (1 in sq) (1 g)	5	tr	tr
cheese	14 (0.5 oz)	71	1	4
cheese low sodium	1 (1 in sq) (1 g)	5	tr	tr
cheese low sodium	14 (0.5 oz)	71	1	4
cheese w/ peanut butter filling	1 (0.24 oz)	34	tr	2
crispbread	3	61	—	2
crispbread rye	1 (0.35 oz)	37	tr	tr
crispbread rye	3	77	—	1
melba toast plain	1 (5 g)	19	tr	tr
melba toast pumpernickel	1 (5 g)	19	tr	tr
melba toast rye	1 (5 g)	19	tr	tr
melba toast wheat	1 (5 g)	19	tr	tr
milk	1 (0.42 oz)	55	tr	2
oyster cracker	1 (1 g)	4	tr	tr
peanut butter sandwich	1 (7 g)	34	tr	2
rusk toast	1 (0.35 oz)	41	tr	1
rye w/ cheese filling	1 (0.24 oz)	34	tr	2
rye wafers plain	2 (0.9 oz)	84	tr	tr
rye wafers seasoned	1 (0.8 oz)	84	tr	2
saltines	1 (3 g)	13	tr	tr
saltines low salt	1 (3 g)	13	tr	tr
snack cracker	1 (3 g)	15	tr	1
snack cracker low salt	1 (3 g)	15	tr	1
snack cracker w/ cheese filling	1 (7 g)	33	tr	2
soup cracker	1 (1 g)	4	tr	tr
water biscuits	3	92	—	3
wheat w/ cheese filling	1 (0.24 oz)	35	tr	2
wheat w/ peanut butter filling	1 (0.24 oz)	35	tr	2
wheat thins	1 (2 g)	9	tr	tr

FOOD	PORTION	CALS.	SAT. FAT	FAT
wheat thins	7 (0.5 oz)	67	1	3
wheat thins low salt	7 (0.5 oz)	67	1	3
whole wheat	1 (4 g)	18	tr	1
whole wheat low salt	1 (4 g)	18	tr	1
zwieback	3.5 oz	374	—	4

CRANBERRIES
CANNED

FOOD	PORTION	CALS.	SAT. FAT	FAT
Cranberry Sauce Jellied (Ocean Spray)	2 oz	90	0	0
Cranberry Sauce Jellied Old Fashioned (S&W)	½ cup	90	0	0
CranFruit Cranberry Raspberry Sauce (Ocean Spray)	2 oz	100	0	0
CranFruit Cranberry Strawberry Sauce (Ocean Spray)	2 oz	100	0	0
CranFruit Cranberry Orange Sauce (Ocean Spray)	2 oz	100	0	0
Whole Berry Sauce (Ocean Spray)	2 oz	90	0	0
cranberry sauce sweetened	½ cup	209	—	tr

FRESH

FOOD	PORTION	CALS.	SAT. FAT	FAT
Ocean Spray	½ cup	25	0	0
chopped	1 cup	54	—	tr

JUICE

FOOD	PORTION	CALS.	SAT. FAT	FAT
Apple & Eve	6 fl oz	100	0	0
Ocean Spray Cocktail	8 fl oz	140	0	0
Ocean Spray Cocktail Reduced Calorie	8 fl oz	50	0	0
Ocean Spray Lightstyle Cranberry Juice Cocktail Low Calorie	8 fl oz	40	0	0
Seneca Cranberry Juice Cocktail frzn, as prep	8 fl oz	140	0	0
Smucker's Juice Sparkler	10 oz	140	—	tr
Tropicana Twister Ruby Red	1 bottle (10 fl oz)	150	0	0
Tropicana Twister Ruby Red	8 fl oz	120	0	0
Veryfine	8 oz	160	0	0
cranberry juice cocktail	1 cup	147	—	tr

FOOD	PORTION	CALS.	SAT. FAT	FAT
cranberry juice cocktail	6 oz	108	—	tr
cranberry juice coctail low calorie	6 oz	33	0	0
cranberry juice cocktail, frzn	12 oz can	821	0	0
cranberry juice cocktail, frzn, as prep	6 oz	102	0	0

CRANBERRY BEANS
CANNED
cranberry beans	1 cup	216	tr	1

DRIED
Bean Cuisine	½ cup	115	—	1
cooked	1 cup	240	tr	1

CRAYFISH
cooked	3 oz	97	tr	1
raw	3 oz	76	tr	1
raw	8	24	tr	tr

CREAM
(see also SOUR CREAM, SOUR CREAM SUBSTITUTES, WHIPPED TOPPINGS)

LIQUID
Half & Half (Farmland)	2 tbsp	40	2	3
Light Cream (Farmland)	2 tbsp	30	2	3
half & half	1 tbsp	20	1	2
half & half	1 cup	315	17	28
heavy whipping	1 tbsp	52	3	6
light coffee	1 tbsp	29	2	3
light coffee	1 cup	496	29	46
light whipping	1 tbsp	44	3	5

WHIPPED
heavy whipping	1 cup	411	55	44
light whipping	1 cup	345	46	37

CREAM CHEESE
NEUFCHATEL
Philadephia Brand Light Spreadery	1 oz	80	4	7
Neufchatel w/ Classic Ranch Flavor	1 oz	70	4	7
Neufchatel w/ French Onion	1 oz	70	4	6
Neufchatel w/ Garden Vegetables	1 oz	70	3	6

FOOD	PORTION	CALS.	SAT. FAT	FAT
Neufchatel w/ Garlic & Herb	1 oz	70	4	6
Neufchatel w/ Strawberries	1 oz	70	3	5
WisPride Garden Vegetable Cup	2 tbsp (1.1 oz)	60	3	5
WisPride Garlic & Herb Cup	2 tbsp (1.1 oz)	60	3	5
neufchatel	1 oz	74	4	7
neufchatel	1 pkg (3 oz)	221	13	20
REDUCED CALORIE				
Alpine Lace Fat Free Garden Vegetable	2 tbsp (1 oz)	30	tr	tr
Alpine Lace Fat Free Garlic & Herbs	2 tbsp (1 oz)	30	tr	tr
Friendship NY Style Reduced Fat	2 tbsp (1 oz)	50	2	3
Healthy Choice Fat Free	1 oz	25	0	0
Healthy Choice Fat Free Soft Garlic & Herb	1 oz	25	0	0
Healthy Choice Fat Free Soft Strawberry	1 oz	35	0	0
Philadelphia Brand Light	1 oz	60	3	5
Weight Watchers	2 tbsp	35	—	2
REGULAR				
Fleur De Lait	2 tbsp (1 oz)	100	6	10
Bermuda Onion & Chives	2 tbsp (0.9 oz)	90	5	8
Cinnamon Raisin	2 tbsp (0.9 oz)	90	5	8
Date Nut Rum	2 tbsp (0.9 oz)	90	5	8
Fresh Cut Garden Vegetable	2 tbsp (0.9 oz)	80	5	8
Garden Vegetable	2 tbsp (0.9 oz)	80	5	8
Garlic & Spice	2 tbsp (0.9 oz)	90	6	9
Herb & Sprice	2 tbsp (0.9 oz)	90	6	9
Irish Creme	2 tbsp (0.9 oz)	100	5	9
Lemon	2 tbsp (0.9 oz)	90	4	7
Lox	2 tbsp (0.9 oz)	90	5	8
Maindarin Orange	2 tbsp (0.9 oz)	90	5	7
Peach	2 tbsp (0.9 oz)	90	5	7
Pineapple	2 tbsp (0.9 oz)	90	5	8
Strawberry	2 tbsp (0.9 oz)	90	5	8
Toasted Onion	2 tbsp (0.9 oz)	90	6	9
Wildberry	2 tbsp (0.9 oz)	90	5	7

FOOD	PORTION	CALS.	SAT. FAT	FAT
Fresh Cut				
Bac'n & Horseradish	2 tbsp (0.9 oz)	90	5	9
Bermuda Onion & Chives	2 tbsp (0.9 oz)	90	5	8
Date, Nut & Rum	2 tbsp (0.9 oz)	90	5	9
Garlic & Spice	2 tbsp (0.9 oz)	90	6	9
Herb & Spice	2 tbsp (0.9 oz)	90	6	9
Lox	2 tbsp (0.9 oz)	90	5	8
Peaches & Cream	2 tbsp (0.9 oz)	90	5	7
Strawberry	2 tbsp (0.9 oz)	90	5	8
Philadelphia Brand	1 oz	100	6	10
Philadelphia Brand With Chives	1 oz	90	5	9
Philadelphia Brand With Pimentos	1 oz	90	5	9
Ultra Delight				
Cheddar Cream Cheese	2 tbsp (0.9 oz)	60	3	4
Chive	2 tbsp (0.9 oz)	60	3	4
Garlic	2 tbsp (0.9 oz)	60	3	4
Mixed Berry	2 tbsp (0.9 oz)	70	3	4
Nacho	2 tbsp (0.9 oz)	60	3	4
Salsa	2 tbsp (0.9 oz)	60	3	4
Shrimp	2 tbsp (0.9 oz)	60	3	4
Strawberry	2 tbsp (0.9 oz)	60	3	4
Vegetable	2 tbsp (0.9 oz)	50	3	4
cream cheese	1 oz	99	6	10
cream cheese	1 pkg (3 oz)	297	19	30
SOFT				
Heluva Good Cheese	1 tbsp (1 oz)	100	6	10
Philadelphia Brand	1 oz	100	5	10
Philadelphia Brand w/ Chives & Onions	1 oz	100	5	9
Philadelphia Brand w/ Herb & Garlic	1 oz	100	5	9
Philadelphia Brand w/ Olives & Pimento	1 oz	90	5	8
Philadelphia Brand w/ Pineapple	1 oz	90	5	8
Philadelphia Brand w/ Smoked Salmon	1 oz	90	5	8
Philadelphia Brand w/ Strawberries	1 oz	90	5	8
WHIPPED				
Philadelphia Brand	1 oz	100	6	10

FOOD	PORTION	CALS.	SAT. FAT	FAT
Philadelphia Brand w/ Chives	1 oz	90	5	8
Philadelphia Brand w/ Onions	1 oz	90	5	8
Philadelphia Brand w/ Smoked Salmon	1 oz	90	5	8

CREAM CHEESE SUBSTITUTES

Better Than Cream Cheese French Onion Tofutti	1 oz	80	2	8
Better Than Cream Cheese Herb & Chive Tofutti	1 oz	80	2	8
Better Than Cream Cheese Plain Tofutti	1 oz	80	2	8

CREAM OF TARTAR

cream of tartar	1 tsp	8	0	0

CREPES

basic crepe, unfilled	1	75	—	2

CRESS

(see also WATERCRESS)

FRESH

garden, cooked	½ cup	16	tr	tr
garden, raw	½ cup	8	tr	tr

CROAKER

FRESH

atlantic, breaded & fried	3 oz	188	3	11
atlantic, raw	3 oz	89	1	3

CROISSANT

All Butter (Sara Lee)	1	170	—	9
All Butter Petite Size (Sara Lee)	1	120	—	6
Colonial Wheat Croissants (Rainbo)	1	300	—	19
Croissant Sandwich Quartet (Pepperidge Farm)	1	170	—	7
Petite All Butter (Pepperidge Farm)	1	120	—	6
apple	1 (2 oz)	145	3	5
cheese	1 (2 oz)	236	5	12
croissant	1 (2 oz)	232	7	12

FOOD	PORTION	CALS.	SAT. FAT	FAT
TAKE-OUT				
w/ egg & cheese	1	369	14	25
w/ egg, cheese & bacon	1	413	15	28
w/ egg, cheese & ham	1	475	17	34
w/ egg, cheese & sausage	1	524	18	38

CROUTONS

Arnold

Crispy Cheddar Romano	0.5 oz	64	—	3
Crispy Cheese Garlic	0.5 oz	60	tr	2
Crispy Fine Herbs	0.5 oz	50	0	1
Crispy Italian	0.5 oz	60	tr	3
Crispy Onion & Garlic	0.5 oz	60	tr	2
Crispy Seasoned	0.5 oz	60	tr	3

Brownberry

Ceasar Salad	0.5 oz	62	—	3
Cheddar Cheese	0.5 oz	63	—	3
Onion And Garlic	0.5 oz	60	—	2
Seasoned	0.5 oz	59	—	2
Toasted	0.5 oz	56	—	1
Kellogg's Croutettes	1 cup (1 oz)	100	0	0

Pepperidge Farm

Cheddar & Romano Cheese	0.5 oz	60	0	2
Cheese & Garlic	0.5 oz	70	1	3
Onion & Garlic	0.5 oz	70	0	3
Seasoned	0.5 oz	70	1	3
Sour Cream & Chive	0.5 oz	70	1	3
plain	1 cup (1 oz)	122	tr	2
seasoned	1 cup (1.4 oz)	186	2	7

CUCUMBER

FRESH

raw	1 (11 oz)	38	tr	tr
raw, sliced	½ cup	7	tr	tr
JARRED				
Rosoff's Salad	3 slices (1 oz)	12	0	0
Schorr's Cucumber Garden Salad	3 slices (1 oz)	12	0	0
TAKE-OUT				
cucumber salad	3.5 oz	50	tr	tr

CUMIN

seed	1 tsp	8	—	tr

FOOD	PORTION	CALS.	SAT. FAT	FAT
CURRANTS				
DRIED				
zante	½ cup	204	tr	tr
FRESH				
black	½ cup	36	tr	tr
JUICE				
black currant nectar	3.5 oz	55	—	0
red currant nectar	3.5 oz	54	—	tr
CUSK				
fresh fillet, baked	3 oz	106	—	1
CUSTARD				
Custard (Royal)	mix for 1 serving	60	—	0
Flan (Jell-O)	½ cup	151	—	4
Flan Caramel Custard (Royal)	mix for 1 serving	60	—	0
Golden Egg Americana (Jell-O)	½ cup	160	—	6
baked	1 cup	305	7	17
custard, as prep from mix	½ cup	161	—	5
zabaglione (home recipe)	½ cup (57.2 g)	135	2	5
CUTTLEFISH				
steamed	3 oz	134	tr	1
DANDELION GREENS				
fresh, cooked	½ cup	17	—	tr
fresh, raw, chopped	½ cup	13	—	tr
DANISH PASTRY				
FROZEN				
Apple (Pepperidge Farm)	1	220	—	8
Apple (Sara Lee)	1	120	—	6
Apple Danish Twist (Sara Lee)	1 slice (1.9 oz)	190	—	10
Apple Free & Light (Sara Lee)	1 slice (2 oz)	130	—	0
Cheese (Pepperidge Farm)	1	240	—	14
Cheese (Sara Lee)	1	130	—	8
Cheese Danish Twist (Sara Lee)	1 slice (1.9 oz)	200	—	12
Cinnamon Raisin (Pepperidge Farm)	1	250	—	11
Cinnamon Raisin (Sara Lee)	1	150	—	8

FOOD	PORTION	CALS.	SAT. FAT	FAT
Raspberry (Pepperidge Farm)	1	220	—	9
Raspberry Danish Twist (Sara Lee)	1 slice (1.9 oz)	200	—	9
READY-TO-EAT				
Apple (Hostess)	1 (3.8 oz)	400	10	22
Apple Fruit Roll (Hostess)	1 (2 oz)	180	2	4
Coffee Cake Raspberry (Hostess)	1 (1.2 oz)	110	1	3
almond	1 (4 ¼ in diam) (2.3 oz)	280	4	16
apple	1 (4 ¼ in diam) (2.5 oz)	264	3	13
cheese	1 (3 oz)	353	5	25
cheese	1 (4 ¼ in diam) (2.5 oz)	266	5	16
cinnamon	1 (3 oz)	349	3	17
cinnamon	1 (4 ¼ in diam) (2.3 oz)	262	4	15
cinnamon nut	1 (4 ¼ in diam) (2.3 oz)	280	4	16
fruit	1 (3.3 oz)	335	3	16
lemon	1 (4½ in diam) (2.5 oz)	264	3	13
plain ring	1 (12 oz)	1305	22	71
raisin	1 (4 ¼ in diam) (2.5 oz)	264	3	13
raisin nut	1 (4 ¼ in diam) (2.3 oz)	280	4	16
raspberry	1 (4 ¼ in diam) (2.5 oz)	264	3	13
strawberry	1 (4 ¼ in diam) (2.5 oz)	264	3	13
REFRIGERATED				
Caramel Danish w/ Nuts (Pillsbury)	1	160	2	8
Cinnamon Raisin Danish w/ Icing (Pillsbury)	1	150	2	7
Orange Danish w/ Icing (Pillsbury)	1	150	2	7

DATES

DRIED

Bordo Diced	2 oz	203	—	1
California Deglet Noor	10	240	—	0

FOOD	PORTION	CALS.	SAT. FAT	FAT
Dole Chopped	½ cup	280	0	0
Dole Pitted	½ cup	280	0	0
Dromedary Chopped	¼ cup	130	0	0
Dromedary Pitted	5	100	0	0
chopped	1 cup	489	—	1
whole	10	228	—	tr

DEER
(*see* VENISON)

DIETING AIDS
(*see* NUTRITIONAL SUPPLEMENTS)

DILL
seed	1 tsp	6	tr	tr
sprigs, fresh	5	0	tr	tr
sprigs, fresh	1 cup	4	tr	tr
weed, dry	1 tsp	3	—	tr

DINNER
(*see also* BEEF DISHES, PASTA DINNERS, POT PIES, ORIENTAL FOOD, SPANISH FOODS, VEAL DISHES)

FROZEN

Armour Ham Steak	11 oz	350	—	13
Armour Classics				
Chicken & Noodles	11 oz	230	—	73
Chicken Fettucini	11 oz	260	—	9
Chicken Mesquite	9.5 oz	370	—	16
Chicken Parmigiana	11.5 oz	370	—	19
Chicken w/ Wine & Mushroom Sauce	10.75 oz	280	—	11
Glazed Chicken	10.75 oz	300	—	16
Meat Loaf	11.25 oz	360	—	17
Salisbury Parmigiana	11.5 oz	410	—	21
Salisbury Steak	11.25 oz	350	—	17
Swedish Meatballs	11.25 oz	330	—	18
Turkey w/ Dressing & Gravy	11.5 oz	320	—	12
Veal Parmigiana	11.25 oz	400	—	22
Armour Lite				
Beef Pepper Steak	11.25 oz	220	—	4
Beef Stroganoff	11.25 oz	250	—	6
Chicken Ala King	11.25 oz	290	—	7
Chicken Burgundy	10 oz	210	—	2
Chicken Marsala	10.5 oz	250	—	7
Chicken Oriental	10 oz	180	—	1

FOOD	PORTION	CALS.	SAT. FAT	FAT
Armour Lite *(cont.)*				
Salisbury Steak	11.5 oz	300	—	11
Shrimp Creole	11.25 oz	260	—	2
Sweet & Sour Chicken	11 oz	240	—	2
Banquet				
Beans & Frankfurters Dinner	10 oz	350	—	14
Beef Platter	9 oz	230	—	63
Boneless Chicken Drumsnacker Platter	7 oz	290	—	12
Boneless Chicken Nugget Platter	6 oz	340	—	16
Boneless Chicken Patti Platter	6.75 oz	310	—	15
Chicken & Dumplings	10 oz	270	—	10
Fish Platter	8 oz	270	—	7
Fried Chicken Dinner	9 oz	520	—	29
Ham Platter	8.25 oz	200	—	5
Italian Style Dinner	9 oz	180	—	2
Meat Loaf Dinner	9.5 oz	340	—	19
Mexican Style Combination Dinner	11 oz	360	—	12
Mexican Style Dinner	11 oz	410	—	17
Noodles & Chicken	10 oz	170	—	4
Salisbury Steak Dinner	9 oz	280	—	13
Southern Fried Chicken Platter	8.75 oz	400	—	16
Spaghetti & Meat Sauce	8.75 oz	160	—	4
Veal Parmagian	9.25 oz	330	—	16
Western Style Dinner	9 oz	300	—	16
White Meat Fried Chicken Platter	8.75 oz	390	—	13
White Meat Hot'n Spicy Fried Chicken Platter	9 oz	440	—	15
Banquet Cookin' Bag				
Chicken Ala King	4 oz	110	—	5
Creamed Chipped Beef	4 oz	100	—	4
Gravy & Salisbury Steak	5 oz	190	—	14
Gravy & Sliced Beef	4 oz	100	—	5
Gravy & Sliced Turkey	5 oz	100	—	6
Turkey Chili	4 oz	80	—	2
Banquet Extra Helping				
Beef Dinner	15.5 oz	430	—	13
Chicken Nuggets w/ Barbeque Sauce	10 oz	540	—	19

FOOD	PORTION	CALS.	SAT. FAT	FAT
Chicken Nuggets w/ Sweet & Sour Sauce	10 oz	540	—	19
Fried Chicken All White Meat	14.25 oz	760	—	38
Fried Chicken Dinner	14.25 oz	790	—	43
Meat Loaf	16.25 oz	640	—	34
Mexican Style Dinner	19 oz	680	—	25
Salisbury Steak Dinner	16.25 oz	590	—	28
Southern Fried Chicken Dinner	13.25 oz	790	—	39
Turkey Dinner	17 oz	460	—	12
Banquet Family Entree				
Beef Stew	7 oz	140	—	5
Dumplings & Chicken	7 oz	280	—	14
Gravy & Salisbury Steak	7 oz	260	—	19
Gravy & Sliced Steak	7 oz	140	—	5
Gravy & Sliced Turkey	6 oz	120	—	6
Mushroom Gravy & Charbroiled Beef Patties	7 oz	260	—	18
Noodles & Beef w/ Gravy	7 oz	180	—	6
Onion Gravy & Beef Patties	7 oz	260	—	19
Veal Parmagian Patties	7 oz	320	—	16
Birds Eye Easy Recipe Beef Burgundy, not prep	½ pkg	120	1	5
Birds Eye Easy Recipe Beef Fajitas, not prep	½ pkg	80	0	3
Budget Gourmet				
Beef Cantonese	1 pkg (9.1 oz)	270	—	9
Beef Pot Roast	1 pkg (10.5 oz)	230	3	7
Beef Stroganoff	1 pkg (8.75 oz)	260	5	10
Chicken And Egg Noodles	1 pkg (10 oz)	440	—	26
Chicken Au Gratin	1 pkg (9.1 oz)	230	5	8
Chicken Breast Parmigiana	1 pkg (11 oz)	270	3	9
Chicken Marsala	1 pkg (9 oz)	260	—	8
Chicken With Fettucini	1 pkg (10 oz)	400	—	21
Chinese Style Vegetables And Chicken	1 pkg (10 oz)	280	1	7
French Recipe Chicken	1 pkg (10 oz)	220	4	9
Glazed Turkey	1 pkg (9 oz)	260	2	5

FOOD	PORTION	CALS.	SAT. FAT	FAT
Budget Gourmet *(cont.)*				
Ham And Asparagus Au Gratin	1 pkg (8.7 oz)	300	7	14
Herbed Chicken Breast With Fettucini	1 pkg (11 oz)	240	2	6
Italian Style Vegetables And Chicken	1 pkg (10.25 oz)	310	2	8
Mandarin Chicken	1 pkg (10 oz)	240	1	5
Mesquite Chicken Breast	1 pkg (11 oz)	250	1	6
Orange Glazed Chicken	1 pkg (9 oz)	270	1	3
Oriental Beef	1 pkg (10 oz)	290	3	8
Oriental Chicken With Vegetables	1 pkg (9 oz)	280	1	6
Pepper Steak With Rice	1 pkg (10 oz)	300	—	8
Roast Chicken With Homestyle Gravy	1 pkg (11 oz)	280	2	8
Roast Sirloin Supreme	1 pkg (9 oz)	320	—	15
Sirloin Salisbury Steak	1 pkg (11 oz)	280	4	9
Sirloin Salisbury Steak	1 pkg (9 oz)	220	3	8
Sirloin Tips And Country Vegetables	1 pkg (10 oz)	290	—	17
Sirloin Cheddar Melt	1 pkg (9.4 oz)	380	—	21
Sirloin Of Beef In Herb Sauce	1 pkg (9.5 oz)	250	3	9
Sirloin Of Beef In Wine Sauce	1 pkg (11 oz)	280	2	8
Special Recipe Sirloin Of Beef	1 pkg (11 oz)	250	3	9
Stuffed Turkey Breast	1 pkg (11 oz)	250	2	6
Swedish Meatballs With Noodles	1 pkg (10 oz)	590	—	38
Sweet And Sour Chicken	1 pkg (10 oz)	340	—	5
Teriyaki Beef	1 pkg (10.75 oz)	260	2	7
Teriyaki Chicken Breast	1 pkg (11 oz)	300	1	8
Dining Light				
Chicken Ala King	9 oz	240	—	7
Chicken w/ Noodles	9 oz	240	—	7
Salisbury Steak	9 oz	200	—	8
Sauce & Swedish Meatballs	9 oz	280	—	10
Healthy Choice				
Beef & Peppers Cantonese	1 meal (11.5 oz)	270	3	5

FOOD	PORTION	CALS.	SAT. FAT	FAT
Beef Pepper Steak Oriental	1 meal (9.5 oz)	250	2	4
Beef Tips Francais	1 meal (9.5 oz)	280	2	5
Beef Tips With Sauce	1 meal (11 oz)	290	3	6
Chicken Cantonese	1 meal (11.25 oz)	210	0	1
Chicken Parmigiana	1 meal (11.5 oz)	300	1	2
Chicken And Vegetables Marsala	1 meal (11.5 oz)	220	0	1
Chicken Bangkok	1 meal (9.5 oz)	270	1	4
Chicken Broccoli Alfredo	1 meal (12.1 oz)	370	3	8
Chicken Dijon	1 meal (11 oz)	280	2	4
Chicken Imperial	1 meal (9 oz)	230	1	4
Chicken Picante	1 meal (11.25 oz)	220	2	2
Chicken Teriyaki	1 meal (12.25 oz)	270	1	2
Choutry Herb Chicken	1 meal (11.25 oz)	270	2	4
Classics Beef Broccoli Beijing	1 meal (12 oz)	330	1	3
Classics Cacciatore Chicken	1 meal (12.5 oz)	260	1	3
Classics Chicken Francesca	1 meal (12.5 oz)	360	2	5
Classics Country Inn Roast Turkey	1 meal (10 oz)	250	1	4
Classics Ginger Chicken Hunan	1 meal (12.6 oz)	350	1	3
Classics Mesquite Beef Barbecue	1 meal (11 oz)	310	2	4
Classics Salisbury Steak	1 meal (11 oz)	260	3	6
Classics Sesame Chicken Shanghai	1 meal (12 oz)	310	1	5
Classics Shrimp And Vegetables Maria	1 meal (12.5 oz)	260	1	2
Country Glazed Chicken	1 meal (8.5 oz)	200	1	2
Country Herbed Chicken	1 meal (11.5 oz)	270	2	4
Country Roast Turkey With Mushroom	1 meal (8.5 oz)	220	1	4
Country Turkey And Pasta	1 meal (12.6 oz)	300	2	4
Homestyle Turkey With Vegetables	1 meal (9.5 oz)	260	1	2
Honey Mustard Chicken	1 meal (9.5 oz)	260	0	2
Lemon Pepper Fish	1 meal (10.7 oz)	290	1	5
Mandarin Chicken	1 meal (10 oz)	280	0	3
Mesquite Chicken BBQ	1 meal (10.5 oz)	320	1	2

FOOD	PORTION	CALS.	SAT. FAT	FAT
Healthy Choice *(cont.)*				
Shrimp Marinara	1 meal (10.5 oz)	220	0	1
Smoky Chicken Barbecue	1 meal (12.75 oz)	380	2	5
Southwestern Glazed Chicken	1 meal (12.5 oz)	300	1	3
Sweet & Sour Chicken	1 meal (11.5 oz)	310	1	5
Traditional Breast Of Turkey	1 meal (10.5 oz)	280	1	3
Traditional Meatloaf	1 meal (12 oz)	320	4	8
Traditional Salisbury Steak	1 meal (11.5 oz)	320	3	6
Traditional Beef Tips	1 meal (11.25 oz)	260	2	5
Yankee Pot Roast	1 meal (11 oz)	280	2	5
Kid Cuisine				
Chicken Nuggets	6.8 oz	360	—	17
Chicken Sandwiches	8.2 oz	470	—	17
Fish Sticks	7 oz	360	—	14
Fried Chicken	7.5 oz	430	—	22
Hot Dogs w/ Buns	6.7 oz	450	—	19
Mexican Style	5.7 oz	290	—	8
Mega Meal Chicken Nuggets	8.4 oz	470	—	20
Mega Meal Fried Chicken	10.8 oz	720	—	41
Mega Meal Hot Dog w/ Bun	8.25 oz	500	—	25
Le Menu				
Beef Sirloin Tips	11.5 oz	400	—	18
Beef Stroganoff	10 oz	430	—	24
Chicken A La King	10.25 oz	330	—	13
Chicken Cordon Bleu	11 oz	460	—	20
Chicken in Wine Sauce	10 oz	280	—	7
Chicken Parmigiana	11.75 oz	410	—	20
Chopped Sirloin Beef	12.25 oz	430	—	24
Ham Steak	10 oz	300	—	11
Pepper Steak	11.5 oz	370	—	13
Salisbury Steak	10.5 oz	370	—	20
Sliced Breast of Turkey w/ Mushroom Gravy	10.5 oz	300	—	7
Sweet & Sour Chicken	11.25 oz	400	—	18
Veal Parmigiana	11.25 oz	390	—	17
Yankee Pot Roast	10 oz	330	—	13

FOOD	PORTION	CALS.	SAT. FAT	FAT
Le Menu Entree LightStyle				
Chicken A La King	8.25 oz	240	—	5
Chicken Dijon	8 oz	240	—	7
Empress Chicken	8.25 oz	210	—	5
Glazed Turkey	8.25 oz	260	—	6
Herb Roast Chicken	7.75 oz	260	—	6
Swedish Meatballs	8 oz	260	—	8
Traditional Turkey	8 oz	200	—	5
Le Menu LightStyle				
Glazed Chicken Breast	10 oz	230	—	3
Herb Roasted Chicken	10 oz	240	—	7
Salisbury Steak	10 oz	280	—	9
Sliced Turkey	10 oz	210	—	5
Sweet & Sour Chicken	10 oz	250	—	7
Turkey Divan	10 oz	260	—	7
Veal Marsala	10 oz	230	—	3
Lean Cuisine				
Baked Chicken	1 pkg (8 oz)	240	1	5
Beef Pot Roast	1 pkg (9 oz)	210	2	7
Chicken Italiano	1 pkg (9 oz)	270	2	6
Chicken And Vegetables	1 pkg (10.5 oz)	240	1	5
Chicken In Peanut Sauce	1 pkg (9 oz)	280	1	6
Chicken In Honey Barbecue Sauce	1 pkg (8.75 oz)	250	1	5
Chicken Marsala	1 pkg (8.1 oz)	180	1	4
Chicken Oriental	1 pkg (9 oz)	260	1	6
Chicken Parmesan	1 pkg (10.9 oz)	220	2	5
Chicken Pie	1 pkg (9.5 oz)	320	3	10
Chicken a l'Orange	1 pkg (8 oz)	260	1	3
Fiesta Chicken	1 pkg (8.5 oz)	240	1	5
Fish Divan	1 pkg (10.4 oz)	210	1	6
Glazed Chicken	1 pkg (8.5 oz)	240	1	6
Homestyle Turkey	1 pkg (9.4 oz)	230	2	5
Honey Mustard Chicken	1 pkg (7.5 oz)	250	1	5
Meatloaf	1 pkg (9.4 oz)	270	4	10
Oriental Beef	1 pkg (9 oz)	250	3	8
Roasted Turkey Breast	1 pkg (9.75 oz)	290	1	40
Salisbury Steak With Macaroni & Cheese	1 pkg (9.5 oz)	200	4	10
Stuffed Cabbage	1 pkg (9.5 oz)	220	2	7
Swedish Meatballs	1 pkg (9.1 oz)	290	3	8
Sweet And Sour Chicken	1 pkg (10.4 oz)	260	1	3

FOOD	PORTION	CALS.	SAT. FAT	FAT
Lean Cuisine *(cont.)*				
Turkey Pie	1 pkg (9.5 oz)	300	2	9
Morton				
Beans & Franks w/ Sauce	8.5 oz	300	—	11
Fish w/ Mashed Potatoes & Carrots	9.25 oz	350	—	12
Glazed Ham	8 oz	230	—	3
Gravy & Charbroiled Beef Patty	9 oz	270	—	12
Gravy & Salisbury Steak	9 oz	270	—	16
Tomato Sauce & Meatloaf	9 oz	280	—	16
Veal Parmagian	8.75 oz	230	—	7
Stouffer's				
Chicken A La King	1 pkg (9.5 oz)	320	3	10
Chicken Divan	1 pkg (8 oz)	210	4	10
Creamed Chicken	1 pkg (6.5 oz)	280	7	20
Creamed Chipped Beef	½ cup (4.5 oz)	150	3	11
Creamed Chipped Beef Over Country Biscuit	1 pkg (9 oz)	460	7	28
Escalloped Chicken & Noodles	1 pkg (10 oz)	440	6	29
Green Pepper Steak	1 pkg (10.5 oz)	330	3	9
Ham And Asparagus Bake	1 pkg (9.5 oz)	520	14	36
Homestyle Baked Chicken	1 pkg (8.9 oz)	270	3	12
Homestyle Beef Pot Roast	1 pkg (8.9 oz)	270	3	10
Homestyle Breaded Chicken Tenders	1 pkg (6.6 oz)	380	3	18
Homestyle Chicken Parmigiana	1 pkg (10.9 oz)	320	2	10
Homestyle Chicken & Noodles	1 pkg (10 oz)	310	5	14
Homestyle Chicken Monterey	1 pkg (9.4 oz)	410	9	20
Homestyle Fish Filet With Macaroni & Cheese	1 pkg (9 oz)	430	5	21
Homestyle Fried Chicien	1 pkg (7.1 oz)	330	4	16
Homestyle Meatloaf	1 pkg (9.9 oz)	380	8	24
Homestyle Roast Turkey	1 pkg (7.9 oz)	280	3	11

FOOD	PORTION	CALS.	SAT. FAT	FAT
Homestyle Salisbury Steak	1 pkg (9.6 oz)	370	6	19
Homestyle Sliced Beef And Potatoes	1 pkg (8.1 oz)	270	3	10
Homestyle Veal Parmigiana	1 pkg (11.9 oz)	420	4	19
Lunch Express Chicken With Garden Vegetables	1 pkg (9.9 oz)	340	3	11
Lunch Express Mandarin Chicken	1 pkg (9.75 oz)	270	1	6
Lunch Express Mexican Style Rice With Chicken	1 pkg (9 oz)	270	2	8
Lunch Express Oriental Beef	1 pkg (6.2 oz)	260	2	8
Lunch Express Rice And Chicken Stir-Fry	1 pkg (9 oz)	280	1	9
Stuffed Pepper	1 pkg (10 oz)	200	2	8
Swedish Meatballs	1 pkg (9.25 oz)	440	8	23
Swanson				
Beans & Franks	10.5 oz	440	—	19
Beef	11.25 oz	310	—	6
Beef in Barbecue Sauce	11 oz	460	—	17
Chopped Sirloin Beef	10.75 oz	340	—	16
Fish 'n' Chips	10 oz	500	—	21
Fried Chicken White Meat	10.25 oz	550	—	25
Loin of Pork	10.75 oz	280	—	12
Macaroni & Beef	12 oz	370	—	15
Meatloaf	10.75 oz	360	—	15
Noodles & Chicken	10.5 oz	280	—	8
Salisbury Steak	10.75 oz	400	—	17
Swedish Meatballs	8.5 oz	360	—	20
Swiss Steak	10 oz	350	—	11
Turkey	8.75 oz	270	—	11
Turkey	11.5 oz	350	—	11
Turkey w/ Dressing & Potatoes Homestyle	9 oz	290	—	11
Veal Parmigiana	12.25 oz	430	—	20
Western Style	11.5 oz	430	—	19
Swanson Homestyle				
Chicken Cacciatore	10.95 oz	260	—	8
Chicken Nibbles	4.25 oz	340	—	20

FOOD	PORTION	CALS.	SAT. FAT	FAT
Swanson Homestyle *(cont.)*				
Fish & Fries	6.5 oz	340	—	16
Fried Chicken	7 oz	390	—	21
Salisbury Steak	10 oz	320	—	16
Scalloped Potatoes And Ham	9 oz	300	—	13
Seafood Creole With Rice	9 oz	240	—	6
Sirloin Tips In Burgundy Sauce	7 oz	160	—	5
Turkey With Dressing & Potatoes	9 oz	290	—	11
Veal Parmigiana	10 oz	330	—	13
Swanson Hungry-Man				
Boneless Chicken	17.75 oz	700	—	28
Chopped Beef Steak	16.75 oz	640	—	37
Fried Chicken Dark Meat	14.25 oz	860	—	45
Fried Chicken White Meat	14.25 oz	870	—	46
Salisbury Steak	16.5 oz	680	—	41
Sliced Beef	15.25 oz	450	—	12
Turkey	17 oz	550	—	18
Veal Parmigiana	18.25 oz	590	—	26
Tyson				
Beef Champignon	1 pkg (10.5 oz)	370	—	15
Chicken Picante	1 pkg (9 oz)	250	—	4
Chicken Supreme	1 pkg (9 oz)	230	—	6
Francais	1 pkg (9.5 oz)	280	—	14
Glazed Chicken With Sauce	1 pkg (9.25 oz)	240	—	4
Grilled Chicken	1 pkg (7.75 oz)	220	—	3
Grilled Italian Chicken	1 pkg (9 oz)	210	—	3
Healthy Portions BBQ Chicken	1 pkg (12.5 oz)	400	—	8
Healthy Portions Chicken Marinara	1 pkg (13.75 oz)	340	—	7
Healthy Portions Herb Chicken	1 pkg (13.75 oz)	340	—	4
Healthy Portions Honey Mustard Chicken	1 pkg (13.75 oz)	390	—	6
Healthy Portions Italian Style Chicken	1 pkg (13.75 oz)	310	—	4
Healthy Portions Mesquite Chicken	1 pkg (13.25 oz)	330	—	5

FOOD	PORTION	CALS.	SAT. FAT	FAT
Healthy Portions Salsa Chicken	1 pkg (13.75 oz)	370	—	6
Healthy Portions Sesame Chicken	1 pkg (13.5 oz)	400	—	6
Honey Roasted Chicken	1 pkg (9 oz)	220	—	4
Kiev	1 pkg (9.25 oz)	450	—	25
Marsala	1 pkg (9 oz)	200	—	4
Mesquite	1 pkg (9 oz)	320	—	8
Picatta	1 pkg (9 oz)	200	—	4
Roasted Chicken	1 pkg (9 oz)	200	—	2
Sweet & Sour	1 pkg (11 oz)	420	—	15
Turkey With Gravy	1 pkg (9.5 oz)	320	—	12
Ultra Slim-Fast				
Beef Pepper Steak	12 oz	270	—	4
Chicken & Vegetable	12 oz	290	—	3
Chicken Fettucini	12 oz	380	—	12
Country Style Vegetable & Beef Tips	12 oz	230	—	5
Mesquite Chicken	12 oz	360	—	1
Roasted Chicken in Mushroom Sauce	12 oz	280	—	6
Shrimp Creole	12 oz	240	—	4
Shrimp Marinara	12 oz	290	—	3
Sweet & Sour Chicken	12 oz	330	—	2
Turkey Medallions in Herb Sauce	12 oz	280	—	6
Weight Watchers				
Barbecue Glazed Chicken	7 oz	200	3	6
Beef Sirloin Tips	7.5 oz	210	3	6
Beef Stroganoff	8.5 oz	280	1	9
Chicken Ala King	9 oz	230	1	4
Chicken Cordon Bleu	7.7 oz	170	1	5
Chicken Kiev	7 oz	190	2	5
Homestyle Chicken & Noodles	9 oz	240	2	7
Imperial Chicken	8.5 oz	210	1	4
London Broil	7.5 oz	110	1	3
Oven Baked Fish	7 oz	150	1	4
Southern Baked Chicken	6.3 oz	170	2	7
Stuffed Turkey Breast	8.5 oz	270	3	8
Veal Patty Parmigiana	8.2 oz	150	1	4

FOOD	PORTION	CALS.	SAT. FAT	FAT
DIP				
Avocado Guacamole (Kraft)	2 tbsp	50	2	4
Bacon Horseradish (Heluva Good Cheese)	2 tbsp (1.1 oz)	60	3	5
Bacon & Horseradish (Breakstone)	2 tbsp	70	3	6
Bacon & Horseradish (Kraft)	2 tbsp	60	3	5
Bacon & Horseradish (Kraft Premium)	2 tbsp	50	3	5
Bacon & Horseradish (Sealtest)	2 tbsp	70	3	6
Bacon & Onion (Breakstone)	2 tbsp	70	3	6
Bacon & Onion (Kraft Premium)	1 tbsp	60	3	5
Blue Cheese (Kraft Premium)	2 tbsp	50	2	4
Bean (Eagle)	1 oz	35	—	2
Black Bean Mild (Guiltless Gourmet)	1 oz	25	0	0
Black Bean Spicy (Guiltless Gourmet)	1 oz	25	0	0
Cheddar Cheese (Frito Lay)	1 oz	45	—	3
Chesapeake Clam Gourmet (Breakstone)	2 tbsp	50	3	4
Clam (Breakstone)	2 tbsp	50	3	4
Clam (Heluva Good Cheese)	2 tbsp (1.1 oz)	50	3	5
Clam (Kraft)	2 tbsp	60	1	4
Clam (Kraft Premium)	2 tbsp	45	2	4
Clam (Sealtest)	2 tbsp	50	3	4
Creamy Cucumber (Kraft Premium)	2 tbsp	50	2	4
Creamy Onion (Kraft Premium)	2 tbsp	45	2	4
Cucumber & Onion (Breakstone)	2 tbsp	50	3	4
Cucumber & Onion (Sealtest)	2 tbsp	50	3	4
Fiesta Bean (Chi Chi's)	2 tbsp (0.9 oz)	35	1	2
Fiesta Cheese (Chi Chi's)	2 tbsp (0.9 oz)	40	1	3
French Onion (Breakstone)	2 tbsp	50	3	5
French Onion (Frito Lay)	1 oz	50	—	4

FOOD	PORTION	CALS.	SAT. FAT	FAT
French Onion (Heluva Good Cheese)	2 tbsp (1.1 oz)	50	3	5
French Onion (Kraft)	2 tbsp	60	2	4
French Onion (Kraft Premium)	2 tbsp	45	2	4
French Onion (Sealtest)	2 tbsp	50	3	4
Green Onion (Kraft)	2 tbsp	60	2	4
Homestyle Onion (Heluva Good Cheese)	2 tbsp (1.1 oz)	60	3	5
Hommus Tahini No Salt Added (Cedar's)	2 tbsp (1 oz)	50	0	2
Hot Bean (Hain)	4 tbsp	70	—	1
Jalapeno Bean (Frito Lay)	1 oz	30	—	1
Jalapeno Bean (Wise)	2 tbsp	25	0	0
Jalapeno Cheddar Gourmet (Breakstone)	2 tbsp	70	3	6
Jalapeno Cheese (Kraft Premium)	1 tbsp	50	3	4
Jalapeno Pepper (Kraft)	2 tbsp	50	2	4
Mexican Bean (Hain)	4 tbsp	60	—	1
Mushroom & Herb Gourmet (Breakstone)	2 tbsp	50	3	4
Nacho Cheese (Kraft Premium)	2 tbsp	55	2	4
Onion Bean (Hain)	4 tbsp	70	—	1
Picante Sauce (Wise)	1 oz	10	—	0
Pinto Bean (Guiltless Gourmet)	1 oz	25	0	0
Ranch (Heluva Good Cheese)	2 tbsp (1.1 oz)	60	3	5
Snyder's (Mustard Pretzel)	2 tbsp (1.2 oz)	90	2	4
Taco (Wise)	2 tbsp	12	0	0
Taco Dip & Sauce (Hain)	4 tbsp	25	—	1
Toasted Onion Gourmet (Breakstone)	2 tbsp	50	3	5

DOCK
fresh, cooked	3.5 oz	20	—	1
fresh, raw, chopped	½ cup	15	—	tr

DOGFISH
raw	3.5 oz	193	—	15

DOLPHINFISH
fresh, baked	3 oz	93	tr	1
fresh fillet, baked	5.6 oz	174	tr	1

FOOD	PORTION	CALS.	SAT. FAT	FAT
DOUGHNUTS				
(*see also* DUNKIN' DONUTS, WINCHELL'S)				
Assorted Regular (Hostess)	1 (1.6 oz)	200	6	11
Cider (Dutch Mill)	1 (2.1 oz)	240	2	10
Cinnamon (Dutch Mill)	1 (1.8 oz)	210	5	11
Cinnamon (Tastykake)	1 (47 g)	180	2	8
Cinnamon Apple (Earth Grains)	1	310	—	17
Cinnamon Family Pack (Hostess)	1 (1 oz)	110	2	5
Cinnamon Swirl (Hostess)	1 (1.6 oz)	180	3	7
Crumb Regular (Hostess)	1 (1 oz)	130	4	8
Crumb Topped (Entenmann's)	1 (2.1 oz)	260	—	12
Devil's Food (Earth Grains)	1	330	—	21
Devil's Food Crumb (Entenmann's)	1 (2.1 oz)	250	—	12
Donut Holes Double-Dipped Chocolate (Dutch Mill)	3 (1.4 oz)	220	6	16
Donut Holes Shootin' Stars (Dutch Mill)	3 (1.4 oz)	190	3	10
Donut Sticks (Little Debbie)	1 pkg (1.6 oz)	210	3	13
Donut Sticks (Little Debbie)	1 pkg (2 oz)	250	4	15
Donut Sticks (Little Debbie)	1 pkg (2.5 oz)	320	5	19
Donut Sticks (Little Debbie)	1 pkg (3 oz)	390	6	23
Double-Dipped Chocolate (Dutch Mill)	1 (2.1 oz)	280	7	17
Frosted Regular (Hostess)	1 (1.4 oz)	180	7	11
Frosted Rich (Tastykake)	1 (57 g)	260	8	16
Frosted Rich Mini (Tastykake)	1 (14 g)	44	2	3
Gem Donettes Cinnamon (Hostess)	6 (3 oz)	320	4	11
Gem Donettes Frosted (Hostess)	6 (3 oz)	390	15	23
Gem Donettes Frosted Strawberry Filled (Hostess)	3 (3 oz)	240	9	13

FOOD	PORTION	CALS.	SAT. FAT	FAT
Gem Donettes Powdered (Hostess)	6 (3 oz)	350	6	16
Gem Donettes Powdered Strawberry Filled (Hostess)	3 (3 oz)	210	4	9
Glazed (Dutch Mill)	1 (2.1 oz)	250	3	12
Glazed Chocolate (Dutch Mill)	1 (2.4 oz)	270	3	11
Glazed Old Fashioned (Earth Grains)	1	310	—	18
Glazed Party (Hostess)	1 (2.3 oz)	260	5	10
Honey Wheat (Tastykake)	1 (57 g)	210	2	8
Honey Wheat Mini (Tastykake)	1 (12 g)	40	0	1
Hostess O's Raspberry Filled Powdered (Hostess)	1 (2.2 oz)	230	4	10
Jumbo Frosted (Hostess)	1 (2 oz)	260	10	16
Jumbo Plain (Hostess)	1 (1.1 oz)	140	4	7
Jumbo Powdered (Hostess)	1 (1.3 oz)	160	5	9
Mini Chocolate (Hostess)	5 (2 oz)	220	0	9
Old Fashion Donuts (Drake's)	1 (1.7 oz)	182	—	8
Old Fashioned Glazed (Hostess)	1 (2.1 oz)	250	5	12
Old Fashioned Glazed Honey Wheat (Hostess)	1 (2.1 oz)	250	5	12
Old Fashioned Plain (Hostess)	1 (1.5 oz)	170	4	9
Orange Glazed (Tastykake)	1 (57 g)	210	3	9
Plain (Dutch Mill)	1 (1.8 oz)	210	5	12
Plain (Tastykake)	1 (47 g)	190	3	10
Plain Regular (Hostess)	1 (1 oz)	120	3	6
Powdered Family Pack (Hostess)	1 (1 oz)	110	3	6
Powdered Old Fashioned (Earth Grains)	1	290	—	19
Powdered Sugar (Tastykake)	1 (46 g)	180	2	9
Powdered Sugar Donut Delites (Drake's)	7 (2.5 oz)	300	—	15
Powdered Sugar Mini (Tastykake)	1 (12 g)	40	0	1

FOOD	PORTION	CALS.	SAT. FAT	FAT
Rich Frosted (Entenmann's)	1 (2 oz)	280	—	18
Sugared (Dutch Mill)	1 (1.8 oz)	220	5	11
cake type, unsugared	1 (1.6 oz)	198	2	11
chocolate, glazed	1 (1.5 oz)	175	3	8
chocolate, sugared	1 (1.5 oz)	175	3	8
chocolate coated	1 (1.5 oz)	204	4	13
creme filled	1 (3 oz)	307	6	21
french cruller, glazed	1 (1.4 oz)	169	2	8
frosted	1 (1.5 oz)	204	4	13
honey bun	1 (2.1 oz)	242	3	14
jelly	1 (3 oz)	289	4	16
old fashioned	1 (1.6 oz)	198	2	11
sugared	1 (1.6 oz)	192	3	10
wheat, glazed	1 (1.6 oz)	162	1	9
wheat, sugared	1 (1.6 oz)	162	1	9
yeast, glazed	1 (2.1 oz)	242	3	14

DRESSING
(*see also* STUFFING/DRESSING)

DRINK MIXERS
(*see also* SODA, MINERAL/BOTTLED WATER)

FOOD	PORTION	CALS.	SAT. FAT	FAT
Bloody Mary Mix (Libby)	6 oz	40	0	0
Bloody Mary Mix Extra Spicy (Tabasco)	8 fl oz	58	tr	tr
Canada Dry Collins Mixer (Canada Dry)	8 fl oz	120	0	0
Canada Dry Sour Mixer (Canada Dry)	8 fl oz	90	0	0
Margarita Mix w/ rum (Bacardi)	8 fl oz	160	0	0
Margarita Mix w/o liquor (Bacardi)	8 fl oz	100	0	0
Pina Colada (Bacardi)	8 fl oz	140	0	0
Rum Runner (Bacardi)	8 fl oz	140	0	0
Schweppes (Collins Mixer)	8 fl oz	100	0	0
Strawberry Daiquiri w/o liquor (Bacardi)	8 fl oz)	140	0	0
Tabasco Bloody Mary Mix (McIlhenny)	8 fl oz	56	tr	tr
whisky sour mix	2 oz	55	0	0

FOOD	PORTION	CALS.	SAT. FAT	FAT

DRUM
FRESH
| freshwater, baked | 3 oz | 130 | 1 | 5 |
| freshwater fillet, baked | 5.4 oz | 236 | 2 | 10 |

DUCK
w/ skin, roasted	½ duck (13.4 oz)	1287	37	108
w/ skin, roasted	6 oz	583	17	49
w/o skin, roasted	3.5 oz	201	4	11
w/o skin, roasted	½ duck (7.8 oz)	445	9	25
wild w/ skin, raw	½ duck (9.5 oz)	571	14	41
wild breast w/o skin, raw	½ breast (2.9 oz)	102	1	4

DUMPLING
FROZEN
| Apple Dumpling (Pepperidge Farm) | 1 (3 oz) | 260 | — | 13 |

DURIAN
| fresh | 3.5 oz | 141 | — | 2 |

EEL
fresh, cooked	3 oz	200	3	13
fresh, cooked	1 fillet (5.6 oz)	375	5	24
raw	3 oz	156	2	10

EGG
(*see also* EGG DISHES, EGG SUBSTITUTES)
CHICKEN
fried w/ margarine	1	91	2	7
frozen	1	75	2	5
frozen	1 cup	363	8	24
hard cooked	1	77	2	5
hard cooked, chopped	1 cup	210	4	14
poached	1	74	2	5
raw	1	75	2	5
scrambled plain	2	200	6	15
scrambled w/ whole milk & margarine	1	101	2	7
scrambled w/ whole milk & margarine	1 cup	365	8	27
white only	1	17	0	0
white only	1 cup	121	0	0

OTHER POULTRY
| duck, raw | 1 | 130 | 3 | 10 |
| goose, raw | 1 | 267 | 5 | 19 |

FOOD	PORTION	CALS.	SAT. FAT	FAT
quail, raw	1	14	tr	1
turkey, raw	1	135	3	9

EGG DISHES
FROZEN
Chefwich

FOOD	PORTION	CALS.	SAT. FAT	FAT
Cheese Omelet	5 oz	380	—	17
Ham & Cheese Omelet	5 oz	340	—	14
Sausage & Cheese Omelet	5 oz	400	—	19
Western Style Omelet	5 oz	350	—	13
Downyflake				
Scrambled Eggs With Ham And Hash Browns	1 pkg (6.25 oz)	360	—	26
Scrambled Eggs With Ham And Pecan Twirl	1 pkg (6.25 oz)	470	—	28
Scrambled Eggs With Hash Browns And Sausage	1 pkg (6.25 oz)	420	—	34
Scrambled Eggs With Sausage And Pecan Twirl	1 pkg (6.25 oz)	510	—	33
Great Starts				
Egg, Sausage & Cheese	5.5 oz	460	—	28
Omelets With Cheese And Ham	7 oz	390	—	29
Reduced Cholesterol Eggs With Mini Oatbran Muffins	4.75 oz	250	—	12
Scrambled Eggs With Cheese & Cinnamon Pancakes	3.4 oz	290	—	23
Scrambled Eggs & Bacon With Home Fries	5.6 oz	340	—	26
Scrambled Eggs & Home Fries	4.6 oz	260	—	19
Scrambled Eggs & Sausage With Hash Browns	6.5 oz	430	—	34
Kid Cuisine Egg Patties w/ Cheese	4.8 oz	200	—	10
Kid Cuisine Scrambled Eggs	4.1 oz	270	—	17

FOOD	PORTION	CALS.	SAT. FAT	FAT
Quaker Scrambled Eggs Cheddar Cheese & Fried Potatoes	1 pkg (5.9 oz)	250	—	13
Quaker Scrambled Eggs & Sausage With Hash Browns	1 pkg (5.7 oz)	290	—	20
Quaker Scrambled Eggs & Sausage With Pancakes	1 pkg (5.2 oz)	270	—	14
Weight Watchers Garden Vegetable Omelet Sandwich	1 (3.6 oz)	210	—	6
Weight Watchers Ham And Cheese Handy Omelet	4 oz	180	—	5
HOME RECIPE				
deviled	2 halves	145	3	13
TAKE-OUT				
egg sandwich w/ cheese & ham	1	348	7	16
salad	½ cup	307	6	28
sandwich w/ cheese	1	340	7	19
scotch egg	1 (4.2 oz)	301	—	21

EGG SUBSTITUTES

FOOD	PORTION	CALS.	SAT. FAT	FAT
Egg Beaters	¼ cup	25	0	0
Egg Beaters Cheese Omelette	½ cup	110	2	5
Egg Beaters Vegetable Omelette	½ cup	50	0	0
Egg Watchers	2 oz	50	—	2
Healthy Choice Cholesterol Free Egg	¼ cup (2 oz)	25	0	0
Morningstar Farms				
Better'n Eggs	¼ cup (57 g)	30	0	0
Scrambler Links Muffins	1 pkg (4 oz)	220	—	10
Scramblers	¼ cup (57 g)	60	—	3
Scramblers Cheese Home Fries	1 pkg (5 oz)	210	—	9
Scramblers Sandwich w/ Cheese	1 (3.5 oz)	220	—	7
Scramblers Sandwich w/ Pattie	1 (4.5 oz)	300	—	12
Scramblers Sandwich w/ Pattie, Cheese	1 (5 oz)	350	—	15
Scramblers Links Hash Browns	1 pkg (5 oz)	240	—	13

FOOD	PORTION	CALS.	SAT. FAT	FAT
Second Nature No Cholesterol	2 fl oz	60	tr	2
Second Nature No Fat	2 fl oz	40	0	0
Second Nature No Fat With Garden Vegetables	2.5 fl oz	40	0	0
Simply Eggs	1.75 fl oz	35	tr	1
frozen	¼ cup	96	1	7
frozen	1 cup	384	5	27
liquid	1.5 oz	40	tr	2
liquid	1 cup	211	2	8
powder	0.7 oz	88	1	3
powder	0.35 oz	44	tr	1

EGGNOG

Borden	4 fl oz	160	—	9
Borden Light	½ cup	130	—	2
eggnog	1 qt	1368	45	76
eggnog	1 cup	342	11	19
eggnog flavor mix, as prep w/ milk	9 oz	260	5	8

EGGPLANT

CANNED

Caponata (Progresso)	2 tbsp (1 oz)	30	0	2

FRESH

cubed, cooked	½ cup	13	tr	tr
raw, cut up	½ cup (1.4 oz)	11	tr	tr
slices, cooked	4 (7 oz)	38	0	0
whole peeled raw	1 (1 lb)	117	tr	1

FROZEN

Parmigiana (Mrs. Paul's)	5 oz	240	—	16

TAKE-OUT

Baba Ghannouj	¼ cup	55	—	4

ELDERBERRIES

fresh elderberries	1 cup	105	—	1
juice	3.5 oz	38	0	0

ELK

roasted	3 oz	124	1	2

ENDIVE

fresh	3.5 oz	9	—	tr
raw, chopped	½ cup	4	tr	tr

FOOD	PORTION	CALS.	SAT. FAT	FAT
ENGLISH MUFFIN				
FROZEN				
Great Starts Egg, Beefsteak & Cheese	5.9 oz	360	—	20
Great Starts Egg, Canadian Bacon & Cheese	4.1 oz	290	—	15
Weight Watchers Sandwich w/ Egg, Ham & Cheese	1 (4 oz)	230	3	8
HOME RECIPE				
cinnamon raisin	1	186	—	3
english muffin	1	158	—	2
honey bran	1	153	—	3
whole wheat	1	167	—	tr
READY-TO-EAT				
Arnold Extra Crisp	1	130	0	1
Arnold Sourdough	1	130	0	1
Matthew's 9 Grain & Nut	1	140	—	4
Matthew's Cinnamon Raisin	1	160	—	2
Matthew's Golden White	1	140	—	4
Matthew's Whole Wheat	1	150	—	2
Pepperidge Farm Cinnamon Apple	1	140	—	1
Pepperidge Farm Cinnamon Chip	1	160	—	3
Pepperidge Farm Cinnamon Raisin	1	150	—	2
Pepperidge Farm Plain	1	140	—	1
Pepperidge Farm Sourdough	1	135	—	1
Roman Meal	1 (2.2 oz)	135	tr	1
Shop 'n Save	1	130	—	1
Tastykake	1 (57 g)	130	—	1
Tastykake Cinnamon Raisin	1 (64 g)	150	—	1
Tastykake Sourdough	1 (57 g)	130	—	1
Thomas' Honey Wheat	1	128	—	1
Thomas' Oat Bran	1	116	—	1
Thomas' Raisin Cinnamon	1	151	—	1
Thomas' Regular	1	130	—	1
Thomas' Sandwich Size	1 (92 g)	210	1	2
Thomas' Sourdough	1	131	—	1
Wonder	1 (2 oz)	120	0	1
Wonder Raisin Rounds	1 (2.1 oz)	150	0	2
Wonder Sourdough	1 (2 oz)	120	0	1

FOOD	PORTION	CALS.	SAT. FAT	FAT
apple cinnamon	1	138	tr	2
granola	1	155	tr	1
mixed grain	1	155	tr	1
plain	1	134	tr	1
plain toasted	1	133	tr	1
raisin cinnamon	1	138	tr	2
sourdough	1	134	tr	1
wheat	1	127	tr	1
whole wheat	1	134	tr	1
REFRIGERATED				
Roman Meal	½ muffin (1.1 oz)	66	tr	tr
Roman Meal Honey Nut Oat Bran	½ muffin (1.1 oz)	81	tr	1
TAKE-OUT				
w/ butter	1	189	2	6
w/ cheese & sausage	1	394	10	24
w/ egg, cheese & bacon	1	487	12	31
w/ egg, cheese & canadian bacon	1	383	9	20

EPPAW

FOOD	PORTION	CALS.	SAT. FAT	FAT
raw	½ cup	75	—	1

FALAFEL

FOOD	PORTION	CALS.	SAT. FAT	FAT
MIX				
Near East, as prep	3 patties (3.7 oz)	310	0	2
TAKE-OUT				
falafel	1 (1.2 oz)	57	tr	3
falafel	3 (1.8 oz)	170	1	9

FAST FOODS
(see individual names)

FAT
(see also BUTTER, BUTTER BLENDS, BUTTER SUBSTITUTES, MARGARINE, OIL)

FOOD	PORTION	CALS.	SAT. FAT	FAT
Chicken Fat Rendered (Empire)	1 tbsp (0.5 oz)	120	4	13
Crisco	1 tbsp	110	3	12
Crisco Butter Flavor	1 tbsp	110	3	12
Crisco Sticks	1 tbsp (0.4 oz)	110	3	12
Crisco Sticks Butter Flavor	1 tbsp (0.4 oz)	110	3	12
Wesson Shortening	1 tbsp	100	3	12
beef, cooked	1 oz	193	8	20
beef, suet	1 oz	242	15	27
beef, tallow	1 tbsp (13 g)	115	6	13
chicken	1 cup	1846	61	205

FOOD	PORTION	CALS.	SAT. FAT	FAT
chicken	1 tbsp	115	4	13
cocoa butter	1 tbsp	120	8	14
duck	1 tbsp	115	4	13
goose	1 tbsp	115	4	13
lamb, new zealand, raw	1 oz	182	10	19
lard	1 tbsp (13 g)	115	5	13
lard	1 cup (205 g)	1849	80	205
nutmeg butter	1 tbsp	120	12	14
pork, cooked	1 oz	200	8	21
pork, cured, roasted	1 oz	167	—	18
pork, cured, uncooked	1 oz	164	—	17
pork backfat	1 oz	230	—	25
salt pork	1 oz	212	8	23
shortening	1 tbsp	113	3	13
shortening	1 cup	1812	41	205
turkey	1 tbsp	115	4	13
ucuhuba butter	1 tbsp	120	12	14

FAVA BEANS
CANNED
Progresso	½ cup	90	—	tr

FEIJOA
fresh	1 (1.75 oz)	25	—	tr
puree	1 cup	119	—	2

FENNEL
fresh, bulb	1 (8.2 oz)	72	—	tr
fresh, sliced	1 cup	27	—	tr
seed	1 tsp	7	tr	tr

FENUGREEK
seed	1 tsp	12	—	tr

FIBER
(*see also* PECTIN)
Natural Delta Fiber	½ cup (1 oz)	20	—	tr

FIGS
CANNED
Kadota Figs Whole Fancy (S&W)	½ cup	100	0	0
in heavy syrup	3	75	tr	tr
in light syrup	3	58	tr	tr
water pack	3	42	—	tr

DRIED
California	½ cup (3.5 oz)	200	—	1

FOOD	PORTION	CALS.	SAT. FAT	FAT
cooked	½ cup	140	tr	1
whole	10	477	tr	2
FRESH				
fig	1 med	50	tr	tr

FILBERTS

FOOD	PORTION	CALS.	SAT. FAT	FAT
dried, blanched	1 oz	191	1	19
dried, unblanched	1 oz	179	1	18
dry roasted, unblanched	1 oz	188	1	19
oil roasted, unblanched	1 oz	187	1	18

FISH

(*see also individual names*, FISH SUBSTITUTES)

FOOD	PORTION	CALS.	SAT. FAT	FAT
CANNED				
Holmes Finest Kippered Snacks, drained	1 can (3.2 oz)	135	1	8
Port Clyde				
Fish Steaks In Louisiana Hot Sauce	1 can (3.75 oz)	150	2	9
Fish Steaks In Mustard Sauce	1 can (3.75 oz)	140	1	7
Fish Steaks In Soybean Oil With Hot Chilies drained	1 can (3.3 oz)	155	2	8
Fish Steaks In Soybean Oil, drained	1 can (3.3 oz)	220	4	17
Progresso Mixed Seafood Sauce	½ cup	110	tr	6
Progresso Seafood	½ cup	190	9	15
FRESH				
roe	3.5 oz	39	tr	2
FROZEN				
Cajun Cookin' Seafood Gumbo	17 oz	330	—	7
Gorton's				
Crispy Batter Dipped Fillets	2	290	8	19
Crispy Batter Sticks	4	260	6	18
Crunch Fillets	2	230	3	13
Crunchy Sticks	4	210	4	13
Light Recipe Lightly Breaded Fish Fillets	1 fillet	180	3	8
Light Recipe Tempura Fillets	1 fillet	200	4	14
Microwave Fillets	2	340	12	26

FOOD	PORTION	CALS.	SAT. FAT	FAT
Microwave Crispy Batter Large Cut Fillets	1	320	—	21
Microwave Entree Fillets In Herb Butter	1 pkg	190	5	8
Microwave Larger Cut Fillets	1	320	10	22
Microwave Larger Cut Ranch Fillet	1	330	—	21
Microwave Sticks	6	340	7	22
Potato Crisp Fillets	2	300	6	20
Potato Crisp Sticks	4	260	5	16
Value Pack Portions	1 portion	180	—	11
Value Pack Sticks	4	190	—	9
Mrs. Paul's				
40 Crunchy Fish Sticks	4 (2.75 oz)	200	—	10
Batter Dipped Fish Fillets	2 fillets	330	—	17
Battered Fish Portions	2 portions	300	—	19
Battered Fish Sticks	4 sticks	210	—	12
Combination Seafood Platter	9 oz	600	—	33
Crispy Crunchy Breaded Fish Portions	2 portions	230	—	15
Crispy Crunchy Breaded Fish Sticks	4 sticks	140	—	6
Crispy Crunchy Fish Fillets	2 fillets	220	—	9
Crispy Crunchy Fish Sticks	4 sticks	190	—	8
Crunchy Batter Fish Fillets	2 fillets	280	—	14
Fish Cakes	2	190	—	7
Light Fillets In Butter Sauce	1 fillet	140	—	6
Light Seafood Entrees Fish Dijon	8¾ oz	200	2	5
Light Seafood Entrees Fish Florentine	8 oz	220	—	8
Light Seafood Entrees Fish Mornay	9 oz	230	4	10
Microwave Buttered Fillet	1 fillet	80	—	4
Microwave Fillet Sandwich	1	280	—	15
Microwave Fillets	1 fillet	280	—	19

FOOD	PORTION	CALS.	SAT. FAT	FAT
Mrs. Paul's *(cont.)*				
Microwave Fish Sticks	5	290	—	20
Van De Kamp's				
Battered Fish Fillets	1	170	2	10
Battered Fish Sticks	4	160	2	9
Breaded Fish Fillets	2	280	3	18
Breaded Fish Sticks	4	200	2	12
Breaded Fish Sticks Value Pack	4	170	2	10
Crispy Microwave Fillets	1 piece	140	2	9
Crispy Microwave Fish Sticks	3 pieces	130	1	7
Crispy Microwave Large Fillets	1 piece	290	3	17
breaded fillet	1 (2 oz)	155	2	7
sticks	1 stick (1 oz)	76	1	3
MIX				
Beer Batter Fry (Golden Dipt)	1 oz	100	0	0
Cajun Style Fish Fry (Golden Dipt)	⅔ oz	60	0	0
Fish & Chips Batter Mix (Golden Dipt)	1.25 oz	120	0	0
Fish Fry (Golden Dipt)	⅔ oz	60	0	0
Seafood Frying Mix (Golden Dipt)	⅔ oz	60	0	0
Tempura Batter Mix (Golden Dipt)	1 oz	100	0	0
TAKE-OUT				
fish cake	1 (4.7 oz)	166	2	7
kedgeree	5.6 oz	242	—	11
sandwich w/ tartar sauce	1	431	5	55
sandwich w/ tartar sauce, cheese	1	524	8	29
stew	1 cup (7.9 oz)	157	2	4
taramasalata	3.5 oz	446	—	46
FISH PASTE				
fish paste	2 tsp	15	—	1
FISH SUBSTITUTES				
LaLoma Ocean Platter, mix not prep	¼ cup (16 g)	50	0	0
Worthington Fillets	2 (85 g)	180	—	9
Worthington Tuna	2 oz (57 g)	100	—	7

FOOD	PORTION	CALS.	SAT. FAT	FAT
FLATFISH				
FRESH				
cooked	3 oz	99	tr	1
cooked	1 fillet (4.5 oz)	148	tr	2
TAKE-OUT				
battered & fried	3.2 oz	211	3	11
breaded & fried	3.2 oz	211	3	11
FLAX				
Seeds (Arrowhead)	3 tbsp (1 oz)	140	1	10
FLOUNDER				
FROZEN				
Crunchy Batter Fillets (Mrs. Paul's)	2 fillets	220	—	9
Fishmarket Fresh (Gorton's)	5 oz	110	—	1
Flounder Primavera (King & Prince)	6 oz	180	—	9
Flounder Del Rey (King & Prince)	4.5 oz	163	—	8
Light Fillets (Mrs. Paul's)	1 fillet	240	—	10
Light Fillets (Van De Kamp's)	1 piece	260	2	12
Microwave Entree Stuffed (Gorton's)	1 pkg	350	7	18
Natural Fillets (Van De Kamp's)	4 oz	100	0	2
FLOUR				
50/50 Flour (Hodgson Mill)	¼ cup (1 oz)	100	0	1
All Purpose (Ballard)	1 cup	400	—	1
All Purpose (Ceresota)	1 cup	390	—	1
All Purpose (Gold Medal)	1 cup	400	—	1
All Purpose (Heckers)	1 cup	390	—	1
All Purpose (Pillsbury Best)	1 cup	400	—	1
All Purpose (Red Band)	1 cup	390	—	1
All Purpose (White Deer)	1 cup	400	—	1
All Purpose Unbleached (Pillsbury Best)	1 cup	400	0	1
Best for Bread (Hodgson Mill)	¼ cup (1 oz)	100	0	0
Bohemian Style Rye & Wheat (Pillsbury Best)	1 cup	400	—	1

FOOD	PORTION	CALS.	SAT. FAT	FAT
Bread (Pillsbury Best)	1 cup	400	—	2
Buckwheat (Arrowhead)	⅓ cup (1.6 oz)	160	0	1
Drifted Snow (General Mills)	1 cup	400	—	1
Kamut (Arrowhead)	¼ cup (1.2 oz)	110	0	1
La Pina (Gold Medal)	1 cup	390	—	1
Oat Blend (Gold Medal)	1 cup	390	—	3
Oat Bran Blend (Hodgson Mill)	¼ cup (1 oz)	110	0	1
Oat Bran Flour (Hodgson Mill)	¼ cup (1 oz)	110	1	2
Pastry (Arrowhead)	⅓ cup (1.1 oz)	100	0	1
Rye (Hodgson Mill)	¼ cup (1 oz)	90	0	1
Rye Medium (Pillsbury Best)	1 cup	400	—	2
Rye Stone Ground (Robin Hood)	1 cup	360	—	2
Rye Whole Grain (Arrowhead)	¼ cup (1.6 oz)	160	0	1
Seasoned Flour (Hodgson Mill)	¼ cup (1 oz)	90	0	0
Self-Rising (Aunt Jemima)	¼ cup	109	—	tr
Self-Rising (Ballard)	1 cup	380	—	1
Self-Rising (Gold Medal)	1 cup	380	—	1
Self-Rising (Pillsbury Best)	1 cup	380	—	1
Self-Rising (Red Band)	1 cup	380	—	1
Self-Rising (Robin Hood)	1 cup	380	—	1
Shake & Blend (Pillsbury Best)	2 tbsp	50	0	0
Softasilk (General Mills)	¼ cup	100	—	0
Spelt (Arrowhead)	¼ cup (1.2 oz)	100	0	1
Teff (Arrowhead)	¼ cup (1.4 oz)	140	0	1
Unbleached (Gold Medal)	1 cup	400	—	1
Unbleached (Robin Hood)	1 cup	400	—	1
Unbleached (Pillsbury Best)	1 cup	400	—	1
Unbleached White (Arrowhead)	2 oz	200	—	1
White (Hodgson Mill)	¼ cup (1 oz)	100	0	0
Whole Grain Wheat (Arrowhead)	¼ cup (1.6 oz)	160	0	1
Whole Wheat (Arrowhead)	¼ cup (1.2 oz)	130	0	1
Whole Wheat (Ceresota)	1 cup	400	—	2
Whole Wheat (Gold Medal)	1 cup	390	—	2
Whole Wheat (Heckers)	1 cup	400	—	2

FOOD	PORTION	CALS.	SAT. FAT	FAT
Whole Wheat (Hodgson Mill)	¼ cup (1 oz)	100	0	1
Whole Wheat (Pillsbury Best)	1 cup	400	—	2
Whole Wheat Blend (Gold Medal)	1 cup	370	—	2
Wondra	1 cup	400	—	1
corn, masa	1 cup	416	tr	4
corn, whole grain	1 cup	422	tr	5
cottonseed lowfat	1 oz	94	tr	tr
peanut, defatted	1 cup	196	tr	tr
peanut, lowfat	1 cup	257	2	13
potato	1 cup (6.3 oz)	628	tr	1
rice, brown	1 cup	574	tr	4
rice, white	1 cup	578	tr	2
rye, dark	1 cup	415	tr	3
rye, light	1 cup	374	tr	1
rye, medium	1 cup	361	tr	2
sesame, lowfat	1 oz	95	tr	tr
triticale whole grain	1 cup	440	tr	2
white, all-purpose	1 cup	455	tr	1
white, self-rising	1 cup	442	tr	1
white bread	1 cup	495	tr	2
white cake	1 cup	395	tr	tr
whole wheat	1 cup	407	tr	2

FRANKFURTER
(see HOT DOG)

FRENCH BEANS
DRIED

cooked	1 cup	228	tr	1

FRENCH FRIES
(see POTATOES)

FRENCH TOAST
FROZEN

Aunt Jemima	3 oz	166	1	4
Aunt Jemima Cinnamon Swirl	3 oz	171	1	4
Downyflake	2	270	—	12
Downyflake Extra Thick	1	150	—	9
Downyflake Texas Style & Sausage	1 pkg (4.25 oz)	400	—	24

FOOD	PORTION	CALS.	SAT. FAT	FAT
Great Starts				
Cinnamon Swirl With Sausage	5.5 oz	390	—	21
French Toast With Sausage	5.5 oz	380	—	21
Mini French Toast With Sausage	2.5 oz	190	—	9
Oatmeal French Toast With Lite Links	4.65 oz	310	—	13
Healthy Starts French Toast With LeanLinks	6.5 oz	400	—	13
Kid Cuisine	4.11 oz	260	—	12
Quaker French Toast Sticks & Syrup	1 pkg (5.2 oz)	400	—	20
Quaker French Toast Wedges & Sausage	1 pkg (5.3 oz)	360	—	17
Weight Watchers French Toast With Cinnamon	2 slices (3 oz)	160	1	5
Weight Watchers French Toast With Links	4.5 oz	270	—	11
french toast	1 slice (2 oz)	126	1	4
HOME RECIPE				
as prep w/ 2% milk	1 slice	149	2	7
as prep w/ whole milk	1 slice	151	2	7
TAKE-OUT				
w/ butter	2 slices	356	8	19

FROG'S LEGS

frog leg, as prep w/ seasoned flour & fried	1 (0.8 oz)	70	—	5

FROSTING
(see CAKE)

FRUCTOSE
(see also SUGAR, SUGAR SUBSTITUTES)

Estee	1 pkg (3 g)	10	0	0
Estee	1 tsp (4 g)	15	0	0

FRUIT DRINKS
(see also LEMONADE)

FROZEN
Dole

Country Raspberry 100% Juice Blend as prep	8 fl oz	140	0	0

FOOD	PORTION	CALS.	SAT. FAT	FAT
Mountain Cherry 100% Juice Blend as prep	8 fl oz	120	0	0
Orchard Peach 100% Juice Blend as prep	8 fl oz	140	0	0
Pineapple Grapefruit as prep	8 fl oz	130	0	0
Pineapple Passion Banana as prep	8 fl oz	120	0	0
Pineapple Orange Banana as prep	8 fl oz	130	0	0
Pineapple Orange Guava as prep	8 fl oz	120	0	0
Pineapple Orange as prep	8 fl oz	120	0	0
Tropical Fruit as prep	8 fl oz	140	0	0
Five Alive Berry Citrus	8 fl oz	120	0	0
Five Alive Citrus	9 fl oz	120	0	0
Five Alive Tropical Citrus	8 fl oz	120	0	0
Minute Maid				
Berry Punch	8 fl oz	130	0	0
Citrus Punch	8 fl oz	120	0	0
Fruit Punch	8 fl oz	120	0	0
Limeade	8 fl oz	100	0	0
Pineapple Orange	8 fl oz	120	0	0
Tropical Punch	8 fl oz	120	0	0
Seneca Cranberry Apple Juice Cocktail	6 oz	110	0	0
Seneca Raspberry Cranberry Juice Cocktail	6 oz	110	0	0
Tree Top Apple Citrus, as prep	6 oz	90	0	0
Tree Top Apple Cranberry, as prep	6 oz	100	0	0
Tree Top Apple Grape, as prep	6 oz	100	0	0
Tree Top Apple Pear, as prep	6 oz	90	0	0
Tree Top Apple Raspberry, as prep	6 oz	80	0	0
citrus juice drink, as prep	1 cup	114	0	0
citrus juice drink, not prep	12 oz	684	tr	tr
fruit punch, not prep	1 can (12 oz)	678	tr	tr
fruit punch, as prep w/ water	1 cup	113	tr	tr
limeade	1 can (6 oz)	408	tr	tr

FOOD	PORTION	CALS.	SAT. FAT	FAT
limeade, as prep w/ water	1 cup	102	tr	tr
MIX				
Crystal Light				
Berry Blend Sugar Free	8 oz	3	0	0
Fruit Punch Sugar Free	8 oz	3	0	0
Lemon-Lime	8 oz	4	0	0
Tropic Quencher	8 oz	5	0	0
Kool-Aid				
Lemon-Lime	8 oz	98	0	0
Purplesaurus Rex	8 oz	98	0	0
Rainbow Punch	8 oz	98	0	0
Raspberry	8 oz	98	0	0
Sharkleberry Fin	8 oz	98	0	0
Strawberry	8 oz	98	0	0
Sugar Free Berry Blue	8 oz	3	0	0
Sugar Free Berry Punch	8 oz	3	0	0
Sugar Free Purplesaurus Rex	8 oz	3	0	0
Sugar Free Rainbow Punch	8 oz	4	0	0
Sugar Free Sharkleberry Fin	8 oz	3	0	0
Sugar Free Tropical Punch	8 oz	3	0	0
Sugar Sweetened Mountain Berry Punch	8 oz	98	0	0
Sugar Sweetened Purplesaurus Rex	8 oz	84	0	0
Sugar Sweetened Rainbow Punch	8 oz	84	0	0
Sugar Sweetened Sharkleberry Fin	8 oz	84	0	0
Sugar Sweetened Sunshine Punch	8 oz	83	0	0
Sugar Sweetened Surfin' Berry Punch	8 oz	79	0	0
Sugar Sweetened Tropical Punch	8 oz	84	0	0
Tropical Punch	8 oz	98	0	0
Unsweetened Berry Blue	8 oz	98	0	0
Wylers Drink Mix	8 oz	2	0	0
Unsweetened Bunch O' Berries				

FOOD	PORTION	CALS.	SAT. FAT	FAT
Wylers Drink Mix Unsweetened Pink	8 fl oz	3	0	0
Wylers Drink Mix Unsweetened Tropical Punch	8 oz	2	0	0
fruit punch, as prep w/ water	9 oz	97	0	0
READY-TO-DRINK				
Apple & Eve				
Apple Grape	6 fl oz	120	0	0
Cranberry Grape	6 fl oz	100	0	0
Fruit Punch	6 fl oz	78	0	0
Raspberry Cranberry	6 fl oz	90	0	0
BAMA Fruit Punch	8.45 fl oz	130	0	0
Boku White Grape Raspberry (McCain)	16 fl oz	120	0	0
Bright & Early Fruit Punch Frozen	8 fl oz	130	0	0
Chiquita Orange Banana	6 fl oz	90	—	0
Crystal Geyser Juice Squeeze				
Citrus Grape	1 bottle (12 fl oz)	145	0	0
Orange & Passion Fruit	1 bottle (12 fl oz)	130	0	0
Passion Fruit & Mango	1 bottle (12 fl oz)	125	0	0
Wild Berry	1 bottle (12 fl oz)	130	0	0
Dole				
Pineapple Passion Banana	6 fl oz	100	0	0
Pineapple Orange	6 fl oz	90	0	0
Pineapple Orange Banana	6 fl oz	100	0	0
Pineapple Orange Guava	6 fl oz	100	0	0
Five Alive				
Citrus	6 fl oz	90	0	0
Citrus	1 bottle (16 fl oz)	120	0	0
Citrus	1 can (11.5 fl oz)	170	0	0
Citrus Chilled	8 fl oz	120	0	0
Hawaiian Punch				
Fruit Juicy Red	6 fl oz	90	—	0
Island Fruit Cocktail	6 fl oz	90	—	0
Lite Fruit Juicy Red	6 fl oz	60	—	0
Tropical Fruits	6 fl oz	90	—	0
Very Berry	6 fl oz	90	—	0
Wild Fruit	6 fl oz	90	—	0

FOOD	PORTION	CALS.	SAT. FAT	FAT
Hi-C				
Boppin' Berry Box	8.45 fl oz	140	0	0
Boppin' Berry	8 fl oz	130	0	0
Double Fruit Box	8.45 fl oz	130	0	0
Double Fruit Cooler	8 fl oz	130	0	0
Ecto Cooler	1 can (11.5 fl oz)	180	0	0
Ecto Cooler	8 fl oz	130	0	0
Ecto Cooler Box	8.45 fl oz	130	0	0
Fruit Punch	1 can (11.5 fl oz)	190	0	0
Fruit Punch	8 fl oz	130	0	0
Fruit Punch Box	8.45 fl oz	140	0	0
Fruity Bubble Gum	8 fl oz	120	0	0
Fruity Bubble Gum Box	8.45 fl oz	130	0	0
Hula Punch	1 can (11.5 fl oz)	170	0	0
Hula Punch	8 fl oz	120	0	0
Hula Punch Box	8.45 fl oz	120	0	0
Jammin' Apple Box	8.45 fl oz	130	0	0
Stompin' Banana Berry	8 fl oz	130	0	0
Stompin' Banana Berry Box	8.45 fl oz	130	0	0
Wild Berry	8 fl oz	120	0	0
Wild Berry Box	8.45 fl oz	130	0	0
Juice Works Appleberry	6 fl oz	100	—	0
Juicy Juice				
Apple Grape	1 box (8.45 fl oz)	120	0	0
Berry	1 bottle (6 fl oz)	90	0	0
Berry	1 box (8.45 fl oz)	130	0	0
Cherry	1 box (8.45 fl oz)	130	0	0
Punch	1 bottle (6 fl oz)	100	0	0
Punch	1 box (8.45 fl oz)	140	0	0
Tropical	1 bottle (6 fl oz)	110	0	0
Tropical	1 box (8.45 fl oz)	150	0	0
Kern's				
Apple Strawberry Nectar	6 fl oz	110	0	0
Apricot Pineapple Nectar	6 fl oz	110	0	0
Banana Pineapple Nectar	6 fl oz	110	0	0
Coconut Pineapple Nectar	6 fl oz	140	0	0
Orange Banana Nectar	6 fl oz	110	0	0
Strawberry Banana Nectar	6 fl oz	110	0	0
Tropical Nectar	6 fl oz	110	0	0

FOOD	PORTION	CALS.	SAT. FAT	FAT
Kool-Aid Koolers				
Mountainberry Punch	1 pkg (8.45 fl oz)	142	0	0
Rainbow Punch	1 pkg (8.45 fl oz)	135	0	0
Sharkleberry Fin	1 pkg (8.45 fl oz)	140	0	0
Tropical Punch	1 pkg (8.45 fl oz)	132	0	0
Libby Strawberry Banana Nectar	1 can (11.5 fl oz)	220	0	0
Mauna La'i				
Island Guava Hawaiian Guava Fruit Juice Drink	8 fl oz	130	0	0
Mango & Hawaiian Guava Fruit Juice Drink	8 fl oz	130	0	0
Paradise Guava Hawaiian Guava & Passion Fruit Juice Drink	8 fl oz	130	0	0
Minute Maid				
Berry Punch Box	8.45 fl oz	130	0	0
Berry Punch Chilled	8 fl oz	130	0	0
Citrus Punch Chilled	8 fl oz	130	0	0
Fruit Punch Box	8.45 fl oz	120	0	0
Fruit Punch Chilled	8 fl oz	120	0	0
Grape Punch Chilled	8 fl oz	130	0	0
Juices To Go Citrus Punch	1 bottle (10 fl oz)	160	0	0
Juices To Go Citrus Punch	1 can (11.5 fl oz)	180	0	0
Juices To Go Concord Punch	1 bottle (10 fl oz)	160	0	0
Juices To Go Concord Punch	1 bottle (16 fl oz)	130	0	0
Juices To Go Concord Punch	1 can (11.5 fl oz)	180	0	0
Juices To Go Fruit Punch	1 bottle (10 fl oz)	160	0	0
Juices To Go Fruit Punch	1 bottle (16 fl oz)	120	0	0
Juices To Go Fruit Punch	1 can (11.5 fl oz)	180	0	0
Juices To Go Orange Blend	1 bottle (10 fl oz)	150	0	0
Juices To Go Orange Blend	1 can (11.5 fl oz)	170	0	0

FOOD	PORTION	CALS.	SAT. FAT	FAT
Minute Maid *(cont.)*				
Naturals Apple Cranberry	8 fl oz	170	0	0
Naturals Concord Medley	8 fl oz	130	0	0
Naturals Fruit Medley	8 fl oz	120	0	0
Naturals Orange Grape Medley	8 fl oz	120	0	0
Naturals Tropical Medley	8 fl oz	120	0	0
Tropical Punch Box	8.45 fl oz	130	0	0
Tropical Punch Chilled	8 fl oz	120	0	0
Mott's				
Apple Cranberry Blend	10 fl oz	180	0	0
Apple Cranberry From Concentrate as prep	8 fl oz	120	0	0
Apple Grape From Concentrate as prep	8 fl oz	120	0	0
Apple Raspberry Blend	10 fl oz	140	0	0
Apple Raspberry From Concentrate	8.45 fl oz	120	0	0
Fruit Basket Apple Raspberry Juice Cocktail as prep	8 fl oz	130	0	0
Fruit Basket Tropical Blend Juice Cocktail as prep	8 fl oz	120	0	0
Fruit Punch From Concentrate	10 fl oz	170	0	0
Fruit Punch From Concentrate	8.45 fl oz	120	0	0
Grape Apple	10 fl oz	170	0	0
Pineapple Orange	10 fl oz	170	0	0
Ocean Spray				
Cran-Blueberry	8 fl oz	160	0	0
Cran-Cherry	6 fl oz	160	0	0
Cran-Grape	8 fl oz	170	0	0
Cran-Raspberry	8 fl oz	140	0	0
Cran-Raspberry Reduced Calorie	8 fl oz	50	0	0
Cran-Strawberry	8 fl oz	140	0	0
Cranapple	8 fl oz	160	0	0
Cranapple Reduced Calorie	8 fl oz	50	0	0

FOOD	PORTION	CALS.	SAT. FAT	FAT
Cranicot	8 fl oz	160	0	0
Crantastic	8 fl oz	150	0	0
Fruit Punch	8 fl oz	130	0	0
Lightstyle Cran-Grape Low Calorie	8 fl oz	40	0	0
Lightstyle Cran-Raspberry Low Calorie	8 fl oz	40	0	0
Refreshers Citrus Cranberry Juice Drink	8 fl oz	140	0	0
Refreshers Citrus Peach Juice Drink	8 fl oz	120	0	0
Refreshers Orange Cranberry Juice Drink	8 fl oz	130	0	0
Ruby Red & Tangerine Grapefruit Juice Cocktail	8 fl oz	130	0	0
Odwalla				
Blackberry Fruitshake	8 fl oz	160	0	0
Boyzenberry Mango	8 fl oz	140	0	0
C Monster	16 fl oz	300	0	0
Guanaba Dabba Doo!	8 fl oz	130	0	0
Lotta Colada	8 fl oz	160	—	3
Mango Tango	8 fl oz	150	—	3
Mo Beta	16 fl oz	280	—	1
Raspberry Smoothie	8 fl oz	140	0	0
Strawberry Banana Smoothie	8 fl oz	100	0	0
Strawberry Go Man Go	8 fl oz	100	—	1
Super Protein	16 fl oz	400	—	6
S&W Apricot Pineapple Nectar	6 fl oz	120	0	0
S&W Apricot Pineapple Nectar Diet	6 fl oz	80	0	0
Sipps				
Fruit Punch	8.45 oz	130	—	0
Lemon Lime Cooler	8.45 oz	130	—	0
Mixed Berry	8.45 oz	130	—	0
Sunshine Punch	8.45 oz	130	—	0
Smucker's Apple Cranberry Juice	8 oz	120	0	0
Smucker's Orange Banana Juice	8 oz	120	0	0
Sunny Delight	6 fl oz	90	—	0

FOOD	PORTION	CALS.	SAT. FAT	FAT
Tang Mixed Fruit	8.45 fl oz	137	0	0
Tree Top				
Apple Citrus	6 fl oz	90	0	0
Apple Cranberry	6 fl oz	100	0	0
Apple Grape	6 fl oz	100	0	0
Apple Pear	6 fl oz	90	0	0
Apple Raspberry	6 fl oz	80	0	0
Tropicana				
Berry Punch	8 fl oz	120	0	0
Citrus Punch	1 bottle (10 fl oz)	180	0	0
Citrus Punch	8 fl oz	140	0	0
Cranberry Punch	1 bottle (10 fl oz)	170	0	0
Cranberry Punch	1 can (11.5 fl oz)	200	0	0
Cranberry Punch	8 fl oz	140	0	0
Fruit Punch	1 bottle (10 fl oz)	150	0	0
Fruit Punch	1 can (11.5 fl oz)	170	0	0
Fruit Punch	1 container (10 fl oz)	160	0	0
Fruit Punch	8 fl oz	130	0	0
Orange Pineapple	1 bottle (10 fl oz)	130	0	0
Orange Pineapple	8 fl oz	110	0	0
Pineapple Punch	1 bottle (10 fl oz)	160	0	0
Pineapple Punch	8 fl oz	120	0	0
Season's Best Cranberry Medley	8 fl oz	120	0	0
Tropicana Tropics				
Apple Cranberry Kiwi	8 fl oz	120	0	0
Orange Strawberry Banana	8 fl oz	110	0	0
Orange Kiwi Passion	8 fl oz	100	0	0
Orange Peach Mango	8 fl oz	110	0	0
Orange Pineapple	8 fl oz	110	0	0
Pineapple Passion	8 fl oz	120	0	0
Tropicana Twister				
Apple Raspberry Blackberry	1 bottle (10 fl oz)	150	0	0
Apple Raspberry Blackberry	1 can (11.5 fl oz)	180	0	0
Apple Raspberry Blackberry	8 fl oz	120	0	0
Cranberry Raspberry Strawberry	1 bottle (10 fl oz)	160	0	0
Cranberry Raspberry Strawberry	8 fl oz	120	0	0

FOOD	PORTION	CALS.	SAT. FAT	FAT
Orange Strawberry Banana	1 container (10 fl oz)	140	0	0
Orange Cranberry	1 bottle (10 fl oz)	140	0	0
Orange Cranberry	1 container (10 fl oz)	140	0	0
Orange Cranberry	8 fl oz	120	0	0
Orange Peach	1 bottle (10 fl oz)	140	0	0
Orange Peach	1 can (11.5 fl oz)	160	0	0
Orange Peach	8 fl oz	120	0	0
Orange Raspberry	1 bottle (10 fl oz)	140	0	0
Orange Raspberry	8 fl oz	120	0	0
Strawberry Banana	1 bottle (10 fl oz)	140	0	0
Strawberry Banana	1 can (11.5 fl oz)	160	0	0
Strawberry Banana	8 fl oz	120	0	0
Strawberry Guava	1 bottle (10 fl oz)	140	0	0
Strawberry Guava	8 fl oz	110	0	0
Tropicana Twister Light				
Cranberry Raspberry Strawberry	1 container (10 fl oz)	50	0	0
Cranberry Raspberry Strawberry	8 fl oz	45	0	0
Orange Strawberry Banana	1 container (10 fl oz)	45	0	0
Orange Strawberry Banana	1 container (10 fl oz)	45	0	0
Orange Strawberry Banana	8 fl oz	35	0	0
Orange Cranberry	1 container (10 fl oz)	35	0	0
Orange Cranberry	1 container (10 fl oz)	35	0	0
Orange Cranberry	8 fl oz	30	0	0
Orange Raspberry	1 container (10 fl oz)	45	0	0
Orange Raspberry	8 fl oz	35	0	0
Veryfine				
Apple Cherryberry	8 fl oz	130	0	0
Apple Cranberry	8 fl oz	130	0	0
Apple Raspberry	8 fl oz	110	0	0
Fruit Punch	8 fl oz	130	0	0
Guava Strawberry	8 fl oz	120	0	0
Lemon & Lime	8 fl oz	120	0	0
Papaya Punch	8 fl oz	120	0	0
Passionfruit Orange	8 fl oz	110	0	0

FOOD	PORTION	CALS.	SAT. FAT	FAT
Veryfine *(cont.)*				
Pineapple Orange	8 fl oz	130	0	0
White House Apple Cherry	6 fl oz	90	0	0
cranberry apple drink	6 oz	123	—	0
cranberry apricot drink	6 oz	118	0	0
fruit punch	6 oz	87	0	tr
orange & apricot	1 cup	128	tr	tr
orange & grapefruit juice	1 cup	107	tr	tr
pineapple & grapefruit	1 cup	117	tr	tr
pineapple & orange drink	1 cup	125	0	0

FRUIT, MIXED
(see also individual names)

FOOD	PORTION	CALS.	SAT. FAT	FAT
CANNED				
Chunky Mixed Diet (S&W)	½ cup	40	0	0
Chunky Mixed Lite (Libby)	½ cup (4.3 oz)	60	0	0
Chunky Mixed Natural Style (S&W)	½ cup	90	0	0
Chunky Mixed Unsweetened (S&W)	½ cup	40	0	0
Fruit Cocktail (Hunt's)	4 oz	90	—	tr
Fruit Cocktail Diet (S&W)	½ cup	40	0	0
Fruit Cocktail Heavy Syrup (S&W)	½ cup	90	0	0
Fruit Cocktail Natural Lite (S&W)	½ cup	60	0	0
Fruit Cocktail Natural Style (S&W)	½ cup	90	0	0
Fruit Cocktail Unsweetened (S&W)	½ cup	40	0	0
Tropical Fruit Salad (Dole)	½ cup	70	—	tr
fruit cocktail in heavy syrup	½ cup	93	tr	tr
fruit cocktail juice pack	½ cup	56	tr	tr
fruit cocktail water pack	½ cup	40	tr	tr
fruit salad in heavy syrup	½ cup	94	tr	tr
fruit salad in light syrup	½ cup	73	tr	tr
fruit salad juice pack	½ cup	62	tr	tr
fruit salad water pack	½ cup	37	tr	tr
mixed fruit in heavy syrup	½ cup	92	tr	tr
tropical fruit salad in heavy syrup	½ cup	110	tr	tr
DRIED				
Fruit'n Nut Mix (Planters)	1 oz	150	2	9

FOOD	PORTION	CALS.	SAT. FAT	FAT
mixed	11 oz pkg	712	tr	1
FROZEN				
Applesauce Strawberry (Dole)	1 pkg (4 oz)	60	0	0
Burst O' Berries (Big Valley)	⅔ cup (4.9 oz)	70	0	0
California Tropics (Big Valley)	⅔ cup (4.9 oz)	60	0	0
Cup A Fruit (Big Valley)	1 pkg (4 oz)	50	0	0
Mixed (Big Valley)	4.9 oz	60	0	0
Mixed Fruit (Birds Eye)	½ cup	120	0	0
mixed fruit sweetened	1 cup	245	tr	tr

FRUIT SNACKS

FOOD	PORTION	CALS.	SAT. FAT	FAT
Brock				
Beauty And The Beast	1 pkg (0.9 oz)	90	0	0
Cinderella	1 pkg (0.9 oz)	90	0	0
Dinosaurs	1 pkg (0.9 oz)	90	0	0
Ninja Trolls	1 pkg (0.9 oz)	90	0	0
Sharks	1 pkg (0.9 oz)	90	0	0
Fruit Bites Jungle Pals	1 pkg (0.9 oz)	90	—	1
Fruit By The Foot Cherry	1	80	—	2
Fruit By The Foot Grape	1	80	—	2
Fruit By The Foot Strawberry	1	80	—	2
Fruit Roll-Ups				
Cherry	1 (0.5 oz)	50	—	tr
Crazy Colors	1 (0.5 oz)	50	—	tr
Fruit Punch	1 (0.5 oz)	50	—	tr
Grape	1 (0.5 oz)	50	—	tr
Raspberry	1 (0.5 oz)	50	—	tr
Strawberry	1 (0.5 oz)	50	—	tr
Garfield And Friends				
1–2 Punch	1 pkg	100	—	1
Cat Cooler	1 pkg	100	—	1
Fat Cat Funnies	1 (0.5 oz)	50	—	tr
Fruit Party	1 (0.5 oz)	50	—	tr
Very Strawberry	1 pkg	100	—	1
Hanna Barbera Flintstones	1 pkg (1 oz)	100	—	0
Hanna Barbera Jetsons	1 pkg (1 oz)	100	—	0
Hanna Barbera Yo Yogi!	1 pkg (1 oz)	100	—	0
Health Valley				
Bakes Apple	1 bar	100	—	3
Bakes Date	1 bar	100	—	3

FOOD	PORTION	CALS.	SAT. FAT	FAT
Health Valley *(cont.)*				
Bakes Raisin	1 bar	100	—	3
Fat Free Fruit Bars 100% Organic Apple	1 bar	140	—	tr
Fat Free Fruit Bars 100% Organic Apricot	1 bar	140	—	tr
Fat Free Fruit Bars 100% Organic Date	1 bar	140	—	tr
Fat Free Fruit Bars 100% Organic Raisin	1 bar	140	—	tr
Fruit & Fitness Bars	2 bars	200	—	5
Oat Bran Bakes Apricot	1 bar	100	—	3
Oat Bran Bakes Fig & Nut	1 bar	110	—	3
Oat Bran Jumbo Fruit Bars Almond & Date	1 bar	170	—	5
Oat Bran Jumbo Fruit Bars Raisin & Cinnamon	1 bar	160	—	2
Rice Bran Jumbo Fruit Bars Almond & Date	1 bar	160	—	5
Shark Bites & Berry Bears Assorted Fruit	1 pkg	100	—	tr
Shark Bites & Berry Bears Fruit Punch	1 pkg	100	—	tr
Squeezit				
Berry B. Wild	1 (6.75 oz)	90	0	0
Chucklin' Cherry	1 (6.75 oz)	90	0	0
Grumpy Grape	1 (6.75 oz)	90	0	0
Mean Green Puncher	1 (6.75 oz)	90	0	0
Silly Billy Strawberry	1 (6.75 oz)	90	0	0
Smarty Arty Orange	1 (6.75 oz)	90	0	0
Sunbelt				
Fruit Boosters Apple	1 (1.3 oz)	130	0	2
Fruit Boosters Blueberry	1 (1.3 oz)	130	0	2
Fruit Boosters Strawberry	1 (1.3 oz)	130	0	2
Fruit Jammers	1 (1 oz)	100	1	1
Sunkist				
Fruit Flippits Cherry	0.8 oz	107	—	4
Fruit Flippits Strawberry	0.8 oz	107	—	4
Fruit Roll Apricot	1	76	—	1
Fruit Roll Cherry	1	75	—	tr
Fruit Roll Grape	1	76	—	tr

FOOD	PORTION	CALS.	SAT. FAT	FAT
Fruit Roll Raspberry	1	75	—	tr
Fruit Roll Strawberry	1	74	—	tr
Fun Fruit Animals	0.9 oz	100	—	1
Fun Fruit Dinosaurs Strawberry	0.9 oz	100	—	1
Fun Fruit Galactic Gems	0.9 oz	100	—	1
Fun Fruit Mario Nintendo	0.9 oz	100	—	tr
Fun Fruit Meteorites	0.9 oz	100	—	1
Fun Fruit Spooky Fruit	1 pkg	100	—	1
Fun Fruit Strawberry	0.9 oz	100	—	1
Fun Fruit Wacky Players	0.9 oz	100	—	1
Surf's Up! Sun Splash	1 pkg	100	—	1
Surf's Up! Tutti Frutti	1 pkg	100	—	1
Thunder Jets Assorted Fruit Squadron	1 pkg	100	—	1
Thunder Jets Mach 1 Fruit Mix	1 pkg	100	—	1
Tiny Toons Bunch Of Berries	1 pkg (0.9 oz)	100	—	1
Tiny Toons Fruit Assortment	1 pkg (0.9 oz)	100	—	1
Tiny Toons Paaaarrrty Punch	1 pkg (0.9 oz)	100	—	1
Weight Watchers Apple	½ oz	50	0	tr
Weight Watchers Cinnamon	½ oz	50	0	tr
Weight Watchers Peach	½ oz	50	0	tr
Weight Watchers Strawberry	½ oz	50	0	tr

GARBANZO
(see CHICKPEAS)

GARLIC

clove	1	4	tr	tr
powder	1 tsp	9	—	tr

GEFILTE FISH
READY-TO-USE

Manischewitz	1 piece	107	—	4
Manischewitz Gefiltefish & Pike	1 piece	99	—	4
Manischewitz Gefiltefish & Pike Sweet	1 piece	129	—	4
Manischewitz Homestyle	1 piece	111	—	4

FOOD	PORTION	CALS.	SAT. FAT	FAT
Manischewitz Sweet	1 piece	132	—	4
sweet	1 piece (1.5 oz)	35	tr	1

GELATIN
DRINKS

FOOD	PORTION	CALS.	SAT. FAT	FAT
Orange Flavored Drinking Gelatin w/ Nutrasweet (Knox)	1 envelope	39	—	tr

MIX

FOOD	PORTION	CALS.	SAT. FAT	FAT
Apple (Royal)	½ cup	80	0	0
Apricot (Jell-O)	½ cup	82	tr	tr
Blackberry (Jell-O)	½ cup	82	tr	tr
Blackberry (Royal)	½ cup	80	0	0
Black Cherry (Jell-O)	½ cup	82	tr	tr
Black Raspberry (Jell-O)	½ cup	82	tr	tr
Cherry (D-Zerta)	½ cup	8	0	0
Cherry (Royal)	½ cup	80	0	0
Cherry Sugar Free (Diamond Crystal)	½ cup	8	—	tr
Cherry Sugar Free (Jell-O)	½ cup	9	0	0
Cherry Sugar Free (Royal)	½ cup	8	0	0
Concord Grape (Jell-O)	½ cup	82	tr	tr
Concord Grape (Royal)	½ cup	80	0	0
Fruit Punch (Royal)	½ cup	80	0	0
Hawaiian Pineapple Sugar Free (Jell-O)	1 pop	8	—	tr
Kosher-Jel (Emes)	½ cup (4 fl oz)	60	0	0
Kosher-Jel Plain (Emes)	1 tbsp (7 g)	21	0	0
Lemon (D-Zerta)	½ cup	8	0	0
Lemon (Jell-O)	½ cup	81	tr	tr
Lemon (Royal)	½ cup	80	0	0
Lemon Sugar Free (Diamond Crystal)	½ cup	8	—	tr
Lemon Sugar Free (Jell-O)	½ cup	8	0	0
Lemon-Lime (Royal)	½ cup	80	0	0
Lime (D-Zerta)	½ cup	9	0	0
Lime (Jell-O)	½ cup	82	tr	tr
Lime (Royal)	½ cup	80	0	0
Lime Sugar Free (Diamond Crystal)	½ cup	8	—	tr
Lime Sugar Free (Jell-O)	½ cup	9	0	0
Lime Sugar Free (Royal)	½ cup	8	0	0
Mixed Berry (Royal)	½ cup	80	0	0
Mixed Fruit (Jell-O)	½ cup	81	tr	tr

FOOD	PORTION	CALS.	SAT. FAT	FAT
Mixed Fruit Sugar Free (Jell-O)	½ cup	8	0	0
Orange (D-Zerta)	½ cup	80	0	0
Orange (Jell-O)	½ cup	82	tr	tr
Orange (Royal)	½ cup	80	0	0
Orange Sugar Free (Diamond Crystal)	½ cup	8	0	0
Orange Sugar Free (Jell-O)	½ cup	8	0	0
Orange Sugar Free (Royal)	½ cup	10	0	0
Peach (Royal)	½ cup	80	0	0
Peach Sugar Free (Jell-O)	½ cup	8	—	tr
Pineapple (Royal)	½ cup	80	0	0
Raspberry (D-Zerta)	½ cup	8	0	0
Raspberry (Royal)	½ cup	80	0	0
Raspberry Sugar Free (Diamond Crystal)	½ cup	8	—	tr
Raspberry Sugar Free (Jell-O)	½ cup	8	0	0
Raspberry Sugar Free (Royal)	½ cup	8	0	0
Strawberry (D-Zerta)	½ cup	8	0	0
Strawberry (Royal)	½ cup	80	0	0
Strawberry Sugar Free (Diamond Crystal)	½ cup	8	—	tr
Strawberry Sugar Free (Jell-O)	½ cup	9	0	0
Strawberry Sugar Free (Royal)	½ cup	8	0	0
Strawberry Banana Sugar Free (Jell-O)	½ cup	9	0	0
Strawberry Banana Sugar Free (Royal)	½ cup	8	0	0
Strawberry-Orange (Royal)	½ cup	80	0	0
Triple Berry Sugar Free (Jell-O)	½ cup	8	—	tr
Tropical Fruit (Royal)	½ cup	80	0	0
Wild Strawberry (Jell-O)	½ cup	81	tr	tr
fruit flavored	½ cup	70	0	0
low calorie	½ cup	8	0	0
GIBLETS				
capon, simmered	1 cup (5 oz)	238	3	8
chicken, floured, fried	1 cup (5 oz)	402	6	19
chicken, simmered	1 cup (5 oz)	228	2	7
turkey, simmered	1 cup (5 oz)	243	2	7

FOOD	PORTION	CALS.	SAT. FAT	FAT
GINGER				
ground	1 tsp	6	tr	tr
root, fresh	¼ cup	17	tr	tr
root, fresh	5 slices	8	tr	tr
root, fresh, sliced	¼ cup	17	tr	tr
GINKGO NUTS				
canned	1 oz	32	tr	tr
dried	1 oz	99	tr	tr
raw	1 oz	52	tr	tr
GIZZARDS				
chicken, simmered	1 cup (5 oz)	222	2	5
turkey, simmered	1 cup (5 oz)	236	2	6
GOAT				
roasted	3 oz	122	1	3
GOOSE				
FRESH				
w/ skin, roasted	6.6 oz	574	13	41
w/ skin, roasted	½ goose (1.7 lbs)	2362	53	170
w/o skin, roasted	5 oz	340	7	18
w/o skin, roasted	½ goose (1.3 lbs)	1406	27	75
GOOSEBERRIES				
fresh	1 cup	67	tr	1
CANNED				
in light syrup	½ cup	93	tr	tr
GRANOLA				
(see also CEREAL)				
BARS				
Fi-Bar Coconut	1	120	1	4
Fi-Bar Peanut Butter	1	130	1	4
Grist Mill				
Chewy Apple Cinnamon	1 (1 oz)	120	1	4
Chewy Chocolate Chip	1 (1 oz)	130	1	4
Chewy Chunky Nut And Raisin	1 (1 oz)	130	2	6
Chewy Peanut Butter	1 (1 oz)	130	1	5
Chewy Peanut Butter Chocolate	1 (1 oz)	130	1	4
Chocolate Snack Chocolate Chip	1 (1.2 oz)	180	5	10

FOOD	PORTION	CALS.	SAT. FAT	FAT
Chocolate Snack Nutty Fudge	1 (1.3 oz)	190	5	11
Crunchy Cinnamon	1 (0.8 oz)	110	1	5
Crunchy Oats 'N Honey	1 (0.8 oz)	110	1	5
Hershey Chocolate Covered Chocolate Chip	1 (1.2 oz)	170	—	8
Hershey Chocolate Covered Cocoa Creme	1 (1.2 oz)	180	—	9
Hershey Chocolate Covered Cookies & Creme	1 (1.2 oz)	170	—	8
Hershey Chocolate Covered Peanut Butter	1 (1.2 oz)	180	—	10
Kudos Chocolate Chip	1 bar (1 oz)	130	3	5
Kudos Nutty Fudge	1 bar (1 oz)	130	3	5
Kudos Peanut Butter	1 bar (1 oz)	130	3	5
Nature Valley				
Cinnamon	1	120	1	5
Oat Bran Honey Graham	1	110	tr	4
Oats 'N Honey	1	120	1	5
Peanut Butter	1	120	1	6
Rice Bran Cinnamon Graham	1	90	tr	4
New Trail Chocolate Covered Cookies & Creme	1	200	—	11
Quaker Chewy Chocolate Chip	1	128	2	5
Quaker Chewy Chunky Nut & Raisin	1	131	1	6
Quaker Chewy Cinnamon Raisin	1	128	1	5
Quaker Chewy Honey & Oats	1	125	1	4
Quaker Chewy Peanut Butter	1	128	1	5
Quaker Chewy Peanut Butter Chocolate Chip	1	131	2	6
Quaker Dipps Caramel Nut	1	148	3	6
Quaker Dipps Chocolate Chip	1	139	3	6
Quaker Dipps Chocolate Fudge	1	160	—	8
Quaker Dipps Peanut Butter	1	170	3	9

FOOD	PORTION	CALS.	SAT. FAT	FAT
Quaker Dipps Peanut Butter Chocolate Chip	1	174	—	10
Quaker Dipps Rocky Road	1	140	—	7
Sunbelt Chewy Chocolate Chip	1 (1.8 oz)	220	4	10
Sunbelt Chewy Oats & Honey	1 (1 oz)	130	2	5
Sunbelt Chewy w/ Almonds	1 (1 oz)	130	2	7
Sunbelt Chewy w/ Raisins	1 (1.2 oz)	150	2	6
Sunbelt Fudge Dipped Chewy Chocolate Chip	1 (1.5 oz)	190	4	8
Sunbelt Fudge Dipped Chewy Macaroon	1 (1.4 oz)	200	7	13
Sunbelt Fudge Dipped Chewy Macaroon	1 bar (2 oz)	280	9	17
Sunbelt Fudge Dipped Chewy w/ Peanuts	1 bar (1.5 oz)	210	3	12
Sunbelt Fudge Dipped Chewy w/ Peanuts	1 (2 oz)	270	4	15
CEREAL				
Erewhon Date Nut	1 oz	130	—	6
Erewhon Honey Almond	1 oz	130	—	6
Erewhon Maple	1 oz	130	—	5
Erewhon Spiced Apple	1 oz	130	—	6
Erewhon Sunflower Crunch	1 oz	130	—	4
Erewhon w/ Bran	1 oz	130	—	6
Good Shepherd				
Crunchy	1 oz	130	—	5
Honey Almond	1 oz	120	—	4
Organic 5 Grain Muesli	1 oz	160	—	3
Organic Brown Rice	1 oz	130	—	4
Organic Wheat Free	1 oz	90	—	3
Organic Wheat Free Apple Cinnamon	1 oz	125	—	4
Organic Wheat Free Blueberry Amaranth	1 oz	110	—	1
Organic Wheat Free Strawberry Amaranth	1 oz	110	—	1
Grist Mill Low Fat With Raisins	⅔ cup (1.9 oz)	220	1	3
Kellogg's Low Fat	⅓ cup (1 oz)	110	0	2
Kellogg's Low Fat With Raisins	⅓ cup (1.1 oz)	120	0	2

FOOD	PORTION	CALS.	SAT. FAT	FAT
Nature Valley Cinnamon & Raisin	⅓ cup	120	—	4
Nature Valley Fruit & Nut	⅓ cup (1 oz)	130	—	5
Nature Valley Toasted Nut	⅓ cup (1 oz)	130	—	5
Post Hearty	¼ cup (1 oz)	128	—	4
Quaker Sun Country 100% Natural w/ Almonds	¼ cup	130	1	5
Quaker Sun Country 100% Natural w/ Raisins & Dates	¼ cup	123	1	5
Quaker Sun Country w/ Raisins	¼ cup	125	1	5
Sunbelt Banana Nut	1.9 oz	250	4	9
Sunbelt Fruit & Nut	1.9 oz	230	3	7
Sunbelt Low Fat	1.9 oz	200	1	3
Granola	¼ cup	138	1	8

GRAPEFRUIT
CANNED

FOOD	PORTION	CALS.	SAT. FAT	FAT
Sections in Light Syrup (S&W)	½ cup	80	0	0
Sections Natural Style (S&W)	½ cup	40	0	0
Sections Unsweetened (S&W)	½ cup	40	0	0
juice pack	½ cup	46	tr	tr
unsweetened	1 cup	93	tr	tr
water pack	½ cup	44	tr	tr

FRESH

FOOD	PORTION	CALS.	SAT. FAT	FAT
Chiquita Ruby Red	½	40	—	0
Dole	½	50	—	0
Ocean Spray Pink	½ med	50	0	0
Ocean Spray White	½ med	45	0	0
pink	½	37	tr	tr
pink sections	1 cup	69	tr	tr
red	½	37	tr	tr
red sections	1 cup	69	tr	tr
white	½	39	tr	tr
white sections	1 cup	76	tr	tr

JUICE

FOOD	PORTION	CALS.	SAT. FAT	FAT
Crystal Geyser Juice Squeeze	1 bottle (12 fl oz)	150	0	0
Minute Maid Frozen	8 fl oz	100	0	0

FOOD	PORTION	CALS.	SAT. FAT	FAT
Minute Maid *(cont.)*				
Juices To Go	1 bottle (10 fl oz)	120	0	0
Juices To Go	1 bottle (16 fl oz)	100	0	0
Juices To Go	1 can (11.5 fl oz)	140	0	0
Juices To Go Pink Cocktail	1 bottle (10 fl oz)	140	0	0
Juices To Go Pink Cocktail	1 bottle (16 fl oz)	110	0	0
Juices To Go Pink Juice Cocktail	8 fl oz	160	0	0
Mott's From Concentrate as prep	8 fl oz	120	0	0
Ocean Spray				
100%	8 oz	100	0	0
Lightstyle Pink Grapefruit Juice Cocktail Low Calorie	8 fl oz	40	0	0
Pink Grapefruit Juice Cocktail	8 oz	110	0	0
Ruby Red Grapefruit Drink	8 oz	130	0	0
Odwalla	8 fl oz	90	0	0
S&W Unsweetened	6 oz	80	0	0
Tree Top	6 oz	80	0	0
Tropicana	1 container (6 fl oz)	80	0	0
Tropicana	8 fl oz	90	0	0
Ruby Red	1 container (10 fl oz)	120	0	0
Ruby Red	8 fl oz	100	0	0
Season's Best	1 bottle (10 fl oz)	110	0	0
Season's Best	1 bottle (7 fl oz)	80	0	0
Season's Best	1 can (11.5 fl oz)	120	0	0
Season's Best	8 fl oz	90	0	0
Twister Pink	1 can (11.5 fl oz)	160	0	0
Twister Pink	1 container (10 fl oz)	140	0	0
Twister Pink	8 fl oz	110	0	0
Twister Light Pink	1 container (10 fl oz)	50	0	0
Twister Light Pink	8 fl oz	40	0	0
Veryfine 100%	8 oz	101	0	0
Veryfine Pink Grapefruit	8 oz	120	0	0
fresh	1 cup	96	tr	tr
frzn, as prep	1 cup	102	tr	tr

FOOD	PORTION	CALS.	SAT. FAT	FAT
frzn, not prep	6 oz	302	tr	1
sweetened	1 cup	116	tr	tr

GRAPES

CANNED

FOOD	PORTION	CALS.	SAT. FAT	FAT
Thompson Seedless Premium (S&W)	½ cup	100	0	0
thompson seedless in heavy syrup	½ cup	94	tr	tr
thompson seedless water pack	½ cup	48	tr	tr

FRESH

FOOD	PORTION	CALS.	SAT. FAT	FAT
Dole	1½ cup	85	—	0
grapes	10	36	tr	tr

JUICE

FOOD	PORTION	CALS.	SAT. FAT	FAT
Bama	8.45 oz	120	0	0
Bright & Early Frozen	8 fl oz	140	0	0
Hawaiian Punch	6 oz	90	—	0
Hi-C	1 can (11.5 fl oz)	180	0	0
Hi-C	8 fl oz	130	0	0
Hi-C Box	8.45 fl oz	130	0	0
Juice Works	6 oz	100	—	0
Juicy Juice	1 bottle (6 fl oz)	90	0	0
Juicy Juice	1 box	130	0	0
Kool-Aid	8 oz	98	0	0
Kool-Aid Sugar Free	8 oz	3	0	0
Kool-Aid Sugar Sweetened	8 oz	80	0	0
Minute Maid Chilled	8 fl oz	130	0	0
Minute Maid Grape Punch Frozen	8 fl oz	130	0	0
Mott's Drink	10 fl oz	170	0	0
Mott's Fruit Basket Grape Juice Cocktail as prep	8 fl oz	130	0	0
S&W Concord Unsweetened	6 oz	100	0	0
Seneca				
Blush Grape Juice frzn, as prep	8 fl oz	170	0	0
Fortified With Vitamin C frzn, as prep	8 fl oz	170	0	0
Sweetened frzn, as prep	8 fl oz	140	0	0
White Grape Juice frzn, as prep	8 fl oz	140	0	0
Sippin' Pak 100% Pure	8.45 fl oz	130	0	0
Sipps Grape	8.45 oz	130	—	0

FOOD	PORTION	CALS.	SAT. FAT	FAT
Tang Fruit Box	8.45 oz	131	0	0
Tree Top	6 oz	120	0	0
Tree Top Sparkling Juice	6 oz	120	0	0
Tropicana Season's Best	8 fl oz	160	0	0
Veryfine 100%	8 oz	153	0	0
Veryfine Grape Drink	8 oz	130	0	0
Wylers Drink Mix Unsweetened	8 oz	2	0	0
bottled	1 cup	155		tr
frzn, sweetened, as prep	1 cup	128		tr
frzn, sweetened, not prep	6 oz	386		1
grape drink	6 oz	84		0

GRAVY
(see also SAUCE)

CANNED

FOOD	PORTION	CALS.	SAT. FAT	FAT
Aus Jus (Franco-American)	2 oz	10	—	0
Beef (Franco-American)	2 oz	25	—	1
Chicken (Franco-American)	2 oz	45	—	4
Chicken Giblet (Franco-American)	2 oz	30	—	2
Cream (Franco-American)	2 oz	35	—	2
Gravymaster	¼ tsp	3	0	0
Mushroom (Franco-American)	2 oz	25	—	1
Pork (Franco-American)	2 oz	40	—	3
Turkey (Franco-American)	2 oz	30	—	2
au jus	1 cup	38	tr	tr
beef	1 cup	124	3	6
beef	1 can (10 oz)	155	3	7
chicken	1 cup	189	3	14
mushroom	1 cup	120	1	6
turkey	1 cup	122	1	5

DRY

FOOD	PORTION	CALS.	SAT. FAT	FAT
Bournvita	2 heaping tsp	34	—	1
Bovril	1 heaping tsp	9	—	0
Brown (Hain)	¼ pkg	16	0	0
Brown (Pillsbury)	¼ cup	15	0	0
Chicken (Diamond Crystal)	2 oz	30	—	1
Chicken (Pillsbury)	¼ cup	25	—	1
Chicken Gravy Quik, as prep (LaLoma)	2 tsp	45	—	4
Country Quik Gravy, as prep (LaLoma)	2 tsp	10	—	tr
Home Style (Pillsbury)	¼ cup	15	0	0

FOOD	PORTION	CALS.	SAT. FAT	FAT
Marmite	1 heaping tsp	9	—	0
Mushroom Quik Gravy, as prep (LaLoma	2 tsp	10	—	tr
Oil-Less Roux And Gravy Mix (Cajun King)	3.5 oz	394	—	4
Onion Quik Gravy, as prep (LaLoma)	2 tsp	10	—	tr
au jus, as prep w/ water	1 cup	32	1	1
brown, as prep w/ water	1 cup	75	1	2
chicken, as prep	1 cup	83	1	2
mushroom, as prep	1 cup	70	1	1
onion, as prep w/ water	1 cup	77	tr	1
pork, as prep	1 cup	76	1	2
turkey, as prep	1 cup	87	1	2

GREAT NORTHERN BEANS
CANNED

FOOD	PORTION	CALS.	SAT. FAT	FAT
Allen	½ cup (4.5 oz)	100	0	1
Green Giant	½ cup	80	—	1
Hanover	½ cup	110	—	0
Trappey's With Sausage Trappey	½ cup (4.5 oz)	100	1	1
great northern	1 cup	300	tr	1

DRIED

FOOD	PORTION	CALS.	SAT. FAT	FAT
Bean Cuisine	½ cup	115	—	1
cooked	1 cup	210	tr	1

GREEN BEANS
CANNED

FOOD	PORTION	CALS.	SAT. FAT	FAT
Almondine (Green Giant)	½ cup	45	0	3
Cut				
(Allen)	½ cup (4.2 oz)	30	0	1
(Alma)	½ cup (4.2 oz)	30	0	1
(Crest Top)	½ cup (4.2 oz)	30	0	1
(GaBelle)	½ cup (4.2 oz)	30	0	1
(Green Giant)	½ cup	16	0	0
(Hanover)	½ cup	20	—	0
(Owatonna)	½ cup	20	—	0
(Seneca)	½ cup	20	0	0
(Sunshine)	½ cup (4.2 oz)	30	0	1
No Added Salt (Allen)	½ cup (4.2 oz)	15	0	0
Cuts Natural Pack (Seneca)	½ cup	20	0	0
Dilled (S&W)	½ cup	60	0	0
French (Green Giant)	½ cup	16	0	0

FOOD	PORTION	CALS.	SAT. FAT	FAT
French (Owatonna)	½ cup	20	0	0
French (Seneca)	½ cup	20	0	0
French Natural Pack (Seneca)	½ cup	20	0	0
French Style (Allen)	½ cup (4.2 oz)	25	0	0
French Style Premium Blue Lake (S&W)	½ cup	20	0	0
Green Beans & Wax Beans (S&W)	½ cup	20	0	0
Italian (Allen)	½ cup (4.2 oz)	35	0	1
Italian (Sunshine)	½ cup (4.2 oz)	35	0	1
Kitchen Sliced (Green Giant)	½ cup	16	0	0
Shell Outs (Allen)	½ cup (4.5 oz)	30	0	0
Whole (Seneca)	½ cup	20	0	0
Whole Fancy Stringless (S&W)	½ cup	20	0	0
Whole Vertical Pack (S&W)	½ cup	20	0	0
FROZEN				
Cut (Birds Eye)	½ cup	25	0	tr
Cut (Fresh Like)	3.5 oz	29	—	tr
Cut (Hanover)	½ cup	20	0	0
Cut Beans (Southland)	3 oz	25	—	0
Cut in Butter Sauce (Green Giant)	½ cup	30	tr	1
Farm Fresh Whole (Birds Eye)	¾ cup	30	0	0
French (Southland)	3 oz	25	0	0
French Cut (Birds Eye)	½ cup	25	0	0
French Style Blue Lake (Hanover)	½ cup	25	—	0
Green Giant	½ cup	14	0	0
Harvest Fresh Cut (Green Giant)	½ cup	16	0	0
In Sauce French Green Beans With Toasted Almonds (Birds Eye)	½ cup	50	tr	2
Italian (Birds Eye)	½ cup	31	0	tr
Italian (Fresh Like)	3.5 oz	35	—	tr
Italian Cut (Hanover)	½ cup	35	0	0
One Serve in Butter Sauce (Green Giant)	1 pkg	60	tr	2
Polybag Cut (Birds Eye)	½ cup	25	0	0

FOOD	PORTION	CALS.	SAT. FAT	FAT
Polybag Deluxe Whole (Birds Eye)	½ cup	20	0	0
Polybag French Cut (Birds Eye)	½ cup	25	0	0
Whole (Fresh Like)	3.5	29	—	tr
Whole Blue Lake (Hanover)	½ cup	30	—	0
Whole Deluxe (Birds Eye)	½ cup	45	0	0
SHELF STABLE				
Cut (Pantry Express)	½ cup	12	0	0

GROUNDCHERRIES
fresh	½ cup	37	—	tr

GROUPER
FRESH				
cooked	3 oz	100	tr	1
cooked	1 fillet (7.1 oz)	238	1	3
raw	3 oz	78	tr	1

GUAVA
guava sauce	½ cup	43	tr	tr
fresh	1	45	tr	1
JUICE				
Kern's Nectar	6 oz	110	0	0
Libby's Nectar	1 can (11.5 oz)	110	0	0

GUINEA HEN
w/ skin, raw	½ hen (12.1 oz)	545	—	22
w/o skin, raw	½ hen (9.3 oz)	292	—	7

HADDOCK
FRESH				
cooked	3 oz	95	tr	1
cooked	1 fillet (5.3 oz)	168	tr	1
raw	3 oz	74	tr	1
roe, raw	3½ oz	130	—	2
FROZEN				
Batter-Dipped (Van De Kamp's)	2 pieces	250	3	15
Breaded Fillets (Van De Kamp's)	2 pieces	270	3	16
Crunchy Batter Fillets (Mrs. Paul's)	2 fillets	190	—	5

FOOD	PORTION	CALS.	SAT. FAT	FAT
Fishmarket Fresh (Gorton's)	5 oz	110	—	1
Light Fillets (Mrs. Paul's)	1 fillet	220	—	9
Light Fillets (Van De Kamp's)	1 piece	240	2	11
Microwave Entree in Lemon Butter (Gorton's)	1 pkg	360	10	21
SMOKED				
smoked	3 oz	99	tr	1
smoked	1 oz	33	tr	tr

HAKE
raw	3.5 oz	84	—	1

HALIBUT
FRESH				
atlantic & pacific, cooked	½ filled (5.6 oz)	223	1	5
atlantic & pacific, cooked	3 oz	119	tr	2
atlantic & pacific, raw	3 oz	93	tr	2
greenland, baked	3 oz	203	2	15
greenland, baked	5.6 oz	380	5	28
FROZEN				
Battered (Van De Kamp's)	2 pieces	150	1	6

HAM
(*see also* HAM DISHES, LUNCHEON MEATS/COLD CUTS, PORK, TURKEY)

Alpine Lace Boneless Cooked	2 slices (2 oz)	60	1	2
Armour Golden Star Boneless	1 oz	33	—	1
Armour Golden Star Canned	1 oz	32	—	tr
Armour Lower Salt 93% Fat Free	1 oz	35	—	1
Armour Lower Salt Boneless	1 oz	34	—	1
Armour Star Boneless	1 oz	41	—	2
Armour Star Canned	1 oz	34	—	1
Armour Star Speedy Cut	1 oz	44	—	3
Armour 1877 Boneless	1 oz	42	—	2
Black Label Chopped	2 oz	140	4	11
Carl Buddig	1 oz	50	—	3
Carl Buddig Honey Ham	1 oz	50	1	3
Hansel 'n Gretel Baked Virginia	1 oz	34	—	1

FOOD	PORTION	CALS.	SAT. FAT	FAT
Hansel 'n Gretel Black Forest	1 oz	32	—	1
Hansel 'n Gretel Cappy	1 oz	31	—	1
Hansel 'n Gretel Cooked Fresh	1 oz	33	—	1
Hansel 'n Gretel Deluxe	1 oz	31	—	1
Hansel 'n Gretel Honey Valley	1 oz	31	—	1
Hansel 'n Gretel Jalapeno	1 oz	25	—	1
Hansel 'n Gretel Lessalt	1 oz	30	—	1
Hansel 'n Gretel Lessalt Virginia	1 oz	32	—	1
Hansel 'n Gretel Light	1 oz	27	—	1
Hansel 'n Gretel Travane	1 oz	31	—	1
Healthy Choice				
Cooked	3 slices (2.2 oz)	70	1	2
Deli-Thin Baked With Natural Juice	1.9 oz	60	1	2
Deli-Thin Variety Pack	2.2. oz	70	1	2
Honey With Natural Juices	1.9 oz	60	1	2
Smoked	3 slices (2.2 oz)	70	1	2
Smoked With Natural Juices	1.9 oz	60	1	2
Hillshire				
Brown Sugar	1 oz	40	—	2
Cooked Ham	1 oz	30	—	1
Deli Select Baked Ham	1 slice	10	—	tr
Deli Select Brown Sugar Baked	1 slice	10	—	tr
Deli Select Cajun Ham	1 slice	10	—	tr
Deli Select Honey Ham	1 slice	10	—	tr
Deli Select Lower Salt	1 slice	10	—	tr
Deli Select Smoked Ham	1 slice	10	—	tr
Flavor Pack 90–99% Fat Free Brown Sugar Baked	1 slice (0.6 oz)	20	—	tr
Flavor Pack 90–99% Fat Free Honey Ham	1 slice (0.6 oz)	20	—	tr
Flavor Pack 90–99% Fat Free Smoked	1 slice (0.6 oz)	20	—	tr
Genuine Baked	1 oz	35	—	1
Honey Ham	1 oz	40	—	2
Lower Salt	1 oz	30	—	1

FOOD	PORTION	CALS.	SAT. FAT	FAT
Hillshire *(cont.)*				
Lunch 'N Munch Cooked Ham/Swiss/ Snickers Hi-C	1 pkg (4.25 oz + 6 fl oz)	470	—	21
Lunch 'N Munch Cooked Ham/Swiss/ Oreo	1 pkg (4.125 oz)	370	—	21
Lunch 'N Munch Cooked Ham/Swiss	1 pkg (4.5 oz)	360	—	22
Lunch 'N Munch Honey Ham/Cheddar/ Snickers/Hi-C	1 pkg (4.25 oz + 6 fl oz)	500	—	23
Hormel				
Black Label Canned (refrigerated)	3 oz	100	2	5
Black Label Canned (shelf stable)	3 oz	110	2	5
Canned Chunk	2 oz	90	2	6
Cure 81 Half Ham	3 oz	100	2	5
Curemaster	3 oz	80	1	3
Deli Cooked	1 oz	29	—	1
Deviled Ham	4 tbsp (2 oz)	150	4	12
Ham & Cheese Patties	1 patty (2 oz)	190	6	17
Light & Lean	3 oz	90	1	3
Light & Lean 97	3 oz	90	1	3
Light & Lean 97 Cuts	16 pieces (1 oz)	35	1	1
Light & Lean 97 Sliced	1 slice (1 oz)	25	1	1
Patties	1 patty (2 oz)	180	6	17
Primissimo Proscuitti	1 oz	70	2	5
Supreme Cut Canned	1 oz	31	—	1
Jones Family Ham	1 slice	40	—	2
Jones Ham Slices	1 slice	30	—	1
Krakus	1 oz	25	—	1
Louis Rich				
Carving Board Baked With Natural Juices	2 slices (1.6 oz)	45	0	1
Carving Board Honey With Natural Juices	2 slices (1.6 oz)	50	1	2
Carving Board Honey With Natural Juices Carved Thin	6 slices (2.1 oz)	70	1	2
Carving Board Smoked Cooked With Natural Juices	1 slice (1.6 oz)	50	1	2

FOOD	PORTION	CALS.	SAT. FAT	FAT
Dinner Slices Baked	1 slice (3.3 oz)	80	1	2
Oscar Mayer				
Baked	3 slices (2.2. oz)	60	1	1
Boiled	3 slices (2.2 oz)	60	1	3
Chopped	1 slice (1 oz)	50	1	4
Deli-Thin Boiled	4 slices (1.8 oz)	50	1	2
Deli-Thin Honey Ham	4 slices (1.8 oz)	60	1	2
Deli-Thin Smoked	4 slices (1.8 oz)	50	1	2
Dinner Slice	3 oz	90	1	3
Dinner Steaks	1 (2 oz)	60	1	2
Ham and Cheese Loaf	1 slice (1 oz)	70	3	5
Healthy Favorites Baked	4 slices (1.8 oz)	50	0	1
Healthy Favorites Honey Ham	4 slices (1.8 oz)	50	1	2
Healthy Favorites Smoked, Cooked	4 slices (1.8 oz)	50	1	2
Honey Ham	3 slices (2.2 oz)	70	1	3
Lower Sodium	3 slices (2.2 oz)	70	1	3
Lunchables Cookies/ Ham/Swiss	1 pkg (4.2 oz)	360	8	19
Lunchables Dessert Choc. Pudding/Ham/ American	1 pkg (6.2 oz)	390	9	20
Lunchables Ham/ Cheddar	1 pkg (4.5 oz)	340	11	20
Lunchables Ham/Garden Vegetable Cheese	1 pkg (4.5 oz)	380	9	21
Lunchables Honey Ham/ Herb & Chive Cheese	1 pkg (4.5 oz)	390	9	21
Smoked Cooked	3 slices (2.2 oz)	60	1	3
Russer				
Baked	2 oz	70	1	3
Canadian Brand Maple	2 oz	70	1	2
Chopped	2 oz	130	3	9
Cooked Ham	2 oz	60	1	3
Ham & Cheese Loaf	2 oz	120	2	8
Honey & Maple Cured	2 oz	70	1	2
Honey Cured	2 oz	60	1	3
Hot	2 oz	70	1	2
Lil' Salt Cooked	2 oz	60	1	2
Lil' Salt Smoked	2 oz	60	1	2
Smoked Virginia	2 oz	70	1	3
Spiced	2 oz	160	3	12
Spam Spread (Hormel)	4 tbsp (2 oz)	100	4	11

FOOD	PORTION	CALS.	SAT. FAT	FAT
The Spreadables Ham Salad	¼ can	100	—	6
Underwood Deviled	2.08 oz	220	6	19
Underwood Deviled Light	2.08 oz	120	1	8
Underwood Deviled Smoked	2.08 oz	190	6	18
Weight Watchers Deli Thin Oven Roasted	5 slices (⅓ oz)	12	—	tr
Weight Watchers Deli Thin Oven Roasted Honey Ham	5 slices (⅓ oz)	12	—	tr
Weight Watchers Deli Thin Premium Smoked	5 slices (⅓ oz)	12	—	tr
Weight Watchers Oven Roasted Honey Ham	2 slices (¾ oz)	25	—	1
Weight Watchers Oven Roasted Smoked	2 slices (¾ oz)	25	—	1
Weight Watchers Premium Cooked	2 slices (¾ oz)	25	—	1
boneless (11% fat), roasted	3 oz	151	—	8
boneless extra lean, roasted	3 oz	140	—	7
canned (13% fat)	3 oz	192	4	13
canned (13% fat)	1 oz	54	—	4
canned extra lean	1 oz	41	—	2
canned extra lean	3 oz	142	—	7
canned extra lean (4% fat)	3 oz	116	1	4
center slice, lean & fat	4 oz	229	5	15
center slice, lean only	4 oz	220	—	9
chopped	1 oz	65	2	5
chopped, canned	1 oz	68	2	5
ham & cheese loaf	1 oz	73	4	6
ham & cheese spread	1 oz	69	2	5
ham & cheese spread	1 tbsp	37	1	3
ham salad spread	1 oz	61	1	4
ham salad spread	1 tbsp	32	1	2
minced	1 oz	75	2	6
patties, grilled	1 patty (2 oz)	203	—	18
patties, uncooked	1 (2.3 oz)	206	—	18
sliced, extra lean (5% fat)	1 oz	37	tr	1
sliced, regular (11% fat)	1 oz	52	1	3
steak, boneless, extra lean	1 oz	35	tr	1
whole, lean & fat, roasted	3 oz	207	—	14
whole, lean only, roasted	3 oz	133	—	5

FOOD	PORTION	CALS.	SAT. FAT	FAT
HAM DISHES				
FROZEN				
Handy Pocket Cheese Sauce & Ham (Weight Watchers)	1 (4 oz)	200	2	6
Ovenstuffs Ham/Turkey Deli Melt	1 (4.75 oz)	360	—	15
HOME RECIPE				
croquettes	1 (3.1)	217	5	14
salad	½ cup	287	5	23
TAKE-OUT				
sandwich w/ cheese	1	353	6	15
HAMBURGER				
(see also BEEF)				
FROZEN				
Kid Cuisine Beef Patty Sandwich w/ Cheese	6.25 oz	430	—	22
Kid Cuisine Mega Meal Double Beef Patty Sandwich w/ Cheese	9.1 oz	480	—	20
MicroMagic Cheeseburger	1 pkg (4.75 oz)	450	—	25
MicroMagic Hamburger	1 pkg (4 oz)	350	—	18
White Castle Cheeseburger	1 (2.3 oz)	200	—	11
White Castle Hamburger	1 (2.1 oz)	160	—	8
TAKE-OUT				
double patty w/ bun	1 reg	544	10	28
double patty w/ bun, catsup, mayonnaise, mustard, pickle, onion, tomato	1 lg	540	11	27
double patty w/ bun, catsup, mustard, pickle, onion	1 reg	576	12	32
double patty w/ bun, cheese	1 reg	457	13	28
double patty w/ bun, cheese, catsup, mustard, mayonnaise, pickle, tomato	1 lg	706	18	44
double patty w/ bun, cheese, catsup, pickle, mayonnaise, onion, tomato	1 reg	416	8	21

FOOD	PORTION	CALS.	SAT. FAT	FAT
double patty w/ double bun, catsup, pickle, mayonnaise, onion, tomato	1 reg	649	13	35
double patty w/ double bun, cheese	1 reg	461	10	22
single patty w/ bun	1 reg	275	4	12
single patty w/ bun	1 lg	400	8	23
single patty w/ bun, catsup, mayonnaise, mustard, pickle, onion, tomato	1 reg	279	4	13
single patty w/ bun, cheese	1 reg	320	6	15
single patty w/ bun, cheese	1 lg	608	15	33
single patty w/ bun, cheese, bacon, catsup, mustard, pickle, onion	1 lg	609	16	37
single patty w/ bun, cheese, ham, catsup, mayonnaise, pickle, tomato	1 lg	745	21	48
triple patty w/ bun, catsup, mustard, pickle	1 lg	693	16	41
triple patty w/ bun, cheese	1 lg	769	22	51

HEART

FOOD	PORTION	CALS.	SAT. FAT	FAT
beef, simmered	3 oz	148	1	5
chicken, simmered	1 cup (5 oz)	268	3	11
lamb, braised	3 oz	158	3	7
pork, braised	1 (4.3 oz)	191	—	7
turkey, simmered	1 cup (5 oz)	257	3	9
veal, braised	3 oz	158	2	6

HERBAL TEA
(*see* TEA/HERBAL TEA)

HERBS/SPICES
(*see also individual names*)

FOOD	PORTION	CALS.	SAT. FAT	FAT
Ac'cent Flavor Enhancer	½ tsp	5	0	0
Ac'cent Herbal All Purpose Seasoning	½ tsp	0	0	0
All Purpose Seafood (Golden Dipt)	¼ tsp	2	0	0

FOOD	PORTION	CALS.	SAT. FAT	FAT
Bar-B-Q Shaker (Diamond Crystal)	½ tsp	4	0	0
Blackened Redfish (Golden Dipt)	¼ tsp	2	0	0
Broiled Fish (Golden Dipt)	¼ tsp	2	0	0
Cajun Style Shrimp & Crab (Golden Dipt)	¼ tsp	2	0	0
Chef Seasoning (Diamond Crystal)	1 pkg (.45 oz)	2	—	0
Chef Shaker (Diamond Crystal)	½ tsp	4	—	0
Crab Boil (McIlhenny)	3 oz	378	5	17
French Shaker (Diamond Crystal)	½ tsp	4	—	0
Italian Shaker (Diamond Crystal)	½ tsp	4	—	0
Lemon Pepper Seafood (Golden Dipt)	¼ tsp	8	0	0
Mexican Shaker (Diamond Crystal)	½ tsp	4	—	0
Mrs. Dash Extra Spicy	1 tsp	12	—	tr
Mrs. Dash Garlic & Herb	1 tsp	12	—	tr
Mrs. Dash Lemon & Herb	1 tsp	12	—	tr
Mrs. Dash Low Pepper Blend	1 tsp	12	—	tr
Mrs. Dash Original	1 tsp	12	—	tr
Mrs. Dash Table Blend	1 tsp	12	—	tr
Seasoning Blend Sloppy Joe (Lawry's)	1 pkg	126	—	tr
curry powder	1 tsp	6	—	tr
poultry seasoning	1 tsp	5	—	tr
pumpkin pie spice	1 tsp	6	—	tr

HERRING
CANNED
roe	3.5 oz	118	—	3

FRESH
atlantic, cooked	1 fillet (5 oz)	290	4	17
atlantic, cooked	3 oz	172	2	10
atlantic, raw	3 oz	134	2	8
pacific, baked	3 oz	213	4	15
pacific fillet, baked	5.1 oz	360	6	26
roe, raw	3.5 oz	130	—	2

READY-TO-USE
atlantic, kippered	1 fillet (1.4 oz)	87	1	5

FOOD	PORTION	CALS.	SAT. FAT	FAT
atlantic, pickled	½ oz	39	tr	3

HICKORY NUTS

FOOD	PORTION	CALS.	SAT. FAT	FAT
dried	1 oz	187	2	18

HOMINY

CANNED

FOOD	PORTION	CALS.	SAT. FAT	FAT
Golden (Allen)	½ cup (4.5 oz)	120	0	1
Golden (Uncle William)	½ cup (4.5 oz)	120	0	1
Golden (Van Camp's)	½ cup (4.3 oz)	80	0	1
Mexican (Allen)	½ cup (4.5 oz)	120	0	1
Mexican (Uncle William)	½ cup (4.5 oz)	120	0	1
White (Allen)	½ cup (4.5 oz)	100	0	1
White (Uncle William)	½ cup (4.5 oz)	100	0	1
White (Van Camp's)	½ cup (4.3 oz)	80	0	1
canned	½ cup	57	tr	tr

HONEY

FOOD	PORTION	CALS.	SAT. FAT	FAT
Burleson's Clover	1 tbsp	60	0	0
Burleson's Creamed	1 tbsp	60	0	0
Burleson's Natural	1 tbsp	60	0	0
Burleson's Pure	1 tbsp	60	0	0
Burleson's Raw	1 tbsp	60	0	0
Burleson's Rocky Mountain Clover	1 tbsp	60	0	0
Golden Blossom	1 tsp	20	0	0
Smucker's Single Serving	½ oz	45	—	0
honey	1 cup	1030	0	0
honey	1 tbsp	65	0	0

HONEYDEW

FRESH

FOOD	PORTION	CALS.	SAT. FAT	FAT
Chiquita	1 cup	70	—	0
Dole	⅒ mellon	50	—	0
cubed	1 cup	60	—	tr
wedge	⅒ melon	46	—	tr

FROZEN

FOOD	PORTION	CALS.	SAT. FAT	FAT
Big Valley Balls	¾ cup (4.9 oz)	45	0	0

HORSE

FOOD	PORTION	CALS.	SAT. FAT	FAT
roasted	3 oz	149	2	5

HORSERADISH

FOOD	PORTION	CALS.	SAT. FAT	FAT
Gold's Hot	1 tsp	4	—	tr
Gold's Red	1 tsp	4	0	0
Gold's White	1 tsp	4	—	tr

FOOD	PORTION	CALS.	SAT. FAT	FAT
Hebrew National White	1 tbsp	7	0	0
Heluva Good Cheese (Heluva Good Cheese)	1 tsp (5 g)	0	0	0
Kraft Prepared	1 tbsp	10	0	0
Kraft Horseradish Mustard	1 tbsp	14	0	1
Kraft Cream Style	1 tbsp	12	0	1
Rosoff's Red	1 tbsp (0.5 oz)	8	0	0
Rosoff's White	1 tbsp (0.5 oz)	7	0	0
Sauceworks Horseradish	1 tbsp	50	1	5
Schorr's Red	1 tbsp (0.5 oz)	8	0	0
Schorr's White	1 tbsp (0.5 oz)	7	0	0

HOT CAKES
(see PANCAKES)

HOT DOG
(see also MEAT SUBSTITUTES, SAUSAGE, SAUSAGE SUBSTITUTES)

CHICKEN

FOOD	PORTION	CALS.	SAT. FAT	FAT
Empire	1 (2 oz)	100	2	7
Health Valley Wieners	1	96	—	8
Tyson	1	115	—	10
Tyson Cheese	1	145	—	11
Wampler Longacre	1 (2 oz)	144	—	44
Wampler Longacre	1 (1.6 oz)	115	—	35
chicken	1 (1.5 oz)	116	2	9

MEAT

FOOD	PORTION	CALS.	SAT. FAT	FAT
Armour Lower Salt Jumbo	1	170	—	15
Armour Lower Salt Jumbo Beef	1	170	—	15
Armour Star Jumbo	1	190	—	18
Armour Star Jumbo Beef	1	190	—	18
Chefwich Chili Dog	5 oz	380	—	15
Healthy Choice	1 (1.6 oz)	60	1	2
Healthy Choice Bunsize	1 (2 oz)	70	1	2
Hebrew National				
Beef	1 (1.7 oz)	150	—	14
Cocktail Beef	6 (1.8 oz)	160	—	15
Dinner Beef	1 (4 oz)	350	—	34
Reduced Fat Beef	1 (1.7 oz)	120	—	10
Hillshire				
Franks Bun Size Beef	2 oz	180	—	16
Franks Jumbo Light & Mild	1 link	110	—	8
Lit'l Franks Beef	2 oz	180	—	16
Lit'l Wieners	2 oz	180	—	16

FOOD	PORTION	CALS.	SAT. FAT	FAT
Hillshire *(cont.)*				
Weiners Bun Size	2 oz	180	—	16
Weiners Natural Casing	2 oz	180	—	17
Weiners Light & Mild	1 link	90	—	7
Hormel Big 8	1 (2 oz)	170	7	15
Hormel Light & Lean 97	1 (1.6 oz)	45	1	1
Hormel Light & Lean 97 Beef	1 (1.6 oz)	45	1	1
Nathan's Famous Natural Casing Franks	1	158	—	14
Nathan's Famous Skinless Franks	1	176	—	16
Oscar Mayer Beef	1 (1.6 oz)	150	6	13
Oscar Mayer				
Big & Juicy Hot 'N Spicy	1 (2.7 oz)	220	8	20
Big & Juicy Original	1 (2.7 oz)	240	9	23
Big & Juicy Original Beef	1 (2.7 oz)	230	9	21
Big & Juicy Quarter Pound Beef	1 (4 oz)	350	13	32
Big & Juicy Smokie Links	1 (2.7 oz)	200	7	18
Bun-Length Beef	1 (2 oz)	180	7	17
Cheese	1 (1.6 oz)	150	5	14
Healthy Favorites Turkey And Beef	1 (2 oz)	60	1	2
Light Beef	1 (2 oz)	110	3	8
Weiners Bun-Length Pork & Turkey	1 (2 oz)	180	6	17
Weiners Light Pork, Turkey, Beef	1 (2 oz)	110	3	8
Weiners Pork & Turkey	1 (1.6 oz)	150	5	13
Weiners Little	6 (2 oz)	170	6	16
Russer Lil' Salt Deli Franks	1 (2.67 oz)	160	4	11
Shofar Kosher Beef	1 (1.8 oz)	150	5	14
Shofar Kosher Beef Reduced Fat Reduced Sodium	1 (1.8 oz)	120	4	10
Wrangler Beef	1 (2 oz)	170	6	15
Wrangler Cheese	1 (2 oz)	170	7	15
Wrangler Smoked	1 (2 oz)	170	6	15
beef	1 (2 oz)	180	7	16
beef	1 (1.5 oz)	142	5	13
beef & pork	1 (2 oz)	183	6	17

FOOD	PORTION	CALS.	SAT. FAT	FAT
beef & pork	1 (1.5 oz)	144	5	13
pork cheesefurter smokie	1 (1.5 oz)	141	5	12
TAKE-OUT				
corndog	1	460	5	19
w/ bun, chili	1	297	5	13
w/ bun, plain	1	242	5	15
TURKEY				
Bil Mar Foods Cheese Franks	1 (1.6 oz)	109	—	9
Empire	1 (2 oz)	90	2	6
Health Valley Wieners	1	96	—	8
Louis Rich	1 (1.6 oz)	90	2	7
Louis Rich	1 (1.5 oz)	80	2	6
Louis Rich Bun Length	1 (2 oz)	110	3	8
Louis Rich Turkey Cheese Franks	1 (1.6 oz)	90	3	7
Mr. Turkey Franks	1 (2 oz)	132	—	11
Mr. Turkey Franks	1 (1.6 oz)	106	—	9
Mr. Turkey Franks	1 (0.5 oz)	79	—	7
Wampler Longacre	1 (1.6 oz)	102	—	31
turkey	1 (1.5 oz)	102	—	8

HUMMUS

hummus	⅓ cup	140	1	7
hummus	1 cup	420	3	21

HYACINTH BEANS

dried, cooked	1 cup	228	—	1

ICE CREAM AND FROZEN DESSERT

(see also ICES AND ICE POPS, PUDDING POPS, SHERBET, YOGURT FROZEN)

FOOD	PORTION	CALS.	SAT. FAT	FAT
3 Musketeers				
Single Chocolate	1 (2 fl oz)	160	6	10
Single Vanilla	1 (2 fl oz)	160	6	10
Snack Chocolate	1 (0.72 fl oz)	60	2	4
Snack Vanilla	1 (0.72 fl oz)	60	2	4
All Flavors Avari Creme Glace	1 oz	10	0	0
All Flavors Ice Cream (Bresler's)	3.5 oz	230	—	12
All Flavors Royale Cremes (Bresler's)	4 oz	260	—	16
All Flavors Royale Lites (Bresler's)	4 oz	217	0	0
Almond Praline Light (Edy's)	4 oz	140	2–3	5

FOOD	PORTION	CALS.	SAT. FAT	FAT
American Glory (Sealtest)	½ cup (2.4 oz)	130	4	6
Banana Bob (Good Humor)	1 (3 fl oz)	155	6	7
Banana Cream (Fi-Bar)	1 bar	93	—	tr
Banana-Politan Light (Edy's)	4 oz	110	2–3	4
Berry Berry Berry (Mocha Mix)	½ cup	209	2	6
Berry Swirl Bar Raspberry (Carnation)	1 bar	70	—	3
Berry Swirl Bar Strawberry (Carnation)	1 bar	70	—	3
Black Cherry Free (Sealtest)	½ cup	100	0	0
Black Cherry Fat Free (Borden)	½ cup	90	tr	tr
Black Forest Low-Fat (Healthy Choice)	½ cup (2.5 oz)	120	1	2
Bon Bons Vanilla With Milk Chocolate Coating (Nestle)	5 pieces	200	8	14
Bon Bons Vanilla With Milk Chocolate Coating (Nestle)	8 pieces	330	13	23
Bourdeaux Cherry Chocolate Chip (Healthy Choice)	½ cup (2.5 oz)	110	2	2
Bounty Cherry/Dark (M&M's)	1 (0.84 fl oz)	70	3	5
Bounty Coconut/Dark (M&M's)	1 (0.84 fl oz)	70	3	5
Bounty Coconut/Milk (M&M's)	1 (0.84 fl oz)	70	3	5
Brownie Marble Fudge Light (Breyers)	½ cup (2.6 oz)	150	3	5
Bubble O' Bill (Good Humor)	1 (3.6 fl oz)	170	8	10
Bubble Play (Good Humor)	1	110	1	1
Butter Almond (Breyers)	½ cup	170	6	11
Butter Pecan (Breyers)	½ cup	180	6	12
Butter Pecan (Frusen Gladje)	½ cup	280	9	21
Butter Pecan (Haagen-Dazs)	4 oz	390	9	24
Butter Pecan (Sealtest)	½ cup	160	5	9

FOOD	PORTION	CALS.	SAT. FAT	FAT
Butter Pecan Crunch (Healthy Choice)	½ cup (2.2 oz)	120	1	2
Butter Pecan Light (Edy's)	4 oz	140	2–3	5
Buttered Pecan (Borden)	½ cup	180	—	12
Butterfinger (Nestle)	1 bar (2.5 oz)	170	7	12
Butterfinger (Nestle)	8 nuggets	340	13	24
Cafe Au Lait Light (Edy's)	4 oz	110	2–3	4
Candy Bar Light (Edy's)	4 oz	140	2–3	5
Candy Cane Crunch (Sealtest)	½ cup (2.4 oz)	150	4	6
Candy Center Crunch Classic (Good Humor)	1 (3.1 fl oz)	260	14	19
Cappuccino (Rice Dream)	½ cup	130	—	5
Cappuccino Chocolate Chunk (Healthy Choice)	½ cup (2.2 oz)	120	1	2
Caramel Almond Crunch Bar (Haagen-Dazs)	1	240	7	18
Caramel Nut Sundae Haagen-Dazs	4 oz	310	—	21
Carob (Rice Dream)	½ cup	130	—	5
Carob (Tofu Ice Creme)	4 fl oz	190	—	8
Carob Almond (Rice Dream)	½ cup	140	—	6
Carob Chip (Rice Dream)	½ cup	140	—	6
Carob Chip Mint (Rice Dream)	½ cup	140	—	6
Cheesecake Bar Original (Carnation)	1 bar	120	—	6
Cheesecake Bar Strawberry (Carnation)	1 bar	125	—	6
Cherry & Ice Cream Swirl (Chiquita)	1 bar	80	—	3
Cherry Garcia (Ben & Jerry's)	1 pop (3.7 fl oz)	250	10	18
Cherry Garcia (Ben & Jerry's)	½ cup (4 fl oz)	230	9	16
Cherry Vanilla (Breyer's)	½ cup	150	5	7
Chip Burrrger (Good Humor)	1 (4.7 oz)	320	9	15
Chip Sandwich (Good Humor)	1 (4.7 oz)	320	9	15
Choco Taco (Good Humor)	1 (4.4 fl oz)	320	11	17
Chocolate (Ben & Jerry's)	4 oz	230	8	14
Chocolate (Breyer's)	½ cup (2.6 oz)	160	6	8

FOOD	PORTION	CALS.	SAT. FAT	FAT
Chocolate (Cyrk)	3 oz	209	9	16
Chocolate (Frusen Gladje)	½ cup	240	9	17
Chocolate (Haagen-Dazs)	4 oz	270	8	17
Chocolate (Sealtest)	½ cup (2.4 oz)	140	4	7
Chocolate (Ultra Slim-Fast)	4 oz	100	—	tr
Chocolate American Dream (Edy's)	3 oz	90	—	1
Chocolate Butter Pecan (Sealtest)	½ cup (2.4 oz)	150	5	8
Chocolate Caramel Sundae Light (Simple Pleasures)	4 oz	90	—	tr
Chocolate Chip (Simple Pleasures)	4 oz	150	—	3
Chocolate Chip American Dream (Edy's)	3 oz	100	—	1
Chocolate Chip Cookie Dough (Ben & Jerry's)	1 pop (2.5 fl oz)	240	9	16
Chocolate Chip Cookie Dough (Ben & Jerry's)	½ cup (4 fl oz)	260	10	17
Chocolate Chip Cookie Dough (Breyer's)	½ cup (2.5 oz)	190	7	10
Chocolate Chip Ice Milk (Light N' Lively)	½ cup	120	—	4
Chocolate Chip Ice Milk (Weight Watchers)	½ cup	120	3	4
Chocolate Chip Light (Edy's)	4 oz	120	2–3	4
Chocolate Chip Light (Light N' Lively)	½ cup (2.4 oz)	130	3	4
Chocolate Dark Chocolate Bar (Haagen-Dazs)	1	390	—	27
Chocolate Dip Bar (Weight Watchers)	1 (2 oz)	110	2	7
Chocolate Eclair Classic (Good Humor)	1 (3.1 fl oz)	170	3	9
Chocolate Fat Free (Borden)	½ cup	100	tr	tr
Chocolate Fat Free Frozen Dessert (Weight Watchers)	½ cup	80	0	0
Chocolate Fudge (Ultra Slim-Fast)	4 oz	120	—	tr
Chocolate Fudge Brownie (Ben & Jerry's)	4 oz	250	8	14
Chocolate Fudge Mousse Light (Edy's)	4 oz	130	2–3	5

FOOD	PORTION	CALS.	SAT. FAT	FAT
Chocolate Fudge Swirl Dessert Bar (Sealtest Free)	1	90	0	0
Chocolate Fudge Twirl Ice Milk (Breyers Light)	½ cup	130	3	4
Chocolate Ice Milk (Borden)	½ cup	100	—	2
Chocolate Malted Bars (Carnation)	1 bar	70	—	3
Chocolate Mousse Bar Sugar Free (Weight Watchers)	1 (1.75 oz)	35	0	tr
Chocolate Nutty Bar (Rice Dream)	1	330	—	23
Chocolate Peanut Butter Chocolate Chip Cookie Dough (Ben & Jerry's)	½ cup (4 fl oz)	280	9	18
Chocolate Swirl (Borden)	½ cup	130	—	6
Chocolate Swirl Fat Free Frozen Dessert (Weight Watchers)	½ cup	90	0	0
Chocolate Treat Bar Sugar Free (Weight Watchers)	1 (2.75 oz)	90	0	0
Chunky Monkey (Ben & Jerry's)	4 oz	270	10	19
Classic				
Almond Bar (Good Humor)	1 (3.1 fl oz)	210	8	12
Candy Center Crunch Vanilla (Good Humor)	1	280	17	21
Chip Cookie Sandwich (Good Humor)	1 (4.1 fl oz)	300	8	13
Toasted Almond Bar (Good Humor)	1 (3.1 fl oz)	170	4	9
Vanilla Bar (Good Humor)	1 (3.1 fl oz)	190	8	10
Cocoa-Fudge 'N Cream (Fi-Bar)	1 bar	93	—	tr
Cocoa Marble Fudge (Rice Dream)	½ cup	140	—	6
Coconut Chocolate (Sealtest)	½ cup (2.4 oz)	160	6	8
Coffee (Breyers)	½ cup (2.6 oz)	150	5	8
Coffee (Haagen-Dazs)	4 oz	270	8	17
Coffee (Sealtest)	½ cup (2.4 oz)	140	4	7

FOOD	PORTION	CALS.	SAT. FAT	FAT
Coffee (Simple Pleasures)	4 oz	120	—	tr
Coffee Heath Bar Crunch (Ben & Jerry's)	½ cup (4 oz)	270	11	19
Coffee Light (Light N' Lively)	½ cup (2.4 oz)	110	2	3
Combo Cup (Good Humor)	1 (6.2 fl oz)	200	7	10
Cookies N' Cream (Breyers)	½ cup	170	6	9
Cookies N' Cream (Healthy Choice)	½ cup	120	2	2
Cookies N' Cream (Simple Pleasures)	4 oz	150	—	2
Cookies 'N' Cream American Dream (Edy's)	3 oz	100	—	1
Cool 'N Creamy Amaretto With Chocolate Swirl	1 bar	62	—	2
Cool 'N Creamy Chocolate/Vanilla	1 bar	54	—	2
Cool 'N Creamy Double Chocolate Fudge	1 bar	55	—	2
Cool 'N Creamy Orange/Vanilla	1 bar	31	—	1
Cool Creations Cookies & Cream Sandwich (Nestle)	1 (3.5 oz)	240	4	11
Cool Creations Mini Sandwich (Nestle)	1 (2.3 oz)	110	2	5
Creamee Burrrger (Good Humor)	1 (4.7 oz)	310	12	17
Creamy Lites Bar Chocolate (Carnation)	1 bar	50	—	2
Creamy Lites Bar Strawberry (Carnation)	1 bar	50	—	2
Cupid's Scoops (Sealtest)	½ cup (2.5 oz)	140	4	6
Deep Chocolate (Haagen-Dazs)	4 oz	290	—	14
Deep Chocolate Fudge (Haagen-Dazs)	4 oz	290	—	14
Deluxe Rocky Road (Breyers)	½ cup (2.5 oz)	190	5	9
Dinosaur Bar (Good Humor)	1	110	1	7
Double Fudge Bar (Weight Watchers)	1 (1.75 oz)	60	0	1

FOOD	PORTION	CALS.	SAT. FAT	FAT
Double Fudge Swirl (Healthy Choice)	½ cup (2.2 oz)	120	2	2
Dove Bite Size				
Almond Praline	1 (0.75 fl oz)	80	3	5
Cherry Royale	1 (0.75 fl oz)	70	3	5
Classic Vanilla	1 (0.75 fl oz)	70	3	5
French Vanilla	1 (0.75 fl oz)	70	3	5
Mint Supreme	1 (0.75 fl oz)	80	3	5
Dove Bar				
Almond	1 (3.67 fl oz)	335	12	22
Caramel Pecan	1 (3.67 fl oz)	350	12	35
Chocolate Milk Chocolate	1 (3.67 fl oz)	340	13	21
Coffee Cashew	1 (3.67 fl oz)	335	13	22
Crunchy Cookie	1 (3.8 fl oz)	340	13	21
Peanut	1 (3.8 fl oz)	380	13	25
Vanilla Dark Chocolate	1 (3.8 fl oz)	340	13	22
Vanilla Milk Chocolate	1 (3.8 fl oz)	340	13	21
Dream Pie				
Chocolate (Rice Dream)	1	380	—	19
Mint (Rice Dream)	1	380	—	19
Mocha (Rice Dream)	1	380	—	19
Vanilla (Rice Dream)	1	380	—	19
Dreamy Caramel Cream Light (Edy's)	4 oz	140	2–3	4
Drumstick Cone				
Chocolate (Nestle)	1 (4.6 oz)	340	10	19
Chocolate Dipped	1 (4.6 oz)	340	10	17
Vanilla	1 (4.6 oz)	350	11	20
Vanilla Caramel	1 (4.6. oz)	360	12	20
Vanilla Fudge	1 (4.6 oz)	370	11	21
Dutch Chocolate (Mocha Mix)	½ cup (2.3 oz)	140	2	8
Dutch Chocolate Olde Fashioned Recipe (Borden)	½ cup	130	—	6
English Toffee Crunch Bar (Weight Watchers)	1 (2 oz)	120	5	11
Fat Frog (Good Humor)	3.6 oz	150	7	8
Flintstones Cool Cream (Nestle)	1 (2.75 oz)	90	1	2
Flintstones Push-Up (Nestle)	1 (2.75 oz)	100	1	2

FOOD	PORTION	CALS.	SAT. FAT	FAT
Foster Freeze Vanilla	1 oz	43	—	1
French Vanilla (Breyers)	(2.5 oz)	170	6	10
French Vanilla (Sealtest)	½ cup (2.4 oz)	140	5	8
Fudge Bar (Ultra Slim-Fast)	1	90	—	tr
Fudge Brownie (Healthy Choice)	½ cup (2.2 oz)	120	1	2
Fudge Pop Bar (Haagen-Dazs)	1	210	—	14
Fudge Royale (Sealtest)	½ cup (2.5 oz)	150	4	7
Fun Box Ice Cream Sandwich (Good Humor)	1 (3.1 fl oz)	160	3	5
Heath (Nestle)	1 bar (2.5 oz)	160	8	12
Heath (Nestle)	8 nuggets	180	7	11
Heath Bar Crunch (Ben & Jerry's)	1 pop (2.5 fl oz)	260	10	18
Heath Bar Crunch (Ben & Jerry's)	1 pop (3.7 fl oz)	340	13	23
Heath Bar Crunch (Ben & Jerry's)	½ cup (4 fl oz)	270	12	19
Heath English Toffee (Friendly's)	½ cup (2.7 oz)	190	6	10
Heaven Bars Vanilla Caramel Nut (Carnation)	1 bar	225	—	15
Heaven Bars Vanilla Nut Fudge (Carnation)	1 bar	222	—	15
Heaven Sundae Bars Chocolate Fudge (Carnation)	1 bar	150	—	9
Heaven Sundae Bars Vanilla Fudge (Carnation)	1 bar	150	—	9
Heavenly Hash (Sealtest)	½ cup (2.4 oz)	150	4	7
Heavenly Hash Light (Breyers)	½ cup (2.4 oz)	150	3	5
Heavenly Hash Light (Light N' Lively)	½ cup (2.4 oz)	140	2	4
Heavenly Hash Reduced Fat (Breyers)	½ cup (2.4 oz)	150	3	5
Honey Vanilla (Haagen-Dazs)	4 oz	250	8	16
Ice Cream Sandwich (Good Humor)	1	190	4	8
King Cone (Good Humor)	1 (5.7 fl oz)	300	11	14

FOOD	PORTION	CALS.	SAT. FAT	FAT
King Cone Classic Vanilla (Good Humor)	1 (4.8 oz)	300	6	10
King Cone Strawberry (Good Humor)	1 (5.7 oz)	250	7	10
Klondike Good Humor				
Almond Bar	1 (5.2 fl oz)	310	14	21
Caramel Crunch	1 (5.2 fl oz)	300	13	18
Chocolate Chocolate Bar	1 (5.2 fl oz)	280	14	20
Coffee Bar	1 (5.2 fl oz)	290	14	20
Dark Chocolate Bar	1 (5.2 fl oz)	290	14	20
Gold Bar	1 (5.2 fl oz)	340	12	23
Krispy Bar	1 (5.2 fl oz)	300	13	20
Krunch	1 (3.1 fl oz)	200	9	13
Lite Bar	1 (2.3 fl oz)	110	4	6
Lite Bar Caramel	1 (2.4 fl oz)	120	5	6
Lite Sandwich	1 (2.9 fl oz)	100	2	2
Movie Bites Chocolate	8 pieces (4.6 fl oz)	340	3	26
Movie Bites Vanilla	8 pieces (4.6 fl oz)	320	18	22
Original Bar	1 (5.2 fl oz)	290	14	20
Sandwich Chocolate	1 (5.2 fl oz)	270	6	10
Sandwich Vanilla	1 (5.2 fl oz)	250	6	9
Lemon (Rice Dream)	½ cup	130	—	5
Macadamia Brittle (Haagen-Dazs)	4 oz	280	—	18
Magnum Almond (Good Humor)	1 (4.2 fl oz)	270	7	12
Magnum Chocolate (Good Humor)	1 (4.2 fl oz)	260	8	12
Malt Ball 'N' Fudge Light (Edy's)	4 oz	140	2–3	5
Malt Caramel Cone (Healthy Choice)	½ cup (2.2 oz)	120	1	2
Maple Walnut (Cyrk)	3 oz	299	10	22
Maple Walnut (Sealtest)	½ cup (2.4 oz)	160	5	9
Marble Fudge Light (Edy's)	4 oz	120	2–3	4
Mars Almond Bar	1 (1.85 fl oz)	210	6	14
Milk Chocolate Almond (Ben & Jerry's)	1 pop (2.5 fl oz)	250	10	19
Milk Way Single Chocolate/ Milk	1 (2 fl oz)	210	7	11
Milk Way Single Vanilla/ Dark	1 (2 fl oz)	200	7	12

FOOD	PORTION	CALS.	SAT. FAT	FAT
Milk Way Snack Chocolate/Milk	1 (0.72 fl oz)	70	3	4
Milk Way Snack Vanilla/Dark	1 (0.72 fl oz)	70	3	4
Mint Chocolate Chip (Breyers)	½ cup (2.6 oz)	170	6	10
Mint Chocolate Chip (Cyrk)	3 oz	258	9	18
Mint Chocolate Chip (Healthy Choice)	½ cup (2.2 oz)	120	1	2
Mint Chocolate Chocolate Chip (Simple Pleasures)	4 oz	150	—	2
Mint Cookie (Ben & Jerry's)	½ cup (4 fl oz)	250	9	17
Mixed Berry & Ice Cream Swirl (Chiquita)	1 bar	80	—	3
Mocha Almond Fudge (Breyers)	½ cup (2.7 oz)	190	5	10
Mocha Almond Fudge (Mocha Mix)	½ cup (2.3 oz)	150	2	8
Mocha Almond Fudge American Dream (Edy's)	3 oz	110	—	1
Mocha Almond Fudge Light (Edy's)	4 oz	140	2–3	5
Neapolitan (Mocha Mix)	½ cup (2.3 oz)	140	2	7
Neapolitan Fat Free Frozen Dessert (Weight Watchers)	½ cup	80	0	0
Nestle Crunch (Nestle)				
Chocolate	1 bar (3 oz)	200	9	14
Cones	1 (4.6 oz)	300	10	16
Crunch King	1 (4 oz)	270	14	19
Nuggets	8 pieces	140	5	9
Reduced Fat	1 (2.5 oz)	130	5	7
Vanilla	1 bar (3 oz)	200	9	14
New York Super Fudge (Ben & Jerry's)	1 pop (2.5 fl oz)	330	11	26
New York Super Fudge (Ben & Jerry's)	4 fl oz	290	10	20
New York Super Fudge (Ben & Jerry's)	1 pop (3.7 fl oz)	290	10	20
Number One Bar (Good Humor)	1 (4.1 fl oz)	190	9	11
Old Nat Sundae Cone (Good Humor)	1 (3.9 oz)	230	6	9

FOOD	PORTION	CALS.	SAT. FAT	FAT
ONE-ders Brownies Creme (Weight Watchers)	4 oz	130	—	4
ONE-ders Chocolate Chip (Weight Watchers)	4 oz	120	3	4
ONE-ders Heavenly Hash (Weight Watchers)	4 oz	130	2	3
ONE-ders Pralines 'N Creme (Weight Watchers)	4 oz	130	—	4
ONE-ders Strawberry (Weight Watchers)	4 oz	110	2	3
Orange & Cream Pop (Haagen-Dazs)	1	130	—	6
Orange & Ice Cream Swirl (Chiquita)	1 bar	80	—	3
Orange Vanilla Treat Bar Sugar Free Fat Free (Weight Watchers)	1 (1.75 oz)	30	0	0
Peach (Breyers)	½ cup (2.6 oz)	130	4	6
Peach (Sealtest Free)	½ cup	100	0	0
Peach (Simple Pleasures)	4 oz	120	—	tr
Peach (Ultra Slim-Fast)	4 oz	100	—	tr
Peanut Butter & Chocolate Light (Edy's)	4 oz	130	2–3	5
Peanut Butter Crunch Bar (Haagen-Dazs)	1	270	21	7
Pecan Praline (Simple Pleasures)	4 oz	140	—	2
Pecan Pralines 'N Creme Ice Milk (Weight Watchers)	½ cup	130	3	4
Popsicle Ice Cream Bar (Good Humor)	1 (3.1 fl oz)	160	9	11
Popsicle Ice Cream Sandwich (Good Humor)	1 (3.6 fl oz)	190	4	8
Praline & Caramel (Healthy Choice)	4 oz	130	1	2
Praline Almond Crunch Reduced Fat (Breyers)	½ cup (2.4 oz)	140	3	5
Praline Almond Crunch Light (Light N' Lively)	½ cup (2.4 oz)	130	2	3
Pralines & Caramel (Ultra Slim-Fast)	4 oz	120	—	tr

FOOD	PORTION	CALS.	SAT. FAT	FAT
Rain Forest Crunch (Ben & Jerry's)	4 oz	270	10	21
Raspberries 'N Cream (Fi-Bar)	1 bar	93	—	tr
Raspberry & Ice Cream Swirl (Chiquita)	1 bar	80	—	3
Raspberry Truffle Light (Edy's)	4 oz	110	2–3	5
Rocky Road (Healthy Choice)	½ cup (2.2 oz)	140	1	2
Rocky Road American Dream (Edy's)	3 oz	110	—	1
Rocky Road Light (Edy's)	4 oz	130	2–3	5
Rum Raisin (Haagen-Dazs)	4 oz	250	8	17
Rum Raisin (Simple Pleasures)	4 oz	130	—	tr
Sandwich Giant Neapolitan (Good Humor)	1 (5.2 fl oz)	260	7	10
Sandwich Giant Vanilla (Good Humor)	1 (5.2 fl oz)	240	6	10
Sandwich Vanilla (Breyers)	1 (2.8 oz)	250	9	11
Sidewalk Sundae Bar (Good Humor)	1	280	17	20
Sidewalk Sundae Cone (Good Humor)	1 (4.2 oz)	270	11	14
Sidewalk Sundae Sandwich (Good Humor)	1 (3.1 oz)	160	3	5
Snickers Single	1 (2 fl oz)	220	6	13
Snickers Snack	1 (1 fl oz)	110	3	7
Sprinkle Sandwich (Good Humor)	1 (3.1 fl oz)	180	4	6
Strawberries 'N Cream Old Fashioned Recipe (Borden)	½ cup	130	—	5
Strawberry (Borden)	½ cup	130	—	6
Strawberry (Breyer's)	½ cup	130	4	6
Strawberry (Cyrk)	3 oz	208	9	15
Strawberry (Frusen Gladje)	½ cup	230	10	15
Strawberry (Haagen-Dazs)	4 oz	250	8	15
Strawberry (Rice Dream)	½ cup	130	—	5
Strawberry (Sealtest)	½ cup	130	4	5
Strawberry American Dream (Edy's)	3 oz	70	—	tr
Strawberry & Ice Cream Swirl (Chiquita)	1 bar	80	—	3

FOOD	PORTION	CALS.	SAT. FAT	FAT
Strawberry Bar (Rice Dream)	1	260	—	15
Strawberry Free (Sealtest)	½ cup	100	0	0
Strawberry Ice Milk (Borden)	½ cup	90	—	2
Strawberry Light (Edy's)	4 oz	110	2–3	4
Strawberry Shortcake Classic (Good Humor)	3 oz	160	4	8
Strawberry Swirl (Mocha Mix)	½ cup (2.3 oz)	140	2	6
Sundae Cone (Borden)	1	210	—	12
Sundae Cone (Meadow Gold)	1	210	—	12
Sundae Twist Cup (Good Humor)	1	160	2	3
Swiss Almond Fudge Twirl Reduced Fat (Breyers)	½ cup (2.5 oz)	160	4	6
Swiss Chocolate Candy Almond (Frusen Gladje)	½ cup	270	9	19
Toasted Almond American Dream (Edy's)	3 oz	110	—	1
Toffee Bar Crunch (Breyers)	½ cup (2.5 oz)	180	7	11
Toffee Bar Crunch Light (Light N' Lively)	½ cup (2.4 oz)	130	3	4
Toffee Crunch (Simple Pleasures)	4 oz	130	—	tr
Toffee Fudge Parfait (Breyers Light)	½ cup	150	4	5
Toffee Taco (Good Humor)	1 (4.4 fl oz)	300	10	16
Tofulite	4 oz	150	—	7
Tofutti Frutti Vanilla Apple Orchard	4 fl oz	100	0	0
Triple Chocolate Passion (Sealtest)	½ cup (2.5 oz)	160	5	7
Vanilla (Ben & Jerry's)	½ cup (4 oz)	215	9	16
Vanilla (Breyers)	½ cup (2.6 oz)	150	6	8
Vanilla (Cyrk)	3 oz	209	9	16
Vanilla (Eagle Brand)	½ cup	150	—	9
Vanilla (Frusen Gladje)	½ cup	230	9	17
Vanilla (Haagen-Dazs)	4 oz	260	8	17
Vanilla (Healthy Choice)	4 oz	120	2	2
Vanilla (Mocha Mix)	½ cup (2.3 oz)	140	2	7
Vanilla (Sealtest)	½ cup (2.4 oz)	140	5	7
Vanilla (Simple Pleasures)	4 oz	120	—	tr
Vanilla (Ultra Slim-Fast)	4 oz	90	—	tr

FOOD	PORTION	CALS.	SAT. FAT	FAT
Vanilla Caramel Praline (Breyers)	½ cup (2.6 oz)	190	6	10
Vanilla Chocolate (Breyers)	½ cup (2.5 oz)	160	6	8
Vanilla Chocolate Sandwich (Ultra Slim-Fast)	1	140	—	2
Vanilla Chocolate Strawberry (Breyers)	½ cup (2.5 oz)	150	6	8
Vanilla-Chocolate-Strawberry (Edy's)	4 oz	110	2–3	4
Vanilla Chocolate Strawberry (Sealtest)	½ cup (2.4 oz)	140	4	6
Vanilla Chocolate Strawberry American Dream (Edy's)	3 oz	80	—	1
Vanilla Chocolate Strawberry Light (Breyers)	½ cup (2.4 oz)	120	3	4
Vanilla Chocolate Strawberry Light (Light N' Lively)	½ cup (2.4 oz)	110	2	3
Vanilla Chocolate Chunk (Ben & Jerry's)	½ cup (4 fl oz)	250	11	18
Vanilla Free (Sealtest)	½ cup	100	0	0
Vanilla Fudge Royale Light (Light N' Lively)	½ cup (2.6 oz)	120	2	3
Vanilla Fudge Swirl Light (Simple Pleasures)	4 oz	90	—	tr
Vanilla Light (Light N' Lively)	½ cup (2.4 oz)	110	2	3
Vanilla Light (Simple Pleasures)	4 oz	80	—	tr
Vanilla Milk Chocolate Almond Bar	1	370	—	27
Vanilla Milk Chocolate Bar (Haagen-Dazs)	1	360	—	27
Vanilla Milk Chocolate Bar (Haagen-Dazs)	1	360	—	27
Vanilla Oatmeal Sandwich (Ultra Slim-Fast)	1	150	—	3
Vanilla Olde Fashioned Recipe (Borden)	½ cup	130	—	7
Vanilla Peanut Butter Swirl (Haagen-Dazs)	4 oz	280	8	21
Vanilla Sandwich (Ultra Slim-Fast)	1	140	—	2

FOOD	PORTION	CALS.	SAT. FAT	FAT
Vanilla Sandwich Bar Fat Free (Weight Watchers)	1 (2.5 oz)	130	0	0
Vanilla Swiss Almond (Frusen Gladje)	½ cup	270	9	19
Vanilla Swiss Almond (Rice Dream)	½ cup	140	—	6
Vanilla Swiss Almond (Haagen-Dazs)	4 oz	290	—	19
Vanilla w/ Orange Sherbert (Sealtest)	½ cup (2.7 oz)	130	3	4
Viennetta Chocolate (Good Humor)	1 (4.2 fl oz)	160	7	9
Viennetta Vanilla (Good Humor)	1 (4.2 fl oz)	160	8	10
WWF Bar (Good Humor)	1 (3.7 fl oz)	200	8	10
Wildberry (Rice Dream)	½ cup	130	—	5
Wildberry Cream (Fi-Bar)	1 bar	93	—	tr
X-Men Bar (Good Humor)	1 (3 fl oz)	150	3	6
french vanilla, soft serve	1 cup	377	14	23
french vanilla, soft serve	½ gal	3014	108	180
vanilla, 10% fat	1 cup	269	9	14
vanilla, 10% fat	½ gal	2153	71	115
vanilla, 16% fat	1 cup	349	15	24
vanilla, 16% fat	½ gal	2805	118	190
vanilla ice milk	1 cup	184	4	6
vanilla ice milk	½ gal	1469	28	45
vanilla ice milk, soft serve	1 cup	223	3	5
vanilla ice milk, soft serve	½ gal	1787	23	37
TAKE-OUT				
cone, vanilla light, soft serve	1 (4.6 oz)	164	4	6
gelato chocolate hazelnut	½ cup (5.3 oz)	370	4	29
gelato vanilla	½ cup (3 oz)	211	8	15
sundae, caramel	1 (5.4 oz)	303	5	9
sundae, hot fudge	1 (5.4 oz)	284	5	9
sundae, strawberry	1 (5.4 oz)	269	4	8

ICE CREAM CONES AND CUPS

Comet Cups	1	18	tr	tr
Comet Rainbow Cups	1 (4.5 oz)	16	tr	tr
Comet Sugar Cone	1	50	tr	tr
Comet Waffle Cone	1	70	tr	tr
Dutch Mill Chocolate Covered Wafer Cups	1 (0.5 oz)	80	2	5
Keebler Sugar Cones	1	45	tr	tr

FOOD	PORTION	CALS.	SAT. FAT	FAT
Keebler Vanilla Cups	1	15	tr	tr
sugar cone	1	40	tr	tr
wafer cone	1	17	tr	tr

ICE CREAM TOPPINGS
(*see also* SYRUP)

FOOD	PORTION	CALS.	SAT. FAT	FAT
Butterscotch (Kraft)	1 tbsp	60	0	1
Butterscotch (Smucker's)	2 tbsp	140	—	1
Butterscotch Special Recipe (Smucker's)	2 tbsp	160	—	3
Caramel (Kraft)	1 tbsp	60	0	0
Caramel (Smucker's)	2 tbsp	140	—	1
Chocolate (Kraft)	1 tbsp	50	0	0
Chocolate Fudge (Hershey)	2 tbsp	100	0	4
Chocolate Fudge (Smucker's)	2 tbsp	130	—	1
Chocolate Fudge Magic Shell (Smucker's)	2 tbsp	190	—	15
Chocolate Magic Shell (Smucker's)	2 tbsp	190	—	15
Chocolate Nut Magic Shell (Smucker's)	2 tbsp	200	—	16
Chocolate Shoppe Candy Bar Sprinkles York (Hershey)	2 tbsp (1.1 oz)	170	5	8
Dark Chocolate Special Recipe (Smucker's)	2 tbsp	130	—	1
Hot Caramel (Smucker's)	2 tbsp	150	—	4
Hot Fudge (Kraft)	1 tbsp	70	1	0
Hot Fudge (Smucker's)	2 tbsp	110	—	4
Hot Fudge Light (Smucker's)	2 tbsp	70	—	tr
Hot Fudge Special Recipe (Smucker's)	2 tbsp	150	—	5
Hot Toffee Fudge (Smucker's)	2 tbsp	110	—	4
Marshmallow (Smucker's)	2 tbsp	120	—	0
Marshmallow Creme (Kraft)	1 oz	90	0	0
Peanut Butter Caramel (Smucker's)	2 tbsp	150	—	2
Pecans in Syrup (Smucker's)	2 tbsp	130	—	1
Pineapple (Kraft)	1 tbsp	50	0	0
Pineapple (Smucker's)	2 tbsp	130	0	0

FOOD	PORTION	CALS.	SAT. FAT	FAT
Strawberry (Kraft)	1 tbsp	50	0	0
Strawberry (Smucker's)	2 tbsp	120	0	0
Swiss Milk Chocolate Fudge (Smucker's)	2 tbsp	140	—	1
Walnuts in Syrup (Smucker's)	2 tbsp	130	—	1

ICED TEA
(see TEA/HERBAL TEA)

ICES AND ICE POPS
(see also ICE CREAM AND FROZEN DESSERTS, PUDDING POPS, SHERBET, YOGURT FROZEN)

FOOD	PORTION	CALS.	SAT. FAT	FAT
Ben & Jerry's				
Cherry Pop	1	330	—	24
Lemon Ice	4 oz	105	—	0
Raspberry	4 oz	105	—	0
Strawberry Ice	4 oz	77	—	0
Chiquita				
Fruit & Cream Banana	1 bar	80	—	2
Fruit & Cream Blueberry	1 bar	80	—	1
Fruit & Cream Peach	1 bar	80	—	1
Fruit & Cream Raspberry	1 bar	80	—	1
Fruit & Cream Strawberry	1 bar	80	—	1
Fruit & Cream Strawberry Banana	1 bar	80	—	2
Fruit & Juice Bar Cherry	1 bar (2 oz)	50	—	0
Fruit & Juice Bar Raspberry	1 bar (2 oz)	50	—	0
Fruit & Juice Bar Raspberry Banana	1 bar (2 oz)	50	—	0
Fruit & Juice Bar Strawberry	1 bar (2 oz)	50	—	0
Fruit & Juice Bar Strawberry Banana	1 bar (2 oz)	50	—	0
Cool Creations (Nestle)				
10 Pack	1 pop (2 oz)	60	0	0
Lion King Cone	1 (4 oz)	280	9	14
Mickey Mouse Bar	1 (2.5 oz)	110	3	7
Mickey Mouse Bar	1 (4 oz)	170	4	11
Surprise Pops	1 (2 oz)	60	0	0
Crystal Light				
Berry Blend	1 bar	13	—	0
Cherry	1 bar	13	—	0
Fruit Punch	1 bar	14	—	0
Orange	1 bar	13	—	0

FOOD	PORTION	CALS.	SAT. FAT	FAT
Crystal Light *(cont.)*				
Pina Colada	1 bar	14	—	0
Pineapple	1 bar	14	—	0
Pink Lemonade	1 bar	14	—	0
Raspberry	1 bar	13	—	0
Strawberry	1 bar	13	—	0
Strawberry Daiquiri	1 bar	14	—	0
Cyrk				
Ice Chocolate	4 oz	85	tr	1
Ice Vanilla	4 oz	75	tr	tr
Sorbet Apricot	4 oz	104	tr	tr
Sorbet Apricot Sugar Free	4 oz	36	tr	tr
Sorbet Blueberry	4 oz	77	tr	tr
Sorbet Cherry	4 oz	98	tr	tr
Sorbet Lemon	4 oz	66	0	0
Sorbet Mango	4 oz	83	tr	tr
Sorbet Mango Sugar Free	4 oz	48	tr	tr
Sorbet Pina Colada	4 oz	107	2	3
Sorbet Pina Colada Sugar Free	4 oz	66	2	3
Sorbet Plum	4 oz	90	tr	tr
Sorbet Raspberry	4 oz	88	tr	tr
Sorbet Raspberry Sugar Free	4 oz	35	tr	tr
Sorbet Strawberry	4 oz	79	tr	tr
Sorbet White Peach	4 oz	96	tr	tr
Dole Fruit 'n Juice				
Coconut	1 bar (4 oz)	210	5	7
Lemonade	1 bar (4 oz)	120	0	0
Lime	1 bar (4 oz)	110	0	0
Peach Passion	1 bar (2.5 oz)	70	0	0
Pineapple Coconut	1 bar (4 oz)	140	4	4
Pineapple Orange Banana	1 bar (2.5 oz)	70	0	0
Pineapple Orange Banana	1 bar (4 oz)	110	0	0
Raspberry	1 bar (2.5 oz)	70	0	0
Strawberry	1 bar (2.5 oz)	70	0	0
Strawberry	1 bar (4 oz)	110	0	0
Dole Fruit Juice				
Grape	1 bar (1.75 oz)	45	0	0
No Sugar Added Grape	1 bar (1.75 oz)	25	0	0

FOOD	PORTION	CALS.	SAT. FAT	FAT
No Sugar Added Strawberry	1 bar (1.75 oz)	25	0	0
Raspberry	1 bar (1.75 oz)	45	0	0
Strawberry	1 bar (1.75 oz)	45	0	0
Fi-Bar Juice Bar Lemoney-Lime	1 bar	63	—	tr
Fi-Bar Juice Bar Strawberry Nectar	1 bar	63	—	tr
Fi-Bar Juice Bar Tropical Delight	1 bar	63	—	tr
Flintstones Rock Pops Nestle	1 (3.5 oz)	80	0	0
Frozfruit Strawberry	1 (4 oz)	80	0	0
Frusen Gladje Sorbet Raspberry	½ cup	140	0	0
Good Humor				
Big Stick Cherry Pineapple	1 (3.6 fl oz)	50	0	0
Big Stick Popsicle	1 (3.6 fl oz)	50	0	0
Calippo Cherry	1 (3.8 fl oz)	100	0	0
Calippo Grape Lemon	1 (3.9 fl oz)	90	0	0
Calippo Orange	1 (3.9 fl oz)	90	0	0
Citrus Bites	1 (1.8 fl oz)	35	0	0
Creamsicle Sugar Free	1 (1.8 fl oz)	25	0	0
Creamsicle Bar Orange	1 (2.8 fl oz)	110	2	3
Creamsicle Bar Orange Raspberry	1 (2.6 fl oz)	100	2	3
Creamsicle Pop Orange	1 (1.8 fl oz)	70	1	2
Flintstones Push-Up Yabba Dabba Doo Orange	1 (2.75 fl oz)	90	—	1
Fudgsicle Pop	1 (1.8 fl oz)	60	1	1
Fudgsicle Sugar Free	1 (1.8 fl oz)	40	1	1
Fudgsicle Bar	1 (2.8 fl oz)	90	1	1
Fun Box Fudge Bar	1 (2.3 fl oz)	80	1	1
Fun Box Pops	1 (2 fl oz)	35	0	0
Fun Box Twin Pop Banana	1 (2.6 fl oz)	50	0	0
Fun Box Twin Pop Blue Raspberry	1 (2.6 fl oz)	50	0	0
Fun Box Twin Pop Cherry	1 (2.6 fl oz)	50	0	0
Fun Box Twin Pop Cherry Lemon	1 (2.6 fl oz)	50	0	0

FOOD	PORTION	CALS.	SAT. FAT	FAT
Good Humor *(cont.)*				
Fun Box Twin Pop Orange, Cherry, Grape	1 (2.6 oz)	50	0	0
Fun Box Twin Pop Root Beer	1 (2.6 fl oz)	50	0	0
Garfield Bar	1 (3.9 fl oz)	90	0	0
Great White	1 (3.1 fl oz)	70	—	1
Hyperstripe	1 (2.8 fl oz)	80	0	0
Ice Stripe Cherry Orange	1 (1.5 fl oz)	35	0	0
Ice Stripe Grape Lemon	1 (1.5 fl oz)	35	0	0
Jumbo Jet Star	1 (4.7 fl oz)	80	0	0
Laser Blazer	1 (2.6 oz)	70	0	0
Popsicle All Natural	1 (1.8 fl oz)	45	0	0
Popsicle Orange, Cherry, Grape	1 (1.8 fl oz)	45	0	0
Popsicle Rainbow Pops	1 (1.8 fl oz)	45	0	0
Popsicle Rootbeer, Banana, Lime	1 (1.8 fl oz)	45	0	0
Popsicle Strawberry, Raspberry, Wildberry	1 (1.8 fl oz)	45	0	0
Popsicle Supersicle Firecracker	1 (4.7 fl oz)	90	0	0
Popsicle Supersicle Traffic Signal	1	80	0	0
Popsicle Twin Pop Cherry	1 (2.6 fl oz)	70	0	0
Popsicle Twin Pop Orange, Cherry, Grape, Lime	1 (2.6 fl oz)	70	0	0
Snow Cone	1	60	—	0
Snowfruit Coconut Bar	1 (3.75 fl oz)	150	3	4
Snowfruit Orange Bar	1	140	0	0
Snowfruit Strawberry Bar	1	120	0	0
Snowfruit Tropical Fruit Bar	1	110	0	0
Sugar Free Pop Orange, Cherry, Grape	1 (1.8 fl oz)	15	0	0
Sunkist Orange Juice Bar	1 (3.4 fl oz)	80	—	1
Sunkist Wildberry	1 (3.4 fl oz)	120	—	1
Super Mario Bar	1	120	1	1

FOOD	PORTION	CALS.	SAT. FAT	FAT
Supersicle Cherry Banana	1 (4.7 fl oz)	80	0	0
Supersicle Cherry Cola	1 (4.7 fl oz)	80	0	0
Supersicle Double Fudge	1 (4.7 fl oz)	150	1	2
Supersicle Firecracker Jr.	1	72	0	0
Supersicle Sour Tower	1	80	0	0
Swirl Bubble Gum	1 (2.7 fl oz)	55	0	0
Swirl Cherry Banana	1 (2.7 fl oz)	55	0	0
Torpedo Cherry	1 (1.8 fl oz)	35	0	0
Twister Blue Raspberry, Cherry, Cherry Cola, Cherry	1 (1.8 fl oz)	45	0	0
Twister, Cherry, Lemon, Orange, Lemon	1 (1.8 fl oz)	45	0	0
Vampire's Deadly Secret	1 (2.8 fl oz)	100	0	0
Watermelon Bar	1 (3.6 fl oz)	80	0	0
Haagen-Dazs				
Sorbet & Cream Blueberry	4 oz	190	—	8
Sorbet & Cream Keylime	4 oz	190	—	7
Sorbet & Cream Orange	4 oz	190	—	8
Sorbet & Cream Raspberry	4 oz	180	—	8
Ice All Flavors Bresler's	3.5 oz	120	0	0
Jell-O				
Berry Punch	1 bar	31	—	tr
Lemon Lime	1 bar	33	—	tr
Mixed Berry	1 bar	31	—	tr
Orange	1 bar	31	—	tr
Orange Pineapple	1 bar	31	—	tr
Raspberry	1 bar	29	—	tr
Raspberry Peach	1 bar	29	—	tr
Side By Side Apple Cherry	1 bar	36	—	tr
Side By Side Grape Lemon	1 bar	36	—	tr
Strawberry	1 bar	31	—	tr
Strawberry Banana	1 bar	31	—	tr
Kool-Aid Cherry	1 bar	42	0	0
Kool-Aid Grape	1 bar	42	0	0
Kool-Aid Mountain Berry Punch	1 bar	42	0	0

FOOD	PORTION	CALS.	SAT. FAT	FAT
Lifesavers Ice Pops	1	35	0	0
Lifesavers Ice Pops Sugar Free	1	12	0	0
Sundae Cup Strawberry (Carnation)	1 (3.3 oz)	200	5	8
Tofutti Frutti Apricot Mango Tofutti	4 fl oz	100	0	0
Tofutti Frutti Three Berry Tofutti	4 fl oz	100	0	0
Vitari Passion-Fruit	4 oz	80	—	0
Vitari Peach	4 oz	80	—	0

ICING
(see CAKE)

INSTANT BREAKFAST
(see BREAKFAST DRINKS)

JACKFRUIT
fresh	3.5 oz	70	—	tr

JALAPENO
(see PEPPERS)

JAM/JELLY/PRESERVES
ALL FRUIT

Apple Butter Simply Fruit (Smucker's)	1 tsp	12	0	0
Blueberry Fruit Spread (Pritikin)	1 tsp	14	—	0
Peach Fruit Spread (Pritikin)	1 tsp	14	—	0
Red Raspberry Fruit Spread (Pritikin)	1 tsp	14	—	0
Simply Fruit Spread, All Flavors (Smucker's)	1 tsp	16	0	0
Strawberry Fruit Spread (Pritikin)	1 tsp	14	0	0

REDUCED CALORIE

All Flavors Slenderella Fruit Spread	1 tsp	7	0	0
Apple (Estee)	1 pkg (0.5 oz)	10	0	0
Apple Slice (Estee)	1 tbsp (0.5 oz)	10	0	0
Apricot (Estee)	1 tbsp (0.5 oz)	5	0	0
Apricot Pineapple Preserves (S&W)	1 tsp	4	0	0

FOOD	PORTION	CALS.	SAT. FAT	FAT
Blackberry (Estee)	1 tbsp (0.5 oz)	5	0	0
Blueberry Jam (S&W)	1 tsp	4	0	0
Cherry (Estee)	1 tbsp (0.5 oz)	5	0	0
Concord Grape Jelly (S&W)	1 tsp	4	0	0
Grape (Estee)	1 tbsp (0.5 oz)	10	0	0
Grape Jelly Reduced Calorie (Kraft)	1 tsp	6	0	0
Grape Spread (Weight Watchers)	1 tsp	8	0	0
Imitation Blackberry Jelly Single Serving (Smucker's)	1 pkg (0.4 oz)	4	0	0
Imitation Cherry Jelly Single Serving (Smucker's)	1 pkg (0.4 oz)	4	0	0
Low Sugar Spread, All Flavors (Smucker's)	1 tsp	8	0	0
Orange (Estee)	1 tbsp (0.5 oz)	10	0	0
Orange Marmalade (S&W)	1 tsp	4	0	0
Peach (Estee)	1 tbsp (0.5 oz)	5	0	0
Raspberry Spread (Weight Watchers)	1 tsp	8	0	0
Red Raspberry (Estee)	1 tbsp (0.5 oz)	5	0	0
Red Raspberry Jam (S&W)	1 tsp	4	0	0
Red Tart Cherry Preserves (S&W)	1 tsp	4	0	0
Strawberry (Estee)	1 tbsp (0.5 oz)	10	0	0
Strawberry Jam (S&W)	1 tsp	4	0	0
Strawberry Preserves (Kraft)	1 tsp	6	0	0
Strawberry Spread (Weight Watchers)	1 tsp	8	0	0
REGULAR				
Apple Butter (BAMA)	2 tsp	25	0	0
Apple Butter (White House)	1 oz	50	0	0
Apple Butter Autumn Harvest (Smucker's)	1 tsp	12	0	0
Apple Butter Natural (Smucker's)	1 tsp	12	0	0
Apple Cider Butter (Smucker's)	1 tsp	12	0	0
Apple Jelly (BAMA)	2 tsp	30	0	0

FOOD	PORTION	CALS.	SAT. FAT	FAT
Blueberry Jam (Whistling Wings)	1 oz	50	—	tr
Grape Jelly (BAMA)	2 tsp	30	0	0
Jelly, All Flavors (Home Brands)	2 tsp	35	0	0
Jelly, All Flavors (Kraft)	1 tsp	17	0	0
Jam, All Flavors (Smucker's)	1 tsp	18	0	0
Jelly, Single Serving, All Flavors (Smucker's)	½ oz	38	0	0
Orange Marmalade (Smucker's)	1 tsp	18	0	0
Peach Butter (Smucker's)	1 tsp	15	0	0
Peach Preserves (BAMA)	2 tsp	30	0	0
Preserves, All Flavors (Home Brands)	2 tsp	35	0	0
Preserves, All Flavors (Kraft)	1 tsp	17	0	0
Preserves, All Flavors (Smucker's)	1 tsp	18	0	0
Pumpkin Butter Autumn Harvest (Smucker's)	1 tsp	12	0	0
Raspberry Jam (Whistling Wings)	1 oz	60	—	tr
Red Plum Jam (BAMA)	2 tsp	30	0	0
Strawberry Preserves (BAMA)	2 tsp	30	0	0
apple jelly	3.5 oz	259	0	0
apricot jam	3.5 oz	250	0	0
blackberry jam	3.5 oz	237	0	0
cherry jam	3.5 oz	250	0	0
orange jam	3.5 oz	243	0	0
plum jam	3.5 oz	241	0	0
quince jam	3.5 oz	236	0	0
raspberry jam	3.5 oz	248	0	0
raspberry jelly	3.5 oz	259	0	0
red currant jam	3.5 oz	237	0	0
red currant jelly	3.5 oz	265	0	0
rose hip jam	3.5 oz	250	0	0
strawberry jam	3.5 oz	234	0	0

JAPANESE FOOD
(see ORIENTAL FOOD)

FOOD	PORTION	CALS.	SAT. FAT	FAT
JAVA PLUM				
fresh	1 cup	82	—	tr
fresh	1	5	—	tr
JELLY				
(see JAM/JELLY/PRESERVES)				
JERUSALEM ARTICHOKE				
(see ARTICHOKE)				
JEW'S EAR				
pepeao, dried	½ cup	36	—	tr
pepeao, raw, sliced	1 cup	25	—	tr
JUJUBE				
fresh	3.5 oz	105	—	tr
KALE				
FRESH				
Dole, chopped	½ cup	17	—	1
chopped, cooked	½ cup	21	tr	tr
raw, chopped	½ cup	21	tr	tr
scotch, chopped, cooked	½ cup	18	tr	tr
FROZEN				
chopped, cooked	½ cup	20	tr	tr
KEFIR				
kefir	3.5 oz	66	—	4
KIDNEY				
beef, simmered	3 oz	122	1	3
lamb, braised	3 oz	117	1	3
pork, braised	3 oz	128	—	4
veal, braised	3 oz	139	1	5
KIDNEY BEANS				
CANNED				
B&M Red Baked Beans	8 oz	250	—	7
Friends Red Baked	8 oz	340	2	4
Goya Spanish Style	7.5 oz	140	—	1
Green Giant Dark Red	½ cup	90	0	0
Green Giant Light Red	½ cup	90	0	0
Hanover Dark Red	½ cup	110	—	0
Hanover Light Red In Sauce	½ cup	120	—	0
Hunt's Red	4 oz	100	—	tr

FOOD	PORTION	CALS.	SAT. FAT	FAT
Luck's Seasoned w/ Pork	7.5 oz	220	—	6
Luck's Special Cook Red	7.5 oz	190	—	4
Progresso Red	½ cup	100	—	tr
S&W Dark Red Lite 50% Less Salt	½ cup	120	—	0
S&W Dark Red Premium	½ cup	120	—	1
S&W Water Pack	½ cup	90	0	0
Trappey				
Dark Red	½ cup (4.5 oz)	130	0	1
Light Red	½ cup (4.5 oz)	120	0	1
Light Red With Jalapeno	½ cup (4.5 oz)	110	0	1
With Chili Gravy	½ cup (4.5 oz)	110	0	1
Light Red New Orleans Style With Bacon	½ cup (4.5 oz)	110	1	1
Van Camp's Dark Red	½ cup (4.6 oz)	90	0	0
Van Camp's Light Red	½ cup (4.6 oz)	90	0	0
kidney beans	1 cup	208	tr	1
red	1 cup	216	tr	1
DRIED				
Arrowhead Red	¼ cup (1.6 oz)	160	0	1
Hurst Brand	1.2 oz	120	0	1
california red, cooked	1 cup	219	tr	tr
kidney beans, cooked	1 cup	225	tr	1
red, cooked	1 cup	225	tr	1
royal red, cooked	1 cup	218	tr	tr
SPROUTS				
cooked	1 lb	152	tr	3
raw	½ cup	27	tr	tr

KIWIS

FOOD	PORTION	CALS.	SAT. FAT	FAT
California Kiwifruit Commission	2 (4.9 oz)	90	—	1
Dole	2	90	—	1
fresh	1 med	46	—	tr

KOHLRABI

FOOD	PORTION	CALS.	SAT. FAT	FAT
raw, sliced	½ cup	19	tr	tr
sliced, cooked	½ cup	24	tr	tr

KUMQUATS

FOOD	PORTION	CALS.	SAT. FAT	FAT
fresh	1	12	—	tr

FOOD	PORTION	CALS.	SAT. FAT	FAT

LAMB
(*see also* LAMB DISHES)
FRESH

FOOD	PORTION	CALS.	SAT. FAT	FAT
cubed, lean only, braised	3 oz	190	3	7
cubed, lean only, broiled	3 oz	158	2	6
ground, broiled	3 oz	240	7	17
leg, lean & fat, Choice, roasted	3 oz	219	6	14
loin chop w/ bone lean & fat, Choice broiled	1 chop (2.3 oz)	201	6	15
loin chop w/ bone, lean only, Choice, broiled	1 chop (1.6 oz)	100	2	5
rib chop, lean & fat, Choice, broiled	3 oz	307	11	25
rib chop, lean only, Choice, broiled	3 oz	200	4	11
shank, lean & fat, Choice, braised	3 oz	206	5	11
shank, lean & fat, Choice, roasted	3 oz	191	4	11
shoulder chop, w/ bone, lean & fat, Choice, braised	1 chop (2.5 oz)	244	7	17
shoulder chop, w/ bone, lean only, Choice, braised	1 chop (1.9 oz)	152	3	8
sirloin, lean & fat, Choice, roasted	3 oz	248	7	21

FROZEN

FOOD	PORTION	CALS.	SAT. FAT	FAT
new zealand, lean & fat, cooked	3 oz	259	9	19
new zealand, lean only, cooked	3 oz	175	3	8

LAMB DISHES
TAKE-OUT

FOOD	PORTION	CALS.	SAT. FAT	FAT
curry	¾ cup	345	3	17
moussaka	5.6 oz	312	—	21
stew	¾ cup	124	1	5

LAMB'S QUARTERS
FRESH

FOOD	PORTION	CALS.	SAT. FAT	FAT
chopped, cooked	½ cup	29	tr	1

FOOD	PORTION	CALS.	SAT. FAT	FAT
LECITHIN				
(*see* SOY)				
LEEKS				
freeze dried	1 tbsp	1	0	0
FRESH				
chopped, cooked	¼ cup	8	tr	tr
cooked	1 (4.4 oz)	38	tr	tr
raw	1 (4.4 oz)	76	tr	tr
raw, chopped	¼ cup	16	tr	tr
LEMON				
FRESH				
Dole	1	18	—	0
lemon	1 med	22	—	tr
peel	1 tbsp	0	—	tr
wedge	1	5	—	tr
JUICE				
Realemon	1 oz	6	0	0
bottled	1 tbsp	3	tr	tr
fresh	1 tbsp	4	0	—
frzn	1 tbsp	3	tr	tr
LEMON CURD				
lemon curd made w/ egg	2 tsp	29	—	1
LEMON EXTRACT				
Virginia Dare	1 tsp	22	—	0
LEMONADE				
FROZEN				
Bright & Early	8 fl oz	120	0	0
Minute Maid	8 fl oz	110	0	0
Country Style	8 fl oz	120	0	0
Cranberry Lemonade	8 fl oz	80	0	0
Pink	8 fl oz	120	0	0
Raspberry	8 fl oz	120	0	0
Seneca as prep	8 fl oz	110	0	0
not prep	1 can (6 oz)	397	tr	tr
MIX				
4C Instant, as prep	8 fl oz	80	—	0
Country Time	8 fl oz	82	0	0
Pink	8 fl oz	82	0	0
Pink Sugar Free	8 fl oz	4	0	0
Sugar Free	8 fl oz	4	0	0

FOOD	PORTION	CALS.	SAT. FAT	FAT
Crystal Light	8 fl oz	5	0	0
Kool-Aid	8 fl oz	99	0	0
Pink	8 fl oz	99	0	0
Sugar Free	8 fl oz	4	0	0
Sugar Sweetened Pink	8 fl oz	82	0	0
Wylers Drink Mix	8 oz	3	0	0
Unsweetened Wyler's powder w/ nutrasweet	1 pitcher (67 oz)	40	0	0
powder, as prep w/ water	9 fl oz	113	tr	tr
READY-TO-DRINK				
Crystal Geyser Juice Squeeze Pink	1 bottle (12 fl oz)	140	0	0
Diet Rite Salt/Sodium Free	8 fl oz	2	0	0
Fruitopia	8 fl oz	120	0	0
Kool-Aid Koolers Lemonade Kool-Aid	1 pkg (8.45 fl oz)	120	0	0
Minute Maid				
Chilled	8 fl oz	110	0	0
Cranberry Chilled	8 fl oz	120	0	0
Juices To Go	1 bottle (16 fl oz)	110	0	0
Juices To Go	1 can (11.5 fl oz)	160	0	0
Juices To Go Cranberry Lemonade	1 bottle (16 fl oz)	110	0	0
Juices To Go Raspberry Lemonade	1 bottle (16 fl oz)	120	0	0
Pink Chilled	8 fl oz	110	0	0
Raspberry Chilled	8 fl oz	120	0	0
Mott's	10 fl oz	160	0	0
Nehi Royal Crown	8 fl oz	130	0	0
Newman's Own Roadside Virginia	8 fl oz	100	—	tr
Ocean Spray	8 fl oz	110	0	0
Ocean Spray With Cranberry Juice	8 fl oz	110	0	0
Ocean Spray With Raspberry Juice	8 fl oz	110	0	0
Odwalla Honey	8 fl oz	70	0	0
Odwalla Strawberry	8 fl oz	150	0	0
Royal Mistic Lemonade Limeade	16 fl oz	230	0	0
Royal Mistic Tropical Pink	16 fl oz	230	0	0
Shasta	12 fl oz	146	—	0
Sipps Lemonade	8.45 fl oz	85	—	0
Tropicana	1 can (11.5 oz)	160	0	0

FOOD	PORTION	CALS.	SAT. FAT	FAT
Tropicana	8 fl oz	110	0	0
Twister Orange Cranberry	8 fl oz	130	0	0
Twister Wild Berry	8 fl oz	120	0	0
Veryfine	8 fl oz	120	0	0
Wylers	1 can (6 fl oz)	64	0	0

LENTILS

CANNED

Health Valley Fast Menu Hearty Lentils Garden Vegetables	7.5 oz	150	—	4
Health Valley Fast Menu Organic Lentils With Tofu Weiners	7.5 oz	170	—	5

DRIED

Hurst	1.2 oz	120	0	1
cooked	1 cup	231	tr	1

FROZEN

Natural Touch Lentil Rice Loaf	2.5 in slice (113 g)	200	—	11

SPROUTS

raw	½ cup	40	tr	tr

LETTUCE

Dole Butter Lettuce	1 head	21	—	tr
Dole Iceberg	⅙ med head	20	—	0
Dole Leaf, shredded	1½ cup	12	—	0
Dole Romaine, shredded	1½ cup	18	—	1
bibb	1 head (6 oz)	21	tr	tr
boston	1 head (6 oz)	21	tr	tr
boston	2 leaves	2	tr	tr
iceberg	1 leaf	3	tr	tr
iceberg	1 head (19 oz)	70	tr	1
looseleaf, shredded	½ cup	5	tr	tr
romaine, shredded	½ cup	4	tr	tr

LIMA BEANS

CANNED

Allen Green	½ cup (4.5 oz)	120	0	1
Allen Green and White	½ cup (4.5 oz)	110	1	1
Dennison's w/ Ham	7.5 oz	250	—	7
East Texas Fair Green	½ cup (4.5 oz)	120	0	1
Luck's Small Seasoned w/ Pork	7.5 oz	220	—	7

FOOD	PORTION	CALS.	SAT. FAT	FAT
Luck's Giant Seasoned w/ Pork	7.5 oz	230	—	7
S&W Small Fancy	½ cup	80	0	0
Seneca	½ cup	80	0	0
Trappey Baby Green With Bacon	½ cup (4.5 oz)	120	1	1
large	1 cup	191	tr	tr
lima beans	½ cup	93	tr	tr
DRIED				
baby, cooked	1 cup	229	tr	1
cooked	½ cup	104	tr	tr
large, cooked	1 cup	217	tr	1
FROZEN				
Birds Eye Baby	½ cup	130	0	0
Birds Eye Fordhook	½ cup	100	0	0
Fresh Like Baby	3.5 oz	138	—	1
Green Giant Harvest Fresh	½ cup	80	0	0
Green Giant In Butter Sauce	½ cup	100	1	3
Hanover Baby	½ cup	110	—	0
Hanover Fordhook	½ cup	100	—	0
cooked	½ cup	94	tr	tr
fordhook, cooked	½ cup	85	tr	tr

LIME
fresh lime	1	20	tr	tr
JUICE				
Odwalla Summertime Lime	8 fl oz	90	0	0
Realime	1 oz	6	0	0
bottled	1 tbsp	3	tr	tr
fresh	1 tbsp	4	tr	tr

LING
baked	3 oz	95	—	1
blue, raw	5.3 oz	168	—	1
fillet, baked	5.3 oz	168	—	1

LINGCOD
baked	3 oz	93	tr	1
fillet, baked	5.3 oz	164	tr	2

LIQUOR/LIQUEUR
(*see also* BEER AND ALE, CHAMPAGNE, DRINK MIXERS, MALT, WINE, WINE COOLERS)

anisette	⅔ oz	74	—	0
apricot brandy	⅔ oz	64	—	0

FOOD	PORTION	CALS.	SAT. FAT	FAT
benedictine	⅔ oz	69	—	0
bloody mary	5 oz	116	tr	tr
bourbon & soda	4 oz	105	0	0
coffee liqueur	1.5 oz	174	tr	tr
coffee liqueur w/ cream	1.5 oz	154	5	7
creme de menthe	1.5 oz	186	tr	tr
curacao liqueur	⅔ oz	54	—	0
daiquiri	2 oz	111	0	0
gin	1.5 oz	110	0	0
gin & tonic	7.5 oz	171	0	0
gin ricky	4 oz	150	—	0
manhattan	2 oz	128	0	0
martini	2.5 oz	156	0	0
mint julep	10 oz	210	—	0
old-fashioned	2.5 oz	127	—	0
pina colada	4.5 oz	262	1	3
rum	1.5 oz	97	0	0
screwdriver	7 oz	174	tr	tr
sloe gin fizz	2.5 oz	132	0	0
tequila sunrise	5.5 oz	189	tr	tr
tom collins	7.5 oz	121	0	0
vodka	1.5 oz	97	0	0
whiskey	1.5 oz	105	0	0
whiskey sour	3 oz	123	tr	tr
whiskey sour mix, as prep	3.6 oz	169	0	0
whiskey sour mix, not prep	1 pkg (.6 oz)	64	0	0

LIVER
(see also PÂTÉ)

FOOD	PORTION	CALS.	SAT. FAT	FAT
Beef, raw (Dakota Lean)	3 oz	100	—	1
beef, braised	3 oz	137	2	4
beef, pan-fried	3 oz	184	2	7
chicken, stewed	1 cup (5 oz)	219	3	8
duck, raw	1 (1.5 oz)	60	1	2
goose, raw	1 (3.3 oz)	125	1	4
lamb, braised	3 oz	187	3	7
lamb, fried	3 oz	202	4	11
pork, braised	3 oz	141	1	4
sheep, raw	3.5 oz	131	—	4
turkey, simmered	1 cup (5 oz)	237	3	8
veal, braised	3 oz	140	2	6
veal, fried	3 oz	208	4	10

FOOD	PORTION	CALS.	SAT. FAT	FAT

LOBSTER
CANNED
| Progresso Rock Lobster Sauce | ½ cup | 120 | 1 | 8 |

FRESH
northern, cooked	1 cup	142	tr	1
northern, cooked	3 oz	83	tr	1
northern, raw	1 lobster (5.3 oz)	136	—	1
spiny, steamed	1 (5.7 oz)	233	tr	3
spiny, steamed	3 oz	122	tr	2

FROZEN
| Crawfish Etouffee (Cajun Cookin') | 12 oz | 390 | — | 10 |
| Gulfstream Tails (King & Prince) | 6 oz | 170 | — | 1 |

TAKE-OUT
| newburg | 1 cup | 485 | — | 27 |

LOGANBERRIES
| frzn | 1 cup | 80 | — | tr |

LONGANS
| fresh | 1 | 2 | 0 | 0 |

LOQUATS
| fresh | 1 | 5 | tr | tr |

LOTUS
root, raw, sliced	10 slices	45	tr	tr
root, sliced, cooked	10 slices	59	tr	tr
seeds dried	1 oz	94	tr	1

LOX
(see SALMON)

LUNCHEON MEATS/COLD CUTS
(see also CHICKEN, HAM, MEAT SUBSTITUTES, TURKEY)
Armour Beef Bologna Lower Salt	1 oz	90	—	8
Armour Bologna Lower Salt	1 oz	90	—	8
Armour Salami Lower Salt	1 oz	80	—	7
Carl Buddig Beef	1 oz	40	1	2
Carl Buddig Corned Beef	1 oz	40	1	2
Carl Buddig Pastrami	1 oz	40	0	2

FOOD	PORTION	CALS.	SAT. FAT	FAT
DiLusso Genoa	1 oz	100	4	8
Hansel 'N Gretel Healthy Deli				
Bologna, Beef & Pork	1 oz	41	—	2
Cooked Corn Beef	1 oz	35	—	1
Italian Roast Beef	1 oz	31	—	1
Pastrami Round	1 oz	34	—	1
Regular Roast Beef	1 oz	30	—	tr
St. Paddy's Corned Beef	1 oz	24	—	tr
Hebrew National				
Bologna Lean Chub	2 oz	90	—	6
Bologna Beef	2 oz	180	—	16
Bologna Beef Reduced Fat	2 oz	130	—	12
Bologna Midget	2 oz	180	—	16
Deli Pastrami	2 oz	80	—	3
Deli Express Corned Beef	2 oz	80	—	3
Deli Express Tongue Sliced	2 oz	120	—	9
Salami Lean Chub	2 oz	90	—	6
Salami Beef	2 oz	170	—	14
Salami Beef Reduced Fat	2 oz	110	—	8
Salami Midget	2 oz	170	—	14
Hillshire				
Bologna Large	1 oz	90	—	8
Bologna Ring	1 oz	90	—	8
Brunschweiger	1 oz	95	—	8
Deli Select Bologna Light	1 slice	12	—	1
Deli Select Corned Beef	1 slice	10	—	tr
Deli Select Oven Roasted Cured Beef	1 slice	10	—	tr
Deli Select Pastrami	1 slice	10	—	tr
Deli Select Roast Beef	1 slice	10	—	tr
Deli Select Smoked Beef	1 slice	10	—	tr
Flavor Pack 90–99% Fat Free Bologna Light	1 slice (0.73 oz)	30	—	2
Flavor Pack 90–99% Fat Free Pastrami	1 slice (0.6 oz)	18	—	tr
Lunch 'N Munch Bologna/American/ Snickers	1 pkg (4.25 oz)	490	—	34

FOOD	PORTION	CALS.	SAT. FAT	FAT
Lunch 'N Munch Bologna/American/ Snickers/Hi-C	1 pkg (4.25 oz + 6 fl oz)	590	—	34
Lunch 'N Munch Bologna/American	1 pkg (4.5 oz)	480	—	37
Lunch 'N Munch Cotto Salami/Monterey Jack	1 pkg (4.5 oz)	440	—	32
Lunch 'N Munch Pepperoni/American	1 pkg (4.5 oz)	570	—	46
Pepperoni	1 oz	110	—	10
Salami Hard	1 oz	100	—	9
Summer Sausage	2 oz	180	—	16
Summer Sausage Beef	2 oz	190	—	17
Summer Sausage Light	2 oz	150	—	12
Summer Sausage w/ Cheddar Cheese	2 oz	200	—	18
Homeland Hard Salami	1 oz	110	5	10
Hormel				
Liverwurst Spread	4 tbsp (2 oz)	130	4	10
Pepperoni Chunk	1 oz	140	6	13
Pepperoni Sliced	15 slices (1 oz)	140	6	13
Pepperoni Twin	1 oz	140	6	13
Pillow Pack Genoa Salami	4 slices (1.1 oz)	120	4	10
Pillow Pack Pepperoni	1 oz	140	6	13
Pillow Pack Pepperoni	16 slices (1 oz)	140	6	13
Jones Liver Sausage	1 slice	80	—	7
Jones Liver Sausage Chub	1 slice	80	—	7
Oscar Mayer				
Bologna Beef	1 slice (1 oz)	90	4	8
Bologna Garlic	1 slice (1.4 oz)	110	4	12
Bologna Pork, Chicken, & Beef	1 slice (1 oz)	90	3	8
Bologna Wisconsin Made Ring	2 oz	140	6	16
Bologna Light	1 slice (1 oz)	60	2	4
Bologna Light Beef	1 slice (1 oz)	60	2	4
Braunschweiger	1 slice (1 oz)	100	3	9
Braunschweiger	2 oz	190	6	17
Braunschweiger German Brand	2 oz	200	6	18
Cotto Salami	2 slices (1.6 oz)	100	4	8
Cotto Salami Beef	2 slices (1.6 oz)	90	3	7
Genoa Salami	3 slices (1 oz)	100	3	9

FOOD	PORTION	CALS.	SAT. FAT	FAT
Oscar Mayer *(cont.)*				
Hard Salami	3 slices (1 oz)	100	3	9
Head Cheese	1 slice (1 oz)	50	2	4
Healthy Favorites Bologna	2 slices (1.6 oz)	45	0	1
Honey Loaf	1 slice (1 oz)	35	0	1
Liver Cheese	1 slice (1.3 oz)	120	4	10
Lunchables Bologna/ American	1 pkg (4.5 oz)	450	15	34
Lunchables Deluxe Turkey/Ham	1 pkg (5.1 oz)	360	10	19
Lunchables Dessert Jello/Honey Turkey/ Cheddar	1 pkg (5.7 oz)	320	9	16
Lunchables Fun Pack Bologna/Wild Cherry	1 pkg (11.2 oz)	530	14	29
Lunchables Fun Pack Ham/Fruit Punch	1 pkg (11.2 oz)	450	10	20
Lunchables Ham/Swiss	1 pkg (4.5 oz)	320	8	17
Lunchables Pepperoni/ American	1 pkg (4.5 oz)	480	17	36
Lunchables Salami/ American	1 pkg (4.5 oz)	430	15	32
Luncheon Loaf Spiced	1 slice (1 oz)	70	2	5
Machiach Brand Salami Beef	2 slices (1.6 oz)	120	5	10
New England Brand Sausage	2 slices (1.6 oz)	60	1	3
Old Fashioned Loaf	1 slice (1 oz)	60	2	5
Olive Loaf	1 slice (1 oz)	70	2	5
Peppered Loaf	1 slice (1 oz)	39	1	2
Pickle And Pimiento Loaf	1 slice (1 oz)	70	2	6
Salami For Beer	1 slices (1.6 oz)	110	3	9
Sandwich Spread	2 oz	140	4	10
Summer Sausage	2 slices (1.6 oz)	140	5	13
Summer Sausage Beef	2 slices (1.6 oz)	140	5	12
Russer				
Bologna	2 oz	180	7	15
Bologna Wunderbar German Brand	2 oz	190	6	16
Bologna Beef	2 oz	180	7	15
Bologna Garlic	2 oz	180	6	16
Bologna Italian Brand Sweet Red Pepper	2 oz	180	6	15

FOOD	PORTION	CALS.	SAT. FAT	FAT
Bologna Jalapeno Pepper	2 oz	170	6	14
Braunschweiger	2 oz	170	6	14
Cooked Salami	2 oz	120	3	8
Dutch Brand	2 oz	130	3	8
Hot Cooked Salami	2 oz	110	3	7
Italian Brand Loaf	2 oz	130	3	8
Jalapeno Loaf With Monterey Jack Cheese	2 oz	160	5	13
Kielbasa Loaf	2 oz	120	3	8
Olive Loaf	2 oz	160	5	13
P & P Loaf	2 oz	160	5	13
Pepper Loaf	2 oz	90	2	3
Polish Loaf	2 oz	140	4	10
Russer Lil' Salt				
Bologna	2 oz	120	3	8
Bologna, Beef	2 oz	120	4	8
Braunschweiger	2 oz	120	3	8
Cooked Salami	2 oz	90	3	5
Old Fashioned Loaf	2 oz	90	3	4
P & P Loaf	2 oz	100	3	6
Shofar Salami Beef	2 oz	160	6	15
Spam	2 oz	170	6	16
Spam Less Salt	2 oz	170	6	16
Spam Lite	2 oz	110	3	8
Underwood Liverwurst	2.08 oz	180	—	15
Weight Watchers Bologna	2 slices (¾ oz)	35	—	2
barbecue loaf, pork & beef	1 oz	49	1	3
beerwurst, beef	1 slice (4 × ⅛ in)	75	3	7
beerwurst, beef	1 slice (2¾ × ⅟₁₆ in)	20	1	2
beerwurst, pork	1 slice (4 × ⅛ in)	55	1	4
beerwurst, pork	1 slice (2¾ × ⅟₁₆ in)	14	tr	1
berliner, pork & beef	1 oz	65	2	4
blood sausage	1 oz	95	3	9
bologna, beef	1 oz	88	3	8
bologna, beef & pork	1 oz	89	3	8
bologna, pork	1 oz	70	2	6
braunschweiger, pork	1 oz	102	3	9
braunschweiger, pork	1 slice (2½ × ¼ in)	65	2	6
corned beef loaf	1 oz	43	1	2
dried beef	1 oz	47	—	1

FOOD	PORTION	CALS.	SAT. FAT	FAT
dried beef	5 slices (21 g)	35	—	tr
dutch brand loaf, pork & beef	1 oz	68	2	5
headcheese, pork	1 oz	60	1	5
honey loaf, pork & beef	1 oz	36	tr	1
honey roll sausage, beef	1 oz	42	2	14
lebanon bologna, beef	1 oz	60	2	4
liver cheese, pork	1 oz	86	3	7
liverwurst, pork	1 oz	92	3	8
luncheon meat, beef	1 oz	87	3	7
luncheon meat, pork & beef	1 oz	100	9	3
luncheon meat, pork, canned	1 oz	95	3	9
luncheon sausage, pork & beef	1 oz	74	2	6
luxury loaf, pork	1 oz	40	tr	1
mortadella, beef & pork	1 oz	88	3	7
mother's loaf, pork	1 oz	80	2	6
new england brand sausage, pork & beef	1 oz	46	1	2
olive loaf, pork	1 oz	67	2	5
peppered loaf, pork & beef	1 oz	42	1	2
pepperoni, pork & beef	1 (9 oz)	1248	40	110
pepperoni, pork & beef	1 slice (.2 oz)	27	1	2
pickle & pimiento loaf, pork	1 oz	74	2	6
picnic loaf, pork & beef	1 oz	66	2	5
salami, cooked, beef & pork	1 oz	71	2	6
salami, hard, pork & beef	1 pkg (4 oz)	472	13	39
salami, hard, pork & beef	1 slice (⅓ oz)	42	1	3
salami, hard, pork	1 pkg (4 oz)	460	13	38
salami, hard, pork	1 slice (⅓ oz)	41	1	4
sandwich spread pork & beef	1 tbsp	35	1	3
sandwich spread pork & beef	1 oz	67	2	5
summer sausage thuringer cervelat	1 oz	98	3	8
TAKE-OUT				
submarine w/ salami, ham, cheese, lettuce, tomato, onion, oil	1	456	7	19

FOOD	PORTION	CALS.	SAT. FAT	FAT
LUPINES				
dried, cooked	1 cup	197	1	5
LYCHEES				
fresh	1 cup	6	—	tr
MACADAMIA NUTS				
Candy Glazed (Mauna Loa)	1 oz	170	—	14
Chocolate Covered (Mauna Loa)	1 oz	170	—	13
Honey Roasted (Mauna Loa)	1 oz	200	—	17
Macadamia Nut Brittle (Mauna Loa)	1 oz	150	—	8
Roasted & Salted (Mauna Loa)	1 oz	210	—	21
dried	1 oz	199	3	21
oil roasted	1 oz	204	3	22
MACARONI				
(*see* PASTA)				
MACE				
ground	1 tsp	8	tr	1
MACKEREL				
CANNED				
Jack (Empress)	4 oz	140	—	8
jack	1 cup	296	4	12
jack	1 can (12.7 oz)	563	7	23
FRESH				
atlantic, cooked	3 oz	223	4	15
atlantic, raw	3 oz	174	3	12
jack, baked	3 oz	171	2	9
jack fillet, baked	6.2 oz	354	5	18
king, baked	3 oz	114	tr	2
king fillet, baked	5.4 oz	207	1	4
pacific, baked	3 oz	171	2	9
pacific fillet, baked	6.2 oz	354	5	18
spanish, cooked	3 oz	134	2	5
spanish, cooked	1 fillet (5.1 oz)	230	3	9
spanish, raw	3 oz	118	2	5

FOOD	PORTION	CALS.	SAT. FAT	FAT
MALT				
Bartles & Jaymes Malt Cooler				
Berry	12 fl oz	210	0	0
Berry Light	12 fl oz	140	0	0
Black Cherry	12 fl oz	190	0	0
Mandarin Lemon	12 fl oz	210	0	0
Margarita	12 fl oz	250	0	0
Original	12 fl oz	180	0	0
Peach	12 fl oz	200	0	0
Pina Colada	12 fl oz	270	0	0
Planter's Punch	12 fl oz	220	0	0
Red Sangria	12 fl oz	190	0	0
Strawberry	12 fl oz	200	0	0
Strawberry Daiquiri	12 fl oz	220	0	0
Tropical	12 fl oz	220	0	0
Olde English	12 oz	163	0	0
Schaefer	12 oz	165	0	0
Schlitz	12 oz	177	0	0
nonalcoholic	12 oz	32	0	0
MALTED MILK				
Carnation Chocolate	3 heaping tsp (21 g)	79	—	tr
Carnation Original	3 heaping tsp (21 g)	90	—	2
Kraft Instant Chocolate	3 tsp	90	—	1
Kraft Instant Natural	3 tsp	90	—	2
chocolate flavor powder	3 heaping tsp (¾ oz)	79	tr	1
chocolate, as prep w/ milk	1 cup	229	6	9
natural flavor powder	3 heaping tsp (¾ oz)	87	1	2
natural flavor, as prep w/ milk	1 cup	237	6	10
MAMMY APPLE				
fresh	1	431	—	4
MANGO				
fresh	1	135	tr	1
JUICE				
Kern's Nectar	6 oz	100	0	0
Libby's Nectar	1 can (11.5 fl oz)	210	0	0

FOOD	PORTION	CALS.	SAT. FAT	FAT
MARGARINE				
(*see also* BUTTER BLENDS, BUTTER SUBSTITUTES)				
REDUCED CALORIE				
Fleischmann's Diet	1 tbsp	50	1	6
Fleischmann's Extra Light Corn Oil Spread	1 tbsp	50	1	6
Mazola Diet	1 tbsp	50	1	6
Mazola Diet	1 cup	815	16	93
Mazola Light Corn Oil Spread	1 tbsp	50	1	6
Mazola Light Corn Oil Spread	1 cup	835	15	94
Parkay Diet Soft	1 tbsp	50	1	6
Smart Beat	1 tbsp	25	tr	3
Smart Beat Unsalted	1 tbsp	25	tr	3
Weight Watchers Extra Light Sweet Unsalted Tub	1 tbsp	50	1	6
Weight Watchers Extra Light Tub	1 tbsp	50	1	6
Weight Watchers Light Stick	1 tbsp	60	1	7
diet	1 tsp	17	tr	2
diet	1 cup	800	18	90
REGULAR				
Blue Bonnet	1 tbsp	100	2	11
Fleischmann's	1 tbsp	100	2	11
Fleischmann's Light Corn Oil Stick	1 tbsp	80	1	8
Fleischmann's Sweet Unsalted	1 tbsp	100	2	11
Hain Safflower	1 tbsp	100	2	11
Hain Safflower Unsalted	1 tbsp	100	2	11
Krona	1 tbsp	100	—	11
Land O'Lakes Spread	1 tbsp	90	2	10
Land O'Lakes Spread With Sweet Cream	1 tbsp (0.5 oz)	90	2	10
Land O'Lakes Spread With Sweet Cream Unsalted	1 tbsp (0.5 oz)	90	2	10
Mazola	1 cup (229 g)	1650	32	184
Mazola	1 tbsp (14 g)	100	2	11
Mazola Unsalted	1 cup	1635	32	184
Mazola Unsalted	1 tbsp	100	2	11
Mother's	1 tbsp	100	—	11

FOOD	PORTION	CALS.	SAT. FAT	FAT
Mother's Unsalted	1 tbsp	100	—	11
Nucanola	1 tbsp (14 g)	90	1	10
Parkay	1 tbsp	100	2	11
Promise	1 tbsp	90	—	10
corn	1 stick (4 oz)	815	15	91
corn	1 tsp	34	1	4
salted	1 stick (4 oz)	815	18	91
salted	1 tsp	39	1	4
unsalted	1 stick (4 oz)	809	17	91
unsalted	1 tsp	34	1	4
SOFT				
Blue Bonnet	1 tbsp	100	2	11
Chiffon	1 tbsp	90	1	10
Chiffon Stick	1 tbsp	100	2	11
Chiffon Unsalted	1 tbsp	90	2	10
Fleischmann's	1 tbsp	100	2	11
Fleischmann's Light Corn Oil Spread	1 tbsp	80	1	8
Fleischmann's Sweet Unsalted	1 tbsp	100	2	11
Hain Safflower	1 tbsp	100	2	11
Hollywood Soft Spread	1 tbsp	90	1	10
I Can't Believe It's Not Butter!	1 tbsp	90	—	10
Land O'Lakes Spread Tub	1 tbsp (0.5 oz)	80	2	8
Land O'Lakes Spread w/ Sweet Cream Tub	1 tbsp (0.5 oz)	80	2	8
Mother's Salted	1 tbsp	100	—	11
Mother's Unsalted	1 tbsp	100	—	11
Parkay Soft	1 tbsp	100	2	11
Parkay Spread	1 tbsp	60	1	7
corn	1 tsp	34	1	4
corn	1 cup	1626	21	183
safflower	1 tsp	34	tr	4
safflower	1 cup	1626	31	183
soybean, salted	1 tsp	34	1	4
soybean, salted	1 cup	1626	31	183
soybean, unsalted	1 tsp	34	1	4
soybean, unsalted	1 cup	1626	31	182
tub, salted	1 tsp	34	1	4
tub, salted	1 cup	1626	31	183
tub, unsalted	1 tsp	34	1	4
tub, unsalted	1 cup	1626	31	182

FOOD	PORTION	CALS.	SAT. FAT	FAT
SQUEEZE				
Parkay Squeeze	1 tbsp	90	2	10
soybean & cottonseed	1 tsp	34	1	4
WHIPPED				
Blue Bonnet Whipped Spread	1 tbsp	80		9
Chiffon	1 tbsp	70	1	8
Fleischmann's Lightly Salted	1 tbsp	70	2	7
Fleischmann's Unsalted	1 tbsp	70	2	7
Miracle Brand	1 tbsp	60	1	7
Miracle Brand Stick	1 tbsp	70	1	7
Parkay	1 tbsp	70	1	7
Parkay Stick	1 tbsp	70	1	7
MARJORAM				
dried	1 tsp	2	—	tr
MARSHMALLOW				
Campfire (Borden)	2 lg	40	0	0
Campfire Miniature (Borden)	24	40	0	0
Funmallows (Kraft)	1	30	0	0
Funmallows Miniature (Kraft)	10	18	0	0
Jet-Puffed (Kraft)	1	25	0	0
Marshmallow Fluff	1 heaping tsp (18 g)	59	—	tr
Miniature (Kraft)	10	18	0	0
marshmallow	1 oz	90	0	0
MATZO				
American Matzo (Manischewitz)	1	115	—	2
Daily Thin Tea (Manischewitz)	1	103	0	tr
Dietetic (Streit's)	1 (1 oz)	100	0	0
Dietetic Thins (Manischewitz)	1	91	—	tr
Egg Dark Chocolate Coated (Manischewitz)	½ matzo (1 oz)	97	2	3
Egg Milk Chocolate Coated (Horowitz Margareten)	1 oz	97	3	4
Egg n' Onion (Manischewitz)	1	112	tr	tr

FOOD	PORTION	CALS.	SAT. FAT	FAT
Lightly Salted (Streit's)	1 (1 oz)	110	0	1
Matzo Ball Mix 50% Less Salt (Goodman's)	2 tbsp (0.5 oz)	50	0	0
Matzo Ball Mix, as prep (Goodman's)	2 tbsp (0.5 oz)	60	0	0
Matzo Cracker Miniatures (Manischewitz)	10	90	—	tr
Matzo Farfel (Manischewitz)	1 cup	180	—	1
Matzo Meal (Manischewitz)	1 cup	514	—	1
Matzoh Meal (Streit's)	¼ cup (1 oz)	110	0	1
Passover (Manischewitz)	1	129	—	tr
Passover (Streit's)	1 (1 oz)	110	0	1
Passover Egg (Manischewitz)	1	132	—	2
Passover Egg Matzo Crackers (Manischewitz)	10	108	—	2
Salted Thin (Manischewitz)	1	100	—	tr
Unsalted (Manischewitz)	1	110	0	tr
Unsalted (Streit's)	1 (0.9 oz)	100	0	1
Wheat Matzo Crackers (Manischewitz)	10	90	—	1
Whole Wheat (Streit's)	1 (1 oz)	110	0	1
Whole Wheat w/ Bran (Manischewitz)	1	110	0	1
egg	1 (1 oz)	111	tr	1
egg & onion	1 (1 oz)	111	tr	1
plain	1 (1 oz)	112	tr	tr
whole wheat	1 (1 oz)	99	tr	tr

MAYONNAISE

(*see also* MAYONNAISE TYPE SALAD DRESSING, RELISH)

REDUCED CALORIE

FOOD	PORTION	CALS.	SAT. FAT	FAT
Best Foods Cholesterol Free Reduced Calorie	1 cup (233 g)	760	11	75
Best Foods Cholesterol Free Reduced Calorie	1 tbsp (15 g)	50	1	5
Best Foods Light	1 cup (233 g)	760	14	78
Best Foods Light	1 tbsp (15 g)	50	1	5
Diamond Crystal	1 tbsp	50	—	5
Hain Canola	1 tbsp	60	0	5
Hain Light Low Sodium	1 tbsp	60	1	6
Hellmann's Light Reduced Calorie	1 cup	760	14	78

FOOD	PORTION	CALS.	SAT. FAT	FAT
Hellmann's Light Reduced Calorie	1 tbsp (15 g)	50	1	5
Hellmann's Cholesterol Free Reduced Calorie	1 cup (233 g)	760	11	75
Hellmann's Cholesterol Free Reduced Calorie	1 tbsp (15 g)	50	1	5
Kraft Free	1 tbsp	12	0	0
Kraft Light	1 tbsp	50	1	5
Smart Beat Canola Oil	1 tbsp	40	tr	4
Smart Beat Corn Oil	1 tbsp	40	tr	4
Weight Watchers Fat Free	1 tbsp	12	0	0
Weight Watchers Light	1 tbsp	50	1	5
Weight Watchers Low Sodium	1 tbsp	50	1	1
reduced calorie	1 cup	556	8	46
reduced calorie	1 tbsp	34	1	3
REGULAR				
BAMA	1 tbsp	100	—	11
Bennett's	1 tbsp	110	—	12
Best Foods Real	1 cup	1570	26	175
Best Foods Real	1 tbsp	100	2	11
Hain				
Canola	1 tbsp	100	1	11
Cold Processed	1 tbsp	110	2	12
Eggless No Salt Added	1 tbsp	110	2	12
Real No Salt Added	1 tbsp	110	2	12
Safflower	1 tbsp	110	1	12
Hellmann's	1 cup	1570	26	173
Hellmann's Real	1 tbsp	100	2	11
Hollywood	1 tbsp	110	1	12
Hollywood Canola	1 tbsp	100	3	11
Hollywood Safflower	1 tbsp	100	1	12
Kraft Real Mayonnaise	1 tbsp	100	2	12
Kraft Sandwich Spread	1 tbsp	50	1	5
McIlhenny Spicy	1 tbsp (0.5 oz)	108	3	12
Mother's	1 tbsp	100	—	11
mayonnaise	1 cup	1577	26	175
mayonnaise	1 tbsp	99	2	11
sandwich spread	1 tbsp	60	1	5

MAYONNAISE TYPE SALAD DRESSING

(see also MAYONNAISE, RELISH)

REDUCED CALORIE

Miracle Whip Free	1 tbsp	20	0	0

FOOD	PORTION	CALS.	SAT. FAT	FAT
Miracle Whip Light	1 tbsp	45	1	4
Smart Beat	1 tbsp	12	0	0
Weight Watchers Fat Free Whipped Dressing	1 tbsp	16	0	0
reduced calorie w/o cholesterol	1 cup	1084	17	107
reduced calorie w/o cholesterol	1 tbsp	68	1	7
REGULAR				
BAMA	1 tbsp	50	—	4
Bright Day Dressing	1 tbsp	60	—	6
Miracle Whip	1 tbsp	70	1	7
Miracle Whip Coleslaw Dressing	1 tbsp	70	1	6
Spin Blend	1 tbsp	60	1	5
Spin Blend Cholesterol Free	1 tbsp	40	1	4
home recipe	1 cup	400	7	24
home recipe	1 tbsp	25	1	2
mayonnaise type salad dressing	1 cup	916	12	78
mayonnaise type salad dressing	1 tbsp	57	5	5

MEAT STICKS

DRIED

FOOD	PORTION	CALS.	SAT. FAT	FAT
Tombstone Beef Jerky	1	35	0	0
Tombstone Beef Sticks	1	110	5	10
Tombstone Snappy Sticks	1	110	5	10

MEAT SUBSTITUTES

(*see also* BACON SUBSTITUTES, CHICKEN SUBSTITUTES, SAUSAGE SUBSTITUTES, TURKEY SUBSTITUTES)

FOOD	PORTION	CALS.	SAT. FAT	FAT
Better Than Burger? Sovex	½ cup (1.9 oz)	165	1	2
Harvest Direct TVP				
Beef Chunks	3.5 oz	280	tr	1
Beef Chunks Flavored	3.5 oz	250	tr	1
Beef Ground	3.5 oz	280	tr	1
Beef Ground Flavored	3.5 oz	250	tr	1
Beef Strips	3.5 oz	280	tr	1
Jaclyn's Salisbury Steak Style Dinner	11 oz	260	—	8
Jaclyn's Sirloin Strips Style Dinner	12 oz	290	—	6

FOOD	PORTION	CALS.	SAT. FAT	FAT
Ken & Robert's Veggie Burger	1 (62 g)	110	0	2
Knox Mountain Farm Wheat Balls Mix	1 serv (⅒ pkg)	110	—	1
LaLoma				
Big Franks	1 (51 g)	110	—	6
Corn Dogs	1 (71 g)	190	—	8
Dinner Cuts	2 pieces (99 g)	110	—	1
Griddle Steaks	1 piece (54 g)	140	—	7
Nuteena	½ in slice (65 g)	160	—	12
Patty Mix	¼ cup (16 g)	50	0	0
Redi-Burger	½ in slice (68 g)	130	—	6
Sandwich Spread	3 tbsp (48 g)	70	—	4
Savory Dinner Loaf Mix, not prep	¼ cup (16 g)	50	0	0
Savory Meatballs	7 (70 g)	190	—	8
Sizzle Burger	1 patty (71 g)	220	—	12
Sizzle Franks	2 (68 g)	170	—	13
Swiss Steak	1 piece (92 g)	170	—	10
Tender Bits	4 pieces (57 g)	80	—	3
Tender Rounds	6 pieces (73 g)	120	—	4
Vege-Burger	½ cup (108 g)	110	—	2
Vita-Burger Chunk	¼ cup (21 g)	70	0	0
Vita-Burger Granules	3 tbsp (21 g)	70	0	0
Lightlife				
American Grill	2.75 oz	110	1	3
Barbecue Grill	2.75 oz	130	1	6
Smart Deli Slices	2 slices (1.5 oz)	44	0	0
Smart Dogs	1 (1.5 oz)	40	0	0
Smart Dogs To Go	1 (5 oz)	115	0	0
Tofu Pups	1 (1.5 oz)	92	—	5
Vegetarian Sloppy Joe	4.3 oz	130	1	6
Midland Harvest Burger n' Loaf				
Chili w/o Beans	0.8 oz	90	1	3
Herbs & Spice	3.2 oz	140	1	5
Italian	3.2 oz	140	1	5
Original	3.2 oz	140	1	5
Sloppy Joe w/o Sauce	0.8 oz	80	1	2
Taco	2.7 oz	90	tr	2
Morningstar Farms				
Breaded Cutlet	1 patty (71 g)	230	—	14
Deli Franks	1 (35 g)	90	—	6
Sandwich Burger Pattie w/ Cheese	1 (4.75 oz)	370	—	17

FOOD	PORTION	CALS.	SAT. FAT	FAT
Morningstar Farms *(cont.)*				
Sandwich Pattie Biscuit	1 (3.5 oz)	280	—	11
Natural Touch				
Dinner Entree	1 patty (85 g)	230	—	14
Garden Pattie	1 (67 g)	120	—	4
Loaf Mix, as prep	4 oz	180	—	7
Okara Pattie	1 (64 g)	160	—	10
Stroganoff Mix, as prep	4 oz	90	—	3
Taco Mix, as prep	2 tbsp	90	—	2
Spring Creek Soysage	1 patty (1.6 oz)	63	—	tr
White Wave Meatless				
Healthy Franks	1 (1.5 oz)	90	0	2
Jumbo Franks	1 (3 oz)	170	1	3
Sandwich Slices Beef	2 slices (1.6 oz)	90	0	0
Sandwich Slices Bologna	2 slices (1.6 oz)	120	2	8
Sandwich Slices Pastrami	2 slices (1.6 oz)	90	0	0
Worthington				
Beef Style Meatless	4 slices (70 g)	130	—	6
Bolono	2 slices (38 g)	60	—	2
Choplets	2 slices (92 g)	100	—	2
Corn Beef Sliced	4 slices (57 g)	120	—	6
Country Stew	9.5 oz (270 g)	220	—	10
Dinner Roast	2 oz	120	—	8
FriPats	1 (64 g)	180	—	12
Granburger, not prep	6 tbsp (33 g)	110	—	1
Multigrain Cutlet	2 slices (92 g)	90	—	2
Non-Meat Balls	3 (54 g)	100	—	6
Numete	½ in slice (68 g)	150	—	11
Prime Stakes	1 piece (92 g)	160	—	10
Prosage Patties	2 (76 g)	210	—	14
Prosage Roll	2⅜ in slice (70 g)	180	—	12
Protose	½ in slice (76 g)	180	—	8
Salami Meatless	2 slices (38 g)	70	—	4
Savory Slices	2 slices (56 g)	100	—	6
Smoked Beef Slices	6 slices (56 g)	120	—	6
Stakelets	1 piece (71 g)	150	—	8
Veelets	1 patty (71 g)	230	—	14
Vegetable Skallops	½ cup (85 g)	90	—	2
Vegetable Skallops No Added Salt	½ cup (85 g)	80	—	1
Vegetable Steaks	2.5 pieces (90 g)	110	—	2
Vegetarian Burger	½ cup (113 g)	150	—	4

FOOD	PORTION	CALS.	SAT. FAT	FAT
Vegetarian Burger No Added Salt	½ cup (113 g)	150	—	4
Vegetarian Beef Pie	1 (227 g)	360	—	16
Wham	3 slices (68 g)	120	—	7
simulated sausage	1 patty (38 g)	97	1	7
simulated sausage	1 link (25 g)	64	1	5
simulated meat product	1 oz	88	tr	1

MELON
(*see also individual names*)

FRESH
Chiquita Cantalene	1 cup	60	—	0
Chiquita Honey Mist	1 cup	80	—	0

FROZEN
Mixed (Big Valley)	¾ cup (4.9 oz)	40	0	0
melon balls	1 cup	55	—	tr

MILK
(*see also* CHOCOLATE, COCOA, MILK DRINKS)

CANNED
Carnation Evaporated	2 tbsp	40	2	3
Carnation Evaporated Lowfat	2 tbsp	25	—	1
Carnation Evaporated Skim	½ cup (4 fl oz)	100	—	tr
Carnation Sweetened Condensed	2 tbsp	130	2	3
Eagle Sweetened Condensed	⅓ cup	320	—	9
Pet Evaporated	½ cup	170	—	10
Pet Evaporated Filled	½ cup	150	1	8
Pet Evaporated Light Skim	½ cup	100	—	tr
condensed, sweetened	1 oz	123	2	3
condensed, sweetened	1 cup	982	17	27
evaporated	½ cup	169	6	10
evaporated, skim	½ cup	99	tr	tr

DRIED
Carnation, Nonfat	⅓ cup dry	80	—	tr
Nutra/Balance Lactose Reduced, as prep	8 oz	80	—	tr
Sanalac, as prep	8 oz	80	—	tr
buttermilk	1 tbsp	25	tr	tr
nonfat instantized	1 pkg (3.2 oz)	244	tr	tr

LIQUID, LOWFAT
1%	1 cup	102	2	3

FOOD	PORTION	CALS.	SAT. FAT	FAT
1%	1 qt	409	6	10
1% protein fortified	1 cup	119	2	3
1% protein fortified	1 qt	477	7	12
2%	1 cup	121	3	5
2%	1 qt	485	12	19
Borden Acidophilus 1%	8 fl oz	100	—	2
Borden Golden Churn Lowfat Buttermilk	8 fl oz	120	—	4
Borden Hi-Protein 2%	8 fl oz	140	—	5
CalciMilk	8 fl oz	102	2	3
Easylac 1% (Farmland)	8 fl oz	100	—	2
Farmland 1% (Farmland)	8 fl oz	100	2	3
Farmland 2% (Farmland)	8 fl oz	130	3	5
Friendship Buttermilk	8 oz	120	3	4
Lactaid 1%	1 cup	102	2	3
Viva 2%	8 fl oz	120	—	5
buttermilk	1 cup	99	1	2
buttermilk	1 qt	396	5	9
LIQUID, REGULAR				
Borden	8 fl oz	150	—	8
Borden Hi-Calcium	8 fl oz	150	—	8
Farmland Cholesterol Reduced	8 oz	150	—	8
Farmland 2% (Farmland)	8 fl oz	150	5	8
buffalo	3.5 oz	112	5	8
camel	3.5 oz	80	—	4
donkey	3.5 oz	43	—	1
goat	1 cup	168	7	10
goat	1 qt	672	26	40
human	1 cup	171	5	11
indian buffalo	1 cup	236	11	17
low sodium	1 cup	149	5	8
mare	3.5 oz	49	—	2
sheep	1 cup	264	11	17
whole	1 cup	150	5	8
LIQUID, SKIM				
Borden	8 fl oz	90	—	1
Borden Skim-line	8 fl oz	100	—	1
Easylac Nonfat (Farmland)	8 fl oz	90	—	0
Farmland	8 fl oz	80	0	0
Farmland Skim Plus	8 fl oz	100	—	tr
Lactaid Nonfat	8 fl oz	86	tr	tr
Viva	8 fl oz	90	tr	—
Weight Watchers	1 cup	90	—	tr

FOOD	PORTION	CALS.	SAT. FAT	FAT
skim	1 cup	86	tr	tr
skim	1 qt	342	1	2
skim, protein fortified	1 cup	100	tr	1
skim, protein fortified	1 qt	400	2	2

MILK DRINKS
(*see also* BREAKFAST DRINKS, CHOCOLATE, COCOA)

FOOD	PORTION	CALS.	SAT. FAT	FAT
Bosco Chocolate Milk	1 cup (8 fl oz)	230	—	8
Chocolate Lowfat Dutch Brand Borden	8 fl oz	180	—	5
Chocolate Milk (Meadow Gold)	1 cup	210	—	8
Chocolate Milk 1% (Lactaid)	8 fl oz	158	2	3
Chocolate Milk 2% (Hershey)	1 cup	190	—	5
Quik Banana Lowfat Milk (Nestle)	8 oz	190	—	4
Quik Chocolate (Nestle)	.75 oz	90	—	1
Quik Chocolate, as prep w/ 2% milk (Nestle)	8 oz	210	—	5
Quik Chocolate, as prep w/ skim milk (Nestle)	8 oz	170	—	1
Quik Chocolate, as prep w/ whole milk (Nestle)	8 oz	230	—	9
Quik Chocolate Lowfat Milk (Nestle)	8 oz	200	—	5
Quik Lite Ready to Drink Chocolate Lowfat (Nestle)	8 oz	130	—	5
Quik Ready to Drink Chocolate (Nestle)	8 oz	230	—	9
Quik Ready to Drink Strawberry (Nestle)	8 oz	230	—	8
Quick Strawberry (Nestle)	¾ oz	80	—	0
Quik Strawberry, as prep w/ 2% milk (Nestle)	8 oz	200	—	5
Quik Strawberry, as prep w/ skim milk (Nestle)	8 oz	160	—	0
Quik Strawberry, as prep w/ whole milk (Nestle)	8 oz	220	—	8
Quik Strawberry Lowfat Milk (Nestle)	8 oz	200	—	4
Quik Sugar Free Chocolate (Nestle)	1 heaping tsp	18	—	tr

FOOD	PORTION	CALS.	SAT. FAT	FAT
Quik Sugar Free Chocolate, as prep w/ 2% milk (Nestle)	8 oz	140	—	5
Quik Syrup Chocolate (Nestle)	1⅓ tbsp	100	—	1
Quik Syrup Chocolate, as prep w/ 2% milk (Nestle)	8 oz	220	—	5
Quik Syrup Chocolate, as prep w/ skim milk (Nestle)	8 oz	220	—	9
Quik Syrup Chocolate, as prep w/ whole milk (Nestle)	8 oz	240	—	9
Quik Syrup Strawberry (Nestle)	1⅓ tbsp	100	—	0
Quik Syrup Strawberry, as prep w/ 2% milk (Nestle)	8 oz	220	—	5
Quik Syrup Strawberry, as prep w/ skim milk (Nestle)	8 oz	180	—	0
Quik Syrup Strawberry, as prep w/ whole milk (Nestle)	8 oz	240	—	8
Quik Vanilla Lowfat Milk (Nestle)	8 oz	200	—	4
Whole Chocolate Milk (Hershey)	8 oz	210	—	9
chocolate milk	1 cup	208	5	8
chocolate milk	1 qt	833	21	34
chocolate milk 1%	1 cup	158	2	3
chocolate milk 1%	1 qt	630	6	10
chocolate milk 2%	1 cup	179	3	5
strawberry flavor mix, as prep w/ whole milk	9 oz	234	5	8

MILK SUBSTITUTES
(*see also* COFFEE WHITENERS)

Better Than Milk				
Carob	8 fl oz	130	—	5
Chocolate	8 fl oz	125	—	5
Light	8 fl oz	80	—	tr
Natural	8 fl oz	90	—	5
Edensoy	8.45 fl oz	140	1	4

FOOD	PORTION	CALS.	SAT. FAT	FAT
Edensoy Extra	8.45 fl oz	140	1	4
First Alternative	8 fl oz	80	tr	2
Health Valley Soo Moo	1 cup	120	—	6
Health Valley				
Rice Dream				
Carob Lite	8 fl oz	150	—	3
Chocolate	8 fl oz	190	—	3
Organic Original Lite	8 fl oz	130	—	2
Vanilla Lite	8 fl oz	130	—	2
Spring Creek Honey Vanilla	1 oz	23	—	5
Spring Creek Original	1 oz	21	—	5
Spring Creek Plain	1 oz	15	—	5
Vegelicious	8 fl oz	100	—	2
Vitamite	8 fl oz	100	—	5
Vitasoy				
Carob Supreme	8 fl oz	150	—	4
Cocoa Light	8 fl oz	140	1	2
Cocoa Rich	8 fl oz	160	—	4
Original Creamy	8 fl oz	100	—	5
Original Light	8 fl oz	90	1	2
Vanilla Delite	8 fl oz	150	—	4
Vanilla Light	8 fl oz	110	1	2
Westsoy Cocoa Lite	8 fl oz	140	tr	2
Westsoy Plain Lite	8 fl oz	100	tr	2
Westsoy Vanilla Lite	8 fl oz	110	tr	2
imitation milk	1 cup	150	2	8
imitation milk	1 qt	600	33	33

MILKFISH
baked	3 oz	162	—	7

MILKSHAKE
Chocolate (Frostee)	1 cup	200	—	8
Chocolate (MicroMagic)	1 (10.5 oz)	290	—	8
Chocolate Fudge	1 pkg	70	—	tr
(Weight Watchers)				
Milk Way Shake	1 (10 fl oz)	390	10	16
Orange Sherbert	1 pkg	70	—	tr
(Weight Watchers)				
Strawberry (Frostee)	1 cup	180	—	7
chocolate	10 oz	360	7	11
chocolate thick shake	10.6 oz	356	5	8
strawberry	10 oz	319	—	8
vanilla	10 oz	314	5	8
vanilla thick shake	11 oz	350	6	10

FOOD	PORTION	CALS.	SAT. FAT	FAT

MILLET

FOOD	PORTION	CALS.	SAT. FAT	FAT
cooked	½ cup	143	tr	1

MINERAL/BOTTLED WATER

FOOD	PORTION	CALS.	SAT. FAT	FAT
Artesia	7 oz	0	—	0
Artesia Almund	7 oz	0	—	0
Artesia Cranberi	7 oz	0	—	0
Artesia Lemin	7 oz	0	—	0
Artesia Orange	7 oz	0	—	0
Canada Dry Sparkling Water	8 fl oz	0	0	0
Crystal Geyser Sparkling Lemon	6 oz	0	0	0
Crystal Geyser Sparkling Mineral	6 oz	0	0	0
Crystal Geyser Sparkling Natural Wild Cherry	6 oz	0	0	0
Crystal Geyser Sparkling Orange	6 oz	0	0	0
Diamond Spring	1 qt (liter)	0	—	0
Evian	1 liter	0	0	0
Glenpatrick Spring Pure Irish	8 oz	0	—	0
LaCroix Sparkling				
Berry	12 fl oz	0	0	0
Lemon	12 fl oz	0	0	0
Lime	12 fl oz	0	0	0
Orange	12 fl oz	0	0	0
Regular	12 fl oz	0	0	0
Mountain Valley	1 qt (liter)	0	—	0
San Pellegrino	1 liter (33.8 oz)	0	0	0
Saratoga Sparkling	8 oz	0	0	0

MISO

FOOD	PORTION	CALS.	SAT. FAT	FAT
miso	½ cup	284	1	8

MOCHA

FOOD	PORTION	CALS.	SAT. FAT	FAT
Bavarian Mint Mocha (Hills Bros.)	6 oz	50	—	1
Bavarian Mint Mocha Sugar Free (Hills Bros.)	6 oz	35	—	1
Cafe Mocha (Hills Bros.)	6 oz	50	—	1
Cafe Mocha (MJB Co.)	6 oz	50	—	1
Cherry Mocha (MJB Co.)	6 oz	50	—	1
Fudge Mocha Sugar Free (MJB Co.)	6 oz	40	—	2

FOOD	PORTION	CALS.	SAT. FAT	FAT
Mint Mocha (MJB Co.)	6 oz	50	—	1
Mint Mocha Sugar Free (MJB Co.)	6 oz	35	—	1
Swiss Mocha (Hills Bros.)	6 oz	40	—	2
Vanilla Mocha Sugar Free (MJB Co.)	6 oz	40	—	2

MOLASSES

Brer Rabbit Dark	2 tbsp	110	0	0
Brer Rabbit Light	2 tbsp	110	0	0
McIlhenny	1 tbsp (0.7 oz)	66	tr	tr
blackstrap	2 tbsp	85	0	0
molasses	2 tbsp	85	0	0

MONKFISH

baked	3 oz	82	—	2

MOOSE

roasted	3 oz	114	tr	1

MOTH BEANS

cooked	1 cup	207	tr	1

MOUSSE

FROZEN

Chocolate (Sara Lee)	1 Slice (2.7 oz)	260	—	17
Chocolate (Weight Watchers)	1 (2.5 oz)	160	tr	3
Chocolate (Sara Lee)	1 (3 oz)	170	—	8
Light Classics Strawberry (Sara Lee)	1 slice (53.8 g)	180	—	11
Praline Pecan (Weight Watchers)	1 (2.71 oz)	180	1	4
San Francisco Chocolate (Pepperidge Farm)	1	490	18	34

HOME RECIPE

crab	¼ cup	364	—	20
orange	½ cup	87	—	5

MIX

Chocolate Fudge Rich and Luscious (Jell-O)	½ cup	145	—	6
Chocolate Mousse (Weight Watchers)	½ cup	70	—	3
Chocolate Mousse No Bake (Royal)	⅛ pie	130	0	4
Dark Chocolate, as prep (Knorr)	½ cup	90	—	5

FOOD	PORTION	CALS.	SAT. FAT	FAT
Milk Chocolate, as prep (Knorr)	½ cup	90	—	5
Unflavored Mousse Mix, as prep (Knorr)	½ cup	80	—	5
White Chocolate Almond Mousse, as prep (Weight Watchers)	½ cup	70	—	3
White Chocolate Mousse Mix, as prep (Knorr)	½ cup	80	—	4

MUFFIN
FROZEN

FOOD	PORTION	CALS.	SAT. FAT	FAT
Almond & Date Oat Bran Fancy Fruit (Health Valley)	1	180	—	4
Apple Oat Bran (Sara Lee)	1	190	—	6
Apple Spice (Sara Lee)	1	220	—	8
Apple Spice Fat Free (Health Valley)	1	140	—	tr
Banana Fat Free (Health Valley)	1	130	—	tr
Banana Nut (Pepperidge Farm)	1	170	—	6
Banana Nut (Weight Watchers)	1 (2.5 oz)	170	—	5
Blueberry (Pepperidge Farm)	1	170	—	7
Blueberry (Sara Lee)	1	200	—	8
Blueberry (Weight Watchers)	1 (2.5 oz)	170	—	5
Blueberry Free & Light (Sara Lee)	1	120	—	0
Cheese Streusel (Sara Lee)	1	220	—	11
Chocolate Chunk (Sara Lee)	1	220	—	8
Cholesterol Free Multi-Grain Muesli (Pepperidge Farm)	1	200	1	8
Cholesterol Free Oat Bran w/ Apple (Pepperidge Farm)	1	190	1	7
Cholesterol Free Raisin Bran (Pepperidge Farm)	1	170	1	6
Cinnamon Swirl (Pepperidge Farm)	1	190	1	6

FOOD	PORTION	CALS.	SAT. FAT	FAT
Corn (Pepperidge Farm)	1	180	1	7
Golden Corn (Sara Lee)	1	240	—	13
Oat Bran (Sara Lee)	1	210	—	8
Oat Bran Fancy Fruit Blueberry (Health Valley)	1	140	—	4
Oat Bran Fancy Fruit Raisin (Health Valley)	1	180	—	5
Raisin Bran (Sara Lee)	1	220	—	7
Raisin Spice Fat Free (Health Valley)	1	140	—	tr
Rice Bran Fancy Fruit Raisin (Health Valley)	1	210	—	7
HOME RECIPE				
blueberry as prep with 2% milk	1 (2 oz)	163	1	6
blueberry as prep with whole milk	1 (2 oz)	165	1	6
corn as prep w/ 2% milk	1 (2 oz)	180	1	7
corn as prep w/ whole milk	1 (2 oz)	183	2	7
plain as prep w/ 2% milk	1 (2 oz)	169	1	7
plain as prep w/ whole milk	1 (2 oz)	172	1	7
wheat bran as prep w/ 2% milk	1 (2 oz)	161	1	7
wheat bran as prep w/ whole milk	1 (2 oz)	164	2	7
MIX				
Apple Cinnamon (Betty Crocker)	1	120	1	4
Apple Cinnamon No Cholesterol Recipe (Betty Crocker)	1	110	1	2
Apple Cinnamon as prep (Jiffy)	1	190	3	7
Banana Nut (Betty Crocker)	1	120	1	5
Banana Nut as prep (Jiffy)	1	180	4	7
Banana Nut No Cholesterol Recipe (Betty Crocker)	1	110	1	4
Blueberry Streusel Bake Shop (Betty Crocker)	1	210	—	8
Blueberry as prep (Jiffy)	1	190	4	7
Bran (Arrowhead)	⅓ cup (1.4 oz)	150	0	2

FOOD	PORTION	CALS.	SAT. FAT	FAT
Bran With Dates as prep (Jiffy)	1	170	3	6
Cinnamon Streusel (Betty Crocker)	1	200	2	9
Corn as prep (Jiffy)	1	180	2	4
Corn Muffin (Dromedary)	1	120	—	4
Corn Muffin (Flako)	1	120	—	4
Honey Date as prep (Jiffy)	1	170	2	5
Oat Bran (Betty Crocker)	1	190	2	8
Oat Bran Apple Cinnamon (Hain)	1	140	—	3
Oat Bran Banana Nut (Hain)	1	140	—	4
Oat Bran Raspberry Spice (Hain)	1	140	—	3
Oat Bran No Cholesterol Recipe (Betty Crocker)	1	180	2	7
Oat Bran Wheat Free (Arrowhead)	⅓ cup (1.5 oz)	160	2	4
Oatmeal as prep (Jiffy)	1	180	2	7
Twice The Blueberries (Betty Crocker)	1	120	1	4
Twice The Blueberries No Cholesterol Recipe (Betty Crocker)	1	110	1	3
Wild Blueberry (Betty Crocker)	1	120	1	4
Wild Blueberry Light (Betty Crocker)	1	70	—	tr
Wild Blueberry Light No Cholesterol Recipe (Betty Crocker)	1	70	—	tr
Wild Blueberry No Cholesterol Recipe (Betty Crocker)	1	110	tr	3
blueberry	1 (1.75 oz)	149	1	4
corn	1 (1.75 oz)	160	1	5
wheat bran as prep	1 (1.75 oz)	138	1	5
READY-TO-EAT				
Apple Cinnamon (Weight Watchers)	1 (2.5 oz)	200	2	5
Apple Oat Bran (Dutch Mill)	1 (2 oz)	180	1	5
Banana Walnut (Dutch Mill)	1 (2 oz)	220	1	6

FOOD	PORTION	CALS.	SAT. FAT	FAT
Blueberry (Entenmann's)	1 (2 oz)	200	—	8
Bran'nola (Arnold)	1 (2.3 oz)	160	0	1
Carrot (Dutch Mill)	1 (2 oz)	190	2	7
Corn (Dutch Mill)	1 (2 oz)	190	3	6
Cranberry Orange (Dutch Mill)	1 (2 oz)	170	3	6
Lemon Poppy Seed (Weight Watchers)	1 (2.5 oz)	200	2	5
Mini Apple Cinnamon (Hostess)	5 (2 oz)	260	3	16
Mini Banana Nut (Hostess)	5 (2 oz)	260	2	16
Mini Blueberry (Hostess)	5 (2 oz)	240	2	13
Mini Chocolate Chip (Hostess)	5 (2 oz)	260	5	15
Muffin Loaf Blueberry (Hostess)	1 (3.8 oz)	440	3	19
Oat Bran (Hostess)	1 (1.5 oz)	160	1	8
Oat Bran Banana Nut (Hostess)	1 (1.5 oz)	150	1	6
Raisin (Arnold)	1 (2.3 oz)	160	0	1
Raisin Bran (Dutch Mill)	1 (2 oz)	230	3	5
blueberry	1 (2 oz)	158	1	4
corn	1 (2 oz)	174	1	5
oat bran wheat free	1 (2 oz)	154	1	4
toaster type blueberry	1	103	tr	3
toaster type corn	1	114	1	4
toaster type wheat bran w/ raisins	1 (36 g)	106	1	3

MULBERRIES

fresh	1 cup	61	—	1

MULLET

striped, cooked	3 oz	127	1	4
striped, raw	3 oz	99	1	3

MUNG BEANS

DRIED

cooked	1 cup	213	tr	1

SPROUTS

canned	½ cup	8	tr	tr
cooked	½ cup	13	tr	tr
raw	½ cup	16	tr	tr
stir-fried	½ cup	31	tr	tr

FOOD	PORTION	CALS.	SAT. FAT	FAT
MUNGO BEANS				
dried, cooked	1 cup	190	tr	1
MUSHROOMS				
CANNED				
Button (Empress)	2 oz	14	0	0
Button Sliced (Empress)	2 oz	14	0	0
Mushrooms (B In B)	¼ cup	12	0	0
Mushrooms (Seneca)	¼ cup	35	0	0
Mushrooms w/ Garlic (B In B)	¼ cup	12	0	0
Oriental Straw Mushrooms (Green Giant)	¼ cup	12	0	0
Pieces & Stems (Empress)	2 oz	14	0	0
Pieces & Stems (Green Giant)	¼ cup	12	0	0
Sliced (Green Giant)	¼ cup	12	0	0
Straw Mushrooms Broken (Empress)	2 oz	10	0	0
Whole (Green Giant)	¼ cup	12	0	0
chanterelle	3.5 oz	12	—	1
pieces	½ cup	19	tr	tr
whole	1 (.4 oz)	3	tr	tr
DRIED				
chanterelle	3.5 oz	89	—	2
shiitake	4 (½ oz)	44	tr	tr
FRESH				
chanterelle	3½ oz	11	—	tr
enoki, raw	1	2	tr	tr
morel	3.5 oz	9	—	tr
raw	1 (½ oz)	5	tr	tr
raw, sliced	½ cup	9	tr	tr
shitake, cooked	4 (2.5 oz)	40	tr	tr
sliced, cooked	½ cup	21	tr	tr
whole, cooked	1 (.4 oz)	3	tr	tr
FROZEN				
Breaded (Empire)	7 (2.8 oz)	90	0	1
Fresh Like	3.5 oz	28	—	tr
MUSKRAT				
roasted	3 oz	199	—	10
MUSSELS				
FRESH				
blue, cooked	3 oz	147	1	4

FOOD	PORTION	CALS.	SAT. FAT	FAT
blue, raw	1 cup	129	1	3
blue, raw	3 oz	73	tr	2

MUSTARD

FOOD	PORTION	CALS.	SAT. FAT	FAT
Blanchard & Blandchard	1 tsp (5 g)	0	0	0
Estee Sodium Free	1 pkg (0.5 oz)	5	—	1
Grey Poupon Country Dijon	1 tsp	6	0	0
Grey Poupon Dijon	1 tsp	6	0	0
Grey Poupon Parisian	1 tsp	6	0	0
Gulden's Diablo	1 tsp	8	0	0
Gulden's Mild	1 tsp	6	0	0
Gulden's Spicy Brown	1 tsp	8	0	0
Hain Stone Ground	1 tbsp	14	—	1
Hain Stone Ground No Salt Added	1 tbsp	14	—	1
Heinz Mild Yellow	1 tbsp	8	0	tr
Heinz Spicy Brown	1 tbsp	14	—	1
Kosciuszko Spicy Brown (Plochman's)	1 tsp	11	—	1
Kraft Horseradish	1 tbsp	14	0	1
Kraft Pure Prepared	1 tbsp	4	0	1
McIlhenny Coarse Ground	1 tsp (0.2 oz)	4	tr	tr
McIlhenny Spicy	1 tsp (0.2 oz)	6	tr	tr
Plochman's Dijon	1 tsp (5 g)	7	—	1
Plochman's Spoonable Salad	1 tsp (5 g)	4	—	tr
Plochman Squeeze Salad	1 tsp (5 g)	4	—	tr
Plochman's Stone Ground	1 tsp (5 g)	6	—	tr
Russer Deli	1 tsp (5 g)	4	0	0
dry mustard seed yellow	1 tsp	15	tr	1
yellow, ready-to-use	1 tsp	5	tr	tr

MUSTARD GREENS
CANNED

FOOD	PORTION	CALS.	SAT. FAT	FAT
Allen	½ cup (4.1 oz)	25	0	1
Allen	½ cup (4.1 oz)	30	0	1
Sunshine	½ cup (4.1 oz)	25	0	1
Sunshine	½ cup (4.1 oz)	30	0	1
FRESH				
chopped, cooked	½ cup	11	tr	tr
raw, chopped	½ cup	7	tr	tr
FROZEN				
chopped, cooked	½ cup	14	tr	tr

FOOD	PORTION	CALS.	SAT. FAT	FAT
NATTO				
natto	½ cup	187	1	10
NAVY BEANS				
CANNED				
Allen	½ cup (4.5 oz)	110	0	1
Hanover	½ cup	100	—	0
Luck's Seasoned w/ Pork	7.5 oz	230	—	7
Trappey With Bacon And Jalapeno	½ cup (4.5 oz)	110	1	2
Trappey With Bacon	½ cup (4.5 oz)	110	1	2
navy	1 cup	296	tr	1
DRIED				
cooked	1 cup	259	1	tr
SPROUTS				
cooked	3.5 oz	78	—	1
raw	½ cup	35	—	tr
NECTARINE				
Dole	1	70	—	1
fresh	1	67	—	1
NEUFCHATEL CHEESE				
(see CREAM CHEESE)				
NON-DAIRY CREAMERS				
(see COFFEE WHITENERS)				
NON-DAIRY WHIPPED TOPPINGS				
(see WHIPPED TOPPINGS)				
NOODLES				
(see also PASTA DINNERS)				
CANNED				
Van Camp's Noodle Weenee	1 can (8 oz)	230	2	8
DRY				
Chinese (Azumaya)	4 oz	293	—	1
Chow Mein Narrow (La Choy)	½ cup	150	1	8
Chow Mein Wide (La Choy)	½ cup	150	1	8
Egg (Creamette)	2 oz	221	—	3
Egg (Golden Grain)	2 oz	210	1	2
Egg (Mueller's)	2 oz (57 g)	220	—	3
Egg (San Giorgio)	2 oz	210	—	3

FOOD	PORTION	CALS.	SAT. FAT	FAT
Egg Fine uncooked (Noodles By Leonardo)	1 cup (2 oz)	210	1	2
Egg Medium uncooked (Noodles By Leonardo)	1 cup (2 oz)	210	1	2
Egg Wide uncooked (Noodles By Leonardo)	1 cup (2 oz)	210	1	2
Egg, not prep (Creamette)	2 oz	220	—	3
Japanese (Azumaya)	4 oz	289	—	1
No Yolks (Shofar)	2 oz	210	0	0
Noodle Trio (Mueller's)	2 oz (57g)	220	—	2
Rice (La Choy)	½ cup	130	—	5
Veggie Egg, uncooked (Hodgson Mill)	2 oz	200	1	2
Whole Wheat Spinach Egg, uncooked (Hodgson Mill)	2 oz	190	1	2
Whole Wheat Egg, uncooked (Hodgson Mill)	2 oz	190	1	2
cellophane	1 cup	492	tr	tr
chow mein	1 cup	237	2	14
egg	1 cup (38g)	145	tr	2
egg, cooked	1 cup	212	tr	2
japanese soba	2 oz	192	tr	2
japanese soba, cooked	½ cup	56	tr	tr
japanese somen	2 oz	203	tr	tr
japanese somen, cooked	½ cup	115	tr	tr
spinach/egg	1 cup	145	tr	2
spinach/egg, cooked	1 cup	211	3	3
DRY MIX				
Kraft Egg Noodle w/ Chicken Dinner, as prep	¾ cup	240	2	9
La Choy Ramen Noodles Beef, as prep	1 cup	200	1	8
La Choy Ramen Noodles Chicken, as prep	1 cup	200	1	7
Lipton Noodles & Sauce				
Alfredo, as prep	½ cup	131	—	3
Beef, as prep	½ cup	120	—	2
Butter, as prep	½ cup	142	—	4
Butter & Herb, as prep	½ cup	136	—	3
Carbonara Alfredo	½ cup	126	—	3
Cheese, as prep	½ cup	136	—	2
Chicken, as prep	½ cup	125	—	2
Chicken Broccoli	½ cup	124	—	2

FOOD	PORTION	CALS.	SAT. FAT	FAT
Lipton Noodles & Sauce *(cont.)*				
Creamy Chicken	½ cup	125	—	2
Parmesan, as prep	½ cup	138	—	4
Romanoff	½ cup	136	—	3
Sour Cream & Chive, as prep	½ cup	142	—	3
Stroganoff, as prep	½ cup	110	—	2
Tomato Alfredo	½ cup	126	—	3
Minute Microwave Chicken Flavored	½ cup	157	2	5
Minute Microwave Parmesan	½ cup	178	3	6
Noodle Roni				
Chicken & Mushroom, as prep	½ cup	160	—	4
Fettuccini, as prep	½ cup	300	—	18
Herb & Butter, as prep	½ cup	160	—	7
Parmesano, as prep	½ cup	240	—	13
Romanoff, as prep	½ cup	240	—	11
Stroganoff, as prep	½ cup	350	—	17
Noodles By Leonardo Macaroni & Cheese, as prep	1 cup (2.5 oz)	250	0	1
Ultra Slim-Fast				
Noodles & Alfredo Sauce	2.3 oz	240	—	4
Noodles & Beef	2.3 oz	230	—	3
Noodles & Cheese	2.3 oz	230	—	4
Noodles & Chicken Sauce	2.3 oz	220	—	3
Noodles & Tomato Herb Sauce	2.3 oz	220	—	3
TAKE-OUT				
noodle pudding	½ cup	132	4	7

NUTMEG
ground	1 tsp	12	1	1

NUTRITIONAL SUPPLEMENTS
(*see also* BREAKFAST BAR, BREAKFAST DRINKS)

FOOD	PORTION	CALS.	SAT. FAT	FAT
DIET				
Dynatrim Dutch Chocolate, as prep w/ 1% milk	8 oz	220	—	4
Dynatrim Strawberry Royale, as prep w/ 1% milk	8 oz	220	—	4

FOOD	PORTION	CALS.	SAT. FAT	FAT
Dynatrim Vanilla, as prep w/ 1% milk	8 oz	220	—	4
Figurines Chocolate	1 bar	100	—	5
Figurines Chocolate Caramel	1 bar	100	—	6
Figurines Chocolate Peanut Butter	1 bar	100	—	6
Figurines S'Mores	1 bar	100	—	5
Figurines Vanilla	1 bar	100	—	5
Nestle Sweet Success				
Bar Chewy Chocolate Brownie	1 (1.6 oz)	120	2	4
Bar Chewy Chocolate Chip	1 (1.6 oz)	120	2	4
Bar Chewy Chocolate Peanut Butter	1 (1.6 oz)	120	2	4
Bar Chewy Chocolate Raspberry	1 (1.6 oz)	120	2	4
Bar Chewy Oatmeal Raisin	1 (1.6 oz)	120	2	4
Chocolate Raspberry Truffle	1 can (10 fl oz)	200	1	3
Chocolate Raspberry, as prep w/ skim milk	9 fl oz	180	1	1
Chocolate Mocha Supreme	1 can (10 fl oz)	200	1	3
Chocolate Mocha Supreme, as prep/ skim milk	9 fl oz	180	1	tr
Classic Chocolate Chip, as prep/skim milk	9 fl oz	180	2	1
Creamy Milk Chocolate	1 can (10 fl oz)	200	1	3
Creamy Milk Chocolate	1 carton (12 fl oz)	220	1	2
Creamy Milk Chocolate, as prep w/ skim milk	9 fl oz	180	1	1
Creamy Vanilla Delight, as prep w/ skim milk	9 fl oz	180	1	tr
Dark Chocolate Fudge	1 can (10 fl oz)	200	1	3
Dark Chocolate Fudge	1 carton (12 fl oz)	220	1	2
Dark Chocolate Fudge, as prep w/ skim milk	9 fl oz	180	1	1
Rich Chocolate Almond	1 can (10 fl oz)	200	1	3
Rich Chocolate Almond	1 carton (12 fl oz)	220	1	2
Rich Chocolate Almond, as prep w/ skim milk	9 fl oz	180	1	tr

FOOD	PORTION	CALS.	SAT. FAT	FAT
Nestle Sweet Success *(cont.)*				
Smooth Vanilla Creme	1 can (10 fl oz)	200	1	3
Sego Lite				
Chocolate	10 fl oz	150	—	3
Dutch Chocolate	10 fl oz	150	—	3
French Vanilla	10 fl oz	150	—	4
Strawberry	10 fl oz	150	—	4
Vanilla	10 fl oz	150	—	4
Sego Very				
Chocolate	10 fl oz	225	—	1
Chocolate Malt	10 fl oz	225	—	1
Strawberry	10 fl oz	225	—	5
Vanilla	10 fl oz	225	—	5
Slim-Fast Nutrition Bar Dutch Chocolate	1	130	—	4
Slim-Fast Nutrition Bar Peanut Butter	1	140	—	6
Slim-Fast Powder Chocolate, as prep w/ skim milk	8 oz	190	—	1
Slim-Fast Powder Chocolate Malt, as prep w/ skim milk	8 oz	190	—	tr
Slim-Fast Powder Strawberry, as prep w/ skim milk	8 oz	190	—	1
Slim-Fast Powder Vanilla, as prep w/ skim milk	8 oz	190	—	1
Ultra Slim-Fast Cafe Mocha, as prep w/ skim milk	8 oz	200	—	tr
Ultra Slim-Fast Chocolate Royale, as prep w/ skim milk	8 oz	200	—	1
Ultra Slim-Fast Crunch Bar Cocoa Almond	1	110	—	3
Ultra Slim-Fast Crunch Bar Cocoa Raspberry	1	100	—	3
Ultra Slim-Fast Crunch Bar Vanilla Almond	1	110	—	4
Ultra Slim-Fast Dutch Chocolate, as prep w/ water	8 oz	220	—	tr

FOOD	PORTION	CALS.	SAT. FAT	FAT
Ultra Slim-Fast French Vanilla, as prep w/ skim milk	8 oz	190	—	tr
Ultra Slim-Fast French Vanilla, as prep w/ water	8 oz	220	—	tr
Ultra Slim-Fast Fruit Juice Mix, as prep w/ fruit juice	8 oz	200	—	tr
Ultra Slim-Fast Pina Colada, as prep w/ skim milk	8 oz	180	—	tr
Ultra Slim-Fast Ready-to-Drink Chocolate Royale	11 oz	230	tr	1
Ultra Slim-Fat Ready-to-Drink Chocolate Royale	12 oz	250	—	1
Ultra Slim-Fast Ready-to-Drink French Vanilla	12 oz	220	tr	1
Ultra Slim-Fast Ready-to-Drink Strawberry Supreme	12 oz	220	—	1
Ultra Slim-Fast Strawberry Supreme, as prep w/ water	8 oz	220	—	tr
Ultra Slim-Fast Strawberry, as prep w/ skim milk	8 oz	190	—	1
REGULAR				
EggPro	4 oz	220	—	4
Fi-Bar Apple	1 (1 oz)	90	—	3
Fi-Bar Cocoa Almond	1	130	—	4
Fi-Bar Cocoa Peanut	1	130	—	4
Fi-Bar Cranberry & Wild Berries	1 (1 oz)	100	—	3
Fi-Bar Lemon	1 (1 oz)	90	—	3
Fi-Bar Mandarin Orange	1 (1 oz)	99	—	4
Fi-Bar Raspberry	1 (1 oz)	100	—	3
Fi-Bar Strawberry	1 (1 oz)	100	—	3
Fi-Bar Treat Yourself Right Almond	1	152	—	6
Fi-Bar Treat Yourself Right Peanutty Butter	1	152	—	5
Fi-Bar Vanilla Almond	1	130	—	4
Fi-Bar Vanilla Peanut	1	130	—	4

FOOD	PORTION	CALS.	SAT. FAT	FAT
Fi-Bar Nuggets Almond Cappuccino Crunch	1 pkg	136	—	6
Fi-Bar Nuggets Almond Butter Crunch	1 pkg	163	—	11
Fi-Bar Nuggets Coconut Almond Crunch	1 pkg	136	—	6
Fi-Bar Nuggets Peanut Butter Crunch	1 pkg	160	—	10
Gookinaid Lemonade	1 cup (8 fl oz)	45	—	0
Malsovit Mealwafers	2	152	—	8
Meal on the Go Apple	1 bar (3 oz)	294	2	5
Meal on the Go Banana w/ Pecans	1 bar (3 oz)	289	—	10
Meal on the Go Original	1 bar (3 oz)	286	—	9
Nutra/Balance Frozen Pudding Butterscotch	4 oz	225	—	8
Nutra/Balance Frozen Pudding Chocolate	4 oz	225	—	8
Nutra/Balance Frozen Pudding Tapioca	4 oz	225	—	8
Nutra/Balance Frozen Pudding Vanilla	4 oz	225	—	8
NutraShake Chocolate	4 oz	200	—	6
NutraShake Strawberry	4 oz	200	—	6
NutraShake Vanilla	4 oz	200	—	6
NutraShake w/ Fibre Strawberry	6 oz	300	—	2
NutraShake w/ Fibre Vanilla	6 oz	300	—	2
Vita-J Apple Juice	11.5 fl oz	8	0	0
Vita-J Fruit Punch	11.5 fl oz	8	0	0
Vita-J Grapefruit Cocktail w/ Raspberry	11.5 fl oz	8	0	0
Vita-J Orange Juice	11.5 fl oz	8	0	0

NUTS, MIXED
(see also INDIVIDUAL NAMES)

FOOD	PORTION	CALS.	SAT. FAT	FAT
Cashews & Peanuts, Honey Roasted (Eagle)	1 oz	170	—	8
Cashews & Peanuts Honey Roasted (Planters)	1 oz	170	2	12
Mixed (Eagle)	1 oz	180	—	16
Mixed Deluxe (Eagle)	1 oz	180	—	17
Mixed Lightly Salted (Planters)	1 oz	170	2	15

FOOD	PORTION	CALS.	SAT. FAT	FAT
Mixed Nuts Deluxe Lightly Salted (Fisher)	1 oz	180	3	16
Mixed Nuts Deluxe Salted (Fisher)	1 oz	180	3	16
Mixed Nuts Oil Roasted 25% More Cashews Lightly Salted (Fisher)	1 oz	180	3	16
Mixed Nuts Oil Roasted 25% More Cashews Salted (Fisher)	1 oz	180	3	16
Mixed With Peanuts (Guy's)	1 oz	180	—	16
Nut & Fruit Pina Colada (Fisher)	1 oz	150	2	10
Nut & Fruit Raisin Cranberry (Fisher)	1 oz	150	2	10
Nut & Fruit Tropical Fruit (Fisher)	1 oz	140	1	8
Nut Toppings Oil Roasted With Peanuts (Fisher)	1 oz	190	3	17
Peanuts & Cashews Honey Roasted (Planters)	1 oz	170	2	12
Peanuts Cashews (Fisher)	1 oz	170	2	13
Tasty Mix (Guy's)	1 oz	130	—	7
dry roasted w/ peanuts	1 oz	169	2	15
dry roasted w/ peanuts, salted	1 oz	169	2	15
oil roasted w/ peanuts	1 oz	175	2	16
oil roasted w/ peanuts, salted	1 oz	175	2	16
oil roasted w/o peanuts	1 oz	175	2	16
oil roasted w/o peanuts, salted	1 oz	175	2	16
OCTOBER BEANS				
CANNED				
Seasoned w/ Pork (Luck's)	7.25 oz	230	—	6
OCTOPUS				
fresh, steamed	3 oz	140	tr	2
OHELOBERRIES				
fresh	1 cup	39	—	tr

FOOD	PORTION	CALS.	SAT. FAT	FAT
OIL				
(see also FAT)				
All Blend (Hain)	1 tbsp	120	2	14
Almond (Hain)	1 tbsp	120	1	14
Apricot Kernel (Hain)	1 tbsp	120	1	14
Avocado (Hain)	1 tbsp	120	1	14
Bertolli Classico	1 tbsp	120	—	14
Bertolli Extra Light	1 tbsp	120	—	14
Bertolli Extra Virgin	1 tbsp	120	—	14
Canola Hain	1 tbsp	120	1	14
Canola Hollywood	1 tbsp	120	1	14
Canola Smart Beat	1 tbsp (14 g)	120	1	14
Canola (Wesson)	1 tbsp	120	1	14
Canola Organic (Hain)	1 tbsp	120	1	14
Coconut (Hain)	1 tbsp	120	12	14
Cooking Spray Lite (Wesson)	0.5 sec spray	0	—	0
Corn (Hain)	1 tbsp	120	2	14
Corn (Wesson)	1 tbsp	120	2	14
Crisco	1 tbsp (0.5 fl oz)	120	2	14
Crisco Corn Canola	1 tbsp (0.5 fl oz)	120	2	14
Crisco Puritan Canola (Procter & Gamble)	1 tbsp (0.5 fl oz)	120	1	14
Flax Seed (Arrowhead)	1 tbsp (0.5 fl oz)	120	1	14
Garlic & Oil (Hain)	1 tbsp	120	3	14
Hazelnut (Arrowhead)	1 tbsp (0.5 fl oz)	120	1	14
Hot chili Sesame (House Of Tsang)	1 tsp (5 g)	45	1	5
Italica	1 tbsp	120	2	9
Mazola	1 tbsp	120	2	14
Mazola	1 cup	1955	29	221
Mazola No Stick	2.5 second spray (0.2 g)	2	tr	tr
Mongolian Fire (House Of Tsang)	1 tsp (5 g)	45	1	5
Olive (Hain)	1 tbsp	120	2	14
Olive (Progresso)	1 tbsp	119	2	14
Olive (Wesson)	1 tbsp	120	2	14
Olive Extra Light (Progresso)	1 tbsp	119	2	14
Olive Extra Virgin (Progresso)	1 tbsp	119	2	14
Orville Redenbacher's	1 tbsp	120	2	14
Pam	1 sec spray (0.266 g)	2	—	t

FOOD	PORTION	CALS.	SAT. FAT	FAT
Pam Butter	1 sec spray (0.266 g)	2	—	tr
Pam Olive Oil	1 sec spray (0.266 g)	2	—	tr
Pam Pump	1 spray (0.43 g)	4	—	tr
Peanut (Hain)	1 tbsp	120	2	14
Peanut (Hollywood)	1 tbsp	120	4	14
Peanut (Planters)	1 tbsp	120	2	14
Pompian	1 tbsp	130	—	14
Popcorn (Planters)	1 tbsp	120	2	13
Pure Sesame (House of Tsang)	1 tsp (5 g)	45	1	5
Rice Bran (Hain)	1 tbsp	120	3	14
Safflower (Hain)	1 tbsp	120	1	14
Safflower (Hollywood)	1 tbsp	120	1	14
Safflower Hi-Oleic (Hain)	1 tbsp	120	1	14
Safflower Organic (Hain)	1 tbsp	120	1	14
Sesame (Hain)	1 tbsp	120	2	14
Singapore Curry (House Of Tsang)	1 tsp (5 g)	45	1	5
Smart Beat	1 tbsp	120	1	14
Soy (Hain)	1 tbsp	120	2	14
Soy (Hollywood)	1 tbsp	120	3	14
Sunflower (Hain)	1 tbsp	120	2	14
Sunflower (Hollywood)	1 tbsp	120	2	14
Sunflower (Wesson)	1 tbsp	120	2	14
Sunflower Organic (Hain)	1 tbsp	120	2	14
Vegetable (Wesson)	1 tbsp	120	2	14
Walnut (Hain)	1 tbsp	120	2	14
Weight Watchers Butter Spray	1-second spray	2	0	tr
Weight Watchers Cooking Spray	1-second spray	2	0	tr
Wok Oil (House of Tsang)	1 tbsp (0.5 oz)	130	3	14
almond	1 tbsp	120	1	14
almond	1 cup	1927	1	218
apricot kernel	1 tbsp	120	1	14
apricot kernel	1 cup	1927	14	218
avocado	1 tbsp	124	2	14
avocado	1 cup	1927	25	218
babassu (palm)	1 tbsp	120	11	14
canola	1 tbsp	124	2	14
canola	1 cup	1927	15	218
coconut	1 tbsp	117	12	14
corn	1 tbsp	120	2	14

FOOD	PORTION	CALS.	SAT. FAT	FAT
corn	1 cup	1927	28	218
cottonseed	1 tbsp	120	4	14
cottonseed	1 cup	1927	56	218
cupu assu	1 tbsp	120	7	14
grapeseed	1 tbsp	120	1	14
hazelnut	1 tbsp	120	1	14
hazelnut	1 cup	1927	1	218
mustard	1 tbsp	124	2	14
mustard	1 cup	1927	25	218
oat	1 tbsp	120	3	14
olive	1 tbsp	119	2	14
olive	1 cup	1909	26	216
palm	1 tbsp	120	7	14
palm	1 cup	1927	107	218
palm kernel	1 tbsp	117	11	14
palm kernel	1 cup	1879	178	218
peanut	1 tbsp	119	2	14
peanut	1 cup	1909	36	216
poppyseed	1 tbsp	120	2	14
pumkinseed	3.5 oz	925	—	100
rice bran	1 tbsp	120	3	14
safflower	1 tbsp	120	1	14
safflower	1 cup	1927	20	218
sesame	1 tbsp	120	2	14
sheanut	1 tbsp	120	6	14
soybean	1 tbsp	120	2	14
soybean	1 cup	1927	31	218
sunflower	1 tbsp	120	1	14
sunflower	1 cup	1927	23	218
teaseed	1 tbsp	120	3	14
tomatoseed	1 tbsp	120	3	14
vegetable soybean & cottonseed	1 tbsp	120	2	14
vegetable soybean & cottonseed	1 cup	1927	2	218
walnut	1 tbsp	120	1	14
walnut	1 cup	1927	20	218
wheat germ	1 tbsp	120	3	14
FISH OIL				
Cod Liver (Hain)	1 tbsp	120	—	14
Cod Liver Cherry (Hain)	1 tbsp	120	—	14
Cod Liver Mint (Hain)	1 tbsp	120	—	14
cod liver	1 tbsp	123	3	14
herring	1 tbsp	123	3	14

FOOD	PORTION	CALS.	SAT. FAT	FAT
menhaden	1 tbsp	123	4	14
salmon	1 tbsp	123	3	14
sardine	1 tbsp	123	4	14
shark	3.5 oz	945	—	100
whale	3.5 oz	945	—	100

OKRA
CANNED
Cocktail Hot (Trappey)	2 pieces (1 oz)	8	tr	tr
Cocktail Mild (Trappey)	1 pieces (1 oz)	9	tr	tr
Creole Cumbo (Trappey)	½ cup (4.2 oz)	35	0	0
Cut (Allen)	½ cup (4.4 oz)	25	0	0
Cut (Trappey)	½ cup (4.4 oz)	25	0	0
Pickled (McIlhenny)	2 pieces (1 oz)	7	tr	tr

FRESH
raw	8 pods	36	tr	tr
raw, sliced	½ cup	19	tr	tr
sliced, cooked	8 pods	27	tr	tr
sliced, cooked	½ cup	25	tr	tr

FROZEN
Cut (Fresh Like)	3.5 oz	26	—	tr
Cut (Hanover)	½ cup	25	—	0
Whole (Fresh Like)	3.5 oz	32	—	tr
Whole (Hanover)	½ cup	35	—	0
sliced, cooked	½ cup	34	tr	tr
sliced, cooked	1 pkg (10 oz)	94	tr	1

OLIVES
California Ripe	2 jumbo	188	—	9
California Ripe	3 sm	4	0	tr
Olive Appetizer (Progresso)	½ cup	180	3	21
Olive Condite (Progresso)	½ cup	130	2	14
Ripe Extra Large (S&W)	3.5 oz	163	—	18
Ripe Pitted Large (S&W)	3.5 oz	163	—	18
Salad Olives (Progresso)	½ cup	120	2	15
Spanish Green (Tee Pee)	2 oz	98	—	10
green	3 extra lg	15	tr	2
green	4 med	15	tr	2
ripe	1 sm	4	tr	tr
ripe	1 lg	5	tr	tr
ripe	1 jumbo	7	tr	1
ripe	1 colossal	12	tr	1

FOOD	PORTION	CALS.	SAT. FAT	FAT
ONION				
CANNED				
Lightly Spiced Cocktail Onions (Vlasic)	1 oz	4	0	0
Whole Small (S&W)	½ cup	35	0	0
chopped	½ cup	21	tr	tr
whole	1 (2.2 oz)	12	tr	tr
DRIED				
flakes	1 tbsp	16	tr	tr
powder	1 tsp	7	—	tr
FRESH				
Antioch Farms Vidalia	1 med	60	—	0
Dole	1 med	60	—	0
Dole Green, chopped	1 tbsp	2	—	tr
chopped, cooked	½ cup	47	tr	tr
raw, chopped	1 tbsp	4	tr	tr
raw, chopped	½ cup	30	tr	tr
scallions, raw, chopped	1 tbsp	2	tr	tr
scallions, raw, sliced	½ cup	16	tr	tr
welsh, raw	3.5 oz	34	tr	tr
FROZEN				
Chopped (Ore Ida)	¾ cup (3 oz)	25	0	0
Chopped (Southland)	2 oz	15	—	0
Crispy Onion Rings (Mrs. Paul's)	2.5 oz	190	—	12
Diced (Fresh Like)	3.5 oz	29	—	0
Onion Ringers (Ore Ida)	6 pieces (3 oz)	240	3	14
Polybag Whole Small (Birds Eye)	½ cup	30	0	0
Small With Cream Sauce (Birds Eye)	½ cup	100	1	3
Whole (Fresh Like)	3.5 oz	37	—	tr
chopped, cooked	1 tbsp	4	tr	tr
chopped, cooked	½ cup	30	tr	tr
rings	7 (2.5 oz)	285	6	19
rings, cooked	2 (0.7 oz)	81	2	5
whole, cooked	3.5 oz	28	0	tr
TAKE-OUT				
fried	½ cup (7.5 oz)	176	6	11
rings, breaded & fried	8–9	275	7	16
OPOSSUM				
roasted	3 oz	188	—	9

FOOD	PORTION	CALS.	SAT. FAT	FAT

ORANGE
CANNED

FOOD	PORTION	CALS.	SAT. FAT	FAT
Mandarin Natural Style (S&W)	½ cup	60	0	0
Mandarin Oranges (Empress)	5.5 oz	100	0	0
Mandarin Oranges from Japan (Empress)	5.5 oz	35	0	0
Mandarin Segments (Dole)	½ cup	70	—	tr
Mandarin Selected Sections in Heavy Syrup (S&W)	½ cup	76	0	0
Mandarin Unsweetened (S&W)	½ cup	28	0	0
Pineapple Mandarin Orange Segments (Dole)	½ cup	60	—	tr

FRESH

FOOD	PORTION	CALS.	SAT. FAT	FAT
Dole	1	50	—	0
california valencia	1	59	tr	tr
california navel	1	65	tr	tr
florida	1	69	tr	tr
peel	1 tbsp	6	tr	tr
sections	1 cup	85	tr	tr

JUICE

FOOD	PORTION	CALS.	SAT. FAT	FAT
BAMA	8.45 oz	120	0	0
Bright & Early Chilled	8 fl oz	120	0	0
Bright & Early Frozen	8 fl oz	120	0	0
Hawaiian Punch	6 oz	100	—	0
Hi-C	1 can (11.5 fl oz)	180	0	0
Hi-C	8 fl oz	130	0	0
Hi-C Box	8.45 fl oz	130	0	0
Juice Works	6 oz	90	—	0
Kool-Aid Orange	8 oz	98	0	0
Kool-Aid Sugar Sweetened Orange	8 oz	79	0	0
Kool-Aid Koolers	1 (8.45 fl oz)	115	0	0
Libby	6 fl oz	80	0	0
Minute Maid				
Box	8.45 fl oz	120	0	0
Calcium Rich Chilled	8 fl oz	120	0	0
Calcium Rich Frozen	8 fl oz	120	0	0
Chilled	8 fl oz	110	0	0
Country Style Chilled	8 fl oz	110	0	0
Country Style Frozen	8 fl oz	110	0	0

FOOD	PORTION	CALS.	SAT. FAT	FAT
Minute Maid *(cont.)*				
Juices To Go	1 bottle (10 fl oz)	140	0	0
Juices To Go	1 bottle (16 fl oz)	110	0	0
Juices to Go	1 can (11.5 fl oz)	160	0	0
Orange Punch Box	8.45 fl oz	130	0	0
Premium Choice Chilled	8 fl oz	110	0	0
Pulp Free Chilled	8 fl oz	110	0	0
Pulp Free Frozen	8 fl oz	110	0	0
Reduced Acid Frozen	8 fl oz	110	0	0
Mott's From Concentrate	10 fl oz	130	0	1
Ocean Spray	8 fl oz	120	0	0
Odwalla	8 fl oz	110	—	1
S&W 100% Unsweetened	½ cup	83	0	0
S&W 100% Unsweetened	6 oz	83	0	0
Sippin' Pak 100% Pure	8.45 fl oz	110	0	0
Sipps Orange	8.45 oz	130	—	0
Tang Tropical Orange	8.45 fl oz	146	0	0
Tang Breakfast Crystals Sugar Free, as prep	6 oz	5	0	0
Tang Breakfast Crystals, as prep	6 oz	86	0	0
Tang Fruit Box	8.45 oz	127	0	0
Tree Top	6 oz	90	0	0
Tropicana	1 container (10 fl oz)	130	0	0
Tropicana	1 container (6 fl oz)	80	0	0
Tropicana	1 container (8 fl oz)	110	0	0
Tropicana	8 fl oz	110	0	0
Tropicana				
Season's Best	1 bottle (10 fl oz)	130	0	0
Season's Best	1 bottle (7 fl oz)	90	0	0
Season's Best	1 can (11.5 fl oz)	140	0	0
Season's Best	8 fl oz	110	0	0
Season's Best Calcium	8 fl oz	110	0	0
Season's Best Homestyle	8 fl oz	110	0	0
Season's Best Vitamin	8 fl oz	110	0	0
frzn, as prep	6 fl oz	110	0	0
Veryfine 100%	8 oz	121	0	0
Veryfine Orange Drink	8 oz	140	0	0
canned	1 cup	104	tr	tr
chilled	1 cup	110	tr	1
fresh	1 cup	111	tr	tr

FOOD	PORTION	CALS.	SAT. FAT	FAT
frzn, as prep	1 cup	112	tr	tr
frzn, not prep	6 oz	339	tr	tr
mandarin orange	3.5 oz	47	—	tr
orange drink	6 oz	94	0	0

ORANGE EXTRACT
Virginia Dare	1 tsp	22	—	0

OREGANO
ground	1 tsp	5	tr	tr

ORGAN MEATS
(see BRAINS, GIBLETS, GIZZARD, HEART, KIDNEY, LIVER, SWEETBREADS)

ORIENTAL FOOD
(see also DINNER, NOODLES, RICE)

FOOD	PORTION	CALS.	SAT. FAT	FAT
CANNED				
Chun King Divider Pak				
Beef Chow Mein	8 oz	110	—	2
Beef Chow Mein	7 oz	100	—	2
Beef Pepper Oriental	7 oz	110	—	4
Chicken Chow Mein	7 oz	110	—	4
Chicken Chow Mein	8 oz	120	—	4
Pork Chow Mein Mein	7 oz	120	—	4
Shrimp Chow Mein	7 oz	100	—	2
Chun King Stir-Fry Entree				
Chow Mein w/ Beef	6 oz	290	—	19
Chow Mein w/ Chicken	6 oz	220	—	11
Egg Foo Yung	5 oz	140	—	8
Pepper Steak	6 oz	250	—	17
Sukiyaki	6 oz	290	—	19
La Choy Bi-Pack				
Beef Pepper	¾ cup	80	—	2
Chow Mein Chicken	¾ cup	80	1	3
Chow Mein Pork	¾ cup	80	tr	4
Chow Mein Shrimp	¾ cup	70	tr	1
Sweet & Sour Chicken	¾ cup	120	tr	2
Teriyaki Chicken	¾ cup	85	1	2
La Choy Dinner Chow Mein Chicken	¾ pkg	300	8	17
La Choy Entree				
Beef Pepper Oriental	¾ cup	100	2	4
Chow Mein Beef	¾ cup	40	1	2
Chow Mein Chicken	¾ cup	70	1	4
Chow Mein Meatless	¾ cup	25	tr	tr
Chow Mein Shrimp	¾ cup	35	tr	1

FOOD	PORTION	CALS.	SAT. FAT	FAT
La Choy Entree *(cont.)*				
Sweet & Sour Chicken	¾ cup	240	1	2
Sweet & Sour Pork	¾ cup	250	1	4
chow mein chicken	1 cup	95	tr	tr
FRESH				
Won Ton Wraps (Azumaya)	1 (8 g)	23	—	tr
egg roll wrapper	1	83	tr	tr
wonton wrappers	1	23	tr	tr
FROZEN				
Benihana Oriental Lites Chicken in Spicy Garlic Sauce	9 oz	270	—	4
Birds Eye Chicken Teriyaki Easy Recipe, not prep	½ pkg	160	1	4
Birds Eye Chinese Stir Fry Internationals not prep	3.3 oz	35	0	0
Birds Eye Oriental Beef Easy Recipe not prep	½ pkg	100	1	7
Chun King				
Beef Pepper Oriental	13 oz	319	—	3
Chicken Chow Mein	13 oz	370	—	6
Crunchy Walnut Chicken	13 oz	310	—	5
Egg Rolls, Chicken	1 (3.6 oz)	220	—	8
Egg Rolls, Meat & Shrimp	1 (3.6 oz)	220	—	8
Egg Rolls, Shrimp	1 (3.6 oz)	200	—	6
Fried Rice w/ Chicken	8 oz	260	—	4
Fried Rice w/ Pork	8 oz	270	—	6
Imperial Chicken	13 oz	300	—	1
Restaurant Style Egg Rolls, Pork	1 (3 oz)	180	—	6
Sweet & Sour Pork	13 oz	400	—	5
Dining Light Chicken Chow Mein	9 oz	180	—	2
Egg Rolls Large (Empire)	1 (3 oz)	190	1	6
Egg Rolls Miniature (Empire)	6 (4.8 oz)	280	2	8
Japanese Stir Fry International, not prep (Birds Eye)	3.3 oz	30	0	0
La Choy				
Almond Chicken Egg Roll Restaurant Style	1 (3 oz)	120	—	3
Chicken Snack Egg Roll	2	90	—	3

FOOD	PORTION	CALS.	SAT. FAT	FAT
Lobster Snack Egg Roll	1 (1.45 oz)	75	—	2
Meat & Shrimp Snack Egg Roll	(1.45 oz)	180	—	3
Pork Egg Roll Restaurant Style	1 (3 oz)	150	—	5
Shrimp Egg Roll Restaurant Style	1 (3 oz)	130	—	4
Shrimp Snack Egg Roll	1 (1.45 oz)	75	—	2
Sweet & Sour Chicken Egg Roll Restaurant Style	1 (3 oz)	150	—	4
Lean Cuisine Chicken Chow Mein w/ Rice	1 pkg (9 oz)	210	1	5
Stir Fry Kit With Yoshida Oriental Sauce (Tyson)	10.6 oz	330	—	10
Stouffer's Chicken Chow Mein With Rice	1 pkg (10.6 oz)	260	1	4
Stouffer's Chicken Oriental	1 pkg (9.75 oz)	320	2	9
Stouffer's Teriyaki Stir-Fry	1 pkg (9 oz)	260	1	5
Tyson Sweet & Sour Kit With Sweet & Sour Sauce	14.85 oz	440	—	9
Worthington Vegetarian Egg Rolls	1 (85 g)	160	—	6
HOME RECIPE				
chop suey w/ beef & pork	1 cup	300	4	17
chow mein chicken	1 cup	255	4	10
MIX				
Kikkoman Chow Mein Seasoning	1⅛ oz pkg	98	—	tr
Kikkoman Teriyaki Baste & Glaze	1 tbsp	24	—	tr
La Choy Dinner Classics Egg Foo Yung	2 patties + 3 oz sauce	170	2	7
La Choy Dinner Classics Pepper Steak	¾ cup	180	3	9
La Choy Dinner Classics Sweet & Sour	¾ cup	310	1	6
TAKE-OUT				
chicken teriyaki	¾ cup	399	6	27
chop suey w/ pork	1 cup	375	8	29
chow mein pork	1 cup	425	8	24
chow mein shrimp	1 cup	221	1	10
fried rice	6.6 oz	249	—	6

FOOD	PORTION	CALS.	SAT. FAT	FAT
fried rice w/ egg	6.7	395	—	20
wonton	1 cup	205	1	3
wonton, fried	½ cup (1 oz)	111	1	8

OYSTERS
CANNED

FOOD	PORTION	CALS.	SAT. FAT	FAT
Bumble Bee Whole	½ cup (3.5 oz)	100	1	4
Empress Whole	4 oz	100	—	4
S&W Fancy Whole	2 oz	95	—	3
eastern	1 cup	170	2	6
eastern	3 oz	58	1	2

FRESH

FOOD	PORTION	CALS.	SAT. FAT	FAT
eastern, raw	6 med	58	1	2
eastern, raw	1 cup	170	2	6
eastern, cooked	6 med	58	1	2
eastern, cooked	3 oz	117	1	4
pacific, raw	1 med	41	tr	1
pacific, raw	3 oz	69	tr	2
steamed	1 med	41	tr	1
steamed	3 oz	138	1	4

FROZEN

FOOD	PORTION	CALS.	SAT. FAT	FAT
Carnation Jumbo or Extra Select Breaded Oysters (King & Prince)	3.5 oz	130	—	2

TAKE-OUT

FOOD	PORTION	CALS.	SAT. FAT	FAT
battered & fried	6 (4.9 oz)	368	5	18
breaded & fried	4 (4.9 oz)	368	5	18
eastern, breaded & fried	6 med	173	3	11
eastern, breaded & fried	3 oz	167	3	11
oysters rockefeller	3	66	—	2
stew	1 cup	278	10	18

PANCAKE/WAFFLE SYRUP
(*see also* SYRUP)

FOOD	PORTION	CALS.	SAT. FAT	FAT
Alaga Breakfast	2 tbsp	108	—	0
Alaga Butter Lite	2 tbsp	54	—	0
Alaga Honey Flavor	2 tbsp	124	—	0
Alaga Lite	2 tbsp	54	—	0
Aunt Jemima	2 tbsp	110	0	0
Aunt Jemima Butter Lite	2 tbsp	50	0	0
Aunt Jemima Lite	2 tbsp	50	0	0
Brer Rabbit Dark	2 tbsp	120	0	0
Brer Rabbit Light	2 tbsp	120	0	0
Estee Lite Maple	¼ cup (2.4 oz)	8	0	0
Golden Griddle	1 tbsp (21 g)	50	0	0

FOOD	PORTION	CALS.	SAT. FAT	FAT
Golden Griddle	1 cup (321 g)	885	0	0
Karo	1 tbsp (21 g)	60	0	0
Log Cabin Country Kitchen	1 oz	103	0	0
Log Cabin Lite	1 oz	49	0	tr
Tastee	2 tbsp	121	—	0
Tastee Maple	2 tbsp	113	—	0
Weight Watchers	1 tbsp	25	0	0
Whitfield White Label	2 tbsp	121	—	0
Whitfield Yellow Label	2 tbsp	125	—	0
Whitfield Yellow Label Butter Flavor	2 tbsp	117	—	0
Whitfield Yellow Label Maple Flavor	2 tbsp	117	—	0
low calorie	1 tbsp	12	0	0
maple	2 tbsp	122	0	0

PANCAKES

FROZEN

FOOD	PORTION	CALS.	SAT. FAT	FAT
Blueberry (Aunt Jemima)	3.48 oz	220	1	4
Blueberry (Kid Cuisine)	3.47 oz	210	—	9
Blueberry Microwave (Pillsbury)	3	250	—	4
Buttermilk (Aunt Jemima)	3.48 oz	210	1	3
Buttermilk (Kid Cuisine)	4.17 oz	180	—	4
Buttermilk (Weight Watchers)	2 (2.5 oz)	140	—	3
Buttermilk Batter, as prep (Aunt Jemima)	3.6 oz	180	1	2
Buttermilk Microwave (Pillsbury)	3	260	—	4
Harvest Wheat Microwave (Pillsbury)	3	240	—	4
Lite Buttermilk (Aunt Jemima)	3.48 oz	140	—	3
Lite Pancakes & Lite Links (Quaker)	1 pkg (6 oz)	310	—	10
Lite Pancakes & Lite Syrup (Quaker)	1 pkg (6 oz)	260	—	3
Original (Aunt Jemima)	3.48 oz	211	—	4
Original Batter, as prep (Aunt Jemima)	3.6 oz	183	1	2
Original Microwave (Pillsbury)	3	240	—	4
Pancakes & Sausages (Downyflake)	1 pkg (5.5 oz)	430	—	23

FOOD	PORTION	CALS.	SAT. FAT	FAT
Pancakes & Sausages (Great Starts)	6 oz	460	—	22
Pancakes & Sausages (Quaker)	1 pkg (6 oz)	420	—	16
Pancakes/Links (Morningstar Farms)	1 pkg (4 oz)	240	8	—
Pancakes w/ Bacon (Great Starts)	4.5 oz	400	—	20
Pancakes w/ Lean Links (Healthy Starts)	6 oz	360	—	8
Pancakes w/ Links (Weight Watchers)	4 oz	220	—	10
Regular (Downyflake)	3	280	—	9
Rolled Pancakes w/ Apples (Kid Cuisine)	3.85 oz	210	—	7
Silver Dollar Pancakes & Sausage (Great Starts)	3.75 oz	310	—	4
Whole Wheat Pancakes & Lite Links (Great Starts)	5.5 oz	350	—	16
buttermilk	1 (4" diam) (1.3 oz)	83	tr	1
plain	1 (4" diam) (1.3 oz)	83	tr	1
HOME RECIPE				
blueberry	1 (4" diam)	84	4	1
plain	1 (4" diam)	86	1	4
MIX				
Apple Cinnamon Shake 'N Pour (Bisquick)	3 (4" diam)	240	—	3
Blueberry (Hungry Jack)	3 (4" diam)	320	—	15
Blueberry Shake 'N Pour Bisquick	3 (4" diam)	270	—	3
Buckwheat Hodgson Mill	½ cup (1.8 oz)	160	0	1
Buckwheat Pancake & Waffle Mix (Aunt Jemima)	3 (4" diam)	230	—	8
Buttermilk (Betty Crocker)	3 (4" diam)	240	—	11
Buttermilk (Hungry Jack)	3 (4" diam)	240	—	11
Buttermilk Complete (Hungry Jack)	3 (4" diam)	180	—	1
Buttermilk Complete Packets (Hungry Jack)	3 (4" diam)	180	—	3
Buttermilk Complete Pancake & Waffle Mix (Aunt Jemima)	3 (4" diam)	230	—	3

FOOD	PORTION	CALS.	SAT. FAT	FAT
Buttermilk Pancake & Waffle Mix (Aunt Jemima)	3 (4" diam)	220	—	8
Buttermilk Shake 'N Pour (Bisquick)	3 (4" diam)	250	3	—
Complete Pancake & Waffle Mix (Aunt Jemima)	3 (4" diam)	250	—	4
Extra Lights (Hungry Jack)	3 (4" diam)	210	—	7
Extra Lights Complete (Hungry Jack)	3 (4" diam)	190	—	2
Fast Shake Blueberry (Little Crow)	1 serving (2.5 oz)	251	—	3
Fast Shake Buttermilk (Little Crow)	1 serving (2.5 oz)	258	—	3
Fast Shake Original (Little Crow)	1 serving (2.5 oz)	266	—	4
Multigrain Pancake & Waffle Mix (Arrowhead)	¼ cup (1.2 oz)	120	0	1
Original Pancake & Waffle Mix (Aunt Jemima)	3 (4" diam)	200	—	7
Original Shake 'N Pour (Bisquick)	3 (4" diam)	250	—	3
Pancake Mix Fat Free, as prep (Estee)	4 (4" diam)	180	0	0
Pancake Mix, not prep (Health Valley)	1 oz	100	—	1
Panshakes (Hungry Jack)	3 (4" diam)	250	—	6
Whole Wheat Pancake & Waffle Mix (Aunt Jemima)	3 (4" diam)	270	—	9
buckwheat	1 (4" diam)	62	1	2
buttermilk	1 (4" diam) (1.3 oz)	74	tr	1
plain	1 (4" diam) (1.3 oz)	74	tr	1
sugar free low sodium	1 (3" diam)	44	tr	tr
whole wheat	1 (4" diam)	92	1	3
TAKE-OUT				
buckwheat	1 (4" diam)	55	1	2
potato	1 (4" diam)	78	1	6
w/ butter & syrup	3	519	6	14

PANCREAS
(see SWEETBREADS)

FOOD	PORTION	CALS.	SAT. FAT	FAT
PAPAYA				
FRESH				
Papaya	½ cup	80	—	0
(Produce Marketing Assoc)				
cubed	1 cup	54	tr	tr
papaya	1	117	tr	tr
JUICE				
Goya Nectar	6 oz	110	0	0
Kern's Nectar	6 oz	110	0	0
Libby's Nectar	6 oz	110	0	0
nectar	1 cup	142	tr	tr
PAPRIKA				
paprika	1 tsp	6	tr	tr
PARSLEY				
Dole, chopped	1 tbsp	10	tr	tr
dry	1 tsp	1	tr	tr
dry	1 tbsp	1	tr	tr
fresh, chopped	½ cup	11	tr	tr
PARSNIPS				
FRESH				
cooked	1 (5.6 oz)	130	tr	tr
cooked, sliced	½ cup	63	tr	tr
raw, sliced	½ cup	50	tr	tr
PASSION FRUIT				
purple	1	18	tr	tr
purple juice	1 cup	126	tr	tr
yellow juice	1 cup	149	tr	tr
PASTA				
(*see also* NOODLES, PASTA DINNERS, PASTA SALAD)				
DRY				
Bowties Egg (San Giorgio)	2 oz	210	—	3
Capellini (Pomi)	2 oz	210	—	1
Capellini (San Giorgio)	2 oz	210	—	1
Capellini uncooked (Noodles By Leonardo)	½ cup (2 oz)	200	0	1
Dinosaurs (Mueller's)	2 oz (57 g)	210	—	1
Egg (Prince)	2 oz	221	1	3
Elbow Macaroni (San Giorgio)	2 oz	210	—	1
Elbow Macaroni, not prep (Creamette)	2 oz	210	—	1

FOOD	PORTION	CALS.	SAT. FAT	FAT
Elbow Style (Weight Watchers)	2 oz	160	—	1
Elbows (Ronzoni)	¾ cup (2 oz)	210	—	1
Elbows uncooked (Noodles By Leonardo)	½ cup (2 oz)	200	0	1
Fettuccine Egg (San Giorgio)	2 oz	210	—	3
Fettuccini Florentine (San Giorgio)	2 oz	210	—	3
Fettucini (Ronzoni)	¾ cup (2 oz)	210	—	1
Fettucini uncooked (Noodles By Leonardo)	½ cup (2 oz)	200	0	1
Fusilli (Ronzoni)	¾ cup (2 oz)	210	—	1
Jungle Animals (Mueller's)	2 oz (57 g)	210	—	1
Lasagna No Boil (DeFino)	1 oz	102	—	tr
Lasagna Spinach Whole Wheat (Health Valley)	2 oz	170	—	1
Lasagna Whole Wheat (Health Valley)	2 oz	170	—	1
Lasagne (Mueller's)	2 oz (57 g)	210	—	1
Lasagne (Ronzoni)	¾ cup (2 oz)	210	—	1
Lasagne (San Giorgio)	2 oz	210	—	1
Linguine uncooked (Noodles By Leonardo)	½ cup (2 oz)	200	0	1
Linguini (San Giorgio)	2 oz	210	—	1
Linguini Egg (Creamette)	2 oz	221	—	3
Manicotti (Ronzoni)	¾ cup (2 oz)	210	—	1
Manicotti (San Giorgio)	2 oz	210	—	1
Monsters (Mueller's)	2 oz (57 g)	210	—	1
Mostaccioli (Ronzoni)	¾ cup (2 oz)	210	—	1
Mostaccioli Rigati (San Giorgio)	2 oz	210	—	1
Outer Space (Mueller's)	2 oz	210	—	1
Pasta				
(Anthony)	2 oz	210	0	1
(Gioia)	2 oz	210	0	1
(Golden Grain)	2 oz	203	tr	1
(Luxury)	2 oz	210	0	1
(Merlino's)	2 oz	210	0	1
(Penn Dutch)	2 oz	210	0	1
(Prince)	2 oz	210	0	1
(Red Cross)	2 oz	210	0	1
(Ronco)	2 oz	210	0	1
(Vimco)	2 oz	210	0	1
Radiatori (La Molisana)	2 oz	230	—	1

FOOD	PORTION	CALS.	SAT. FAT	FAT
Rainbow (Prince)	2 oz	210	0	1
Ribbon Pasta Whole Wheat (Pritikin)	2 oz	220	—	2
Ribbons No Boil (DeFino)	2 oz	204	—	2
Rigatoni (Ronzoni)	¾ cup (2 oz)	210	—	1
Rigatoni (San Giorgio)	2 oz	210	—	1
Rigatoni uncooked (Noodles By Leonardo)	½ cup (2 oz)	200	0	1
Rotelle (Creamette)	2 oz	210	—	1
Rotelle uncooked (Ronzoni)	¾ cup (2 oz)	210	—	1
Rotini (San Giorgio)	2 oz	210	—	1
Rotini, uncooked (Noodles By Leonardo)	½ cup (2 oz)	200	0	1
Rotini, uncooked (Ronzoni)	¾ cup (2 oz)	210	—	1
Rotini Rainbow (Creamette)	2 oz	210	—	1
Shells (San Giorgio)	2 oz	210	—	1
Shells, uncooked (Noodles By Leonardo)	½ cup (2 oz)	200	0	1
Shells, uncooked (Ronzoni)	¾ cup (2 oz)	210	—	1
Shells Jumbo (Ronzoni)	¾ cup (2 oz)	210	—	1
Spaghetti (Mueller's)	2 oz (57 g)	210	—	1
Spaghetti (San Giorgio)	2 oz	210	—	1
Spaghetti, not prep (Creamette)	2 oz	210	—	1
Spaghetti, uncooked (Noodles By Leonardo)	½ cup (2 oz)	200	0	1
Spaghetti, uncooked (Ronzoni)	¾ cup (2 oz)	210	—	1
Spaghetti Amaranth (Health Valley)	2 oz	170	—	1
Spaghetti Egg (Creamette)	2 oz	221	—	3
Spaghetti Oat Bran (Health Valley)	2 oz	120	—	1
Spaghetti Spinach Whole Wheat (Health Valley)	2 oz	170	—	1
Spaghetti Thin (Creamette)	2 oz	210	—	1
Spaghetti Wheels (Hanover)	½ cup	90	—	0
Spaghetti Whole Wheat (Delverde)	2 oz	206	1	1

FOOD	PORTION	CALS.	SAT. FAT	FAT
Spaghetti Whole Wheat (Health Valley)	2 oz	170	—	1
Spaghetti Whole Wheat (Pritikin)	2 oz	220	—	2
Spaghetti Whole Wheat Spinach, uncooked (Hodgson Mill)	2 oz	190	1	2
Spaghettini (Weight Watchers)	2 oz	160	—	1
Spaghettini, uncooked (Noodles By Leonardo)	½ cup (2 oz)	200	0	1
Spinach Egg (Prince)	2 oz	220	—	3
Spinach Ribbons, not prep (Creamette)	2 oz	210	—	1
Teddy Bears (Mueller's)	2 oz (57 g)	210	—	1
Thin Spaghetti (San Giorgio)	2 oz	210	—	1
Tubettini (Ronzoni)	¾ cup (2 oz)	210	—	1
Twists Tri Color (Mueller's)	2 oz (57 g)	210	—	1
Veggie Bows, uncooked (Hodgson Mill)	2 oz	200	0	1
Veggie Rotini, uncooked (Hodgson Mill)	2 oz	200	0	1
Veggie Wagon Wheels, uncooked (Hodgson Mill)	2 oz	200	0	1
Vermicelli (San Giorgio)	2 oz	210	—	1
Vermicelli, uncooked (Noodles By Leonardo)	½ cup (2 oz)	200	0	1
Whole Wheat Spirals, uncooked (Hodgson Mill)	2 oz	190	1	1
Ziti (Creamette)	2 oz	210	—	1
Ziti Cut (San Giorgio)	2 oz	210	—	1
corn, cooked	1 cup	176	tr	1
elbows	1 cup	389	tr	2
elbows, cooked	1 cup	197	tr	tr
protein-fortified, cooked	1 cup	188	tr	tr
shells	1 cup	389	tr	2
shells, cooked	1 cup	197	tr	tr
spaghetti	2 oz	211	tr	tr
spaghetti, cooked	1 cup	197	tr	tr
spaghetti, protein-fortified, cooked	1 cup	229	tr	tr

FOOD	PORTION	CALS.	SAT. FAT	FAT
spinach spaghetti	2 oz	212	tr	tr
spinach spaghetti, cooked	1 cup	183	tr	tr
spirals	1 cup	389	tr	2
spirals, cooked	1 cup	197	tr	tr
vegetable	1 cup	308	tr	tr
vegetable, cooked	1 cup	171	tr	tr
whole wheat	1 cup	365	tr	1
whole wheat, cooked	1 cup	174	tr	tr
whole wheat spaghetti	2 oz	198	tr	tr
whole wheat spaghetti, cooked	1 cup	174	tr	tr
FRESH				
Angel's Hair (Contadina)	1¼ cup (2.8 oz)	240	1	3
Fettuccine (Contadina)	1¼ cup (2.9 oz)	250	1	4
Fettuccine Cholesterol Free (Contadina)	1 cup (2.9 oz)	240	0	3
Linguine (Contadina)	1¼ cup (3 oz)	260	1	4
Linguine Cholesterol Free (Contadina)	1¼ cup (3.1 oz)	250	0	3
Ravioli Beef And Garlic (Contadina)	1¼ cup (4 oz)	350	5	14
Ravioli Cheese (Contadina)	1 cup (3.1 oz)	280	6	12
Ravioli Chicken And Rosemary (Contadina)	1¼ cup (4 oz)	330	4	12
Ravioli Light Cheese (Contadina)	1 cup (3.1 oz)	240	2	5
Ravioli Light Garden Vegetable (Contadina)	1¼ cup (3.8 oz)	290	4	6
Tagliatelli Spinach (Contadina)	1¼ cup (3.1 oz)	270	1	4
Tortellini Spinach Three Cheese (Contadina)	¾ cup (3.1 oz)	280	3	5
Tortelloni Cheese (Contadina)	¾ cup (3 oz)	260	3	6
Tortelloni Cheese And Basil (Contadina)	1 cup (4 oz)	360	4	11
Tortelloni Chicken And Prosciutto (Contadina)	1 cup (3.8 oz)	360	4	13
Tortelloni Chicken And Vegetable (Contadina)	¾ cup (2.9 oz)	260	2	7
Tortelloni Light Garlic And Cheese (Contadina)	1 cup (3.6 oz)	280	3	5
Tortelloni Spicy Italian Sausage And Bell Pepper (Contadina)	1 cup (3.6 oz)	330	4	10

FOOD	PORTION	CALS.	SAT. FAT	FAT
plain made w/ egg, cooked	2 oz	75	tr	tr
spinach made w/ egg, cooked	2 oz	74	tr	tr
HOME RECIPE				
made w/ egg, cooked	2 oz	74	tr	tr
made w/o egg, cooked	2 oz	71	tr	tr

PASTA DINNERS
(*see also* DINNER, PASTA SALAD)
CANNED
Chef Boyardee

FOOD	PORTION	CALS.	SAT. FAT	FAT
ABC's & 1, 2, 3's in Cheese Flavor Sauce	7.5 oz	180	tr	1
ABC's & 1, 2, 3's w/ Mini Meatballs	7.5 oz	260	4	11
Beef Ravioli	7.5 oz	190	2	4
Beefaroni	7.5 oz	220	1	7
Cheese Ravioli in Meat Sauce	7.5 oz	200	—	3
Dinosaurs in Cheese Flavor Sauce	7.5 oz	180	tr	1
Dinosaurs w/ Meatballs	7.5 oz	240	3	9
Elbows in Beef Sauce	7.5 oz	210	—	7
Lasagna	7.5 oz	230	—	9
Lasagna in Garden Vegetable Sauce	7.5 oz	170	tr	1
Macaroni & Cheese	7.5 oz	180	tr	5
Microwave Main Meal Beans & Pasta	10.5 oz	200	tr	1
Microwave Main Meal Beef Ravioli Suprema	10.5 oz	290	—	4
Microwave Main Meal Cheese Ravioli Suprema	10.5 oz	290	—	4
Microwave Main Meal Fettuccine	10.5 oz	290	4	9
Microwave Main Meal Lasagna	10.5 oz	290	—	8
Microwave Main Meal Meat Tortellini	10.5 oz	220	2	4
Microwave Main Meal Noodles w/ Chicken	10.5 oz	170	—	1
Microwave Main Meal Peas & Pasta	10.5 oz	190	tr	2

FOOD	PORTION	CALS.	SAT. FAT	FAT
Chef Boyardee *(cont.)*				
Microwave Main Meal Spaghetti Suprema	10.5 oz	200	—	7
Microwave Main Meal Zesty Macaroni	10.5 oz	290	—	8
Microwave Main Meal Ziti In Sauce	10.5 oz	210	tr	tr
Pasta Rings & Meatballs	7.5 oz	220	3	8
Rigatoni	7.5 oz	210	—	6
Rings & Franks	7.5 oz	190	2	5
Shells In Mushroom Sauce	7.5 oz	170	tr	1
Shells In Meat Sauce	7.5 oz	210	—	6
Spaghetti & Meat Balls	7 oz	230	—	7
Tic Tac Toes in Cheese Flavor Sauce	7.5 oz	170	0	1
Tic Tac Toes w/ Mini Meatballs	7.5 oz	250	3	10
Turtles In Sauce	7.5 oz	160	—	1
Turtles w/ Meatballs	7.5 oz	210	3	8
Dinty Moore American Classics Lasagna With Meat & Sauce	1 bowl (10 oz)	260	2	4
Dinty Moore Noodles & Chicken	1 can (7.5 oz)	180	2	8
Franco-American				
Beef RavioliO's in Meat Sauce	½ can (7.5 oz)	250	—	8
CircusO's Pasta in Tomato & Cheese Sauce	½ can (7.38 oz)	170	—	2
CircusO's Pasta w/ Meatballs in Tomato Sauce	½ can (7.38 oz)	210	—	8
Macaroni & Cheese	½ can (7.38 oz)	170	—	6
Spaghetti in Tomato Sauce w/ Cheese	½ can (7.38 oz)	180	—	2
Spaghetti w/ Meatballs in Tomato Sauce	½ can (7.38 oz)	220	—	8
SpaghettiO's in Tomato & Cheese Sauce	½ can (7.38 oz)	170	—	2
SpaghettiO's w/ Meatballs	½ can (7.38 oz)	220	—	9
SpaghettiO's w/ Sliced Franks	½ can (7.38 oz)	220	—	9

FOOD	PORTION	CALS.	SAT. FAT	FAT
SportyO's in Tomato & Cheese Sauce	½ can (7.5 oz)	170	—	2
SportyO's Pasta w/ Meatballs in Tomato Sauce	½ can (7.38 oz)	210	—	8
TeddyO's in Tomato & Cheese Sauce	½ can (7.5 oz)	170	—	2
TeddyO's Pasta w/ Meatballs	½ can (7.38 oz)	210	—	8
Hormel				
Lasagna	1 can (7.5 oz)	250	7	14
Micro Cup Meals Lasagna	1 cup (7.5 oz)	230	2	7
Micro Cup Meals Lasagna & Beef Tomato Sauce	1 cup	359	7	19
Micro Cup Meals Macaroni & Beef With Vegetables	1 cup	285	3	8
Micro Cup Meals Macaroni And Cheese	1 cup (7.5 oz)	260	6	11
Micro Cup Meals Noodles & Chicken	1 cup (10.4 oz)	250	3	11
Micro Cup Meals Noodles & Chicken	1 cup (7.5 oz)	180	2	8
Micro Cup Meals Ravioli Tomato Sauce	1 cup (7.5 oz)	260	5	10
Micro Cup Meals Spaghetti & Meat Sauce	1 cup (7.5 oz)	220	2	5
Spaghetti & Meatballs	1 can (7.5 oz)	210	4	7
Kid's Kitchen (Hormel)				
Cheezy Mac & Beef	1 cup (7.5 oz)	250	3	7
Microwave Meals Beefy Macaroni	1 cup (7.5 oz)	190	3	6
Microwave Meals Macaroni & Cheese	1 cup (7.5 oz)	260	6	11
Microwave Meals Mini Ravioli	1 cup (7.5 oz)	240	3	7
Microwave Meals Spaghetti Rings & Meatballs	1 cup (7.5 oz)	250	3	7
Noodle Rings & Chicken	1 cup (7.5 oz)	150	2	5
Spaghetti Rings & Franks	1 cup (7.5 oz)	230	3	6

FOOD	PORTION	CALS.	SAT. FAT	FAT
Top Shelf Italian Lasagna	1 bowl (10 oz)	350	8	15
Top Shelf Spaghetti With Meat Sauce	1 bowl (10 oz)	240	3	5
Van Camp's Spaghetti Weenee	1 can (8 oz)	230	2	8
DRY MIX				
Golden Grain Macaroni & Cheese	½ cup	310	—	15
Hain				
Pasta & Sauce Creamy Parmesan	¼ pkg	150	—	3
Pasta & Sauce Creamy Swiss	¼ pkg	170	—	4
Pasta & Sauce Fettuccine Alfredo	¼ pkg	180	—	4
Pasta & Sauce Italian Herb	¼ pkg	110	—	2
Pasta & Sauce Primavera	¼ pkg	140	—	4
Pasta & Sauce Tangy Cheddar	¼ pkg	180	—	6
Kraft Dinomac Macaroni & Cheese Dinner	¾ cup	310	3	14
Kraft Egg Noodle & Cheese Dinner	¾ cup	340	4	17
Kraft Macaroni & Cheese Deluxe Dinner	¾ cup	260	4	8
Kraft Macaroni & Cheese Dinner	¾ cup	290	3	13
Kraft Macaroni & Cheese Dinner Family Size	¾ cup	290	3	13
Kraft Mild American Style Spaghetti Dinner	1 cup	300	2	7
Kraft Pasta & Cheese Fettuccini Alfredo	½ cup	180	3	9
Kraft Pasta & Cheese 3-Cheese w/ Vegetables	½ cup	180	3	8
Kraft Pasta & Cheese Cheddar Broccoli	½ cup	180	3	8
Kraft Pasta & Cheese Chicken w/ Herbs	½ cup	170	2	7
Kraft Pasta & Cheese Parmesan	½ cup	180	2	8
Kraft Pasta & Cheese Sour Cream w/ Chives	½ cup	180	2	8

FOOD	PORTION	CALS.	SAT. FAT	FAT
Kraft Spaghetti w/ Meat Sauce Dinner	1 cup	360	4	14
Kraft Spirals Macaroni & Cheese Dinner	¾ cup	340	4	18
Kraft Tangy Italian Style Spaghetti Dinner	1 cup	310	2	8
Kraft Teddy Bears Macaroni & Cheese Dinner	¾ cup	310	3	14
Kraft Wild Wheels Macaroni & Cheese Dinner	¾ cup	310	3	14
Lipton Pasta & Sauce				
Cheddar Broccoli	½ cup	132	—	2
Creamy Garlic	½ cup	144	—	3
Creamy Mushroom	½ cup	143	—	3
Herb Tomato	½ cup	130	—	tr
Minute Microwave Cheddar Cheese Broccoli And Pasta, as prep	½ cup	160	3	5
Nile Spice Pasta'n Sauce Mediterranean	1 pkg	210	3	5
Nile Spice Pasta'n Sauce Parmesan	1 pkg	200	2	3
Nile Spice Pasta'n Sauce Primavera	1 pkg	200	3	4
Terrazza Pasta E Fagioli, as prep	½ cup	150	—	3
Ultra Slim-Fast Macaroni & Cheese	2.3 oz	230	—	3
Uncle Ben Country Inn				
Pasta And Sauce Angel Hair Parmesan	1 serv (2.2 oz)	245	—	5
Pasta And Sauce Broccoli & White Cheddar	1 serv (2.2 oz)	240	—	5
Pasta And Sauce Butter & Herb	1 serv (2 oz)	230	—	6
Pasta And Sauce Creamy Garlic	1 serv (2.4 oz)	261	—	5
Pasta And Sauce Fettuccine Alfredo	1 serv (2.2 oz)	310	—	6
Pasta And Sauce Herb Linguine	1 serv (2.2 oz)	240	—	3
Pasta And Sauce Mushroom Fettuccine	1 serv (2.2 oz)	250	—	6

FOOD	PORTION	CALS.	SAT. FAT	FAT
Uncle Ben Country Inn *(cont.)*				
Pasta And Sauce Vegetable Alfredo	1 serv (2.2 oz)	240	—	5
Velveeta Bits of Bacon Shells & Cheese Dinner	½ cup	240	5	10
Velveeta Shells & Cheese Dinner	¾ cup	210	4	8
Velveeta Touch of Mexico Shells & Cheese Dinner	½ cup	210	4	8
FROZEN				
Banquet				
Family Entree Chicken & Vegetable Primavera	7 oz	140	—	3
Lasagne w/ Meat Sauce	7 oz	270	—	10
Macaroni & Cheese	6.5 oz	290	—	14
Macaroni & Cheese	9 oz	240	—	8
Macaroni & Cheese	7 oz	260	—	11
Mostaccioli w/ Meat Sauce	7 oz	170	—	3
Spaghetti & Meat Sauce	8.75 oz	160	—	4
Banquet Cookin' Bag Chicken & Vegetables Primavera	4 oz	100	—	2
Banquet Entree Spaghetti w/ Meat Sauce	8.5 oz	220	—	8
Birds Eye Easy Recipe Chicken Primavera, not prep	½ pkg	80	1	3
Birds Eye Easy Recipe Chicken Alfredo, not prep	½ pkg	160	1	7
Budget Gourmet				
Cheese Manicotti	1 pkg (10 oz)	440	—	24
Cheese Ravioli	1 pkg (9.5 oz)	290	6	13
Cheese Tortellini	1 pkg (5.5 oz)	200	—	8
Italian Sausage Lasagna	1 pkg (10 oz)	430	—	23
Lasagne w/ Meat Sauce	1 pkg (9.4 oz)	290	4	11
Macaroni & Cheese	1 pkg (5.75 oz)	230	—	12
Pasta Alfredo w/ Broccoli	1 pkg (5.5 oz)	210	—	10
Penne Pasta With Chunky Tomato Sauce And Italian Sausage	1 pkg (10 oz)	320	2	9

FOOD	PORTION	CALS.	SAT. FAT	FAT
Rigatoni In Cream Sauce With Broccoli And Chicken	1 pkg (10.8 oz)	290	3	7
Spaghetti With Chunky Tomato And Meat Sauce	1 pkg (10 oz)	300	2	8
Three Cheese Lasagne	1 pkg	390	—	18
Ziti in Marinara Sauce	1 pkg	200	—	9
Dining Light Cheese Cannelloni	9 oz	310	—	9
Dining Light Cheese Lasagna	9 oz	260	—	6
Dining Light Fettuccini	9 oz	290	—	12
Dining Light Lasagne	9 oz	240	—	5
Dining Light Spaghetti	9 oz	220	—	8
Formagg Penne Pasta Alfredo	⅔ cup (5 oz)	190	0	2
Formagg Penne Pasta Primavera	⅔ cup (5 oz)	190	0	2
Formagg Vegetable Pasta & Ceasar Italian Garden	⅔ cup (5 oz)	190	0	2
Green Giant Garden Gourmet				
Creamy Mushroom	1 pkg	220	6	11
Pasta Dijon	1 pkg	260	9	17
Pasta Florentine	1 pkg	230	5	9
Rotini Cheddar	1 pkg	230	6	10
Green Giant One Serve				
Cheese Tortellini	1 pkg	260	3	9
Macaroni & Cheese	1 pkg	230	4	9
Pasta Marinara	1 pkg	180	tr	5
Pasta Parmesan w/ Green Peas	1 pkg	170	2	5
Green Giant Pasta Accents				
Creamy Cheddar	½ cup	100	2	5
Garden Herb	½ cup	80	tr	3
Garlic Seasoning	½ cup	110	2	5
Pasta Primavera	½ cup	110	2	5
Healthy Choice				
Cheese Ravioli Parmigiana	1 meal (9 oz)	250	2	4
Chicken Fettuccini Alfredo	1 meal (8.5 oz)	250	1	3
Classics Pasta Shells Marinara	1 meal (12 oz)	360	2	3

FOOD	PORTION	CALS.	SAT. FAT	FAT
Healthy Choice *(cont.)*				
Classics Turkey Fettuccine Alla Crema	1 meal (12.5 oz)	350	2	4
Fettuccini Alfredo	1 meal (8 oz)	240	2	5
Lasagna Roma	1 meal (13.5 oz)	390	2	5
Macaroni & Cheese	1 meal (9 oz)	290	2	5
Spaghetti Bolognese	1 meal (10 oz)	260	1	3
Three Cheese Manicotti	1 meal (11 oz)	310	5	9
Vegetable Pasta Italiano	1 meal (10 oz)	220	0	1
Zucchini Lasagna	1 meal (14 oz)	330	1	2
Kid Cuisine				
Macaroni & Cheese w/ Mini Franks	9 oz	360	—	15
Mega Meal Macaroni & Cheese	12.45 oz	470	—	13
Mini Cheese Ravioli	8.75 oz	290	—	8
Spaghetti w/ Meat Sauce	9.25 oz	310	—	8
Le Menu Manicotti w/ Three Cheeses	11.75 oz	390	—	15
Le Menu LightStyle				
3-Cheese Stuffed Shells	10 oz	280	—	8
Cheese Tortellini	10 oz	230	—	6
Garden Vegetables Lasagna	10.5 oz	260	—	8
Lasagna w/ Meat Sauce	10 oz	290	—	8
Meat Sauce & Cheese Tortellini	8 oz	250	—	8
Spaghetti w/ Beef Sauce & Mushrooms	9 oz	280	—	6
Lean Cuisine				
Angel Hair Pasta	1 pkg (10 oz)	210	1	4
Cheddar Bake With Pasta	1 pkg (9 oz)	220	2	6
Cheese Cannelloni	1 pkg (9.1 oz)	270	4	8
Cheese Ravioli	1 pkg (8.5 oz)	250	3	8
Chicken Fettuccini	1 pkg (9 oz)	270	3	6
Classic Cheese Lasagna	1 pkg (11.5 oz)	290	3	6
Fettucini Alfredo	1 pkg (9 oz)	270	3	7
Fettucini Primavera	1 pkg (10 oz)	260	3	8
Lasagne w/ Meat Sauce	1 pkg (10.25 oz)	270	3	6
Macaroni & Beef	1 pkg (10 oz)	280	2	8
Macaroni & Cheese	1 pkg (9 oz)	270	4	7
Marinara Twist	1 pkg (10 oz)	240	1	3
Rigatoni	1 pkg (9 oz)	180	2	4

FOOD	PORTION	CALS.	SAT. FAT	FAT
Spaghetti & Meatballs	1 pkg (9.5 oz)	290	2	7
Spaghetti w/ Meat Sauce	1 pkg (11.5 oz)	290	2	6
Tuna Lasagna	1 pkg (9.75 oz)	230	2	6
Zucchini Lasagna	1 pkg (11 oz)	240	2	4
Morton Macaroni & Cheese	6.5 oz	290	—	14
Morton Spaghetti & Meat Sauce	8.5 oz	170	—	2
Mrs. Paul's Light Seafood Lasagna Seafood Entree	9.5 oz	290	—	8
Mrs. Paul's Light Seafood Rotini Seafood Entree	9 oz	240	—	6
Mrs. Paul's Seafood Rotini	9 oz	240	2	6
Palmazone Macaroni 'n Cheese	½ pkg (6 oz)	260	—	7
Stouffer's				
Beef Ravioli	1 pkg (9.5 oz)	370	4	14
Cheese Tortellini With Alfredo Sauce	1 pkg (8.9 oz)	550	18	33
Cheese Tortellini With Tomato Sauce	1 pkg (9.25 oz)	290	5	6
Cheese Manocotti	1 pkg (9 oz)	340	7	16
Cheese Ravioli With Tomato Sauce	1 pkg (9.5 oz)	360	5	16
Cheese Shells With Tomato Sauce	1 pkg (9.25 oz)	340	7	16
Fettucini Alfredo	1 pkg (10 oz)	480	17	29
Four Cheese Lasagna	1 pkg (10.75 oz)	410	10	19
Homestyle Chicken Fettucini	1 pkg (10.5 oz)	380	4	15
Lasagna With Meat Sauce	1 cup (7 oz)	260	4	10
Lasagna With Meat Sauce	1 pkg (10.5 oz)	360	5	13
Lunch Express Cheese Lasagna Casserole	1 pkg (9.5 oz)	270	3	7
Lunch Express Cheese Ravioli	1 pkg (8.5 oz)	310	4	12
Lunch Express Chicken Fettucini	1 pkg (10.25 oz)	250	3	6
Lunch Express Chicken Alfredo	1 pkg (9.6 oz)	360	6	17
Lunch Express Fettucini Primavera	1 pkg (10.25 oz)	420	12	25

FOOD	PORTION	CALS.	SAT. FAT	FAT
Stouffer's *(cont.)*				
Lunch Express Lasagna With Meat Sauce	1 pkg (10 oz)	350	5	12
Lunch Express Macaroni & Cheese With Broccoli	1 pkg (10.4 oz)	360	5	19
Lunch Express Macaroni And Cheese And Broccoli	1 pkg (9.5 oz)	240	3	7
Lunch Express Pasta And Chicken Marinara	1 pkg (9.1 oz)	270	2	6
Lunch Express Pasta And Tuna Casserole	1 pkg (9.6 oz)	280	2	6
Lunch Express Pasta And Turkey Dijon	1 pkg (9.9 oz)	270	2	6
Lunch Express Rigatoni With Meat Sauce	1 pkg (10.75 oz)	340	3	12
Lunch Express Spaghetti With Meat Sauce	1 pkg (9.6 oz)	320	4	10
Lunch Express Swedish Meatballs With Pasta	1 pkg (10.25 oz)	530	11	32
Macaroni And Beef	1 pkg (11.5 oz)	340	5	12
Macaroni And Cheese	1 cup (6 oz)	330	6	17
Noodles Romanoff	1 pkg (12 oz)	460	6	23
Spaghetti With Meat Sauce	1 pkg (12.9 oz)	430	5	13
Spaghetti With Meatballs	1 pkg (12.6 oz)	420	15	15
Tuna Noodle Casserole	1 pkg (10 oz)	330	2	14
Turkey Tettrazini	1 pkg (10 oz)	360	3	19
Vegetable Lasagna	1 cup (8 oz)	280	5	12
Vegetable Lasagna	1 pkg (10.5 oz)	370	5	19
Swanson Lasagne w/ Meat Sauce Homestyle	10.5 oz	400	—	15
Swanson Macaroni & Cheese	12.25 oz	370	—	15
Swanson Macaroni & Cheese Homestyle	10 oz	390	—	19
Swanson Spaghetti & Meatballs	12.5 oz	390	—	17
Swanson Spaghetti w/ Italian Style Meatballs Homestyle	13 oz	490	—	18

FOOD	PORTION	CALS.	SAT. FAT	FAT
Tyson Parmigiana	1 pkg (11.25 oz)	380	—	17
Ultra Slim-Fast Pasta Primavera	12 oz	340	—	9
Ultra Slim-Fast Spaghetti w/ Beef & Mushroom Sauce	12 oz	370	—	10
Weight Watchers				
Angel Hair Pasta	10 oz	200	1	4
Baked Cheese Ravioli	9 oz	240	2	6
Cheese Manicotti	9.25 oz	260	3	8
Cheese Tortellini	9 oz	310	1	6
Chicken Fettuccini	8.25 oz	280	3	9
Fettuccini Alfredo	8 oz	230	2	7
Garden Lasagne	11 oz	260	2	7
Italian Cheese Lasagne	11 oz	290	2	6
Lasagne	10.25 oz	240	2	6
Spaghetti w/ Meat Sauce	10 oz	240	1	7
HOME RECIPE				
macaroni & cheese	1 cup	430	10	22
spaghetti w/ meatballs & tomato sauce	1 cup	330	4	12
TAKE-OUT				
lasagna	1 piece (2.5″ × 2.5″)	374	11	21
macaroni & cheese	1 cup	230	5	10
manicotti	¾ cup (6.4 oz)	273	6	12
rigatoni w/ sausage sauce	¾ cup	260	4	12
spaghetti w/ meatballs & cheese	1 cup	407	6	19

PASTA SALAD
FROZEN

FOOD	PORTION	CALS.	SAT. FAT	FAT
Hanover Italian	½ cup	60	—	0
Hanover Milano	½ cup	60	—	0
Hanover Oriental	½ cup	80	—	0
Hanover Primavera	½ cup	50	—	0
MIX				
Kraft Garden Primavera Pasta Salad & Dressing	½ cup	170	2	7
Kraft Homestyle Pasta Salad & Dressing	½ cup	240	2	16
Kraft Light Italian Pasta Salad & Dressing	½ cup	130	1	3

FOOD	PORTION	CALS.	SAT. FAT	FAT
Kraft Light Rancher's Choice Pasta Salad & Dressing	½ cup	170	1	7
Kraft Pasta Salad & Dressing, Broccoli & Vegetables	½ cup	210	2	16
Suddenly Salad				
Classic Pasta, as prep	½ cup	160	—	6
Creamy Macaroni, as prep	½ cup	200	—	10
Creamy Macaroni, as prep low fat recipe	½ cup	140	—	4
Italian Pasta, as prep	½ cup	160	—	6
Pasta Primavera, as prep	½ cup	190	—	10
Pasta Primavera, as prep low fat recipe	½ cup	150	—	5
Tortellini Italiano, as prep	½ cup	160	—	7
TAKE-OUT				
elbow macaroni salad	3.5 oz	160	2	5
italian style pasta salad	3.5 oz	140	1	7
mustard macaroni salad	3.5 oz	190	1	10
pasta salad w/ vegetables	3.5 oz	140	3	4

PASTRY

(see BROWNIE, CAKE, DANISH PASTRY)

PÂTÉ

CANNED

FOOD	PORTION	CALS.	SAT. FAT	FAT
Liver (Sells)	2.08 oz	190	—	16
chicken liver	1 tbsp	109	—	2
chicken liver	1 oz	238	—	4
goose liver, smoked	1 tbsp	60	—	6
goose liver, smoked	1 oz	131	—	12
liver	1 tbsp	41	—	4
liver	1 oz	90	—	8

PEACH

CANNED

FOOD	PORTION	CALS.	SAT. FAT	FAT
Clingstone Halves (S&W)	½ cup	100	0	0
Clingstone Halves Diet (S&W)	½ cup	30	0	0
Clingstone Halves Unsweetened (S&W)	½ cup	30	0	0

FOOD	PORTION	CALS.	SAT. FAT	FAT
Clingstone Sliced Diet (S&W)	½ cup	30	0	0
Clingstone Sliced Unsweetened (S&W)	½ cup	30	0	0
Freestone Halves Diet (S&W)	½ cup	30	0	0
Freestone Halves in Heavy Syrup (S&W)	½ cup	100	0	0
Freestone Slices Diet (S&W)	½ cup	30	0	0
Freestone Slices in Heavy Syrup (S&W)	½ cup	100	0	0
Halves (Hunt's)	4 oz	90	—	tr
Sliced Yellow Cling Natural Style (S&W)	½ cup	90	0	0
Slices (Hunt's)	4 oz	90	—	tr
Yellow Cling Halves Lite (Libby)	½ cup (4.4 oz)	60	0	0
Yellow Cling Natural Lite (S&W)	½ cup	50	0	0
Yellow Cling Sliced Premium in Heavy Syrup	½ cup	100	0	0
Yellow Cling Whole Spiced in Heavy Syrup (S&W)	½ cup	90	0	0
halves in heavy syrup	1 half	60	tr	tr
halves in light syrup	1 half	44	tr	tr
halves juice pack	1 half	34	tr	tr
halves water pack	1 half	18	tr	tr
spiced in heavy syrup	1 fruit	66	tr	tr
spiced in heavy syrup	1 cup	180	tr	tr
DRIED				
Peaches (Mariani)	¼ cup	140	—	0
halves	10	311	tr	1
halves	1 cup	383	tr	1
halves, cooked w/ sugar	½ cup	139	tr	tr
halves, cooked w/o sugar	½ cup	99	tr	tr
FRESH				
Dole	2	70	—	0
peach	1	37	tr	tr
sliced	1 cup	73	tr	tr
FROZEN				
Freestone (Big Valley)	⅔ cup (4.9 oz)	50	0	0
slices, sweetened	1 cup	235	tr	tr

FOOD	PORTION	CALS.	SAT. FAT	FAT
JUICE				
Goya Nectar	6 oz	110	—	0
Kern's Nectar	6 fl oz	110	0	0
Libby's Nectar	6 oz	100	0	0
Mott's Fruit Basket Orchard Peach Juice Cocktail, as prep	8 fl oz	130	0	0
Smucker's	8 oz	120	0	0
nectar	1 cup	134	tr	tr
PEANUT BUTTER				
Arrowhead Creamy	2 tbsp	200	3	15
Arrowhead Crunchy	2 tbsp	200	3	15
BAMA Creamy	2 tbsp	200	—	17
BAMA Crunchy	2 tbsp	200	—	17
BAMA Jelly & Peanut Butter	2 tbsp	150	—	7
Erewhon Chunky, Salted	2 tbsp	190	—	14
Erewhon Chunky, Unsalted	2 tbsp	190	—	14
Erewhon Creamy, Salted	2 tbsp	190	—	14
Erewhon Creamy, Unsalted	2 tbsp	190	—	14
Estee				
Chunky Sodium Free	2 tbsp (1 oz)	190	3	15
Chunky Sodium Free Sorbitol Sweetened	2 tbsp (1 oz)	190	3	15
Creamy Sodium Free	2 tbsp (1 oz)	190	3	15
Creamy Sodium Free Sorbitol Sweetened	2 tbsp (1 oz)	190	3	15
Health Valley Chunky, No Salt	2 tbsp	170	—	14
Health Valley Creamy, No Salt	2 tbsp	170	—	14
Hollywood Creamy	1 tbsp	35	0	3
Hollywood Crunchy	1 tbsp	35	0	3
Hollywood Unsalted	1 tbsp	35	0	3
Home Brand	2 tbsp	210	—	17
Home Brand Natural, Lightly Salted	2 tbsp	210	—	17
Home Brand Natural, Unsalted	2 tbsp	210	—	17
Home Brand No Sugar Added	2 tbsp	180	—	16
Jif Creamy	2 tbsp (1.1 oz)	190	3	16
Jif Extra Crunchy	2 tbsp (1.1 oz)	190	3	16

FOOD	PORTION	CALS.	SAT. FAT	FAT
Peter Pan Creamy	2 tbsp	190	2	16
Peter Pan Creamy, Salt Free	2 tbsp	190	2	17
Peter Pan Crunchy	2 tbsp	190	2	16
Peter Pan Crunchy, Salt Free	2 tbsp	190	2	17
Reese's Peanut Butter Flavored Chips	¼ cup (1.5 oz)	230	—	13
Simply Jif Creamy	2 tbsp (1.1 oz)	180	3	16
Simply Jif Extra Crunchy	2 tbsp (1.1 oz)	180	3	16
Skippy Creamy	1 cup (263 g)	1540	27	135
Skippy Creamy, w/ 2 slices white bread	1 sandwich	340	3	19
Skippy Reduced Fat Creamy	2 tbsp	190	3	12
Skippy Super Chunk	2 tbsp	190	3	17
Skippy Super Chunk	1 cup	1540	27	138
Skippy Super Chunk, w/ 2 slices white bread	1 sandwich	340	3	19
Smucker's Goober Grape	2 tbsp	180	2	10
Smucker's Honey Sweetened	2 tbsp	200	3	16
Smucker's Natural	2 tbsp	200	3	16
Smucker's Natural, No-Salt Added	2 tbsp	200	3	16
Teddie Natural Peanut Butter w/ No Salt Added	2 tbsp	200	—	17
chunky	2 tbsp	188	3	16
chunky	1 cup	1520	25	129
chunky w/o salt	2 tbsp	188	3	16
chunky w/o salt	1 cup	1520	25	129
smooth	2 tbsp	188	3	16
smooth	1 cup	1517	25	128
smooth w/o salt	2 tbsp	188	3	16
smooth w/o salt	1 cup	1517	25	129

PEANUTS

FOOD	PORTION	CALS.	SAT. FAT	FAT
Cocktail Lightly Salted (Planters)	1 oz	170	2	14
Cocktail Unsalted (Planters)	1 oz	170	2	14
Dry Roasted (Frito Lay)	1.2 oz	190	—	16
Dry Roasted (Guy's)	1 oz	170	—	14
Dry Roasted Lightly Salted (Planters)	1 oz	160	2	15

FOOD	PORTION	CALS.	SAT. FAT	FAT
Dry Roasted, Unsalted (Planters)	1 oz	170	2	15
Fresh Roast Lightly Salted (Planters)	1 oz	160	2	14
Fresh Roast Salted (Planters)	1 oz	170	2	14
Honey Roasted (Eagle)	1 oz	170	—	13
Honey Roasted (Planters)	1 oz	170	—	13
Honey Roasted (Weight Watchers)	0.7 oz	100	1	6
Honey Roasted Dry Roasted (Planters)	1 oz	160	2	13
Low Salt (Eagle)	1 oz	170	—	15
Party Peanuts (Fisher)	1 oz	160	—	14
Peanuts (Beer Nuts)	1 oz	180	—	14
Peanuts (Planters)	½-oz bag	80	1	7
Roasted w/ Shell (Lance)	1.75 oz	190	3	15
Salted (Frito Lay)	1 pkg (32 g)	190	3	15
Salted (Lance)	1.13 oz	190	3	15
Salted (Little Debbie)	1 pkg (1.2 oz)	220	3	18
Salted Tube (Lance)	1 pkg (42 g)	240	4	20
Salted-in-Shell, shelled (Fisher)	1 oz	170	2	14
Spanish (Planters)	1 oz	170	5	15
Spanish Raw (Planters)	1 oz	160	2	14
Spanish Roasted (Fisher)	1 oz	180	3	16
Spanish Salted (Guy's)	1 oz	170	—	14
Virginia Fancy (Eagle)	1 oz	90	—	8
cooked	½ cup	102	1	7
dry roasted	1 oz	164	2	14
dry roasted	1 cup	855	10	73
oil roasted	1 oz	163	2	14
oil roasted	1 cup	837	10	71
oil roasted, w/o salt	1 oz	163	2	14
oil roasted, w/o salt	1 cup	837	10	71
spanish, oil roasted	1 oz	162	2	14
spanish, oil roasted w/o salt	1 oz	162	2	14
unroasted	1 oz	159	2	14
valencia, oil roasted	1 oz	165	2	14
valencia, oil roasted	1 cup	848	11	74
valencia, oil roasted, w/o salt	1 oz	165	2	14
valencia, oil roasted, w/o salt	1 cup	848	11	74

FOOD	PORTION	CALS.	SAT. FAT	FAT
virginia, oil roasted	1 oz	161	2	14
virginia, oil roasted	1 cup	826	9	70

PEAR
CANNED

FOOD	PORTION	CALS.	SAT. FAT	FAT
Bartlett Halves in Heavy Syrup (S&W)	½ cup	100	0	0
Bartlett Halves Peeled Unsweetened (S&W)	½ cup	35	0	0
Halves (Hunt's)	4 oz	90	—	tr
Halves Peeled Diet (S&W)	½ cup	35	0	0
Quartered Peeled Diet (S&W)	½ cup	35	0	0
Sliced Lite (Libby)	½ cup (4.3 oz)	60	0	0
Sliced Natural Light Bartlett (S&W)	½ cup	60	0	0
Sliced Natural Style (S&W)	½ cup	80	0	0
halves in heavy syrup	1 half	68	tr	tr
halves in heavy syrup	1 cup	188	tr	tr
halves in light syrup	1 half	45	tr	tr
halves juice pack	1 cup	123	tr	tr
halves water pack	1 half	22	tr	tr

DRIED

FOOD	PORTION	CALS.	SAT. FAT	FAT
Pears (Mariani)	¼ cup	150	—	0
halves	10	459	tr	1
halves	1 cup	472	tr	1
halves, cooked w/ sugar	½ cup	196	tr	tr
halves, cooked w/o sugar	½ cup	163	tr	tr

FRESH

FOOD	PORTION	CALS.	SAT. FAT	FAT
Dole	1	100	—	1
asian	1 (4.3 oz)	51	tr	tr
pear	1	98	tr	1
sliced w/ skin	1 cup	97	tr	1

JUICE

FOOD	PORTION	CALS.	SAT. FAT	FAT
Goya Nectar	6 oz	120	—	0
Kern's Nectar	6 oz	110	0	0
Libby's Nectar	1 can (11.5 fl oz)	220	0	0
nectar	1 cup	149	tr	tr

PEAS
CANNED

FOOD	PORTION	CALS.	SAT. FAT	FAT
Baked Pea Beans (Van De Kamp's)	8 oz	270	—	6
Cream Peas (East Texas Fair)	½ cup (4.4 oz)	120	1	1

FOOD	PORTION	CALS.	SAT. FAT	FAT
Crowder (Allen)	½ cup (4.5 oz)	110	1	1
Crowder (East Texas Fair)	½ cup (4.5 oz)	110	1	1
Crowder (Homefolks)	½ cup (4.5 oz)	110	1	1
Crowder Peas Seasoned w/ Pork (Luck's)	7.5 oz	200	—	7
Early June (Crest Top)	½ cup (4.5 oz)	100	0	1
Early June or Sweet (Owatonna)	½ cup	70	—	0
Field Peas (Sunshine)	½ cup (4.4 oz)	120	1	1
Field Peas with Bacon (Trappey)	½ cup (4.5 oz)	90	1	1
Field Peas w/ Snaps and Bacon (Trappey)	½ cup (4.4 oz)	110	1	1
Lady Peas (Sunshine)	½ cup (4.3 oz)	100	1	1
Lady Peas With Snaps (East Texas Fair)	½ cup (4.3 oz)	100	1	1
Natural Pack (Seneca)	½ cup	60	0	0
Peas 'n Pork (East Texas Fair)	½ cup (4.5 oz)	110	1	2
Pepper Peas (East Texas Fair)	½ cup (4.5 oz)	120	1	1
Petit Pois (S&W)	½ cup	70	0	0
Purple Hull (Allen)	½ cup (4.4 oz)	120	1	1
Purple Hull (East Texas Fair)	½ cup (4.4 oz)	120	1	1
Purple Hull (Homefolks)	½ cup (4.4 oz)	120	1	1
Seneca	½ cup	50	0	0
Small Pea Beans (Friends)	8 oz	360	3	4
Sweet (Green Giant)	½ cup	50	0	0
Sweet (S&W)	½ cup	70	0	0
Sweet Water Pack (S&W)	½ cup	40	0	0
Veri-Green Sweet (S&W)	½ cup	70	0	0
White Acre (East Texas Fair)	½ cup (4.3 oz)	100	1	1
green	½ cup	59	tr	tr
green low sodium	½ cup	59	tr	tr
DRIED				
split, cooked	1 cup	231	tr	1
FRESH				
Dole Sugar Peas	½ cup	30	—	tr
edible-pod, cooked	½ cup	34	tr	tr
green, cooked	½ cup	67	tr	tr
green, raw	½ cup	58	tr	tr

FOOD	PORTION	CALS.	SAT. FAT	FAT
FROZEN				
Chinese Pea Pods (Chun King)	1.5 oz	20	0	0
Green (Birds Eye)	½ cup	80	0	0
Green (Fresh Like)	3.5 oz	85	—	1
Harvest Fresh Early June (Green Giant)	½ cup	60	—	1
Harvest Fresh Sugar Snap (Green Giant)	½ cup	30	0	0
Harvest Fresh Sweet (Green Giant)	½ cup	50	0	0
In Butter Sauce (Birds Eye)	½ cup	80	1	2
In Butter Sauce (Green Giant)	½ cup	80	1	2
Le Suer Early (Green Giant Select)	½ cup	60	0	0
Le Suer Early in Butter Sauce (Green Giant Select)	½ cup	80	tr	2
One Serve in Butter Sauce (Green Giant)	1 pkg	90	tr	2
Petite (Hanover)	½ cup	60	—	0
Polybag Deluxe Tender Tiny (Birds Eye)	½ cup	60	0	0
Snow Pea Pods (La Choy)	½ pkg (3 oz)	35	—	tr
Snow Peas (Hanover)	½ cup	35	—	0
Sugar Snap Deluxe (Birds Eye)	½ cup	45	0	0
Sugar Snap Sweet Peas (Green Giant Select)	½ cup	30	0	0
Sweet (Green Giant)	½ cup	50	—	0
Sweet Peas (Hanover)	½ cup	70	—	0
Tender Tiny Deluxe (Birds Eye)	½ cup	63	0	0
Tiny Green (Fresh Like)	3.5 oz	63	—	tr
edible-pod, cooked	1 pkg (10 oz)	132	tr	1
edible-pod, cooked	½ cup	42	tr	tr
green, cooked	½ cup	63	tr	tr
SHELF STABLE				
Mini Sweet (Green Giant)	½ cup	60	—	tr
SPROUTS				
raw	½ cup	77	tr	tr

FOOD	PORTION	CALS.	SAT. FAT	FAT
TAKE-OUT				
pea & potato curry	1 serving (7 oz)	284	—	22
pea curry	1 serving (4.4 oz)	438	—	42
PECANS				
Halves (Planters)	1 oz	190	2	20
Honey Roasted (Eagle)	1 oz	200	—	19
Pieces (Planters)	1 oz	190	2	20
dried	1 oz	190	2	19
dry roasted	1 oz	187	1	18
dry roasted, salted	1 oz	187	1	18
halves, dried	1 cup	721	6	73
oil roasted	1 oz	195	2	20
oil roasted, salted	1 oz	195	2	20
PECTIN				
(*see also* FIBER)				
Certo	1 tbsp	2	—	0
Slim Set	1 pkg	208	0	0
Slim Set	1 tbsp	3	0	0
Sure-Jell	¼ pkg	38	—	0
Sure-Jell Light	¼ pkg	33	—	0
PEPPER				
Lemon (Ac'cent)	½ tsp	0	0	0
Lemon Pepper (Lawry's)	1 tsp	6	—	tr
Seasoned Ac'cent	½ tsp	0	0	0
black	1 tsp	5	tr	tr
cayenne	1 tsp	6	tr	tr
red	1 tsp	6	tr	tr
white	1 tsp	7	—	tr
PEPPERS				
CANNED				
Banana Mild (Trappey)	3 peppers (1 oz)	6	tr	tr
Banana Sliced Rings (Trappey)	21 slices (1 oz)	6	tr	tr
Cherry Hot (Trappey)	2 peppers (1 oz)	7	tr	tr
Cherry Mild (Trappey)	2 peppers (1 oz)	10	tr	tr
Chilies Diced Green (Chi-Chi's)	2 tbsp (1.2 oz)	10	0	0
Chilies Green Whole (Chi-Chi's)	¾ pepper (1 oz)	10	0	0
Dulcito Italian Pepperonchini (Trappey)	4 peppers (1 oz)	8	tr	tr
Filet (Hebrew National)	¼ pepper (1 oz)	9	0	0

FOOD	PORTION	CALS.	SAT. FAT	FAT
Filet Peppers (Schorr's)	1 oz	9	0	0
Green Chilies Chopped (Old El Paso)	2 tbsp	8	—	tr
Green Chilies Whole (Old El Paso)	1	8	—	tr
Hot Banana Pepper Rings (Vlasic)	1 oz	4	0	0
Hot Cherry (Hebrew National)	⅛ pepper (1 oz)	11	0	0
Hot Cherry (Progresso)	½ cup	190	3	20
Hot Cherry (Vlasic)	1 oz	10	0	0
Hot Cherry Pickled (Progresso)	½ cup	130	2	12
In Vinegar Hot (Trappey)	15 peppers (1 oz)	9	tr	tr
Jalapeno Hot Sliced (Trappey)	21 slices (1 oz)	4	tr	tr
Jalapeno Mexican Hot (Vlasic)	1 oz	8	0	0
Jalapeno Nacho Slices (McIlhenny)	12 slices (1.1 oz)	7	tr	tr
Jalapeno Whole (Trappey)	2 peppers (1 oz)	11	tr	0
Jalapenos Green Wheels (Chi-Chi's)	1 oz	10	0	0
Jalapenos Green Whole (Chi-Chi's)	1 oz	10	0	0
Jalapenos Red Whole (Chi-Chi's)	1 oz	15	0	0
Jalapenos Red Wheels (Chi-Chi's)	1 oz	10	0	0
Mexican Tiny Hot (Vlasic)	1 oz	6	0	0
Mild Cherry (Vlasic)	1 oz	8	0	0
Mild Greek Pepperoncini Salad Peppers (Vlasic)	1 oz	4	0	0
Piccalilli (Progresso)	½ cup	190	3	20
Red Filet (Hebrew National)	¼ pepper (1 oz)	9	0	0
Roasted (Progresso)	½ cup	20	tr	tr
Serano (Trappey)	7 peppers (1 oz)	7	tr	tr
Sweet (Rosoff's)	¼ pepper (1 oz)	9	0	0
Sweet Fried (Progresso)	½ jar	37	tr	tr
Tempero Golden Greek Pepperoncini (Trappey)	4 peppers (1 oz)	7	tr	tr
Torrido Santa Fe Grande (Trappey)	3 peppers (1 oz)	10	tr	tr
Tuscan (Progresso)	½ cup	20	0	0
chili, red hot	1 (2.6 oz)	18	tr	tr

FOOD	PORTION	CALS.	SAT. FAT	FAT
chili, red hot, chopped	½ cup	17	tr	tr
green chili, hot	1 (2.6 oz)	18	tr	tr
green chili, hot, chopped	½ cup	17	tr	tr
green halves	½ cup	13	tr	tr
jalapeno, chopped	½ cup	17	tr	tr
red halves	½ cup	13	tr	tr
DRIED				
green	1 tbsp	1	tr	tr
red	1 tbsp	1	tr	tr
FRESH				
Dole Bell	1 med	25	—	1
chili, red, raw, chopped	½ cup	30	tr	tr
chili, red hot, raw	1 (1.6 oz)	18	tr	tr
green chili, hot, raw	1	18	tr	tr
green chili, hot, raw, chopped	½ cup	30	tr	tr
green, raw, chopped	½ cup	13	tr	tr
green, chopped, cooked	½ cup	19	tr	tr
green, cooked	1 (2.6 oz)	20	tr	tr
green, raw	1 (2.6 oz)	20	tr	tr
red, chopped, cooked	½ cup	19	tr	tr
red, cooked	1 (2.6 oz)	20	tr	tr
red, raw	1 (2.6 oz)	20	tr	tr
red, raw, chopped	½ cup	13	tr	tr
yellow, raw	1 (6.5 oz)	50	tr	tr
yellow, raw	10 strips	14	tr	tr
FROZEN				
Green, Diced (Southland)	2 oz	10	—	0
Sweet Red & Green, Cut (Southland)	2 oz	15	—	0
green, chopped, not prep	1 oz	6	tr	tr
red, chopped, not prep	1 oz	6	tr	tr

PERCH

FOOD	PORTION	CALS.	SAT. FAT	FAT
FRESH				
cooked	1 fillet (1.6 oz)	54	tr	1
cooked	3 oz	99	tr	1
ocean perch, atlantic, cooked	1 fillet (1.8 oz)	60	tr	1
ocean perch, atlantic, cooked	3 oz	103	tr	2
red, raw	3.5 oz	114	tr	4
raw	3 oz	77	tr	1
FROZEN				
Battered (Van De Kamps)	2 pieces	310	4	21

FOOD	PORTION	CALS.	SAT. FAT	FAT
Fishmarket Fresh Ocean Perch (Gorton's)	5 oz	140	—	3
Ocean Perch Light Fillets (Van De Kamp's)	1 piece	280	3	14
Ocean Perch Natural Fillets (Van De Kamp's)	4 oz	130	2	5

PERSIMMONS

FOOD	PORTION	CALS.	SAT. FAT	FAT
dried, japanese	1	93	—	tr
fresh	1	32	—	tr
fresh, japanese	1	118	—	tr

PHEASANT
FRESH

FOOD	PORTION	CALS.	SAT. FAT	FAT
breast w/o skin, raw	½ breast (6.4 oz)	243	2	6
leg w/o skin, raw	1 (3.6 oz)	143	2	5
w/ skin, raw	½ pheasant (14 oz)	723	11	37
w/o skin, raw	½ pheasant (12.4 oz)	470	4	13

PHYLLO

FOOD	PORTION	CALS.	SAT. FAT	FAT
Ekizian Phyllo Dough	½ lb	865	7	17
phyllo dough	1 oz	85	tr	2
sheet	1	57	tr	1

PICKLES

FOOD	PORTION	CALS.	SAT. FAT	FAT
Bread & Butter Chips (Vlasic)	1 oz	30	0	0
Bread & Butter Chunks (Vlasic)	1 oz	25	0	0
Bread 'N Butter Slices (Claussen)	1	7	—	tr
Bread & Butter Stixs (Vlasic)	1 oz	18	0	0
Deli Bread & Butter (Vlasic)	1 oz	25	0	0
Deli Dill Halves (Vlasic)	1 oz	4	0	0
Dill Spears (Claussen)	1	4	—	tr
Garlic (Schorr's)	⅓ pickle (1 oz)	3	0	0
Half Sour (Hebrew National)	½ pickle (1 oz)	4	0	0
Half Sour (Rosoff's)	⅓ pickle (1 oz)	4	0	0
Half Sour (Schorr's)	½ spear (1 oz)	4	0	0
Half Sour (Schorr's)	⅓ pickle (1 oz)	4	0	0

FOOD	PORTION	CALS.	SAT. FAT	FAT
Half Sour Spears (Rosoff's)	½ spear (1 oz)	4	0	0
Half-the-Salt Hamburger Dill Chips (Vlasic)	1 oz	2	0	0
Half-the-Salt Kosher Crunchy Dills (Vlasic)	1 oz	4	0	0
Half-the-Salt Kosher Dill Spears (Vlasic)	1 oz	4	0	0
Half-the-Salt Sweet Butter Chips (Vlasic)	1 oz	30	0	0
Hot & Spicy Garden Mix (Vlasic)	1 oz	4	0	0
Hot N' Sweet (McIlhenny)	4 (1 oz)	42	tr	tr
Kosher (Hebrew National)	⅓ pickle (1 oz)	4	0	0
Kosher (Rosoff's)	⅓ pickle (1 oz)	4	0	0
Kosher Baby Dills (Vlasic)	1 oz	4	0	0
Kosher Barrel Cured Dill (Hebrew National)	1 pkg	23	0	0
Kosher Barrel Cured Hot Dill (Hebrew National)	1 pkg	23	0	0
Kosher Chips (Hebrew National)	3 slices (1 oz)	4	0	0
Kosher Crunchy Dills (Vlasic)	1 oz	4	0	0
Kosher Deli (Schorr's)	½ pickle (1 oz)	4	0	0
Kosher Dill Gherkins (Vlasic)	1 oz	4	0	0
Kosher Dill Spears (Vlasic)	1 oz	4	0	0
Kosher Halves (Claussen)	1 half	9	—	tr
Kosher Halves (Hebrew National)	⅓ pickle (1 oz)	4	0	0
Kosher Halves (Rosoff's)	⅓ pickle (1 oz)	4	0	0
Kosher Halves (Schorr's)	⅓ pickle (1 oz)	4	0	0
Kosher Large (Hebrew National)	⅙ pickle (1 oz)	4	0	0
Kosher Slices (Claussen)	1	1	—	tr
Kosher Snack Chunks (Vlasic)	1 oz	4	0	0
Kosher Spears (Hebrew National)	½ spear (1 oz)	4	0	0
Kosher Spears (Schorr's)	½ spear (1 oz)	4	0	0
Kosher Whole (Claussen)	1	9	—	tr
Kosher Whole (Schorr's)	⅓ pickle (1 oz)	4	0	0
No Garlic Dill Spears (Vlasic)	1 oz	4	0	0
No Garlic Dills (Claussen)	1	17	—	tr

FOOD	PORTION	CALS.	SAT. FAT	FAT
Original Dills (Vlasic)	1 oz	2	0	0
Polish Snack Chunk Dills (Vlasic)	1 oz	4	0	0
Sour Garlic (Hebrew National)	⅓ pickle (1 oz)	3	0	0
Zesty Crunch Dills (Vlasic)	1 oz	4	0	0
Zesty Dill Snack Chunks (Vlasic)	1 oz	4	0	0
Zesty Dill Spears (Vlasic)	1 oz	4	0	0
dill	1 (2.3 oz)	12	tr	tr
dill, low sodium	1 (2.3 oz)	12	tr	tr
dill, low sodium, sliced	1 slice	1	tr	tr
dill, sliced	1 slice	1	tr	tr
gherkins	3.5 oz	21	—	tr
kosher dill	1 (2.3 oz)	12	tr	tr
polish dill	1 (2.3 oz)	12	tr	tr
quick sour	1 (1.2 oz)	4	tr	tr
quick sour, low sodium	1 (1.2 oz)	4	tr	tr
quick sour, sliced	1 slice	1	tr	tr
sweet	1 (1.2 oz)	41	tr	tr
sweet, low sodium	1 (1.2 oz)	41	tr	tr
sweet, sliced	1 slice	7	tr	tr
sweet gherkin	1 sm (½ oz)	20	tr	tr

PIE

(see also PIE CRUST)

CANNED FILLING

FOOD	PORTION	CALS.	SAT. FAT	FAT
Mincemeat Condensed (None Such)	¼ pkg	220	—	2
Mincemeat Old Fashioned (S&W)	½ cup	206	—	2
Mincemeat Ready-to-Use (None Such)	⅓ cup	200	—	1
Mincemeat Read-to-Use w/ Brandy & Rum (None Such)	⅓ cup	220	—	2
Pumpkin Pie Mix (Libby's)	1 cup	210	—	0
pumpkin pie mix	1 cup	282	tr	tr

FROZEN

FOOD	PORTION	CALS.	SAT. FAT	FAT
Apple (Banquet)	1 slice (3.3 oz)	250	—	11
Apple (McMillin's)	4 oz	430	—	23
Apple (Mrs. Smith's)	⅒ of 10 in pie (4.6 oz)	280	3	12
Apple (Mrs. Smith's)	⅙ of 8 in pie (4.3 oz)	270	2	11

FOOD	PORTION	CALS.	SAT. FAT	FAT
Apple (Mrs. Smith's)	⅛ of 9 in pie (4.6 oz)	370	4	18
Apple (Pet-Ritz)	⅙ pie (4.33 oz)	330	—	12
Apple (Weight Watchers)	1 slice (3.5 oz)	165	3	4
Apple Cranberry (Mrs. Smith's)	⅙ of 8 in pie (4.3 oz)	280	2	11
Apple Homestyle (Sara Lee)	1 slice (4 oz)	280	—	12
Apple Homestyle High (Sara Lee)	1 slice (4.9 oz)	400	—	23
Apple Lattice Ready To Serve (Mrs. Smith's)	⅕ of 8 in pie (4.6 oz)	310	3	13
Apple SmartStyle (Mrs. Smith's)	⅙ of 8 in pie (4 oz)	220	1	5
Apple Streusel Free & Light (Sara Lee)	1 slice (2.9 oz)	170	—	2
Banana (Banquet)	1 slice (2.3 oz)	180	—	10
Banana Cream (Mrs. Smith's)	¼ of 8 in pie (3.4 oz)	250	3	9
Banana Cream (Pet-Ritz)	⅙ pie (2.33 oz)	170	—	9
Berry (McMillin's)	4 oz	430	—	23
Berry (Mrs. Smith's)	⅙ of 8 in pie (4.3 oz)	280	2	11
Blackberry (Banquet)	1 slice (3.3 oz)	270	—	11
Blackberry (Mrs. Smith's)	⅙ of 8 in pie (4.3 oz)	280	2	11
Blueberry (Banquet)	1 slice (3.3 oz)	270	—	11
Blueberry (Mrs. Smith's)	⅙ of 8 in pie	260	2	11
Blueberry (Pet-Ritz)	⅙ pie (4.33 oz)	370	—	12
Blueberry Cheese Yogurt SmartStyle (Mrs. Smith's)	¼ of 7 in pie (4.2 oz)	270	3	8
Blueberry Homestyle (Sara Lee)	1 slice (4 oz)	300	—	12
Boston Cream (Mrs. Smith's)	⅛ of 8 in pie (2.4 oz)	170	2	5
Cherry (Banquet)	1 slice (3.3 oz)	250	—	11
Cherry (McMillin's)	4 oz	430	—	24
Cherry (Mrs. Smith's)	1/10 of 10 in pie (4.6 oz)	410	—	18
Cherry (Mrs. Smith's)	⅙ of 8 in pie	270	2	11
Cherry (Mrs. Smith's)	⅛ of 9 in pie (4.6 oz)	320	3	13
Cherry (Pet-Ritz)	⅙ pie (4.33 oz)	300	—	12

FOOD	PORTION	CALS.	SAT. FAT	FAT
Cherry Homestyle (Sara Lee)	1 slice (4 oz)	270	—	13
Cherry Lattice Ready To Serve (Mrs. Smith's)	⅙ of 8 in pie (4.6 oz)	320	3	13
Cherry SmartStyle (Mrs. Smith's)	⅙ of 8 in pie (4 oz)	230	1	4
Cherry Streusel Free & Light (Sara Lee)	1 slice (3.6 oz)	160	—	2
Chocolate (Banquet)	1 slice (2.3 oz)	190	—	10
Chocolate Cream (Mrs. Smith's)	¼ of 8 in pie (3.4 oz)	290	4	14
Chocolate Cream (Pet-Ritz)	⅙ pie (2.33 oz)	190	—	8
Chocolate Mocha (Weight Watchers)	1 (2.75 oz)	180	tr	4
Chocolate Pudding (McMillin's)	4 oz	420	—	21
Coconut (Banquet)	1 slice (2.3 oz)	190	—	11
Coconut Cream (Mrs. Smith's)	¼ of 8 in pie (3.4 oz)	280	4	14
Coconut Cream (Pet-Ritz)	⅙ pie (2.33 oz)	190	—	8
Coconut Custard (Mrs. Smith's)	⅕ of 8 in pie (5 oz)	280	5	12
Coconut Pudding (McMillin's)	4 oz	450	—	26
Dutch Apple (Mrs. Smith's)	⅒ of 10 in pie (4.6 oz)	320	3	12
Dutch Apple (Mrs. Smith's)	⅙ of 8 in pie	310	3	13
Dutch Apple (Mrs. Smith's)	⅙ of 9 in pie (4.5 oz)	300	3	12
Dutch Apple Homestyle (Sara Lee)	1 slice (4 oz)	300	—	12
Egg Custard (Pet-Ritz)	⅙ pie (4.0 oz)	200	—	8
French Silk Cream (Mrs. Smith's)	⅕ of 8 in pie (4.8 oz)	410	6	21
Hearty Pumpkin (Mrs. Smith's)	⅕ of 8 in pie (5.2 oz)	280	3	10
Hyannis Boston Cream Pie (Pepperidge Farm)	1	230	4	10
Lemon (Banquet)	1 slice (2.3 oz)	170	—	9
Lemon (McMillin's)	4 oz	450	—	25
Lemon Cream (Mrs. Smith's)	¼ of 8 in pie (3.4 oz)	270	3	13
Lemon Cream (Pet-Ritz)	⅙ pie (2.33 oz)	190	—	9

FOOD	PORTION	CALS.	SAT. FAT	FAT
Lemon Meringue (Mrs. Smith's)	⅙ of 8 in pie (4.8 oz)	300	2	8
Mince (Mrs. Smith's)	⅙ of 8 in pie (4.3 oz)	300	2	11
Mince (Pet-Ritz)	⅙ pie (4.33 oz)	280	—	9
Mince Homestyle (Sara Lee)	1 slice (4 oz)	300	—	13
Mincemeat (Banquet)	1 slice (3.3 oz)	260	—	11
Mississippi Mud (Pepperidge Farm)	1	310	12	23
Neapolitan Cream (Pet-Ritz)	⅙ pie (2.33 oz)	180	—	10
Peach (Banquet)	1 slice (3.3 oz)	245	—	11
Peach (McMillin's)	4 oz	430	—	24
Peach (Mrs. Smith's)	⅙ of 8 in pie	260	2	11
Peach (Mrs. Smith's)	⅛ of 9 in pie (4.6 oz)	310	3	13
Peach (Pet-Ritz)	⅙ pie (4.33 oz)	320	—	12
Peach Cheese Yogurt SmartStyle (Mrs. Smith's)	¼ of 7 in pie (4.2 oz)	270	3	8
Peach Homestyle (Sara Lee)	1 slice (3.4 oz)	280	—	12
Pecan (Mrs. Smith's)	⅛ of 10 in pie (4.5 oz)	500	4	23
Pecan Homestyle (Sara Lee)	1 slice (3.4 oz)	400	—	18
Pumpkin (Banquet)	1 slice (3.3 oz)	200	—	8
Pumpkin (Mrs. Smith's)	⅙ of 8 in pie (5.2 oz)	270	2	8
Pumpkin (Mrs. Smith's)	⅛ of 10 in pie (5.1 oz)	250	2	8
Pumpkin Homestyle (Sara Lee)	1 slice (4 oz)	240	—	10
Pumpkin Custard (Pet-Ritz)	⅙ pie (4.33 oz)	250	—	9
Raspberry Homestyle (Sara Lee)	1 slice (4 oz)	280	—	13
Red Raspberry (Mrs. Smith's)	⅙ of 8 in pie (4.3 oz)	280	2	11
Strawberry (Banquet)	1 slice (2.3 oz)	170	—	9
Strawberry (McMillin's)	4 oz	400	—	20
Strawberry Banana Yogurt SmartStyle (Mrs. Smith's)	¼ of 7 in pie (4.2 oz)	240	1	5

FOOD	PORTION	CALS.	SAT. FAT	FAT
Strawberry Rhubarb (Mrs. Smith's)	⅕ of 8 in pie (4.8 oz)	520	4	23
Strawberry Rhubarb (Mrs. Smith's)	⅙ of 8 in pie (4.3 oz)	280	2	11
Strawberry Cream (Pet-Ritz)	⅙ pie (2.33 oz)	170	—	9
Strawberry SmartStyle (Mrs. Smith's)	⅕ of 8 in pie (4 oz)	210	1	4
Sweet Potato (Pet-Ritz)	⅙ pie (3.33 oz)	150	—	7
apple	⅛ of 9 in pie (4.4 oz)	297	3	14
blueberry	⅛ of 9 in pie (4.4 oz)	289	2	13
cherry	⅛ of 9 in pie (4.4 oz)	325	3	14
chocolate creme	⅙ of 8 in pie (4 oz)	344	6	22
coconut creme	⅙ of 7 in pie (2.2 oz)	191	5	11
lemon meringue	⅙ of 8 in pie (4.5 oz)	303	2	10
peach	⅙ of 8 in pie (4.1 oz)	261	2	12
HOME RECIPE				
apple	⅛ of 9 in pie (5.4 oz)	411	5	19
banana cream	⅛ of 9 in pie (5.2 oz)	398	6	20
blueberry	⅛ of 9 in pie (5.2 oz)	360	4	18
butterscotch	⅛ of 9 in pie (4.5 oz)	355	5	18
cherry	⅛ of 9 in pie (6.3 oz)	486	5	22
coconut creme	⅛ of 9 in pie (4.7 oz)	396	8	21
custard	⅛ of 9 in pie (4.5 oz)	262	4	11
lemon meringue	⅛ of 9 in pie (4.5 oz)	362	4	16
mince	⅛ of 9 in pie (5.8 oz)	477	4	18
pecan	⅛ of 9 in pie (4.3 oz)	502	5	27
pumpkin	⅛ of 9 in pie (5.4 oz)	316	5	14

FOOD	PORTION	CALS.	SAT. FAT	FAT
vanilla cream	⅙ of 9 in pie (4.4 oz)	350	5	18
MIX				
Banana Cream as prep w/ whole milk (Jell-O)	⅙ of 8 in pie	103	—	3
Boston Cream Classic Dessert (Betty Crocker)	⅛ pie	270	—	6
Chocolate Cream Pie No Bake Dessert (Jell-O)	⅛ pie	260	—	17
Chocolate Mousse (Jell-O)	⅛ pie	259	—	17
Coconut Cream (Jell-O)	⅛ pie	258	—	16
Coconut Cream as prep w/ whole milk (Jell-O)	⅙ of 8 in pie	111	—	4
Key Lime Pie Filling (Royal)	mix for 1 serving	50	0	0
Lemon (Jell-O)	⅙ of 8 in pie	175	—	2
Lemon Meringue No-Bake (Royal)	⅛ pie	210	—	5
Lemon Pie Filling (Royal)	mix for 1 serving	50	0	0
Pumpkin (Jell-O)	⅛ pie	253	—	13
banana cream no-bake	⅛ of 9 in pie (3.2 oz)	231	6	12
chocolate mousse no-bake	⅛ of 9 in pie (3.3 oz)	247	8	15
coconut creme no-bake	⅛ of 9 in pie (3.3 oz)	259	10	17
READY-TO-EAT				
Apple Homestyle (Entenmann's)	1 serving (2.1 oz)	140	—	7
Coconut Custard (Entenmann's)	1 serving (1.8 oz)	140	—	8
coconut custard	⅙ of 8 in pie (3.6 oz)	271	6	14
custard	⅙ of 9 in pie	330	6	17
pecan	⅙ of 8 in pie (4 oz)	452	4	21
pumpkin	⅙ of 8 in pie (3.8 oz)	229	2	10
SNACK				
Apple (Drake's)	1 (2 oz)	210	—	10
Apple (Tastykake)	1 pkg (113 g)	300	3	12
Banana Creme (Tastykake)	1 pkg (120 g)	380	6	16
Blueberry (Drake's)	1 (2 oz)	210	—	10
Blueberry (Tastykake)	1 pkg (113 g)	310	2	9

FOOD	PORTION	CALS.	SAT. FAT	FAT
Cherry (Drake's)	1 (2 oz)	220	—	10
Cherry (Tastykake)	1 pkg (113 g)	300	2	10
Coconut Creme (Tastykake)	1 pkg (113 g)	380	5	20
French Apple (Tastykake)	1 pkg (120 g)	350	2	11
Lemon (Drake's)	1 (2 oz)	210	—	11
Lemon (Tastykake)	1 pkg (113 g)	320	3	13
Lemon Lime (Tastykake)	1 pkg (113 g)	320	3	13
Marshmallow Banana (Little Debbie)	1 pkg (1.4 oz)	160	3	5
Marshmallow Banana (Little Debbie)	1 pkg (2 oz)	240	5	8
Marshmallow Banana (Little Debbie)	1 pkg (2.7 oz)	320	7	11
Marshmallow Chocolate (Little Debbie)	1 pkg (1.4 oz)	160	3	5
Marshmallow Chocolate (Little Debbie)	1 pkg (2 oz)	240	5	9
Marshmallow Chocolate (Little Debbie)	1 pkg (2.7 oz)	320	7	11
Oatmeal Creme (Little Debbie)	1 pkg (1.3 oz)	170	2	8
Oatmeal Creme (Little Debbie)	1 pkg (2.5 oz)	300	2	11
Oatmeal Creme (Little Debbie)	1 pkg (3 oz)	360	3	14
Peach (Tastykake)	1 pkg (113 g)	300	3	12
Pecan (Lance)	1 (38 g)	350	3	15
Pineapple Cheese (Tastykake)	1 pkg (120 g)	340	3	13
Pumpkin (Tastykake)	1 pkg (4 oz)	320	4	14
Raisin Creme (Little Debbie)	1 pkg (1.2 oz)	140	1	5
Raisin Creme (Little Debbie)	1 pkg (2.5 oz)	290	3	12
Strawberry (Tastykake)	1 pkg (113 g)	340	3	11
Tasty Klair (Tastykake)	1 pkg (113 g)	400	4	20
apple	1 (3 oz)	266	7	14
apple fried	1 (6.4 oz)	404	3	21
blueberry fried	1 (6.4 oz)	404	3	21
cherry	1 (3 oz)	266	7	14
cherry fried	1 (6.4 oz)	404	3	21
lemon	1 (3 oz)	266	7	14
lemon fried	1 (6.4 oz)	404	3	21

FOOD	PORTION	CALS.	SAT. FAT	FAT
peach fried	1 (6.4 oz)	404	3	21
strawberry fried	1 (6.4 oz)	404	3	21
PIE CRUST				
(*see also* PIE)				
FROZEN				
Oronoque	⅙ pie (1.23 oz)	170	—	12
Oronoque Deep Dish	⅙ pie (1.41 oz)	200	—	13
Pepperidge Farm Patty Shells	1	210	—	15
Pepperidge Farm Puff Pastry Sheets	¼ sheet	260	—	17
Pet-Ritz				
Deep Dish	⅙ pie (1 oz)	130	—	8
Graham Cracker	⅙ pie (0.83 oz)	110	—	6
Regular	⅙ pie (0.83 oz)	110	—	7
Tart Shells	1	150	—	10
baked	⅛ of 9 in pie (0.6 oz)	82	2	5
baked	9 in shell (4.4 oz)	647	13	41
puff pastry baked	1 shell (1.4 oz)	223	2	15
HOME RECIPE				
9-inch crust	1	900	15	60
baked	⅛ of 9 in crust (0.8 oz)	119	2	8
baked	9 in shell (6.3 oz)	949	15	62
MIX				
Betty Crocker	1/16 pkg	120	2	8
Betty Crocker Sticks	1/16 pkg	120	2	8
Flako	⅙ of 9" pie	250	—	15
Pillsbury Mix	⅙ of 2-crust pie	270	—	17
Pillsbury Stick	⅙ of 2-crust pie	270	—	17
as prep	⅛ of 9 in pie (0.7 oz)	100	2	6
as prep	9 in crust (5.6 oz)	801	12	49
READY-TO-EAT				
Chocolate (Ready Crust)	1 (3 in diam)	110	1	5
Chocolate (Ready Crust)	⅛ of 9 in pie	100	1	5
Graham Generic Label	⅛ pie (0.7 oz)	110	3	5
Graham (Ready Crust)	1 (3 in diam)	110	1	5
Graham (Ready Crust)	⅛ of 9 in pie	100	1	5
Honeymaid Graham (Nabisco)	1 slice (0.75 oz)	110	1	6
Nilla (Nabisco)	1 slice (0.75 oz)	110	1	6

FOOD	PORTION	CALS.	SAT. FAT	FAT
Oreo (Nabisco)	1 slice (0.75 oz)	110	1	6
chocolate cookie crumb, baked	⅛ of 9 in pie (1 oz)	139	2	9
chocolate cookie crumb, baked	9 in crust (7.7 oz)	1130	15	69
chocolate cookie crumb, chilled	⅛ of 9 in pie (1 oz)	142	2	9
chocolate cookie crumb, chilled	9 in crust (7.8 oz)	1127	15	69
graham cracker, baked	⅛ of 9 in pie (1 oz)	148	2	8
graham cracker, baked	9 in crust (8.4 oz)	1181	12	60
graham cracker, chilled	⅛ of 9 in pie (1 oz)	150	2	8
graham cracker, chilled	9 in crust (8.6 oz)	1182	12	60
vanilla wafer cracker crumbs, baked	⅛ of 9 in pie (0.8 oz)	119	2	8
vanilla wafer cracker crumbs, baked	9 in crust (6.1 oz)	937	13	64
vanilla wafer cracker crumbs, chilled	⅛ of 9 in pie (0.8 oz)	117	2	8
vanilla wafer cracker crumbs, chilled	9 in crust (6.2 oz)	934	13	64
REFRIGERATED				
Pillsbury All Ready	⅛ of 2-crust pie	240	—	15
PIEROGI				
FROZEN				
Potato and Cheddar Cheese (Mrs. T's)	1 (1.3 oz)	60	—	tr
Potato and Onion (Mrs. T's)	1 (1.3 oz)	50	—	tr
Potato Cheese (Empire)	3 (4.6 oz)	260	3	6
Potato Cheese (Golden)	3 (4 oz)	250	2	8
Potato Onion (Empire)	3 (4.6 oz)	250	1	5
Potato Onion (Golden)	3 (4 oz)	210	2	6
Sauerkraut (Mrs. T's)	1	60	—	0
TAKE-OUT				
pierogi	¾ cup (4.4 oz)	307	7	19
PIGEON PEAS				
DRIED				
cooked	½ cup	102	tr	tr
cooked	1 cup	204	1	tr

FOOD	PORTION	CALS.	SAT. FAT	FAT
PIGNOLIA				
(*see* PINE NUTS)				
PIG'S EARS AND FEET				
Pickled Feet Hormel	2 oz	80	2	6
Pickled Hocks Hormel	2 oz	110	3	8
ears, frzn, simmered	1 ear (3.7 oz)	183	—	12
feet, pickled	1 oz	58	2	5
feet, pickled	1 lb	923	25	73
feet, simmered	2.5 oz	138	3	9
PIKE				
FRESH				
northern, cooked	3 oz	96	tr	1
northern, cooked	½ fillet (5.4 oz)	176	tr	1
northern, raw	3 oz	75	tr	1
roe, raw	3.5 oz	130	—	2
walleye, baked	3 oz	101	tr	1
walleye, fillet, baked	4.4 oz	147	tr	2
PILLNUTS				
pillnuts, canarytree, dried	1 oz	204	9	23
PIMIENTOS				
Dromedary	1 oz	10	0	0
canned	1 tbsp	3	tr	tr
canned	1 slice	0	0	0
PINE NUTS				
pignolia, dried	1 tbsp	51	1	5
pignolia, dried	1 oz	146	2	14
pinyon, dried	1 oz	161	3	17
PINEAPPLE				
CANNED				
All Cuts Juice Pack (Dole)	½ cup	70	—	tr
All Cuts Syrup Pack (Dole)	½ cup	90	0	tr
Chunk (Empress)	4 oz	70	0	0
Crushed (Empress)	4 oz	70	0	0
Crushed (Libby)	1 cup with juice	140	0	0
Hawaiian Slice in Heavy Syrup (S&W)	½ cup	90	0	0
Hawaiian Slice Juice Pack (S&W)	½ cup	70	0	0
Sliced (Empress)	4 oz	70	0	0

FOOD	PORTION	CALS.	SAT. FAT	FAT
Sliced in Unsweetened Juice (Libby)	1 cup with juice	140	0	0
Sliced Unsweetened (S&W)	½ cup	60	0	0
chunks in heavy syrup	1 cup	199	tr	tr
chunks juice pack	1 cup	150	tr	tr
crushed in heavy syrup	1 cup	199	tr	tr
slices in heavy syrup	1 slice	45	tr	tr
slices in light syrup	1 slice	30	tr	tr
slices juice pack	1 slice	35	tr	tr
slices water pack	1 slice	19	tr	tr
tidbits in heavy syrup	1 cup	199	tr	tr
tidbits in juice	1 cup	150	tr	tr
tidbits in water	1 cup	79	tr	tr
FRESH				
Chiquita	1 cup	90	—	1
Dole	2 slices	90	—	1
diced	1 cup	77	tr	tr
slice	1 slice	42	tr	tr
FROZEN				
chunks sweetened	½ cup	104	tr	tr
JUICE				
Bright & Early Frozen	8 fl oz	120	0	0
Dole 100% frzn as prep	8 oz	90	0	0
Dole refrigerated	6 oz	90	0	0
Minute Maid Box	8.45 fl oz	130	0	0
Minute Maid Frozen	8 fl oz	130	0	0
S&W Unsweetened	6 oz	100	0	0
Tree Top	6 oz	100	0	0
Veryfine 100%	8 oz	125	0	0
canned	1 cup	139	tr	tr
frzn, as prep	1 cup	129	tr	tr
frzn, not prep	6 oz	387	tr	tr
PINK BEANS				
CANNED				
Goya Spanish Style	7.5 oz	140	—	tr
DRIED				
cooked	1 cup	252	tr	1
PINTO BEANS				
CANNED				
Allen	½ cup (4.5 oz)	110	0	1
Brown Beauty	½ cup (4.5 oz)	110	0	1

FOOD	PORTION	CALS.	SAT. FAT	FAT
East Texas Fair	½ cup (4.5 oz)	110	0	1
Gebhardt	4 oz	100	—	tr
Goya Spanish	7.5 oz	140	—	1
Green Giant	½ cup	90	—	1
Green Giant Picante	½ cup	100	—	1
Luck's Seasoned w/ Pork & Onions	7.5 oz	220	—	6
Old El Paso	½ cup	100	0	0
Progresso	½ cup	110	—	tr
Trappey Jalapinto With Bacon	½ cup (4.5 oz)	120	1	1
Trappey With Bacon	½ cup (4.5 oz)	120	1	1
pinto	1 cup	186	tr	1
DRIED				
Arrowhead	¼ cup (1.5 oz)	150	0	1
Hurst	1.2 oz	120	0	1
Hurst with Spanish Seasoning	1.3 oz	120	0	1
cooked	1 cup	235	tr	1
raw	3.5 oz	62	—	1
FROZEN				
cooked	3 oz	152	tr	tr
SPROUTS				
cooked	3.5 oz	22	—	tr
raw	3.5 oz	62	—	1

PINYON
(*see* PINE NUTS)

PISTACHIOS

FOOD	PORTION	CALS.	SAT. FAT	FAT
Dry Roasted (Planters)	1 oz	170	—	15
Lance	1 pkg (32 g)	100	1	8
Red Salted (Planters)	1 oz	170	2	14
Red Tint (Fisher)	1 oz	170	3	15
Shelled (Dole)	1 oz	163	—	14
Shells On (Dole)	1 oz	90	—	7
dried	1 oz	164	2	14
dried	1 cup	739	8	62
dry roasted	1 oz	172	2	15
dry roasted salted	1 oz	172	2	15
dry roasted salted	1 cup	776	9	68

PITANGA

FOOD	PORTION	CALS.	SAT. FAT	FAT
fresh	1	2	—	tr
fresh	1 cup	57	—	1

FOOD	PORTION	CALS.	SAT. FAT	FAT
PIZZA				
DOUGH				
House of Pasta frozen	⅛ of 14 in pie (1.9 oz)	140	0	1
Jiffy as prep	¼ crust	180	3	3
FROZEN				
Celeste				
Canadian Style Bacon	1 (9.25 oz)	550	—	26
Cheese	1 (6.5 oz)	500	—	24
Deluxe	1 (8.25 oz)	600	—	32
Pepperoni	1 (6.75 oz)	540	—	29
Sausage	1 (7.5 oz)	580	—	32
Sausage & Mushroom	1 (9.25 oz)	600	—	32
Supreme	1 (9 oz)	690	—	39
Empire	½ pie (5 oz)	340	7	13
3 Pack	1 (3 oz)	210	4	9
Bagel	1 (2 oz)	150	3	5
English Muffin	1 (2 oz)	130	3	5
Fox Deluxe				
Golden Topping	½ pizza	240	—	11
Hamburger	½ pizza	260	—	12
Pepperoni	½ pizza	250	—	13
Sausage	½ pizza	260	—	13
Sausage & Pepperoni	½ pizza	260	—	13
Healthy Choice				
French Bread Cheese	1 (5.6 oz)	310	2	4
French Bread Sausage	1 (6 oz)	330	2	4
French Bread Supreme	1 (6.35 oz)	340	2	6
French Bread Pepperoni	1 (6 oz)	360	4	9
Jeno's				
4-Pack Cheese	1 pizza	160	—	8
4-Pack Combination	1 pizza	180	—	9
4-Pack Hamburger	1 pizza	180	—	9
4-Pack Pepperoni	1 pizza	170	—	9
4-Pack Sausage	1 pizza	180	—	9
Crisp 'N Tasty Canadian Bacon	½ pizza	250	—	11
Crisp 'N Tasty Cheese	½ pizza	270	—	14
Crisp 'N Tasty Hamburger	½ pizza	290	—	15
Crisp 'N Tasty Pepperoni	½ pizza	280	—	15
Crisp 'N Tasty Sausage	½ pizza	300	—	16
Crisp 'N Tasty Sausage & Pepperoni	½ pizza	300	—	16

FOOD	PORTION	CALS.	SAT. FAT	FAT
Jeno's *(cont.)*				
Microwave Pizza Rolls Pepperoni & Cheese	6	240	—	13
Microwave Pizza Rolls Sausage & Cheese	6	250	—	13
Pizza Rolls Cheese	6	240	—	12
Pizza Rolls Hamburger	6	240	—	13
Pizza Rolls Pepperoni & Cheese	6	230	—	13
Pizza Rolls Sausage & Pepperoni	6	230	—	13
Kid Cuisine				
Cheese	1 (6.85 oz)	380	—	12
Hamburger	6.85 oz	330	—	10
Mega Meal Cheese	1 (9.7 oz)	430	—	7
Lean Cuisine French Bread Cheese	1 pkg (6 oz)	350	4	8
Lean Cuisine French Bread Deluxe	1 pkg (6.1 oz)	350	3	6
Lean Cuisine French Bread Pepperoni	1 pkg (5.25 oz)	330	3	7
MicroMagic				
Deep Dish Combination	1 (6.5 oz)	605	—	34
Deep Dish Pepperoni	1 (6.5 oz)	615	—	32
Deep Dish Sausage	1 (6.5 oz)	590	—	31
Mr. P's				
Combination	½ pizza	260	—	13
Golden Topping	½ pizza	240	—	11
Hamburger	½ pizza	260	—	12
Pepperoni	½ pizza	250	—	13
Sausage	½ pizza	260	—	13
Pappalo's				
French Bread Cheese	1 pizza	360	—	15
French Bread Combination	1 pizza	430	—	21
French Bread Pepperoni	1 pizza	410	—	20
French Bread Sausage	1 pizza	410	—	18
Pan Combination	⅙ pizza	340	—	15
Pan Hamburger	⅙ pizza	310	—	12
Pan Pepperoni	⅙ pizza	330	—	14
Pan Sausage	⅙ pizza	360	—	18
Thin Crust Combination	⅙ pizza	260	—	10
Thin Crust Hamburger	⅙ pizza	240	—	8

FOOD	PORTION	CALS.	SAT. FAT	FAT
Thin Crust Pepperoni	⅙ pizza	270	—	11
Thin Crust Sausage	⅙ pizza	250	—	9
Pepperidge Farm				
Croissant Pastry Cheese	1	430	—	23
Croissant Pastry Deluxe	1	440	—	23
Croissant Pastry Pepperoni	1	420	—	22
Pillsbury Microwave				
Cheese	½ pizza	240	—	10
Combination	½ pizza	310	—	15
French Bread	1 pizza	370	—	15
French Bread Pepperoni	1 pizza	430	—	19
French Bread Sausage	1 pizza	410	—	16
French Bread Sausage & Pepperoni	1 pizza	450	—	21
Pepperoni	½ pizza	300	—	15
Sausage	½ pizza	280	—	13
Stouffer's				
French Bread Bacon Cheddar	1 piece (5.8 oz)	440	7	22
French Bread Cheese	1 piece (5.2 oz)	350	5	14
French Bread Cheeseburger	1 piece (6 oz)	440	9	26
French Bread Deluxe	1 piece (6.2 oz)	440	7	22
French Bread Double Cheese	1 piece (5.9 oz)	420	7	19
French Bread Garden Vegetable	1 piece (5.8 oz)	340	4	12
French Bread Pepperoni	1 piece (5.6 oz)	420	6	20
French Bread Pepperoni & Mushroom	1 piece (6.1 oz)	430	6	21
French Bread Sausage	1 piece (6 oz)	420	5	20
French Bread Sausage & Pepperoni	1 piece (6.25 oz)	460	7	25
French Bread Vegetable Deluxe	1 piece (6.4 oz)	380	17	17
French Bread White Pizza	1 piece (5.1 oz)	460	8	28
Lunch Express Deluxe	1 pkg (6.6 oz)	460	8	25
Lunch Express Double Cheese	1 pkg (5.9 oz)	420	7	19
Lunch Express Pepperoni	1 pkg (5.75 oz)	440	8	23
Lunch Express Sausage	1 pkg (6.5 oz)	460	8	25

FOOD	PORTION	CALS.	SAT. FAT	FAT
Stouffer's *(cont.)*				
Lunch Express Sausage And Pepperoni	1 pkg (6.4 oz)	500	9	27
Tombstone				
Double Top Double Cheese	⅙ pie (4.6 oz)	350	10	19
Double Top Pepperoni With Double Cheese	⅙ pie (4.6 oz)	370	11	21
Double Top Sausage & Pepperoni With Double Cheese	⅙ pie (4.6 oz)	360	10	20
For One ½ Less Fat Cheese	1 pie (6.5 oz)	360	5	10
For One ½ Less Fat Pepperoni	1 pie (6.7 oz)	400	25	20
For One ½ Less Fat Supreme	1 pie (7.7 oz)	400	5	13
For One ½ Less Fat Vegetable	1 pie (7.2 oz)	360	4	10
For One Extra Cheese	1 pie (6.9 oz)	540	14	30
For One Italian Sausage	1 pie (7 oz)	560	14	33
For One Pepperoni	1 pie (6.9 oz)	580	15	35
For One Sausage & Pepperoni	1 pie (7 oz)	590	15	37
For One Supreme	1 pie (7.6 oz)	570	14	34
Tombstone 12 in				
Canadian Bacon Tombstone	⅙ pie (5.4 oz)	370	7	16
Deluxe Tombstone	⅙ pie (4.6 oz)	320	7	16
Extra Cheese Tombstone	⅙ pie (5.1 oz)	370	9	17
Hamburger Tombstone	⅙ pie (5.3 oz)	320	8	16
Light Supreme Tombstone	⅙ pie (4.8 oz)	270	4	9
Light Vegetable Tombstone	⅙ pie (4.6 oz)	240	3	7
Pepperoni Tombstone	⅙ pie (5.3 oz)	340	8	18
Sausage Tombstone	⅙ pie (5.3 oz)	320	8	16
Sausage & Mushroom Tombstone	⅙ pie (4.5 oz)	320	7	16
Sausage & Pepperoni Tombstone	⅙ pie (5.3 oz)	340	8	16
Special Order Four Cheese Tombstone	⅙ pie (5.1 oz)	380	10	18

FOOD	PORTION	CALS.	SAT. FAT	FAT
Special Order Four Meat Tombstone	⅙ pie (4.6 oz)	340	8	17
Special Order Pepperoni Tombstone	⅙ pie (5.3 oz)	420	10	21
Special Order Super Supreme Tombstone	⅙ pie (4.7 oz)	340	8	17
Special Order Three Sausage Tombstone	⅙ pie (4.5 oz)	330	8	16
Supreme Tombstone	⅕ pie (4.6 oz)	330	8	17
ThinCrust Four Meat Tombstone	¼ pie (5.1 oz)	410	12	25
ThinCrust Italian Sausage Tombstone	¼ (5.1 oz)	400	11	24
ThinCrust Pepperoni Tombstone	¼ pie (5 oz)	420	13	27
ThinCrust Supreme Tombstone	¼ pie (5.3 oz)	400	11	24
ThinCrust Taco Tombstone	¼ pie (5.1 oz)	380	11	23
ThinCrust Three Cheese Tombstone	¼ pie (4.8 oz)	380	12	22
Tombstone 9 in				
Deluxe Tombstone	⅓ pie (4.5 oz)	320	7	16
Extra Cheese Tombstone	⅓ pie (5.6 oz)	420	9	19
Hamburger Tombstone	⅓ pie (4.1 oz)	310	7	16
Pepperoni Tombstone	⅓ pie (4.1 oz)	340	8	19
Pepperoni & Sausage Tombstone	⅓ pie (5.3 oz)	360	9	21
Sausage Tombstone	⅓ pie (4.1 oz)	310	7	16
Special Order Four Meat Tombstone	⅙ pie (5.2 oz)	390	9	19
Special Order Pepperoni Tombstone	⅙ pie (4.9 oz)	390	10	20
Special Order Super Supreme Tombstone	⅙ pie (5.4 oz)	390	9	20
Special Order Three Sausage Tombstone	⅙ pie (5 oz)	370	9	18
Totino's				
Microwave Cheese	1 pizza	250	—	8
Microwave Pepperoni	1 pizza	280	—	12
Microwave Sausage	1 pizza	320	—	16
Microwave Sausage Pepperoni Combination	1 pizza	310	—	15

FOOD	PORTION	CALS.	SAT. FAT	FAT
Totino's *(cont.)*				
My Classic Deluxe Cheese	⅙ pizza	210	—	9
My Classic Deluxe Combination	⅙ pizza	270	—	14
My Classic Deluxe Pepperoni	⅙ pizza	260	—	13
Totino's Pan				
Pepperoni	⅙ pizza	330	—	14
Sausage & Pepperoni Combination	⅙ pizza	340	—	15
Sausage	⅙ pizza	320	—	13
Three Cheese	⅙ pizza	290	—	10
Totino's Party				
Bacon	½ pizza	370	—	20
Canadian Bacon	½ pizza	310	—	14
Cheese	½ pizza	340	—	17
Combination	½ pizza	380	—	21
Hamburger	½ pizza	370	—	19
Mexican Style	½ pizza	380	—	21
Pepperoni	½ pizza	370	—	20
Sausage	½ pizza	390	—	21
Vegetable	½ pizza	300	—	13
Totino's Slices				
Cheese	1	170	—	7
Combination	1	200	—	10
Pepperoni	1	190	—	9
Sausage	1	200	—	10
Weight Watchers				
Cheese	1 (6.03 oz)	300	2	7
Deluxe Combination	1 (7.32 oz)	320	2	9
Deluxe French Bread	1 (5.94 oz)	260	1	7
Pepperoni	1 (6.08 oz)	320	2	8
Sausage	1 (6.43 oz)	340	2	11
SAUCE				
Contadina				
Pizza Sauce	¼ cup	35	—	3
Pizza Sauce Flavored With Pepperoni	¼ cup	40	1	3
Pizza Sauce With Italian Cheeses	¼ cup	40	—	3
Pizza Squeeze	¼ cup	35	—	3
Ragu Pizza Quick Traditional	3 tbsp (1.7 oz)	35	—	3

FOOD	PORTION	CALS.	SAT. FAT	FAT
TAKE-OUT				
cheese	⅛ of 12 in pie	140	2	3
cheese	12" pie	1121	12	26
cheese, meat & vegetables	⅛ of 12 in pie	184	2	5
cheese, meat & vegetables	12" pie	1472	12	43
pepperoni	⅛ of 12 in pie	181	2	7
pepperoni	12 in pie	1445	18	56

PLANTAINS

All Natural Plantain Chips (Top Banana)	1 oz	150	—	8
FRESH				
sliced, cooked	½ cup	89	—	tr
uncooked	1	218	—	1
TAKE-OUT				
ripe, fried	2.8 oz	214	—	7

PLUMS

CANNED				
Halves Purple Fancy Unpeeled in Extra Heavy Syrup (S&W)	½ cup	135	0	0
Whole Purple Fancy Unpeeled In Extra Heavy Syrup (S&W)	½ cup	135	0	0
Whole Unpeeled Diet (S&W)	½ cup	52	0	0
purple in heavy syrup	3	119	tr	tr
purple in heavy syrup	1 cup	320	tr	tr
purple in light syrup	3	83	tr	tr
purple in light syrup	1 cup	158	tr	tr
purple juice pack	3	55	tr	tr
purple juice pack	1 cup	146	tr	tr
purple water pack	3	39	tr	tr
purple water pack	1 cup	102	tr	tr
FRESH				
Dole	2	70	—	1
plum	1	36	tr	tr
sliced	1 cup	91	tr	1

POI

| poi | ½ cup | 134 | tr | tr |

POKEBERRY SHOOTS

| Allen | ½ cup (4.1 oz) | 35 | 0 | 1 |

FOOD	PORTION	CALS.	SAT. FAT	FAT
FRESH				
cooked	½ cup	16	—	tr
raw	½ cup	18	—	tr
POLLACK				
atlantic, baked	3 oz	100	tr	1
atlantic fillet, baked	5.3 oz	178	tr	2
FROZEN				
Light Fillets (Mrs. Paul's)	1 fillet (4.5 oz)	240	—	11
POMEGRANATES				
pomegranates	1	104	—	tr
POMPANO				
florida, cooked	3 oz	179	4	10
florida, raw	3 oz	140	3	8
POPCORN				
(see also CHIPS, PRETZELS, SNACKS)				
Barrel O' Fun	1 oz	160	1	12
Baked Curl	1 oz	150	2	9
Caramel Corn	1 oz	115	0	1
Corn Pops	1 oz	190	1	16
White Cheddar Pops	1 oz	170	1	13
Cape Cod	½ oz	80	—	5
Cape Cod Light	½ oz	60	—	3
Cheetos Cheddar Cheese	0.5 oz	80	—	6
Chesters	0.5 oz	70	—	3
Chesters Cheddar Cheese	0.5 oz	80	—	5
Chesters Microwave	3 cups	110	—	7
Chesters Microwave Butter Flavored	3 cups	120	—	7
Chesters Microwave Cheese Flavored	3 cups	110	—	8
Cracker Jack	1 oz	120	—	3
Eagle	½ oz	80	—	6
Estee Caramel No Sugar Added	1 cup (1 oz)	120	0	2
Jiffy Pop				
Bag Butter	3 cups	90	1	5
Bag Lite	3 cups	70	tr	3
Bag Regular	3 cups	100	1	6
Glazed Popcorn Clusters	1 oz	120	tr	4
Microwave Butter	4 cups	140	—	7
Microwave Regular	4 cups	140	—	7

FOOD	PORTION	CALS.	SAT. FAT	FAT
Pan Butter	4 cups	130	—	6
Pan Regular	4 cups	130	—	6
Lance Cheese	1 pkg (25 g)	130	1	8
Lance Plain	1 pkg (25 g)	140	2	9
Lance White Cheddar Cheese	1 pkg (25 g)	140	3	9
Louise's Fat-Free Caramel	1 cup (1 oz)	110	0	0
Louise's Low-Fat Buttered	2½ cups (1 oz)	130	1	3
Louise's Low-Fat Lightly Salted	2¾ cups (1 oz)	130	0	2
Newman's Own Oldstyle Picture Show	3½ cups	80	—	1
Microwave Butter	3 cups	140	—	7
Microwave Light Butter	3 cups	90	1	3
Microwave Light Natural	3 cups	90	1	3
Microwave Natural Butter	3 cups	150	2	8
Microwave No Salt	3 cups	140	2	8
Orville Redenbacher				
Gourmet Hot Air	3 cups	40	—	tr
Gourmet Original	3 cups	80	—	4
Gourmet White	3 cups	80	—	4
Microwave Gourmet	3 cups	100	1	6
Microwave Gourmet Butter	3 cups	100	1	6
Microwave Gourmet Butter Toffee	2½ cups	210	3	12
Microwave Gourmet Caramel	2½ cups	240	3	14
Microwave Gourmet Cheddar Cheese	3 cups	130	2	8
Microwave Gourmet Frozen	3 cups	100	1	6
Microwave Gourmet Frozen Butter	3 cups	100	1	6
Microwave Gourmet Light	3 cups	70	1	3
Microwave Gourmet Light Butter	3 cups	70	1	3
Microwave Gourmet Salt Free	3 cups	100	1	6
Microwave Gourmet Salt Free Butter	3 cups	100	1	6
Microwave Gourmet Sour Cream 'N Onion	3 cups	160	3	12

FOOD	PORTION	CALS.	SAT. FAT	FAT
Pillsbury Microwave Butter	3 cups	210	—	13
Pillsbury Microwave Original	3 cups	210	—	13
Pillsbury Microwave Salt Free	3 cups	170	—	7
Pop Secret				
Butter Flavor	3 cups	100	tr	6
Butter Flavor Singles	6 cups	250	3	16
Natural Flavor	3 cups	100	2	6
Natural Flavor Salt Free	3 cups	100	1	6
Pop Chips	1½ cups (1 oz)	130	1	4
Pop Qwiz Butter Flavor	3 cups	100	1	6
Pop Qwiz Natural Flavor	3 cups	100	2	6
Pop Secret Light				
Butter Flavor	3 cups	70	1	3
Butter Flavor Singles	6 cups	140	1	6
Natural Flavor	3 cups	70	tr	3
Natural Flavor Singles	6 cups	150	1	6
Smartfood Cheddar Cheese	0.5 oz	80	—	5
Smartfood Light Butter	0.5 oz	70	—	3
Snyder's Butter	1 oz	140	—	9
Ultra Slim-Fast Lite N' Tasty	½ oz	60	—	2
Weight Watchers Microwave	1 oz	100	—	1
Weight Watchers Ready-to-Eat Butter	0.7 oz	90	—	3
Weight Watchers Ready-to-Eat White Cheddar Cheese	0.7 oz	90	—	4
Wise Tender Eating	½ oz	70	—	6
Wise w/ Real Premium White Cheddar Cheese	½ oz	70	—	5
air-popped	1 cup	30	tr	tr
popped w/ vegetable oil	1 cup	55	1	3
sugar syrup coated	1 cup	135	tr	1

POPOVER

HOME RECIPE

FOOD	PORTION	CALS.	SAT. FAT	FAT
as prep w/ 2% milk	1 (1.4 oz)	87	1	3
as prep w/ whole milk	1 (1.4 oz)	90	1	3
MIX				
as prep	1 (1.2 oz)	67	tr	2

FOOD	PORTION	CALS.	SAT. FAT	FAT

POPPY SEEDS

| poppy seeds | 1 tsp | 15 | tr | 1 |

PORK

(*see also* BACON, BACON SUBSTITUTES, CANADIAN BACON, HAM, LUNCHEON
MEATS/COLD CUTS, SAUSAGE)

The values for cooked pork may differ slightly from values for raw
pork. When meat is cooked some moisture and fat are lost,
changing the nutritive value slightly. As a rule of thumb, it can be
assumed that a 4-oz. raw portion will equal a 3-oz. cooked portion
of meat.

CANNED

FOOD	PORTION	CALS.	SAT. FAT	FAT
Pickled Tidbits (Hormel)	2 oz	100	3	8
FRESH				
Oscar Mayer Sweet Morsel Pork Shoulder Smoked Boneless	3 oz	180	5	15
blade chop, roasted	1 (3.1 oz)	321	10	27
center loin chop, broiled	1 (3.1 oz)	275	7	24
center loin				
lean & fat, braised	3 oz	301	—	22
lean & fat, pan-fried	3 oz	318	—	26
lean only, broiled	3 oz	196	—	9
lean only, pan-fried	3 oz	226	—	14
lean only, roasted	3 oz	204	—	11
center loin, roasted	3 oz	259	7	18
center loin chop				
lean & fat, braised	1 (2.6 oz)	266	—	19
lean & fat, broiled	1 (3.1 oz)	275	—	19
lean & fat, pan-fried	1 (3.1 oz)	333	—	27
lean & fat, roasted	1 (3.1 oz)	268	—	19
lean only, braised	1 (2.1 oz)	166	—	8
lean only, broiled	1 (2.5 oz)	166	—	8
lean only, pan-fried	1 (2.4 oz)	178	—	11
lean only, roasted	1 (2.4 oz)	180	—	10
ham, fresh				
rump half lean & fat, roasted	3 oz	233	—	23
rump half lean only, roasted	3 oz	187	—	9
shank half, lean & fat, roasted	3 oz	258	—	19

FOOD	PORTION	CALS.	SAT. FAT	FAT
ham, fresh *(cont.)*				
shank half, lean only, roasted	3 oz	183	—	9
whole, lean & fat, roasted	3 oz	250	—	18
whole, lean only, roasted	3 oz	187	—	9
half, lean only, roasted	3 oz	187	—	9
leg, loin & shoulder, lean only, roasted	3 oz	198	—	11
loin				
lean & fat, braised	3 oz	312	—	24
lean & fat, broiled	3 oz	294	—	23
lean only, braised	3 oz	232	—	12
lean only, broiled	3 oz	218	—	13
lean only, roasted	3 oz	204	—	12
loin blade				
lean & fat, braised	3 oz	348	—	29
lean & fat, broiled	3 oz	334	—	29
lean & fat, pan-fried	3 oz	352	—	31
lean & fat, roasted	3 oz	310	—	26
lean only, broiled	3 oz	255	—	18
lean only, pan-fried	3 oz	240	—	17
lean only, roasted	3 oz	238	—	16
loin blade chop				
lean & fat, braised	1 (3.1 oz)	321	—	27
lean & fat, braised	1 (2.4 oz)	275	—	23
lean & fat, pan-fried	1 (3.1 oz)	368	—	33
lean only, braised	1 (1.8 oz)	156	—	10
lean only, broiled	1 (2.1 oz)	177	—	13
lean only, pan-fried	1 (2.2 oz)	175	—	12
lean only, roasted	1 (2.5 oz)	198	—	14
loin chop				
lean & fat, braised	1 (2.3 oz)	267	—	20
lean & fat, braised	1 (2.5 oz)	261	—	20
lean & fat, broiled	1 (2.7 oz)	295	—	23
lean & fat, pan-fried	1 (2.9 oz)	337	—	29
lean & fat, roasted	1 (2.8 oz)	274	—	21
lean & fat, roasted	1 (2.9 oz)	262	—	20
lean only, braised	1 (1.8 oz)	147	—	8
lean only, broiled	1 (2.1 oz)	165	—	10
lean only, pan-fried	1 (2 oz)	157	—	9
lean only, roasted	1 (2.3 oz)	167	7	9
loin w/ fat, roasted	3 oz	271	7	21

FOOD	PORTION	CALS.	SAT. FAT	FAT
lungs, braised	3 oz	84	—	3
pancreas, braised	3 oz	186	—	9
rib chop				
lean & fat, braised	1 (2.2 oz)	246	—	18
lean & fat, broiled	1 (2.6 oz)	264	—	20
lean & fat, pan-fried	1 (2.9 oz)	343	—	29
lean & fat, roasted	1 (2.6 oz)	252	—	19
lean only, braised	1 (1.8 oz)	147	—	8
lean only, broiled	1 (2.1 oz)	162	—	9
lean only, pan-fried	1 (2 oz)	160	—	9
lean only, roasted	1 (2.2 oz)	162	—	9
shoulder blade boston steak				
lean & fat, braised	1 (5.6 oz)	594	—	46
lean & fat, broiled	1 (6.5 oz)	647	—	53
lean & fat, roasted	1 (6.5 oz)	594	—	47
lean only, braised	1 (4.6 oz)	382	—	23
lean only, broiled	1 (5.3 oz)	413	—	28
lean only, roasted	1 (5.5 oz)	404	—	27
shoulder, arm picnic				
cured, lean & fat, roasted	3 oz	238	—	18
cured, lean only, roasted	3 oz	145	—	6
lean & fat, braised	3 oz	293	—	22
lean & fat, roasted	3 oz	281	—	22
lean only, braised	3 oz	211	—	10
lean only, roasted	3 oz	194	—	11
shoulder, blade roll, cured, lean & fat	3 oz	304	9	25
shoulder, boston blade				
lean & fat, braised	3 oz	316	—	24
lean & fat, broiled	3 oz	297	—	24
lean & fat, roasted	3 oz	273	—	21
lean only, braised	3 oz	250	—	15
lean only, broiled	3 oz	233	—	16
lean only, roasted	3 oz	218	—	14
shoulder, whole, roasted	3 oz	277	8	22
shoulder, whole, lean only, roasted	3 oz	207	—	13
sirloin chop				
lean & fat, braised	1 (2.4 oz)	250	—	18
lean & fat, broiled	1 (2.8 oz)	278	—	21
lean & fat, roasted	1 (2.8 oz)	244	—	17
lean only, braised	1 (1.9 oz)	149	—	7

FOOD	PORTION	CALS.	SAT. FAT	FAT
sirloin chop *(cont.)*				
lean only, broiled	1 (2.3 oz)	165	—	9
lean only, roasted	1 (2.5 oz)	175	—	10
spareribs, braised	3 oz	338	10	26
spleen, braised	3 oz	127	1	3
tail, simmered	3 oz	336	—	30
tenderloin, lean only, roasted	3 oz	141	1	4

POSOLE
(*see* HOMINY)

POT PIE
FROZEN

FOOD	PORTION	CALS.	SAT. FAT	FAT
Beef (Morton)	7 oz	430	—	31
Beef (Swanson)	7 oz	370	—	19
Beef Hungry Man (Swanson)	16 oz	610	—	31
Beef Pie (Stouffer's)	1 pkg (10 oz)	450	9	26
Chicken (Empire)	1 (8.1 oz)	440	9	26
Chicken (Swanson)	7 oz	380	—	22
Chicken Homestyle (Swanson)	8 oz	410	—	21
Chicken Hungry Man (Swanson)	16 oz	630	—	35
Chicken Pie (Stouffer's)	1 pkg (10 oz)	520	8	33
Chicken Pie (Stouffer's)	½ pkg (8 oz)	460	30	30
Turkey (Empire)	1 (8.1 oz)	470	5	23
Turkey (Stouffer's)	1 cup (8 oz)	500	8	31
Turkey (Stouffer's)	1 pkg (10 oz)	530	9	33
Turkey (Swanson)	7 oz	380	—	21
Turkey Hungry Man (Swanson)	16 oz	650	—	36
Vegetable Pie w/ Beef (Banquet)	7 oz	510	—	33
Vegetable Pie w/ Beef (Morton)	7 oz	430	—	31
Vegetable Pie w/ Chicken (Banquet)	7 oz	550	—	36
Vegetable Pie w/ Chicken (Morton)	7 oz	420	—	28
Vegetable Pie w/ Turkey (Banquet)	7 oz	510	—	31
Vegetable Pie w/ Turkey (Morton)	7 oz	420	—	28

FOOD	PORTION	CALS.	SAT. FAT	FAT
HOME RECIPE				
beef, baked	⅙ of 9″ pie (7.4 oz)	515	8	30
chicken	⅙ of 9″ pie (8.1 oz)	545	10	31
POTATO				
(*see also* CHIPS)				
CANNED				
Butterfield Diced	⅔ cup (5.7 oz)	100	0	0
Butterfield Sliced	½ cup (5.7 oz)	100	0	0
Butterfield Whole	2½ pieces (5.6 oz)	90	0	0
Hormel Au Gratin & Bacon	1 can (7.5 oz)	250	5	14
Hormel Micro Cup Meals Scalloped Potatoes & Ham	1 cup (10.4 oz)	360	7	23
Hormel Micro Cup Meals Scalloped Potatoes With Ham	1 cup (7.5 oz)	260	5	16
Hormel Scalloped & Ham	1 can (7.5 oz)	260	5	16
Hunt's Whole New	4 oz	70	—	tr
S&W New Potatoes Extra Small	½ cup	45	0	0
Seneca	½ cup	80	0	0
Sunshine Whole	2½ pieces (5.6 oz)	90	0	0
potatoes	½ cup	54	tr	tr
FRESH				
Yukon Gold	1 (5.3 oz)	110	—	0
baked, skin only	1 skin (2 oz)	115	tr	tr
baked w/ skin	1 (6.5 oz)	220	tr	tr
baked w/o skin	1 (5 oz)	145	tr	tr
baked w/o skin	½ cup	57	tr	tr
boiled	½ cup	68	tr	tr
microwaved	1 (7 oz)	212	tr	tr
microwaved w/o skin	½ cup	78	tr	tr
raw w/o skin	1 (3.9 oz)	88	tr	tr
FROZEN				
Au Gratin (Stouffer's)	½ cup (2.25 oz)	130	3	6
Baked Potato Broccoli & Cheese (Weight Watchers)	1	270	6	6
Baked Potato Broccoli & Ham (Weight Watchers)	11.5 oz	280	3	17

FOOD	PORTION	CALS.	SAT. FAT	FAT
Baked Potato Chicken Divan (Weight Watchers)	1	280	2	7
Baked Potato Homestyle Turkey (Weight Watchers)	1	250	2	7
Baked With Broccoli And Cheese (Budget Gourmet)	1 pkg (10.5 oz)	300	4	10
Broccoli & Cheese Over Baked Potato (Stouffer's)	1 pkg (10.1 oz)	320	6	15
Broccoli & Cheese Over Baked Potato Lunch Expree (Stouffer's)	1 pkg (10.25 oz)	250	4	9
Cheddar Broccoli Potatoes (Healthy Choice)	1 meal (10.5 oz)	310	2	5
Cheddar Browns (Ore Ida)	1 patty (3 oz)	90	1	3
Cheddar Cheese & Bacon Over Baked Potato (Stouffer's)	1 pkg (9.4 oz)	380	8	22
Cheddared Potatoes (Budget Gourmet)	1 pkg (5.5 oz)	260	—	16
Cheddared Potatoes w/ Broccoli (Budget Gourmet)	1 pkg (5 oz)	150	—	7
Cottage Fries (Ore Ida)	3 oz	130	1	4
Crispers! (Ore Ida)	3 oz	220	2	13
Crispers! Nacho (Ore Ida)	10 pieces (3 oz)	170	3	9
Crispers! Texas (Ore Ida)	3 oz	170	3	10
Crispy Crowns (Ore Ida)	12 pieces (3 oz)	100	2	11
Crispy Crunchers (Ore Ida)	12 pieces (3 oz)	160	2	9
Deep Fries Crinkle Cuts (Ore Ida)	18 pieces (3 oz)	160	1	7
Deep Fries French Fries (Ore Ida)	22 pieces (3 oz)	160	1	7
Deluxe Cheddar (Lean Cuisine)	1 pkg (10.4 oz)	270	4	10
Dinner Fries Country Style (Ore Ida)	8 pieces (3 oz)	110	1	3
Fast Fries (Ore Ida)	23 pieces (3 oz)	140	2	6
Fast Fries Ranch (Ore Ida)	22 pieces (3 oz)	150	2	7
French Fries (MicroMagic)	1 pkg (3 oz)	290	—	13
Garden Potato Casserole (Healthy Choice)	1 meal (9.25 oz)	200	2	4
Golden Crinkles (Ore Ida)	16 pieces (3 oz)	120	1	4
Golden Fries (Ore Ida)	3 oz	120	1	4
Golden Patties (Ore Ida)	1 (2.5 oz)	140	2	7

FOOD	PORTION	CALS.	SAT. FAT	FAT
Golden Twirls (Ore Ida)	28 pieces (3 oz)	160	1	7
Hash Browns Country Style (Ore Ida)	1 cup (2.6 oz)	60	0	0
Hash Browns Shredded (Ore Ida)	1 patty (3 oz)	70	0	0
Hash Browns Southern Style (Ore Ida)	¾ cup (3 oz)	70	0	0
Hot Tots (Ore Ida)	9 pieces (3 oz)	150	1	6
Mashed Natural Butter (Ore Ida)	½ cup (2.1 oz)	80	1	2
Microwave Crinkle Cuts (Ore Ida)	1 pkg (3.5 oz)	180	2	8
O'Brien Potatoes (Ore Ida)	¾ cup (3 oz)	60	0	0
One Serve Potatoes & Broccoli in Cheese Sauce (Green Giant)	1 pkg	130	2	5
One Serve Potatoes Au Gratin (Green Giant)	1 pkg	200	4	10
Pixie Crinkles (Ore Ida)	33 pieces (3 oz)	140	1	5
Potato Pancakes (Golden)	1 (1.33 oz)	71	0	3
Potato Pancakes Latkes (Empire)	1 (2 oz)	80	2	2
Potato Pancakes Latkes Mini (Empire)	2 (2 oz)	90	1	3
Scalloped (Stouffer's)	½ cup (2.25 oz)	130	1	6
Shoestrings (Ore Ida)	38 pieces (3 oz)	150	1	5
Skinny Fries (MicroMagic)	1 pkg (3 oz)	350	—	15
Snackin' Fries (Ore Ida)	1 pkg (5 oz)	180	4	20
Snackin' Fries Extra Zesty (Ore Ida)	1 pkg (5 oz)	180	4	20
Stuffed Potatoes w/ Cheddar Cheese (Oh Boy!)	1 (6 oz)	130	—	4
Stuffed Potatoes w/ Real Bacon (Oh Boy!)	1 (6 oz)	120	—	3
Tater ABC's (Ore Ida)	10 pieces (3 oz)	190	5	11
Tater Tots (Ore Ida)	9 pieces (3 oz)	160	2	8
Tater Tots w/ Bacon (Ore Ida)	9 pieces (3 oz)	150	2	7
Tater Tots w/ Onion (Ore Ida)	9 pieces (3 oz)	150	2	7
Three Cheese Potatoes (Budget Gourmet)	1 pkg (5.75 oz)	220	—	11
Toaster Hash Browns (Ore Ida)	2 patties (3.5 oz)	190	2	12

FOOD	PORTION	CALS.	SAT. FAT	FAT
Topped Broccoli & Cheese (Ore Ida)	½ (6 oz)	150	2	4
Topped Salsa & Cheese (Ore Ida)	½ (5.5 oz)	160	2	5
Topped Vegetable Primavera (Ore Ida)	1 (6.13 oz)	160	2	5
Twice Baked Butter Flavor (Ore Ida)	1 (5 oz)	200	3	9
Twice Baked Cheddar Cheese (Ore Ida)	1 (5 oz)	190	3	8
Twice Baked Ranch (Ore Ida)	1 (5 oz)	180	2	6
Twice Baked Sour Cream & Chives (Ore Ida)	1 (5 oz)	180	2	6
Waffle Fries (Ore Ida)	15 pieces (3 oz)	140	2	5
Wedges With Skin (Ore Ida)	9 pieces (3 oz)	110	1	3
Zesties! (Ore Ida)	9 pieces (3 oz)	160	2	9
french fries	10	111	2	4
french fries, thick cut	10	109	2	4
hash browns	½ cup	170	4	9
potato puffs	1 puff	16	tr	1
potato puffs	½ cup	138	3	7
HOME RECIPE				
au gratin	½ cup	160	6	9
hash browns	½ cup	163	4	11
mashed	½ cup	111	1	4
o'brien	1 cup	157	2	3
potato dumpling	3.5 oz	334	—	1
potato pancakes	1 (1.3 oz)	101	1	7
scalloped	½ cup	105	3	5
MIX				
Au Gratin, as prep (Betty Crocker)	½ cup	140	—	5
Cheddar 'N Bacon, as prep (Betty Crocker)	½ cup	140	—	5
Cheddar & Bacon Casserole (French's)	½ cup	130	—	5
Cheesy Scalloped, as prep (Betty Crocker)	½ cup	140	—	5
Creamy Italian Scalloped (French's)	½ cup	120	—	3
Creamy Stroganoff (French's)	½ cup	130	—	4

FOOD	PORTION	CALS.	SAT. FAT	FAT
Crispy Top Scalloped w/ Savory Onion (French's)	½ cup	140	—	5
Hash Browns, as prep (Betty Crocker)	½ cup	160	—	6
Hash Browns, as prep w/o salt (Betty Crocker)	½ cup	160	—	6
Homestyle (Betty Crocker)				
American Cheese, as prep	½ cup	140	—	5
Broccoli, Au Gratin, as prep	½ cup	130	—	5
Cheddar Cheese, as prep	½ cup	140	—	5
Cheesy Scalloped, as prep	½ cup	140	—	5
Julienne, as prep (Betty Crocker)	½ cup	130	—	5
Mashed Potato Flakes (Hungry Jack)	½ cup	40	—	7
Mashed, not prep (Country Store)	⅓ cup	70	0	0
Potato Buds, as prep (Betty Crocker)	½ cup	130	—	6
Potato Buds, as prep w/o salt (Betty Crocker)	½ cup	130	—	6
Potatoes & Cheese 2-Cheese (Kraft)	½ cup	130	2	4
Potatoes & Cheese Au Gratin (Kraft)	½ cup	130	2	5
Potatoes & Cheese Broccoli Au Gratin (Kraft)	½ cup	120	2	5
Potatoes & Cheese Scalloped (Kraft)	½ cup	140	2	5
Potatoes & Cheese Scalloped With Ham (Kraft)	½ cup	150	2	5
Potatoes & Cheese Sour Cream With Chives (Kraft)	½ cup	150	2	5
Real Cheese Scalloped (French's)	½ cup	140	—	5
Real Sour Cream and Chives (French's)	½ cup	150	—	7

FOOD	PORTION	CALS.	SAT. FAT	FAT
Scalloped & Ham, as prep (Betty Crocker)	½ cup	160	—	6
Scalloped, as prep (Betty Crocker)	½ cup	140	—	5
Smokey Cheddar, as prep (Betty Crocker)	½ cup	140	—	5
Sour Cream 'N Chive, as prep (Betty Crocker)	½ cup	140	—	5
Spuds Mashed (French's)	½ cup	140	—	7
Tangy Au Gratin (French's)	½ cup	130	—	5
Twice Baked (Betty Crocker)				
Bacon And Cheddar, as prep	½ cup	210	—	11
Herbed Butter, as prep	½ cup	220	—	13
Mild Cheddar With Onion, as prep	½ cup	190	—	10
Sour Cream & Chive, as prep	½ cup	200	—	11
au gratin	4½ oz	127	4	6
instant mashed flakes, as prep w/ whole milk & butter	½ cup	118	4	6
instant mashed flakes, not prep	½ cup	78	tr	tr
instant mashed granules, as prep w/ whole milk & butter	½ cup	114	3	5
instant mashed granules, not prep	½ cup	372	1	1
scalloped	4½ oz	127	4	6
REFRIGERATED				
Simply Potatoes				
Au Gratin	¼ pkg (3 oz)	130	—	8
Hash Browns	⅙ pkg (4 oz)	100	—	tr
Hash Browns Onion	⅙ pkg (4 oz)	120	—	tr
Hash Browns Southwest Style	⅙ pkg (4 oz)	100	—	tr
Mashed	⅙ pkg (4 oz)	90	—	2
Scalloped	¼ pkg (3 oz)	100	—	5
SHELF STABLE				
Augratin (Pantry Express)	½ cup	120	—	5
TAKE-OUT				
au gratin w/ cheese	½ cup	178	4	10

FOOD	PORTION	CALS.	SAT. FAT	FAT
baked, topped w/ cheese sauce	1	475	11	29
baked, topped w/ cheese sauce & bacon	1	451	10	26
baked, topped w/ cheese sauce & broccoli	1	402	9	14
baked, topped w/ cheese sauce & chili	1	481	13	22
baked, topped w/ sour cream & chives	1	394	10	22
curry	1 serving (6 oz)	292	—	16
french fried in vegetable oil	1 reg	235	4	12
french fried in vegetable oil	1 lg	355	6	19
french fried in beef tallow	1 reg	237	6	12
french fried in beef tallow	1 lg	358	9	19
hash browns	½ cup	151	4	9
mashed w/ whole milk & margarine	⅓ cup	66	tr	tr
mustard potato salad	3.5 oz	120	0	6
potato salad	⅓ cup	108	tr	6
potato salad	½ cup	179	2	10
potato salad w/ vegetables	3.5 oz	120	1	3
scalloped	½ cup	127	—	5

POTATO STARCH

FOOD	PORTION	CALS.	SAT. FAT	FAT
Manischewitz	1 cup	570	—	0
potato starch	3.5 oz	335	—	tr

POUT

FRESH

FOOD	PORTION	CALS.	SAT. FAT	FAT
ocean, baked	3 oz	86	tr	1
ocean fillet, baked	4.8 oz	139	1	2

PRESERVES

(see JAM/JELLY/PRESERVES)

PRETZELS

(see also CHIPS, POPCORN, SNACKS)

FOOD	PORTION	CALS.	SAT. FAT	FAT
A & Eagle	1 oz	110	—	2
A & Eagle Beer	1 oz	110	—	2
Barrel O' Fun Mini	1 oz	110	0	1
Barrel O' Fun Sticks	1 oz	110	0	1
Barrel O' Fun Twists	1 oz	110	0	1

FOOD	PORTION	CALS.	SAT. FAT	FAT
Estee				
Dutch Unsalted	2 (1.1 oz)	130	0	1
Nuggets Reduced Sodium	30 (1 oz)	120	0	2
Nuggets Reduced Sodium Ranch	23 (1 oz)	130	1	2
Unsalted	23 (1 oz)	120	0	1
Formagg Pretzel Nuts	1 oz	120	1	4
J&J Soft	1 (2.25 oz)	170	—	0
J&J Soft Bites	5	110	1	0
Lance Twist	1.5 oz	150	0	1
Mister Salty Dutch	1 oz	110	tr	1
Mister Salty Fat Free Sticks	1 oz	100	0	0
Mister Salty Fat Free Twists	1 oz	100	0	0
Mister Salty Mini	1 oz	110	tr	1
Mister Salty Twists	1 oz	110	tr	2
Mister Salty Very Thin Sticks	1 oz	110	tr	1
Mr. Phipps Chips	8 (0.5 oz)	60	tr	1
Mr. Phipps Chips Fat Free	8 (0.5 oz)	50	0	0
Mr. Phipps Chips Lightly Salted	8 (0.5 oz)	60	tr	1
Mr. Phipps Chips Sesame	8	60	tr	2
Quinlan Beers	1 oz	110	1	1
Quinlan Hard Sourdough	1 oz	110	1	2
Quinlan Logs	1 oz	110	1	2
Quinlan Nuggets	1 oz	110	1	2
Quinlan Rods	1 oz	110	1	2
Quinlan Sticks	1 oz	110	1	2
Quinlan Thins	1 oz	110	1	2
Rold Gold				
Bavarian	3 pieces (1 oz)	120	—	2
Pretzels Chips	1 oz	110	—	1
Pretzels Chips Cheese	1 oz	120	—	3
Rods	3 pieces (1 oz)	110	—	2
Snack Mix	½ cup (1 oz)	140	—	6
Sour Dough	1½ pieces (1 oz)	110	—	2
Sticks	50 pieces (1 oz)	110	—	2
Thin Twist	10 pieces (1 oz)	110	—	1
Tiny Twist	15 pieces (1 oz)	110	—	1
Seyfert's Butter Rods	1 oz	110		

FOOD	PORTION	CALS.	SAT. FAT	FAT
Snyder's				
Logs	1 oz	310	0	0
Minis	1 oz	310	0	0
Minis Unsalted	1 oz	310	0	0
Nibblers	1 oz	310	0	0
Oat Bran	1 oz	120	—	1
Old Fashioned Hard	1 oz	111	0	0
Old Fashioned Hard Unsalted	1 oz	100	0	0
Old Tyme	1 oz	310	0	0
Old Tyme Unsalted	1 oz	110	0	0
Rods	1 oz	310	0	0
Sourdough Hard Buttermilk Ranch	1 oz	130	1	5
Sourdough Hard Cheddar Cheese	1 oz	160	1	7
Sourdough Hard Honey Mustard & Onion	1 oz	130	1	5
Stix	1 oz	310	0	0
Very Thins	1 oz	310	0	0
Sunshine California Pretzels	1 oz	110	0	2
Ultra Slim-Fast Lite N' Tasty	1 oz	100	—	tr
Wege Sourdough	1 oz	102	—	tr
Wege Unsalted	1 oz	102	—	tr
Wege Whole Wheat	1 oz	109	—	1
sticks	10	10	tr	tr
twists	1 (0.5 oz)	65	tr	1
twists, thin	10 (2 oz)	240	tr	2

PRICKLY PEAR
fresh	1	42	—	1

PRUNES
CANNED
in heavy syrup	5	90	tr	tr
in heavy syrup	1 cup	245	tr	tr
DRIED				
Mariani Pitted	¼ cup	140	—	1
Mariani Whole	¼ cup	140	—	1
Sunsweet Orange Essence Pitted	6 (1.4 oz)	100	0	0
cooked w/ sugar	½ cup	147	tr	tr

FOOD	PORTION	CALS.	SAT. FAT	FAT
cooked w/o sugar	½ cup	113	tr	tr
dried	10	201	tr	tr
dried	1 cup	385	1	1
JUICE				
S&W Unsweetened	6 oz	120	0	0
canned	1 cup	181	tr	tr

PUDDING
(*see also* CUSTARD, PUDDING POPS)

HOME RECIPE

FOOD	PORTION	CALS.	SAT. FAT	FAT
bread w/ raisins	½ cup	180	2	5
corn	½ cup	97	—	1
corn	⅔ cup	181	4	9
cornstarch	½ cup (4.4 oz)	137	3	5
yorkshire, as prep w/ skim milk	3.5 oz	93	—	4
yorkshire, as prep w/ whole milk	3.5 oz	104	—	5
MIX				
Banana Cream (Royal)	mix for 1 serving	80	0	0
Banana Cream Instant (Royal)	mix for 1 serving	90	0	0
Butterscotch (My*T*Fine)	mix for 1 serving	90	0	0
Butterscotch (Royal)	mix for 1 serving	90	0	0
Butterscotch Instant (Royal)	mix for 1 serving	90	0	0
Cherry Vanilla Instant (Royal)	mix for 1 serving	90	0	0
Chocolate (My*T*Fine)	mix for 1 serving	100	0	0
Chocolate (Royal)	mix for 1 serving	90	0	0
Chocolate Instant (Royal)	mix for 1 serving	110	0	0
Chocolate Instant, as prep w/ skim milk (Weight Watchers)	½ cup	100	—	0
Chocolate Almond (My*T*Fine)	mix for 1 serving	100	0	1
Chocolate Almond Instant (Royal)	mix for 1 serving	120	—	1
Chocolate Chocolate Chip Instant (Royal)	mix for 1 serving	110	0	1
Chocolate Fudge (My*T*Fine)	mix for 1 serving	100	0	1
Chocolate Peanut Butter Instant (Royal)	mix for 1 serving	110	0	1

FOOD	PORTION	CALS.	SAT. FAT	FAT
Chocolate Sugar Free Instant (Royal)	mix for 1 serving	50	—	0
Creme Caramel Flan And Sauce, as prep (Knorr)	½ cup +1 tbsp sauce	190	—	4
Dark 'n Sweet Chocolate (Royal)	mix for 1 serving	90	0	0
Dark 'n Sweet Instant (Royal)	mix for 1 serving	110	0	0
Lemon (My*T*Fine)	mix for 1 serving	90	0	0
Lemon Instant (Royal)	mix for 1 serving	90	0	0
Pistachio Instant (Royal)	mix for 1 serving	90	0	1
Strawberry Instant (Royal)	mix for 1 serving	100	0	0
Toasted Coconut Instant (Royal)	mix for 1 serving	100	—	2
Vanilla (My*T*Fine)	mix for 1 serving	90	0	0
Vanilla (Royal)	mix for 1 serving	80	0	0
Vanilla Chocolate Chip Instant (Royal)	mix for 1 serving	90	0	1
Vanilla Instant (Royal)	mix for 1 serving	90	0	0
Vanilla Instant, as prep w/ skim milk (Weight Watchers)	½ cup	90	—	0
Vanilla Tapioca (My*T*Fine)	mix for 1 serving	80	0	0
MIX WITH 2% MILK				
Banana Instant Sugar Free (Jell-O)	½ cup	84	—	2
Chocolate Instant Sugar Free (Jell-O)	½ cup	92	—	3
Chocolate Sugar Free (Jell-O)	½ cup	91	—	3
Pistachio Instant Sugar Free (Jell-O)	½ cup	94	—	3
Vanilla Instant Sugar Free (Jell-O)	½ cup	82	—	2
MIX WITH SKIM MILK				
Butterscotch w/ Nutrasweet (D-Zerta)	½ cup	68	—	0
Chocolate (D-Zerta)	½ cup	65	—	0
Dietetic (Emes)	½ cup (4 fl oz)	71	—	1
Vanilla w/ Nutrasweet (D-Zerta)	½ cup	69	—	0

FOOD	PORTION	CALS.	SAT. FAT	FAT
MIX WITH WHOLE MILK				
Banana Cream Instant (Jell-O)	½ cup	165	—	4
Butter Pecan Instant (Jell-O)	½ cup	170	—	5
Butterscotch (Jell-O)	½ cup	169	—	4
Butterscotch Instant (Jell-O)	½ cup	164	—	4
Chocolate Instant (Jell-O)	½ cup	176	—	5
Chocolate Fudge Instant (Jell-O)	½ cup	175	—	5
Chocolate Tapioca Americana (Jell-O)	½ cup	169	—	5
Coconut Cream Instant (Jell-O)	½ cup	178	—	6
French Vanilla (Jell-O)	½ cup	169	—	4
French Vanilla Instant (Jell-O)	½ cup	165	—	4
Golden Egg Custard Americana (Jell-O)	½ cup	167	—	6
Lemon Instant (Jell-O)	½ cup	168	—	4
Milk Chocolate Instant (Jell-O)	½ cup	178	—	5
Pineapple Cream Instant (Jell-O)	½ cup	165	—	4
Pistachio Instant (Jell-O)	½ cup	170	—	5
Rice Americana (Jell-O)	½ cup	175	—	4
Vanilla (Jell-O)	½ cup	156	—	4
Vanilla Instant (Jell-O)	½ cup	168	—	4
Vanilla Tapioca Americana (Jell-O)	½ cup	160	—	4
chocolate, instant	½ cup	155	4	4
chocolate, regular	½ cup	150	2	4
rice	½ cup	155	2	4
tapioca	½ cup	145	2	4
vanilla, instant	½ cup	150	2	4
vanilla, regular	½ cup	145	2	4
READY-TO-USE				
Banana (Snack Pack)	4.25 oz	145	1	6
Butterscotch (Snack Pack)	4.25 oz	170	1	6
Butterscotch (Swiss Miss)	4 oz	180	1	6
Butterscotch (Ultra Slim-Fast)	4 oz	100	—	tr
Butterscotch Sugar Free (Diamond Crystal)	½ cup	80	—	tr

FOOD	PORTION	CALS.	SAT. FAT	FAT
Chocolate (Jell-O)	1 (4 oz)	171	—	6
Chocolate (Snack Pack)	4.25 oz	170	1	6
Chocolate (Swiss Miss)	4 oz	180	1	6
Chocolate (Ultra Slim-Fast)	4 oz	100	—	tr
Chocolate Caramel Swirl (Jell-O)	1 (4 oz)	175	—	6
Chocolate Fudge (Snack Pack)	4.25 oz	165	1	6
Chocolate Fudge (Swiss Miss)	4 oz	220	2	6
Chocolate Fudge Light (Swiss Miss)	4 oz	100	—	1
Chocolate Light (Jell-O)	1 (4 oz)	104	—	2
Chocolate Light (Snack Pack)	4.25 oz	100	tr	2
Chocolate Light (Swiss Miss)	4 oz	100	tr	1
Chocolate Marshmallow (Snack Pack)	4.25 oz	165	1	6
Chocolate Sugar Free (Diamond Crystal)	½ cup	70	—	tr
Chocolate Sundae (Swiss Miss)	4 oz	220	2	7
Chocolate Vanilla Light (Jell-O)	1 (4 oz)	104	—	2
Chocolate Vanilla Swirl (Jell-O)	1 (4 oz)	175	—	6
Chocolate Vanilla Swirl (Jell-O)	1 (5.5 oz)	240	—	8
Lemon (Snack Pack)	4.25 oz	150	1	4
Lemon Dream (Imagine Foods)	1 (4 oz)	120	0	0
Milk Chocolate (Jell-O)	1 (4 oz)	173	—	6
Tapioca (Jell-O)	1 (4 oz)	167	—	4
Tapioca (Jell-O)	1 (5.5 oz)	229	—	6
Tapioca (Snack Pack)	4.25 oz	150	1	5
Tapioca (Swiss Miss)	4 oz	160	1	5
Tapioca Light (Snack Pack)	4.25 oz	100	tr	2
Vanilla (Jell-O)	1 (4 oz)	182	—	7
Vanilla (Snack Pack)	4.25 oz	170	1	6
Vanilla (Swiss Miss)	4 oz	190	1	7
Vanilla (Ultra Slim-Fast)	4 oz	100	—	tr
Vanilla Chocolate Parfait Light (Swiss Miss)	4 oz	100	tr	1

FOOD	PORTION	CALS.	SAT. FAT	FAT
Vanilla Chocolate Swirl (Jell-O)	1 (4 oz)	178	—	6
Vanilla Light (Jell-O)	1 (4 oz)	104	—	2
Vanilla Light (Swiss Miss)	4 oz	100	tr	1
Vanilla Parfait (Swiss Miss)	4 oz	180	1	6
Vanilla Sugar Free (Diamond Crystal)	½ cup	80	—	tr
Vanilla Sundae (Swiss Miss)	4 oz	200	2	7
TAKE-OUT				
blancmange	1 serving (4.7 oz)	154	—	5
bread	1 serving (6.7 oz)	564	—	18
queen of puddings	1 serving (4.4 oz)	266	—	10
rice	1 serving (3 oz)	110	—	4
rice w/ raisins	½ cup	246	3	6
tapioca	½ cup	169	3	6

PUDDING POPS

(*see also* ICE CREAM AND FROZEN DESSERTS, PUDDING)

FOOD	PORTION	CALS.	SAT. FAT	FAT
Jell-O				
Chocolate	1 pop	79	—	2
Chocolate/Caramel Swirl	1 pop	74	—	2
Chocolate Fudge	1 pop	79	—	2
Chocolate Peanut Butter Swirl	1 bar	78	—	3
Chocolate Swirl	1 pop	80	—	2
Chocolate/Vanilla Swirl	1 pop	78	—	2
Deluxe Chocolate Covered	1 pop	201	—	10
Deluxe Peanuts and Chocolate	1 bar	185	—	9
Milk Chocolate	1 pop	80	—	2
Vanilla	1 pop	77	—	2

PUMMELO

FOOD	PORTION	CALS.	SAT. FAT	FAT
fresh	1	228	—	tr
sections	1 cup	71	—	tr

PUMPKIN

FOOD	PORTION	CALS.	SAT. FAT	FAT
CANNED				
Libby's Solid Pack	½ cup	60	—	1
Owatonna	½ cup	40	—	1
pumpkin	½ cup	41	tr	tr
FRESH				
cooked, mashed	½ cup	24	tr	tr

FOOD	PORTION	CALS.	SAT. FAT	FAT
flowers, cooked	½ cup	10	tr	tr
flowers, raw	1	0	0	0
leaves, cooked	½ cup	7	tr	tr
leaves, raw	½ cup	4	tr	tr
raw, cubed	½ cup	15	tr	tr
SEEDS				
dried	1 oz	154	2	13
roasted	1 oz	148	2	12
roasted	1 cup	1184	18	96
salted & roasted	1 oz	148	2	12
salted & roasted	1 cup	1184	18	96
whole, roasted	1 oz	127	1	6
whole, roasted	1 cup	285	2	12
whole, salted & roasted	1 oz	127	1	6
whole, salted & roasted	1 cup	285	2	12

PURSLANE

FOOD	PORTION	CALS.	SAT. FAT	FAT
cooked	1 cup	21	—	tr
raw	1 cup	7	—	tr

QUAHOGS
(see CLAMS)

QUAIL
FRESH

FOOD	PORTION	CALS.	SAT. FAT	FAT
breast w/o skin, raw	1 (2 oz)	69	tr	2
w/ skin, raw	1 quail (3.8 oz)	210	4	13
w/o skin, raw	1 quail (3.2 oz)	123	1	4

QUICHE
HOME RECIPE

FOOD	PORTION	CALS.	SAT. FAT	FAT
lorraine	⅛ of 8" pie	600	23	48
TAKE-OUT				
cheese	1 slice (3 oz)	283	—	20
lorraine	1 slice (3 oz)	352	—	25
mushroom	1 slice (3 oz)	256	—	18

QUINCE

FOOD	PORTION	CALS.	SAT. FAT	FAT
fresh	1	53	tr	tr

QUINOA

FOOD	PORTION	CALS.	SAT. FAT	FAT
Arrowhead Quinoa Seeds	¼ cup (1.4 oz)	140	0	2
quinoa	½ cup	318	tr	5

RABBIT

FOOD	PORTION	CALS.	SAT. FAT	FAT
domestic, w/o bone, roasted	3 oz	167	2	7

FOOD	PORTION	CALS.	SAT. FAT	FAT
wild, w/o bone, stewed	3 oz	147	1	3
RACCOON				
roasted	3 oz	217	—	12
RADICCHIO				
raw, shredded	½ cup	5	—	tr
RADISH				
DRIED				
chinese	½ cup	157	tr	tr
daikon	½ cup	157	tr	tr
FRESH				
Dole	7	20	—	0
chinese, raw	1 (12 oz)	62	tr	tr
chinese, raw, sliced	½ cup	8	tr	tr
chinese, sliced, cooked	½ cup	13	tr	tr
daikon, raw	1 (12 oz)	62	tr	tr
daikon, raw, sliced	½ cup	8	tr	tr
daikon, sliced, cooked	½ cup	13	tr	tr
red, raw	10	7	tr	tr
red, sliced	½ cup	10	tr	tr
white icicle, raw	1 (½ oz)	2	tr	tr
white icicle, raw, sliced	½ cup	7	tr	tr
SPROUTS				
raw	½ cup	8	tr	tr
RAISINS				
Cinderella Seedless	½ cup	250	—	0
Dole Golden	½ cup	250	0	0
Dole Seedless	½ cup	250	0	0
golden seedless	1 cup	437	tr	1
seedless	1 tbsp	27	tr	tr
seedless	1 cup	434	tr	1
sultanas	1 oz	88	—	0
RASPBERRIES				
CANNED				
in heavy syrup	½ cup	117	tr	tr
FRESH				
Dole	1 cup	45	—	0
raspberries	1 cup	61	tr	1
raspberries	1 pint	154	tr	2
FROZEN				
Raspberries (Big Valley)	⅔ cup (4.9 oz)	80	0	0

FOOD	PORTION	CALS.	SAT. FAT	FAT
Whole in Lite Syrup (Birds Eye)	½ cup	99	tr	tr
sweetened	1 cup	256	tr	tr
sweetened	1 pkg (10 oz)	291	tr	tr
JUICE				
Crystal Geyser Juice Squeeze Mountain Raspberry	1 bottle (12 fl oz)	135	0	0
Kool-Aid Sugar Free	8 oz	2	0	0
Smucker's	8 oz	120	0	0
Smucker's Juice Sparkler	10 oz	130	—	tr

RED BEANS

CANNED

FOOD	PORTION	CALS.	SAT. FAT	FAT
Allen	½ cup (4.5 oz)	160	0	1
B&M Small Baked	8 oz	223	2	5
Green Giant	½ cup	90	—	1
Small (Hunt's)	½ cup (4.6 oz)	90	—	tr
Van Camp's	½ cup (4.6 oz)	90	0	0

RELISH

FOOD	PORTION	CALS.	SAT. FAT	FAT
Dill (Vlasic)	1 oz	2	0	0
Hamburger (Vlasic)	1 oz	40	0	0
Hot Dog (Vlasic)	1 oz	40	—	1
Hot Piccalilli (Vlasic)	1 oz	35	0	0
India (Vlasic)	1 oz	30	0	0
Jalapeno (Old El Paso)	2 tbsp	16	0	0
Pickle Relish (Claussen)	1 tbsp	14	—	tr
Sandwich Spread (Hellmann's)	1 tbsp	55	1	5
Sweet (Vlasic)	1 oz	30	0	0
cranberry orange	½ cup	246	—	tr
hamburger	1 tbsp	19	tr	tr
hamburger	½ cup	158	tr	1
hot dog	1 tbsp	14	tr	tr
hot dog	½ cup	111	tr	1
piccalilli	1.4 oz	13	—	tr
sweet	1 tbsp	19	tr	tr
sweet	1 cup	159	tr	1

RHUBARB

FOOD	PORTION	CALS.	SAT. FAT	FAT
fresh	½ cup	13	—	tr
frzn	½ cup	60	—	tr
frzn, as prep w/ sugar	½ cup	139	—	tr

FOOD	PORTION	CALS.	SAT. FAT	FAT

RICE
(*see also* BRAN, CEREAL, FLOUR, RICE CAKES, WILD RICE)

BROWN

FOOD	PORTION	CALS.	SAT. FAT	FAT
Arrowhead Basmati	¼ cup (1.5 oz)	150	0	1
Arrowhead Quick Regular	⅓ cup (1.5 oz)	150	0	1
Arrowhead Quick Spanish Style	¼ pkg (1.4 oz)	150	0	1
Arrowhead Quick Vegetable Herb	¼ pkg (1.4 oz)	150	0	1
Arrowhead Quick Wild Rice & Herb	¼ pkg (1.3 oz)	140	0	1
Minute Precooked, as prep	½ cup	121	tr	1
Pritikin Pilaf	½ cup	90	—	tr
Pritikin Spanish	½ cup	100	—	tr
S&W Quick Natural Long Grain	3.5 oz	110	0	0
S&W Quick Natural Long Grain, cooked	3.5 oz	119	0	0
Uncle Ben	1 serv (1.6 oz)	158	1	—
long-grain, cooked	½ cup	109	—	tr
medium-grain, cooked	½ cup	109	tr	tr

CANNED

FOOD	PORTION	CALS.	SAT. FAT	FAT
Old El Paso Spanish	½ cup	70	0	1
Van Camp's Spanish	1 cup	180	1	3

DRY MIX

FOOD	PORTION	CALS.	SAT. FAT	FAT
Chun King Entree Stir Fry	0.25 oz	20	—	0
Goodman's Rice & Vermicelli For Beef	¾ cup	160	0	1
Goodman's Rice & Vermicelli For Chicken	¾ cup	160	0	1
Hain Rice Almondine	½ cup	130	—	5
Hain Rice Oriental 3-Grain Goodness	½ cup	120	—	5
Kikkoman Fried Rice Seasoning Mix	1 oz pkg	91	—	tr
Knorr				
Risotto Milanese w/ Saffron	½ cup	130	—	3
Risotto Tomato	½ cup	110	—	tr
Risotto w/ Mushrooms	½ cup	110	—	tr
Risotto w/ Onion	½ cup	110	—	tr
Risotto w/ Peas & Corn	½ cup	110	—	1

FOOD	PORTION	CALS.	SAT. FAT	FAT
La Choy Chinese Fried Rice	¾ cup	190	tr	1
Lipton Golden Saute Fried Rice Beef	½ cup	124	—	2
Lipton Golden Saute Fried Rice Chicken	½ cup	129	—	2
Lipton Golden Saute Fried Rice Oriental	½ cup	127	—	2
Lipton Rice & Sauce				
Beef	½ cup	119	—	1
Cajun	½ cup	123	—	tr
Cheddar Broccoli	½ cup	125	—	1
Chicken	½ cup	124	—	1
Chicken Broccoli	½ cup	129	—	2
Creamy Chicken	½ cup	142	—	2
Herbs & Butter	½ cup	123	—	2
Long Grain And Wild Rice Original	½ cup	121	—	tr
Mushroom	½ cup	123	—	1
Pilaf	½ cup	122	—	1
Skillet Style Spanish	½ cup	104	0	1
Spanish	½ cup	118	—	1
Lipton Rice Asparagus w/ Hollandaise	½ cup	123	—	tr
Mahatma				
Broccoli & Cheese	1 cup	200	1	2
Jambalaya	1 cup (2 oz)	190	0	1
Long Grain & Wild	1 cup (2 oz)	190	0	1
Pilaf	1 cup (2 oz)	190	0	0
Spanish	1 cup (2 oz)	180	0	1
Yellow Rice Mix	1 cup	190	0	0
Minute				
Fried Rice With Vermicelli as prep	½ cup	158	—	5
Rib Roast With Vermicelli as prep	½ cup	151	—	4
Rice Drumstick With Vermicelli as prep	½ cup	153	—	4
Microwave Broccoli Almondin	½ cup	143	1	4
Microwave Cheddar Cheese Broccoli	½ cup	164	2	5
Microwave French Pilaf	½ cup	133	2	3
Microwave Long Grain Brown And Wild	½ cup	140	2	3

FOOD	PORTION	CALS.	SAT. FAT	FAT
Minute *(cont.)*				
Microwave Rice With Savory Cheese Sauce, as prep	½ cup	162	—	5
Near East Lentil Pilaf, as prep w/ butter	¾ cup (4.9 oz)	180	0	1
Near East Pilaf Chicken Flavor, as prep w/ butter	½ cup	160	—	4
Old El Paso Mexican	½ cup	140	—	2
Rice-A-Roni				
Beef	½ cup	140	—	4
Beef & Mushroom	½ cup	150	—	3
Chicken	½ cup	150	—	3
Chicken & Broccoli	½ cup	150	—	3
Chicken & Mushroom	½ cup	180	—	7
Chicken & Vegetables	½ cup	140	—	3
Fried Rice	½ cup	110	—	5
Herb & Butter	½ cup	130	—	4
Long Grain & Wild, Chicken w/ Almonds	½ cup	140	—	4
Long Grain & Wild, Original	½ cup	130	—	3
Long Grain & Wild, Pilaf	½ cup	130	—	3
Pilaf	½ cup	150	—	4
Risotto	½ cup	200	—	6
Spanish	½ cup	150	—	4
Stroganoff	½ cup	200	—	8
Yellow Rice	½ cup	140	—	4
Success				
Beef Oriental	½ cup	190	0	1
Broccoli & Cheese	½ cup	200	1	2
Brown & Wild	½ cup	190	0	1
Classic Chicken	½ cup	150	0	1
Long Grain & Wild	½ cup	190	0	0
Pilaf	½ cup	200	0	0
Spanish	½ cup	190	0	1
Ultra Slim-Fast Oriental Style	2.3 oz	240	—	1
Ultra Slim-Fast Rice & Chicken Sauce	2.3 oz	240	—	1
Uncle Ben				
Brown & Wild Fast Cooking	1 serv (1.3 oz)	120	—	1
Country Inn Broccoli Almondine	1 serv (1.2 oz)	124	—	2

FOOD	PORTION	CALS.	SAT. FAT	FAT
Country Inn Broccoli And White Cheddar	1 serv (1.2 oz)	131	—	3
Country Inn Broccoli Au Gratin	1 serv (1.1 oz)	116	—	2
Country Inn Chicken Stock	1 serv (1.2 oz)	123	—	1
Country Inn Chicken With Wild Rice	1 serv (1.1 oz)	108	—	1
Country Inn Creamy Chicken & Mushroom	1 serv (1.3 oz)	138	—	3
Country Inn Creamy Chicken & Wild Rice	1 serv (1.3 oz)	135	—	1
Country Inn Green Bean Almondine	1 serv (1.2 oz)	128	—	2
Country Inn Herbed Au Gratin	1 serv (1.2 oz)	119	—	2
Country Inn Homestyle Chicken And Vegetables	1 serv (1.3 oz)	139	—	3
Country Inn Rice Florentine	1 serv (1.2 oz)	212	—	2
Country Inn Vegetable Pilaf	1 serv (1.2 oz)	115	—	1
Long Grain & Wild Chicken Stock Sauce	1 serv (1.3 oz)	133	—	2
Long Grain & Wild Fast Cooking	1 serv (1 oz)	101	—	tr
Long Grain & Wild Garden Vegetable Blend	1 serv (1.3 oz)	128	—	1
Long Grain & Wild Original	1 serv (1 oz)	96	—	tr
FROZEN				
Birds Eye French Style	½ cup	170	1	3
Birds Eye Rice And Broccoli Au Gratin	½ pkg	150	2	4
Birds Eye Rice Pilaf w/ Green Beans	1 pkg (5.5 oz)	230	—	11
Budget Gourmet				
Oriental Rice w/ Vegetables	1 pkg	240	—	12
Green Giant				
Garden Gourmet Asparagus Pilaf	1 pkg	190	2	4
Garden Gourmet Sherry Wild Rice	1 pkg	210	2	4

FOOD	PORTION	CALS.	SAT. FAT	FAT
Green Giant (cont.)				
One Serve Rice 'N Broccoli in Cheese Sauce	1 pkg	180	2	6
One Serve Rice, Peas & Mushrooms w/ Sauce	1 pkg	130	tr	2
Rice Originals Italian Rice & Spinach in Cheese Sauce	½ cup	140	2	4
Rice Originals Pilaf	½ cup	110	tr	1
Rice Originals Rice 'N Broccoli in Cheese Sauce	½ cup	120	1	4
Rice Originals Rice Medley	½ cup	100	tr	1
Rice Originals White & Wild	½ cup	130	tr	2
TAKE-OUT				
pilaf	½ cup	84	1	3
risotto	6.6 oz	426	—	18
spanish	¾ cup	363	10	27
WHITE				
Arrowhead Basmati	¼ cup (1.5 oz)	150	0	0
Minute				
as prep	⅔ cup	141	—	2
Boil In Bag Long Grain as prep	½ cup	94	0	0
Long Grain And Wild as prep	½ cup	149	—	4
Long Grain as prep	⅔ cup	150	—	3
S&W Long Grain, cooked	3.5 oz	106	0	0
Superfino Arborio Rice	½ cup	100	—	0
Uncle Ben Boil-In-Bag	1 serv (0.9 oz)	94	—	tr
Uncle Ben Converted	1 serv (1.2 oz)	123	—	tr
Uncle Ben In An Instant	1 serv (1.1 oz)	111	—	tr
glutinous, cooked	½ cup	116	tr	tr
long-grain, cooked	½ cup	131	tr	tr
long-grain instant, cooked	½ cup	80	tr	tr
long-grain parboiled, cooked	½ cup	100	tr	tr
medium-grain, cooked	½ cup	132	tr	tr
short grain, cooked	½ cup	133	tr	tr
starch	3.5 oz	343	0	0

FOOD	PORTION	CALS.	SAT. FAT	FAT

RICE CAKES
| 7 Grain (Pritikin) | 1 | 35 | 0 | 0 |

Hain
5-Grain	1	40	—	tr
Plain	1	40	—	tr
Plain No Salt Added	1	40	—	tr
Sesame	1	40	—	tr
Sesame No Salt	1	40	—	tr

Hain Mini
Apple Cinnamon	½ oz	60	—	tr
Barbecue	½ oz	70	—	3
Cheese	½ oz	60	—	2
Honey Nut	½ oz	60	—	tr
Nacho Cheese	½ oz	70	—	2
Plain	½ oz	60	—	tr
Plain No Salt Added	½ oz	60	—	tr
Ranch	½ oz	70	—	3
Teriyaki	½ oz	50	—	tr

Lundberg
Organic Lightly Salted	1	60	—	1
Organic Popcorn Lightly Salted	1	60	—	1
Organic Popcorn Unsalted	1	60	—	1
Organic Unsalted	1	60	—	1
Premium Lightly Salted	1	60	—	1
Premium Unsalted	1	60	—	1
Rye With Caraway Lightly Salted	1	59	0	0
Sesame Lightly Salted	1	59	0	0
Plain (Pritikin)	1	35	—	0
Sesame (Pritikin)	1	35	—	0

ROCKFISH
FRESH
pacific, cooked	3 oz	103	tr	2
pacific, cooked	1 filet (5.2 oz)	180	1	3
pacific, raw	3 oz	80	tr	1

ROE
(see also individual fish names)
| baked | 3 oz | 173 | 2 | 7 |
| baked | 1 oz | 58 | 1 | 2 |

FOOD	PORTION	CALS.	SAT. FAT	FAT

ROLL
(*see also* BISCUIT, CROISSANT, ENGLISH MUFFIN, MUFFIN, POPOVER, SCONE)

FROZEN

FOOD	PORTION	CALS.	SAT. FAT	FAT
All Butter Cinnamon Roll w/ Icing (Sara Lee)	1	280	—	11
All Butter Cinnamon Roll w/o Icing (Sara Lee)	1	230	—	11
Cinnamon Roll (Pepperidge Farm)	1 (2.25 oz)	220	—	14
Cinnamon Rolls (Weight Watchers)	1 (2.1 oz)	180	tr	5
HOME RECIPE				
dinner as prep w/ 2% milk	1 (2½ in)	111	1	3
dinner as prep w/ whole milk	1 (2½ in)	112	1	3
raisin & nut	1 (2 oz)	196	1	7
MIX				
German Hard (Natural Ovens)	1 (2.1 oz)	138	0	1
Gourmet Dinner (Natural Ovens)	1 (1 oz)	50	0	1
Hearty Sandwich (Natural Ovens)	1 (1.8 oz)	110	0	1
Hot Roll Mix (Dromedary)	2	239	—	5
Hot Roll Mix (Pillsbury)	2	240	—	4
READY-TO-EAT				
8-inch Francisco (Arnold)	1 (2.5 oz)	210	—	3
Augusto Pan Cubano (Arnold)	1	230	—	3
Bakery Light (Arnold)	1 (1.5 oz)	80	0	<2
Bavarian Cracked Wheat (Bread Du Jour)	1 (1.2 oz)	90	0	1
Big Marty Poppy (Martin's)	1	170	—	2
Big Marty Sesame (Martin's)	1	170	—	2
Bran'nola Buns (Arnold)	1 (1.5 oz)	100	0	1
Brown 'N Serve (Roman Meal)	2 (2 oz)	140	tr	3
Brown 'N Serve Buttermilk (Wonder)	1 (1 oz)	70	0	1
Brown 'N Serve Club (Pepperidge Farm)	1	100	—	1
Brown 'N Serve French (Pepperidge Farm)	½ roll	180	1	2

FOOD	PORTION	CALS.	SAT. FAT	FAT
Brown 'N Serve Hearth (Pepperidge Farm)	1	50	—	1
Brown 'N Serve Wheat (Wonder)	1 (1 oz)	70	0	1
Brown 'N Serve White (Wonder)	1 (1 oz)	70	0	1
Crusty Italian (Bread Du Jour)	1 (1.2 oz)	80	0	1
Dark Bread (Hollywood)	1	40	—	tr
Deli Kaiser (Arnold)	1	170	—	2
Deli Onion (Arnold)	1	170	—	2
Dinner (August Bros)	1	90	—	1
Dinner (Pepperidge Farm)	1	60	0	2
Dinner (Roman Meal)	2 (2 oz)	136	tr	2
Dinner Plain (Arnold)	1 (0.7 oz)	50	0	1
Dinner Sesame (Arnold)	1 (0.7 oz)	50	0	1
Dinner Wheat (Home Pride)	1 (1.9 oz)	160	1	4
Dinner White Light (Wonder)	1 (1 oz)	60	0	1
Dinner County Style Classic (Pepperidge Farm)	1	50	0	1
Dinner Light Pan Special Formula (Hollywood)	1	60	—	tr
Extra Sourdough (Dicarlo's)	1 (1.6 oz)	100	0	1
Finger Poppy Seed (Pepperidge Farm)	1	50	0	2
Finger Sesame Seed (Pepperidge Farm)	1	60	0	2
Frankfurter (Country Kitchen)	1	120	—	2
Frankfurter Dijon (Pepperidge Farm)	1	160	1	5
Frankfurter Side Sliced (Pepperidge Farm)	1	140	1	3
Frankfurter Top Sliced (Pepperidge Farm)	1	140	1	3
Frankfurter w/ Poppy Seeds (Pepperidge Farm)	1	130	1	2
French (Dicarlo's)	1 (1 oz)	70	0	1
French Francisco (Arnold)	1 (2.5 oz)	210	—	3
French Mini Franciso (Arnold)	1	130	—	2

FOOD	PORTION	CALS.	SAT. FAT	FAT
French Petite (Bread Du Jour)	1 (3.5 oz)	230	0	2
French Style (Pepperidge Farm)	1	100	—	1
Hamburger (Arnold)	1	120	—	2
Hamburger (Pepperidge Farm)	1	130	1	2
Hamburger (Roman Meal)	1	113	tr	2
Hamburger (Shop 'n Save)	1	120	—	2
Hamburger (Wonder)	1 (1.5 oz)	110	0	2
Hamburger Light (Wonder)	1	80	0	2
Hamburger Potato Bun (Home Pride)	1 (1.9 oz)	130	0	2
Hamburger Wheat (Wonder)	1 (2.2 oz)	170	0	3
Heat & Serve Butter Crescent (Pepperidge Farm)	1	110	3	6
Heat & Serve Golden Twist (Pepperidge Farm)	1	110	2	5
Hoagie (Martin's)	1	240	—	3
Hoagie Sesame (Martin's)	1	240	—	3
Hoagie Soft (Pepperidge Farm)	1	210	1	5
Hot Dog (Arnold)	1 (1.5 oz)	110	tr	2
Hot Dog (Roman Meal)	1 (1.5 oz)	103	tr	2
Hot Dog (Wonder)	1 (1.5 oz)	110	0	2
Hot Dog Bran'nola (Arnold)	1 (1.5 oz)	110	tr	2
Hot Dog Light (Wonder)	1 (1.5)	80	0	2
Hot Dog New England Style (Arnold)	1	110	—	2
Hot Dog Potato Bun (Home Pride)	1 (1.9 oz)	130	0	2
Italian 8-inch Savoni (Arnold)	1	210	tr	3
Kaiser (August Bros.)	1	170	—	1
Old Fashioned (Pepperidge Farm)	1	50	1	2
Onion (August Bros.)	1	160	—	1
Onion Premium (Arnold)	1 (2.6 oz)	180	—	1
Parker House (Pepperidge Farm)	1	60	0	1
Party (Pepperidge Farm)	1	30	—	1

FOOD	PORTION	CALS.	SAT. FAT	FAT
Party Petite (Arnold)	2	70	tr	2
Potato (Arnold)	1	140	—	2
Potato Dinner (Martin's)	1	100	—	1
Potato Long (Martin's)	1	140	—	1
Potato Party (Martin's)	1	50	—	1
Potato Sandwich (Martin's)	1	140	—	1
Potato Sandwich (Pepperidge Farm)	1	160	1	4
Rye (Bread Du Jour)	1 (1.2 oz)	90	0	2
Salad Roll (Matthew's)	1	110	—	2
Sandwich (Matthew's)	1	110	—	2
Sandwich (Roman Meal)	1 (2.7 oz)	181	tr	3
Sandwich Onion w/ Poppy Seeds (Pepperidge Farm)	1	150	1	3
Sandwich Roll Wheat (Home Pride)	1 (1.9 oz)	160	1	4
Sandwich Salad (Pepperidge Farm)	1	110	4	4
Sandwich Soft Sesame (Arnold)	1	130	—	3
Sandwich Whole Wheat 100% Stoneground (Martin's)	1	160	—	2
Sandwich w/ Sesame Seeds (Pepperidge Farm)	1	140	1	3
Sesame Cubano (Augusto Bros)	1	170	—	1
Sliced Light Special Formula (Hollywood)	1	80	—	tr
Soft Family (Pepperidge Farm)	1	100	1	2
Sourdough (Bread Du Jour)	1 (2.2 oz)	140	0	2
Sourdough Brown 'N Serve (Arnold)	1 (1 oz)	100	—	1
Sourdough Francisco (Arnold)	1 (1 oz)	100	—	1
Sourdough French (Pepperidge Farm)	1	100	—	1
Sub Old Country (Levy)	1	180	—	2
Tea Dinner Rolls (Wonder)	1 (1.5 oz)	80	0	1
Wheat Old Fashioned (Arnold)	2	80	—	3

FOOD	PORTION	CALS.	SAT. FAT	FAT
White (Home Pride)	2 (1.6 oz)	130	1	4
brown & serve	1 (1 oz)	85	tr	2
cheese	1 (2.3 oz)	238	4	12
cinnamon raisin	1 (2¾ in)	223	3	10
dinner	1 (1 oz)	85	tr	2
egg	1 (2½ in)	107	1	2
french	1 (1.3 oz)	105	tr	2
hamburger	1 (1.5 oz)	123	1	2
hamburger multi-grain	1 (1.5 oz)	113	1	2
hamburger reduced calorie	1 (1.5 oz)	84	tr	1
hard	1 (3½ in)	167	tr	2
hot cross bun	1	202	—	4
hotdog	1 (1.5 oz)	123	1	2
hotdog multi-grain	1 (1.5 oz)	113	1	2
hotdog reduced calorie	1 (1.5 oz)	84	tr	1
kaiser	1 (3½ in)	167	tr	2
oat bran	1 (1.2 oz)	78	tr	2
rye	1 (1 oz)	81	tr	1
submarine	1 (4.7 oz)	155	tr	2
wheat	1 (1 oz)	77	tr	2
whole wheat	1 (1 oz)	75	tr	1
REFRIGERATED				
Pillsbury Best Quick Cinnamon w/ Icing	1	110	1	5
Pillsbury Butterflake	1	140	1	5
Pillsbury Crescent	1	100	1	6
cinnamon w/ frosting	1	109	1	4
crescent	1 (1 oz)	98	1	4

ROMAN BEANS
CANNED

Progresso	½ cup	110	—	tr

ROSE APPLE

fresh	3.5 oz	32	—	tr

ROSE HIP

fresh	3.5 oz	91	0	0

ROSELLE

fresh	1 cup	28	—	tr

ROSEMARY

dried	1 tsp	4	—	tr

ROUGHY

orange, baked	3 oz	75	tr	1

FOOD	PORTION	CALS.	SAT. FAT	FAT
RUTABAGA				
Diced (Sunshine)	½ cup (4.2 oz)	30	0	0
fresh, cooked, mashed	½ cup	41	tr	tr
fresh, raw, cubed	½ cup	25	tr	tr
SABLEFISH				
FRESH				
baked	3 oz	213	3	17
fillet, baked	5.3 oz	378	6	30
SMOKED				
sablefish	1 oz	72	1	6
sablefish	3 oz	218	4	17
SAFFLOWER				
(see also OIL)				
seeds, dried	1 oz	147	1	11
SAFFRON				
saffron	1 tsp	2	—	tr
SAGE				
ground	1 tsp	2	tr	tr
SALAD				
(see also PASTA SALAD)				
MIX				
Dole				
Caesar Salad	½ pkg (3.5 oz)	170	2	14
Classic Blend	3.5 oz	25	0	1
Coleslaw Blend	3.5 oz	30	0	1
French Blend	3.5 oz	25	0	1
Italian Blend	3.5 oz	25	0	1
Salad-In-A-Minute Oriental	3.5 oz	110	1	7
Salad-In-A-Minute Spinach	3.5 oz	180	2	9
Fresh Express European Mix	1½ cups (3 oz)	20	0	0
Suddenly Salad Caesar, as prep	½ cup	170	—	8
Suddenly Salad Ranch And Bacon, as prep	½ cup	210	—	11
Suddenly Salad Ranch And Bacon, as prep low fat recipe	½ cup	160	—	5

FOOD	PORTION	CALS.	SAT. FAT	FAT
TAKE-OUT				
chef w/o dressing	1½ cup	386	13	28
tossed w/o dressing	1½ cup	32	0	tr
tossed w/o dressing	¾ cup	16	0	0
tossed w/o dressing w/ cheese & egg	1½ cup	102	3	6
tossed w/o dressing w/ chicken	1½ cup	105	tr	2
tossed w/o dressing w/ pasta & seafood	1½ cup	380	3	21
tossed w/o dressing w/ shrimp	1½ cup	107	tr	2
waldorf	½ cup	79	2	6

SALAD DRESSING

FOOD	PORTION	CALS.	SAT. FAT	FAT
HOME RECIPE				
french	1 tbsp	88	2	10
vinegar & oil	1 tbsp	72	2	8
MIX				
Good Seasons				
Bleu Cheese & Herbs, as prep	1 tbsp	72	—	8
Buttermilk Farm, as prep	1 tbsp	58	—	6
Cheese Garlic, as prep	1 tbsp	72	—	8
Cheese Italian, as prep	1 tbsp	72	—	8
Classic Dill, as prep	1 tbsp	28	tr	tr
Garlic & Herbs, as prep	1 tbsp	84	—	9
Italian, as prep	1 tbsp	71	—	8
Italian Lite, as prep	1 tbsp	27	—	3
Italian No Oil, as prep	1 tbsp	7	0	0
Lemon & Herbs, as prep	1 tbsp	71	—	8
Lite Cheese Italian, as prep	1 tbsp	27	—	3
Lite Ranch, as prep	1 tbsp	29	—	2
Lite Zesty Italian, as prep	1 tbsp	26	—	3
Mild Italian, as prep	1 tbsp	73	—	8
Zesty Italian, as prep	1 tbsp	71	—	8
Hain No Oil				
Bleu Cheese	1 tbsp	14	—	1
Buttermilk	1 tbsp	11	—	tr
Caesar	1 tbsp	6	—	tr

FOOD	PORTION	CALS.	SAT. FAT	FAT
French	1 tbsp	12	—	0
Garlic & Cheese	1 tbsp	6	—	tr
Herb	1 tbsp	2	—	0
Italian	1 tbsp	2	—	0
1000 Island	1 tbsp	12	—	0
READY-TO-USE				
Catalina	1 tbsp	15	0	1
Catalina French	1 tbsp	60	1	5
Creamy French (Estee)	2 tbsp (1 oz)	10	0	0
Diamond Crystal Blue Cheese	1 tbsp	20	—	1
Diamond Crystal Home Style	1 tbsp	20	—	1
Diamond Crystal Thousand Island	1 tbsp	20	—	1
Estee				
Blue Cheese	2 tbsp (1 oz)	15	—	1
Creamy French Fat Free	1 pkg (0.5 oz)	5	0	0
Creamy Garlic	2 tbsp (1 oz)	60	0	0
Creamy Garlic Fat Free	1 pkg (0.5 oz)	5	0	0
Creamy Italian	2 tbsp (1 oz)	15	—	1
Fat Free Thousand Island	1 pkg (0.5 oz)	5	0	0
Italian	2 tbsp (1 oz)	5	0	0
Italian Fat Free	1 pkg (0.5 oz)	0	0	0
Low Fat Blue Cheese	1 pkg (0.5 oz)	5	—	0
Thousand Island	2 tbsp (1 oz)	10	0	0
Hain				
1000 Island	1 tbsp	50	—	5
Creamy Caesar	1 tbsp	60	—	6
Creamy Caesar Low Salt	1 tbsp	60	—	6
Creamy French	1 tbsp	60	—	6
Creamy Italian	1 tbsp	80	—	8
Creamy Italian No Salt Added	1 tbsp	80	—	8
Cucumber Dill	1 tbsp	80	—	8
Dijon Vinaigrette	1 tbsp	50	—	5
Garlic & Sour Cream	1 tbsp	70	—	7
Honey & Sesame	1 tbsp	60	—	5
Italian Cheese Vinaigrette	1 tbsp	55	—	6
Old Fashioned Buttermilk	1 tbsp	70	—	7
Poppyseed Rancher's	1 tbsp	60	—	7

FOOD	PORTION	CALS.	SAT. FAT	FAT
Hain (cont.)				
Savory Herb No Salt Added	1 tbsp	90	—	10
Swiss Cheese Vinaigrette	1 tbsp	60	—	7
Traditional Italian	1 tbsp	80	—	8
Traditional Italian No Salt Added	1 tbsp	60	—	6
Hain Canola				
Garden Tomato	1 tbsp	60	—	6
Italian	1 tbsp	50	—	5
Spicy French Mustard	1 tbsp	50	—	5
Tangy Citrus	1 tbsp	50	—	5
Healthy Sensation				
Blue Cheese	1 tbsp	19	tr	1
French	1 tbsp	21	tr	1
Honey Dijon	1 tbsp	26	tr	1
Italian	1 tbsp	7	0	tr
Ranch	1 tbsp	15	tr	tr
Thousand Island	1 tbsp	20	tr	tr
Italian	1 tbsp	7	0	tr
Herb Magic				
Cucumber Creamy Reduced Calorie	1 tbsp	8	—	0
Herb Basket Reduced Calorie	1 tbsp	6	—	0
Italian Reduced Calorie	1 tbsp	4	—	0
Sweet & Sour Reduced Calorie	1 tbsp	18	—	0
Thousand Island Reduced Calorie	1 tbsp	8	—	0
Vinaigrette Reduced Calorie	1 tbsp	6	—	0
Zesty Tomato Reduced Calorie	1 tbsp	14	—	0
Hollywood				
Caesar	1 tbsp	70	1	7
Creamy French	1 tbsp	70	1	7
Creamy Italian	1 tbsp	90	1	9
Dijon Vinaigrette	1 tbsp	60	1	6
Italian	1 tbsp	90	1	9
Italian Cheese	1 tbsp	80	1	8
Old Fashion Buttermilk	1 tbsp	75	1	8
Poppy Seed Rancher's	1 tbsp	75	1	8
Thousand Island	1 tbsp	60	1	6

FOOD	PORTION	CALS.	SAT. FAT	FAT
Kraft				
Bacon & Tomato	1 tbsp	70	1	7
Bacon & Tomato Reduced Calorie	1 tbsp	30	0	2
Bacon Creamy	1 tbsp	30	0	2
Blue Cheese Chunky	1 tbsp	60	1	6
Buttermilk Creamy	1 tbsp	80	1	8
Buttermilk Creamy Reduced Calorie	1 tbsp	30	0	3
Chunky Blue Cheese Reduced Calorie	1 tbsp	30	1	2
Coleslaw	1 tbsp	70	1	6
Creamy Garlic	1 tbsp	50	1	5
Creamy Italian w/ Real Sour Cream	1 tbsp	50	1	5
Cucumber Creamy	1 tbsp	70	1	8
Free French Nonfat	1 tbsp	26	0	0
Free Italian Nonfat	1 tbsp	6	0	0
Free Ranch Nonfat	1 tbsp	16	0	0
Free Thousand Island Nonfat	1 tbsp	20	0	0
French	1 tbsp	60	0	6
Golden Caesar	1 tbsp	70	1	7
House Italian	1 tbsp	60	1	3
House Italian Reduced Calorie	1 tbsp	30	0	2
Italian Creamy Reduced Calorie	1 tbsp	25	0	2
Italian Oil-Free	1 tbsp	4	0	0
Miracle French	1 tbsp	70	1	6
Oil & Vinegar	1 tbsp	70	1	7
Onion & Chives Creamy	1 tbsp	70	—	7
Presto Italian	1 tbsp	70	1	7
Red Wine Vinegar & Oil	1 tbsp	50	1	4
Russian Creamy	1 tbsp	60	1	5
Russian Reduced Calorie	1 tbsp	30	0	1
Russian w/ Pure Honey	1 tbsp	60	1	5
Thousand Island	1 tbsp	60	1	5
Thousand Island & Bacon	1 tbsp	60	1	6
Thousand Island Reduced Calorie	1 tbsp	20	0	1
Zesty Italian	1 tbsp	50	1	5
Zesty Italian Reduced Calorie	1 tbsp (0.5 fl oz)	90	2	9

FOOD	PORTION	CALS.	SAT. FAT	FAT
Newman's Own Ranch	1 tbsp (0.5 fl oz)	90	2	9
Ott's Famous Chef	1 tbsp	40	—	3
Ott's Italian Chef	1 tbsp	80	—	9
Pritikin				
Creamy Italian	1 tbsp	12	—	0
French	1 tbsp	10	—	0
Italian	1 tbsp	6	—	0
Ranch	1 tbsp	18	—	0
Russian	1 tbsp	12	—	0
Vinaigrette	1 tbsp	10	—	0
Zesty Tomato	1 tbsp	18	—	0
Rancher's Choice	1 tbsp	90	1	6
Rancher's Choice Creamy	1 tbsp	30	0	3
Roka Blue Cheese	1 tbsp	60	1	6
Roka Blue Cheese	1 tbsp	15	1	1
Reduced Calorie				
S&W				
Blue Cheese Low	1 tbsp	25	—	2
Calorie				
Cucumber Creamy Low	1 tbsp	25	—	2
Calorie				
French Low Calorie	1 tbsp	18	0	0
Italian Creamy Low	1 tbsp	10	—	1
Calorie				
Italian No-Oil	1 tbsp	2	0	0
Russian Low Calorie	1 tbsp	25	—	1
Thousand Island Low	1 tbsp	25	—	2
Calorie				
Seven Seas				
Buttermilk	1 tbsp	80	1	8
Buttermilk Ranch Light	1 tbsp	50	1	5
Free Ranch Nonfat	1 tbsp	16	0	0
Free Red Wine Vinegar	1 tbsp	6	0	0
Nonfat				
French Creamy	1 tbsp	60	1	6
French Light	1 tbsp	35	0	3
Herb & Spice	1 tbsp	60	1	6
Italian Creamy	1 tbsp	70	1	7
Thousand Island	1 tbsp	50	1	5
Creamy				
Thousand Island Light	1 tbsp	30	0	2
Seven Seas Viva				
Free Italian Nonfat	1 tbsp	4	0	0
Herbs & Spices! Light	1 tbsp	30	0	3

FOOD	PORTION	CALS.	SAT. FAT	FAT
Italian	1 tbsp	50	1	5
Italian! Light	1 tbsp	30	0	3
Ranch	1 tbsp	80	1	8
Ranch! Light	1 tbsp	50	1	5
Red Wine Vinegar & Oil	1 tbsp	70	1	7
Red Wine! Vinegar & Oil Light	1 tbsp	45	1	4
Ultra Slim-Fast French	1 tbsp	20	—	tr
Ultra Slim-Fast Italian	1 tbsp	6	—	tr
W. J. Clark				
Ginger Orange Vinaigrette	1 tbsp	73	1	7
Herbs and Romano	1 tbsp	67	tr	6
Lemon Peppercorn	1 tbsp	72	1	7
Lime Cilantro Vinaigrette	1 tbsp	73	1	8
Poppy Seed	1 tbsp	75	tr	6
Sweet Pepper Basil	1 tbsp	69	tr	7
Tarragon Honey Mustard	1 tbsp	66	tr	6
Walden Farms				
Bleu Cheese	1 tbsp	27	tr	2
Creamy Italian With Parmesan	1 tbsp	35	tr	3
French	1 tbsp	33	tr	2
Italian	1 tbsp	9	tr	tr
Italian No Sugar Added	1 tbsp	6	tr	tr
Italian Sodium Free	1 tbsp	9	tr	tr
Ranch	1 tbsp	35	tr	2
Thousand Island	1 tbsp	24	tr	2
Weight Watchers				
Caesar	1 pkg (¾ oz)	6	0	0
Caesar	1 tbsp	4	0	0
Cucumber Creamy	1 tbsp	18	0	0
Italian	1 pkg (¾ oz)	8	—	tr
Italian	1 tbsp	6	—	tr
Italian Creamy	1 tbsp	12	0	0
Peppercorn Creamy	1 tbsp	8	0	0
Ranch Creamy	1 pkg (¾ oz)	35	—	tr
Ranch Creamy	1 tbsp	25	—	tr
Russian	1 tbsp	50	1	5
Thousand Island	1 tbsp	50	1	5
Wishbone				
Blue Cheese Chunky	1 tbsp	73	1	8

FOOD	PORTION	CALS.	SAT. FAT	FAT
Wishbone *(cont.)*				
Blue Cheese Chunky Lite	1 tbsp	40	1	4
Caesar With Olive Oil Lite	1 tbsp	28	tr	3
Dijon Vinaigrette Classic	1 tbsp	57	1	6
Dijon Vinaigrette Classic Lite	1 tbsp	30	—	3
French Deluxe	1 tbsp	57	1	5
French Fat Free	1 tbsp	6	0	tr
French Lite	1 tbsp	30	tr	3
French Red	1 tbsp	64	1	6
French Red Lite	1 tbsp	17	—	tr
French Sweet 'N Spicy	1 tbsp	61	1	6
French Sweet 'N Spicy Lite	1 tbsp	17	—	tr
Italian	1 tbsp	45	1	5
Italian Creamy	1 tbsp	54	1	6
Italian Creamy Lite	1 tbsp	26	tr	2
Italian Lite	1 tbsp	6	0	tr
Italian Robusto	1 tbsp	46	1	5
Olive Oil Italian Classic	1 tbsp	33	tr	3
Olive Oil Italian Classic Lite	1 tbsp	20	—	2
Olive Oil Vinaigrette	1 tbsp	30	tr	3
Olive Oil Vinaigrette Lite	1 tbsp	16	tr	1
Ranch	1 tbsp	76	1	8
Ranch Lite	1 tbsp	42	1	4
Red Wine Vinaigrette Olive Oil Lite	1 tbsp	20	tr	2
Red Wine Olive Oil Vinaigrette	1 tbsp	34	1	3
Russian	1 tbsp	54	tr	3
Russian Lite	1 tbsp	21	—	tr
Thousand Island	1 tbsp	66	1	6
Thousand Island Lite	1 tbsp	22	—	1
blue cheese	1 tbsp	77	2	8
french	1 tbsp	67	2	6
french reduced calorie	1 tbsp	22	tr	1
italian	1 tbsp	69	1	7
italian reduced calorie	1 tbsp	16	tr	2
russian	1 tbsp	76	1	8
russian reduced calorie	1 tbsp	23	tr	1
sesame seed	1 tbsp	68	1	7
thousand island	1 tbsp	59	1	6

FOOD	PORTION	CALS.	SAT. FAT	FAT
thousand island reduced calorie	1 tbsp	24	tr	2

SALMON
CANNED
Bumble Bee

FOOD	PORTION	CALS.	SAT. FAT	FAT
Keta	3.5 oz	160	2	8
Pink	3.5 oz	160	2	8
Pink Skinless & Boneless	3.25 oz	120	1	5
Red	3.5 oz	180	2	10
Red Skinless & Boneless	3.25 oz	130	1	6
Deming's Alaska Keta	½ cup	140	—	5
Deming's Alaska Pink	½ cup	140	1	6
Deming's Alaska Red Sockeye	½ cup	170	2	9
Double Q Alaska Pink	½ cup	140	1	6
Humpty Dumpty Alaska Chum	½ cup	140	—	2
Libby's Keta	½ cup (3.8 oz)	140	—	6
Libby's Pink	½ can (3.8 oz)	150	—	7
S&W Bluepack Fancy Diet	½ cup	188	—	11
S&W Red Fancy Sockeye Bluepack	½ cup	190	—	10
chum w/ bone	3 oz	120	1	5
chum w/ bone	1 can (13.9 oz)	521	5	20
pink w/ bone	3 oz	118	1	5
pink w/ bone	1 can (15.9 oz)	631	7	27
sockeye w/ bone	3 oz	130	1	6
sockeye w/ bone	1 can (12.9 oz)	566	6	27

FRESH

FOOD	PORTION	CALS.	SAT. FAT	FAT
atlantic, baked	3 oz	155	1	7
chinook, baked	3 oz	196	3	11
chum, baked	3 oz	131	1	4
coho, cooked	3 oz	157	1	6
coho, cooked	½ fillet (5.4 oz)	286	2	12
pink, baked	3 oz	127	1	4
roe, raw	3.5 oz	207	—	10
sockeye, cooked	3 oz	183	2	9
sockeye, cooked	½ fillet (5.4 oz)	334	3	17
sockeye, raw	3 oz	143	1	7

SMOKED

FOOD	PORTION	CALS.	SAT. FAT	FAT
chinook	3 oz	99	1	4

FOOD	PORTION	CALS.	SAT. FAT	FAT
chinook	1 oz	33	tr	1
TAKE-OUT				
salmon cake	1 (3 oz)	241	7	15

SALSA
(see also MEXICAN FOOD)

FOOD	PORTION	CALS.	SAT. FAT	FAT
Casa Fiesta Chili Salsa	1 oz	9	—	tr
Chi-Chi's				
Hot Chi-Chi	2 tbsp (1 oz)	10	0	0
Mild	2 tbsp (1 oz)	10	0	0
Verde Medium	2 tbsp (1.2 oz)	15	0	0
Verde Mild	2 tbsp (1.2 oz)	15	0	0
Frito Lay Hot	1 oz	12	0	0
Frito Lay Medium	1 oz	12	0	0
Frito Lay Mild	1 oz	12	0	0
Hain Hot	¼ cup	22	0	0
Hain Mild	¼ cup	20	0	0
Heluva Good Cheese Cheese & Salsa	2 tbsp (1.1 oz)	80	5	6
Heluva Good Cheese Thick & Chunky Hot	2 tbsp (1.2 oz)	10	0	0
Heluva Good Cheese Thick & Chunky Mild	2 tbsp (1.2 oz)	10	0	0
Hot Cha Cha Medium	2 tbsp (1 oz)	5	0	0
Newman's Own Bandito Hot	1 tbsp (0.7 oz)	6	—	tr
Newman's Own Bandito Medium	1 tbsp (0.7 oz)	6	—	tr
Newman's Own Bandito Mild	1 tbsp (0.7 oz)	6	—	tr
Old El Paso				
Picante Hot	2 tbsp	10	—	tr
Picante Medium	2 tbsp	10	—	tr
Picante Mild	2 tbsp	10	—	tr
Thick'n Chunky Green Chili	2 tbsp	3	0	0
Thick'n Chunky Hot	2 tbsp	6	—	tr
Thick'n Chunky Medium	2 tbsp	6	—	tr
Thick'n Chunky Mild	2 tbsp	6	—	tr
Thick'n Chunky Salsa Verde	2 tbsp	10	0	tr
Ortega Hot Green Chili	1 tbsp	6	0	0
Ortega Medium Green Chili	1 tbsp	6	0	0
Ortega Mild Green Chili	1 tbsp	8	0	0
Pace Thick & Chunky	2 tbsp (1 fl oz)	12	0	0

FOOD	PORTION	CALS.	SAT. FAT	FAT
Rosarita Chunky Hot	3 tbsp (1.5 oz)	25	—	tr
Rosarita Chunky Medium	3 tbsp (1.5 oz)	25	—	tr
Rosarita Chunky Mild	3 tbsp (1.5 oz)	25	—	tr
Rosarita Taco Salsa Chunky Medium	3 tbsp (1.5 oz)	25	—	tr
Rosarita Taco Salsa Chunky Mild	3 tbsp (1.5 oz)	25	—	tr

SALSIFY
fresh, cooked, sliced	½ cup	46	—	tr
fresh, raw, sliced	½ cup	55	—	tr

SALT/SEASONED SALT
(see also SALT SUBSTITUTES)

Hain Sea Salt	1 tsp	0	0	0
Hain Sea Salt Iodized	1 tsp	0	0	0
Morton				
Garlic	1 tsp	3	—	tr
Iodized	1 tsp	tr	—	0
Kosher	1 tsp	0	—	0
Lite	1 tsp	tr	—	0
Non-Iodized	1 tsp	0	—	0
Seasoned	1 tsp	4	—	tr
Morton Nature's Season Seasoning Blend	1 tsp	3	—	tr
salt	1 tsp	0	0	0

SALT SUBSTITUTES
Morton	1 tsp	tr	—	0
Papa Dash Lite Lite Lite Salt	¼ tsp	1	—	0
Papa Dash Salt Lover's Blend	¼ tsp	tr	—	0

SAPODILLA
fresh	1	140	—	2
fresh, cut up	1 cup	199	—	3

SAPOTES
fresh	1	301	—	1

SARDINES
CANNED

Empress Skinless & Boneless Olive Oil	1 can (3.8 oz)	420	—	38

FOOD	PORTION	CALS.	SAT. FAT	FAT
Empress Skinless & Boneless Soy Oil	1 can (4.4 oz)	500	—	45
In Louisiana Hot Sauce (Port Clyde)	1 can (3.75 oz)	170	2	9
In Mustard Sauce (Holmes)	1 can (3.75 oz)	150	2	9
In Mustard Sauce (Port Clyde)	1 can (3.75 oz)	150	2	9
In Soybean Oil Select Small (Port Clyde)	1 can (3.3 oz)	220	4	17
In Soybean Oil With Hot Chilies (Port Clyde)	1 can (3.3 oz)	155	2	9
In Soybean Oil, drained (Holmes)	1 can (3.3 oz)	220	4	17
In Soybean Oil, drained (Port Clyde)	1 can (3.3 oz)	220	4	17
In Spring Water (Port Clyde)	1 can (3.3 oz)	170	4	10
In Tomato Sauce (Port Clyde)	1 can (3.75 oz)	150	2	9
S&W Norwegian Brisling	1.5 oz	130	—	10
Underwood				
Brisling In Olive Oil	3.75 oz	260	—	20
In Mild Oil, drained	3.75 oz	460	—	42
In Mustard Sauce	3.75 oz	220	—	16
In Soya Oil, drained	3 oz	230	—	18
In Tomato Sauce	3.75 oz	220	—	16
With Tabasco Brand Pepper Sauce, drained	3 oz	220	—	16
Viking's Delight Brisling In Olive Oil	1 can (3.75 oz)	460	—	42
Vikings Delight Brisling In Olive Oil, drained	1 can (3.75 oz)	260	—	20
atlantic in oil w/ bone	2	50	tr	3
atlantic in oil w/ bone	1 can (3.2 oz)	192	1	11
pacific in tomato sauce w/ bone	1	68	1	5
pacific in tomato sauce w/ bone	1 can (13 oz)	658	11	44
FRESH				
raw	3.5 oz	135	—	5

FOOD	PORTION	CALS.	SAT. FAT	FAT

SAUCE
(see also GRAVY, PIZZA, SPAGHETTI SAUCE, TOMATO)

DRY

FOOD	PORTION	CALS.	SAT. FAT	FAT
Au Jus (Knorr)	2 oz	8	—	tr
Bar-B-Q (Diamond Crystal)	2 oz	35	—	1
Bearnaise (Knorr)	2 oz	170	—	17
Brown (Diamond Crystal)	2 oz	15	—	tr
Cheese (Diamond Crystal)	2 oz	50	—	2
Classic Brown Gravy (Knorr)	2 oz	25	—	1
Cream (Diamond Crystal)	2 oz	40	—	1
Demi-Glace (Knorr)	2 oz	30	—	1
Etoufee Seasoning Mix (Cajun King)	3.5 oz	383	—	6
Hollandaise (Knorr)	2 oz	170	—	18
Hunter (Knorr)	2 oz	25	—	tr
Italian (Diamond Crystal)	3 oz	50	—	tr
Jambalaya Seasoning Mix (Cajun King)	3.5 oz	375	—	9
Lyonnaise (Knorr)	2 oz	20	—	tr
Marinade for Meat (Kikkoman)	1-oz pkg	64	—	tr
Mushroom (Knorr)	2 oz	60	—	3
Napoli (Knorr)	4 oz	100	—	3
Pepper (Knorr)	2 oz	20	—	1
Sweet & Sour (Kikkoman)	2.13-oz pkg	228	—	tr
Sweet 'N Sour Entree Mix (Chun King)	3.8 oz	370	—	0
Teriyaki (Kikkoman)	1.5-oz pkg	125	—	tr
bearnaise, as prep w/ milk & butter	1 cup	701	42	68
cheese, as prep w/ milk	1 cup	307	9	17
curry, as prep w/ milk	1 cup	270	6	15
mushroom, as prep w/ milk	1 cup	228	5	10
sour cream, as prep w/ milk	1 cup	509	16	30
stroganoff, as prep	1 cup	271	7	11
sweet & sour, as prep	1 cup	294	tr	tr
teriyaki, as prep	1 cup	131	tr	1
white, as prep	1 cup	241	6	13

JARRED

FOOD	PORTION	CALS.	SAT. FAT	FAT
7 Spice Chili (McIlhenny)	2 tbsp (1.1 fl oz)	16	tr	tr
Alfredo (Progresso)	½ cup	340	19	30

FOOD	PORTION	CALS.	SAT. FAT	FAT
B-B-Q (McIlhenny)	2 tbsp (1.1 oz)	48	tr	2
BBQ Hot & Spicy (Healthy Choice)	2 tbsp (1.1 oz)	25	0	0
BBQ Original (Healthy Choice)	2 tbsp (1.1 oz)	25	0	0
BBQ Dijon Honey (Lawry's)	¼ cup	203	tr	1
BBQ Hickory (Healthy Choice)	2 tbsp (1.1 oz)	25	0	0
Bandito Diavalo Spicy (Newman's Own)	4 oz	70	—	2
Bangkok Padang (House Of Tsang)	1 tbsp (0.6 oz)	45	1	3
Bar-B-Que Honey (Hain)	1 tbsp	14	—	1
Barbecue (Kraft)	2 tbsp	45	0	1
Barbecue (Maull's)	3.5 oz	123	—	2
Barbecue (Ott's)	1 tbsp	14	—	tr
Barbecue Beer Non-Alcoholic (Maull's)	3.5 oz	128	—	2
Barbecue Country Style (Hunt's)	1 tbsp	20	—	tr
Barbecue Garlic (Kraft)	2 tbsp	40	0	0
Barbecus Hickory Smoke (Kraft)	2 tbsp	45	0	1
Barbecue Hickory Smoke Onion Bits (Kraft)	2 tbsp	50	0	1
Barbecue Honey Mustard (Hunt's)	1 tbsp (1.2 oz)	50	—	0
Barbecue Hong Kong (House Of Tsang)	1 tbsp (0.6 oz)	10	0	0
Barbecue Hot (Kraft)	2 tbsp	45	0	1
Barbecue Hot Hickory Smoke (Kraft)	2 tbsp	45	0	1
Barbecue Italian Seasoning	2 tbsp	50	0	1
Barbecue Kansas City Style (Kraft)	2 tbsp	50	0	1
Barbecue New Orleans Style (Hunt's)	1 tbsp	20	—	tr
Barbecue Onion Bits (Kraft)	2 tbsp	50	0	1
Barbecue Original (Hunt's)	2 tbsp	40	0	0
Barbecue Select (Heinz)	1 oz	40	0	0
Barbecue Select Hickory (Heinz)	1 oz	35	0	0

FOOD	PORTION	CALS.	SAT. FAT	FAT
Barbecue Southern Style (Hunt's)	1 tbsp	20	—	tr
Barbecue Sweet-N-Mild (Maull's)	3.5 oz	167	—	2
Barbecue Sweet-N-Smoky (Maull's)	3.5 oz	160	—	tr
Barbecue Texas Style (Hunt's)	1 tbsp	25	—	tr
Barbecue Thick & Rich (Heinz)				
Cajun Style	1 oz	35	0	0
Chunky	1 oz	30	0	0
Hawaiian Style	1 oz	40	0	0
Hickory Smoke	1 oz	35	0	0
Mesquite Smoke	1 oz	30	0	0
Mushroom	1 oz	30	0	0
Old Fashioned	1 oz	35	0	0
Onion	1 oz	30	0	0
Original	1 oz	35	0	0
Texas Hot	1 oz	30	0	0
Barbecue Thick'n Spicy (Kraft)				
Kansas City Style	2 tbsp	60	0	1
Mesquite Smoke	2 tbsp	50	0	1
Original	2 tbsp	50	0	1
With Honey	2 tbsp	60	0	1
Barbecue Western Style (Hunt's)	1 tbsp	20	—	tr
Barbecue w/ Onion Bits (Maull's)	3.5 oz	126	—	2
Cajun Style (Golden Dipt)	1 oz	90	—	8
Cocktail (Heluva Good Cheese)	¼ cup (1.6 oz)	40	0	0
Cocktail (Sauceworks)	1 tbsp	14	0	0
Creole (Golden Dipt)	1 oz	20	—	1
Diable (Escoffier)	1 tbsp	20	0	0
Dijonnaise (Golden Dipt)	1 oz	52	—	4
Duck Sauce Sweet & Sour (La Choy)	1 tbsp	25	—	tr
Enchilada Green (Old El Paso)	2 tbsp	11	0	0
Enchilada Hot (Old El Paso)	¼ cup	30	—	1
Enchilada Mild (Old El Paso)	¼ cup	25	—	1

FOOD	PORTION	CALS.	SAT. FAT	FAT
Enchilada Sauce (Gebhardt)	3 tbsp	25	0	1
French White (Golden Dipt)	1 oz	55	—	4
Ginger Teriyaki Marinade (Golden Dipt)	1 oz	120	—	7
Grilling & Broiling Chardonnay (Knorr)	1.6 oz	50	—	4
Grilling & Broiling Spicy Plum (Knorr)	1.7 oz	60	—	2
Grilling & Broiling Tequilla Lime (Knorr)	1.6 oz	50	—	3
Grilling & Broiling Tuscan Herb (Knorr)	1.6 oz	50	—	4
Hoisin (House of Tsang)	1 tsp (6 g)	15	0	0
Hot Dog (Wolf Brand)	1.25 oz	44	—	2
Hot Dog Chili Sauce (Gebhardt)	2 tbsp	30	—	1
Hot Dog Sauce (Just Rite)	2 oz	60	1	3
Hot Dog Sauce (Gebhardt)	½ tsp	tr	—	tr
Indi-Pep West Indian Style Pepper Sauce (Trappey)	1 tsp (0.1 oz)	1	0	tr
Lemon Butter Dill (Golden Dipt)	1 oz	100	—	9
Lemon Herb Marinade (Golden Dipt)	1 oz	130	—	14
Mandarin Marinade (House of Tsang)	1 tbsp (0.6 oz)	25	0	0
Manwich Mexican	2.5 oz	35	—	1
Mexi Pep Louisiana Hot Sauce (Trappey)	1 tsp (0.1 oz)	tr	0	tr
Microwave Hollandaise (Knorr)	1 oz	50	—	5
Microwave Mandarin Ginger (Knorr)	1.6 oz	50	—	4
Microwave Parmesano (Knorr)	1.6 oz	50	—	4
Microwave Vera Cruz (Knorr)	3.3 oz	70	—	3
Newburg w/ Sherry (Snow's)	⅓ cup	120	—	8
Not-So-Sloppy-Joe Sauce (Hormel)	¼ cup (2.2 oz)	70	0	0
Pepper Sauce (Trappey)	1 tsp (0.2 oz)	1	0	tr
Picante (Pace)	2 tbsp (1 fl oz)	7	0	0
Picante (Tabasco)	2 tbsp (1.5 oz)	17	tr	tr
Picante (Wise)	2 tbsp	12	0	0

FOOD	PORTION	CALS.	SAT. FAT	FAT
Picante Hot (Old El Paso)	2 tbsp	8	—	tr
Picante Medium (Old El Paso)	2 tbsp	8	—	tr
Picante Mild (Old El Paso)	2 tbsp	8	—	tr
Picante Chunky Hot (Old El Paso)	2 tbsp	7	0	0
Picante Chunky Medium (Old El Paso)	2 tbsp	7	0	0
Picante Chunky Mild (Old El Paso)	2 tbsp	7	0	0
Picante Medium (Guiltless Gourmet)	1 oz	6	0	0
Primavera Creamy (Progresso)	½ cup	190	10	17
Red Devil Buffalo Style Hot Sauce (Trappey)	1 tsp (0.1 oz)	1	0	tr
Red Devil Cayenne Pepper Sauce (Trappey)	1 tsp (0.1 oz)	1	0	tr
Rib (Gold's)	1 oz	60	0	0
Saigon Sizzle (House of Tsang)	1 tbsp (0.6 oz)	40	0	1
Seafood Cocktail (Golden Dipt)	1 tbsp	20	0	0
Seafood Cocktail Extra Hot (Golden Dipt)	1 tbsp	20	0	0
Simmer Chef Golden Honey Mustard (Campbell)	½ cup (4 fl oz)	150	0	2
Simmer Chef Hearty Onion & Mushroom (Campbell)	½ cup (4 fl oz)	50	0	1
Sloppy Joe (Manwich)	2.5 oz	40		tr
Spicy Brown Bean (House of Tsang)	1 tsp (6 g)	15	0	0
Steak (Lea & Perrins)	1 oz	40	—	tr
Steak (Mrs. Dash)	1 tbsp	17	—	tr
Stir Fry Classic (House of Tsang)	1 tbsp (0.6 oz)	25	0	1
Stir Fry Sweet & Sour (House Of Tsang)	1 tbsp (0.6 oz)	35	0	0
Stir Fry Szechuan Spicy (House Of Tsang)	1 tbsp (0.6 oz)	20	0	1
Stir Fry (Kikkoman)	1 tbsp	16	—	tr
Sweet & Sour (Kikkoman)	1 tbsp	19	—	tr
Sweet & Sour (La Choy)	1 tbsp	25	—	tr
Sweet & Sour Concentrate (House of Tsang)	1 tsp (6 g)	10	0	0

FOOD	PORTION	CALS.	SAT. FAT	FAT
Sweet 'N Sour (Contadina)	½ cup	150	—	3
Sweet 'N Sour (Sauceworks)	1 tbsp	25	0	0
Tabasco (McIlhenny)	1 tsp	1	tr	tr
Taco Hot (Old El Paso)	2 tbsp	10	—	tr
Taco Medium (Old El Paso)	2 tbsp	10	—	tr
Taco Mild (Old El Paso)	2 tbsp	10	—	tr
Tartar (Best Foods)	1 tbsp (14 g)	70	1	8
Tartar (Bright Day)	1 tbsp	50	—	5
Tartar (Golden Dipt)	1 tbsp	70	—	7
Tartar (Hellman's)	1 tbsp (14 g)	70	1	8
Tartar (Sauceworks)	1 tbsp	50	1	5
Tartar (Weight Watchers)	1 tbsp	35	1	3
Tartar Lite (Golden Dipt)	1 tbsp	50	—	4
Tartar Natural Lemon & Herb (Kraft)	1 tbsp	70	1	8
Teriyaki (Kikkoman)	1 tbsp	15	0	0
Teriyaki Marinade (Lawry's)	2 tbsp	72	tr	tr
Teriyaki Korean (House Of Tsang)	1 tbsp (0.6 oz)	30	0	1
Tomatoes & Jalapenos (Old El Paso)	¼ cup	11	0	tr
Tomatoes & Green Chilies (Old El Paso)	¼ cup	14	—	tr
Welsh Rarebit Cheese (Snow's)	½ cup	170	—	11
Worchestershire (Heinz)	1 tbsp	6	0	0
Worcestershire (Lea & Perrins)	1 tsp	5	—	tr
Worcestershire Chef Magic (Trappey)	1 tsp (0.1 oz)	3	tr	tr
Worcestershire White Wine (Lea & Perrins)	1 tsp	4	—	tr
barbecue	1 cup	188	1	5
teriyaki	1 tbsp	15	0	0
teriyaki	1 oz	30	0	0

SAUERKRAUT

CANNED

FOOD	PORTION	CALS.	SAT. FAT	FAT
Claussen	½ cup	17	—	tr
Hebrew National Gallon Kraut	½ cup	25	0	0

FOOD	PORTION	CALS.	SAT. FAT	FAT
New Kraut (Hebrew National)	½ cup (3.1 oz)	50	—	1
Rosoff's	½ cup (3.2 oz)	50	—	1
S&W	½ cup	25	0	0
Schorr's New Kraut	½ cup (3.2 oz)	50	—	1
Seneca	2 tbsp	5	0	0
SnowFloss Kraut	4 oz	28	—	0
SnowFloss Kraut Bavarian Style	4 oz	64	—	0
Vlasic Old Fashioned	1 oz	4	0	0
canned	½ cup	22	tr	tr
JUICE				
S&W	4 oz	14	0	0

SAUSAGE
(*see also* HOT DOG, SAUSAGE SUBSTITUTES)

FOOD	PORTION	CALS.	SAT. FAT	FAT
Aidells Smoked Chicken And Apple	1 (3.5 oz)	220	5	17
Armour				
Country Sausage Lower Salt	1 oz	110	—	11
Country Sausage Lower Salt Patties	1.5 oz	160	—	16
Country Sausage Lower Salt Links	1 oz	110	—	11
Pork	1 oz	110	—	11
Pork Links	1 oz	110	—	11
Pork Patties	1.5 oz	160	—	16
Bil Mar Foods Breakfast Turkey	1 oz	58	—	4
Bill Mar Foods Smoked	3 oz	142	—	10
Brown & Serve				
Bacon	1	90	—	8
Beef	1	90	—	9
Light	1	60	—	5
Regular	1	100	—	10
Golden Brown				
Beef	1	80	—	7
Light Links	1	60	—	5
Mild	1	100	—	10
Mild Pattie	1	150	—	14
Spicy	1	100	—	9
Hebrew National Beef Knocks	1 (3 oz)	260	—	25

FOOD	PORTION	CALS.	SAT. FAT	FAT
Hebrew National Polish Beef	1 link	240	—	22
Hillshire				
Beer Bratwurst	1 (2 oz)	190	—	17
Bratwurst Fresh	1 (2 oz)	190	—	17
Bratwurst Light Fresh	1 (2 oz)	150	—	11
Bratwurst Spicy	1 (2 oz)	180	—	17
Flavorseal Kielbasa Polska	2 oz	190	—	17
Flavorseal Kielbasa Polska Beef	2 oz	190	—	17
Flavorseal Kielbasa Polska Lite	2 oz	130	—	11
Flavorseal Kielbasa Polska Mild	2 oz	190	—	17
Flavorseal Kielbasa Polska Turkey	2 oz	90	—	5
Flavorseal Smoked	2 oz	190	—	17
Flavorseal Smoked Beef	2 oz	180	—	16
Flavorseal Smoked Beef And Cheddar	2 oz	190	—	15
Flavorseal Smoked Country Recipe	2 oz	180	—	16
Flavorseal Smoked Hot	2 oz	180	—	16
Flavorseal Smoked Lite	2 oz	130	—	11
Flavorseal Smoked Turkey	2 oz	90	—	5
Flavorseal Smoked w/ Italian Seasoning	2 oz	200	—	18
Italian Hot	1 (2 oz)	180	—	17
Italian Hot Light	1 (2 oz)	150	—	11
Italian Mild	1 (2 oz)	190	—	17
Italian Mild Light	1 (2 oz)	150	—	11
Kielbasa Fresh Polska	1 (2 oz)	190	—	17
Kielbasa Fresh Polska Lower Fat	1 (2 oz)	150	—	11
Links 80% Fat Free Cheddar Hots	2 oz	150	—	12
Links 80% Fat Free Kielbasa	2 oz	130	—	10
Links 80% Fat Free Smokies	2 oz	130	—	10
Links Brats Fully Cooked	2 oz	170	—	16

FOOD	PORTION	CALS.	SAT. FAT	FAT
Links Bratwurst Smoked	2 oz	190	—	17
Links Cheddarwurst	2 oz	190	—	17
Links Cheddarwurst Lite	1 link (2.7 oz)	190	—	15
Links Hot	2 oz	190	—	16
Links Hot Beef	2 oz	190	—	17
Links Hot Lite	1 link (2.7 oz)	190	—	15
Links Kielbasa Polska	2 oz	190	—	17
Links Kielbasa Polska Lite	1 link (2.7 oz)	190	—	15
Links Knockwurst Lite	2 oz	180	—	16
Links Lit'l Polskas	2 oz	180	—	16
Links Lit'l Smokies	2 oz	180	—	16
Links Lit'l Smokies Beef	2 oz	180	—	16
Links Lit'l Smokies Cheddar	2 oz	180	—	16
Links Lit'l Smokies Light	2 oz	120	—	8
Links Polish	2 oz	190	—	17
Links Smoked	2 oz	190	—	18
Links Bun Size Cheddarwurst	2 oz	200	—	18
Links Bun Size Kielbasa	2 oz	180	—	16
Links Bun Size Smoked	2 oz	180	—	16
Links Bun Size Smoked Beef	2 oz	180	—	16
Mexican Style	1 (2 oz)	190	—	17
Mexican Style Lower Fat	1 (2 oz)	150	—	11
Hormel Light & Lean 97 Dinner Smoked	2 oz	60	1	2
Hormel Pickled Hot	6 (2 oz)	140	5	11
Hormel Pickled Smoked	6 (2 oz)	140	5	11
Jones				
Cello Beef	1 slice (1 oz)	130	—	13
Cello Hot Country	1 slice (1 oz)	110	—	10
Cello Original	1 slice (1 oz)	100	—	10
Dinner Link	1	280	—	28
Italian	1	160	—	14
Light Link	1	70	—	6
Little Link	1	140	—	14
Patties	1	150	—	14
Scrapple	1 slice (1.5 oz)	90	—	6
Little Sizzlers				
Brown & Serve	2 patties (1.4 oz)	190	6	18

FOOD	PORTION	CALS.	SAT. FAT	FAT
Little Sizzlers *(cont.)*				
Brown & Serve	3 links (2.1 oz)	190	8	22
Heat & Serve Pork cooked	3 links (1.4 oz)	210	7	20
cooked	2 patties (2 oz)	250	8	23
cooked	3 links (1.4 oz)	210	7	20
Louis Rich				
Polska Kielbasa	2 oz	80	2	5
Smoked Sausage With Cheese cooked	1 (1 oz)	47	1	3
Turkey	2.5 oz	110	3	6
Turkey & Cheese Smoked	2 oz	90	2	5
Turkey Links	2 (2 oz)	90	2	6
Turkey Smoked	2 oz	90	2	5
Mr. Turkey Polish Kielbasa	3 oz	177	—	13
Old Smokehouse Summer Sausage	1 oz	110	4	10
Oscar Mayer				
Pork cooked	2 links (1.7 oz)	170	5	15
Smokies Beef	1 (1.5 oz)	120	5	11
Smokies Cheese	1 (1.5 oz)	130	4	12
Smokies Links	1 (1.5 oz)	130	4	12
Smokies Little	6 (2 oz)	170	6	16
Perdue				
Breakfast Links Turkey, cooked	1 (1.3 oz)	40	1	3
Breakfast Patties Turkey, cooked	1 (1.3 oz)	61	1	4
Hot Italian Turkey, cooked	1 (2 oz)	94	2	6
Sweet Italian Turkey, cooked	1 (2 oz)	94	2	6
Shofar Knockwurst Beef	1 (3 oz)	260	9	23
Vienna (Hormel)	2 oz	140	4	13
Vienna Chicken (Hormel)	2 oz	90	3	10
blutwurst, uncooked	3.5 oz	424	—	39
bockwurst, pork & veal, raw	1 link (2.3 oz)	200	7	18
bratwurst pork, cooked	1 link (3 oz)	256	8	22
bratwurst, pork	1 oz	92	3	8
bratwurst pork & beef	1 link (2.5 oz)	226	7	19
country-style pork, cooked	1 link (½ oz)	48	1	4
country-style pork, cooked	1 patty (1 oz)	100	3	8

FOOD	PORTION	CALS.	SAT. FAT	FAT
gelbwurst, uncooked	3.5 oz	363	—	33
italian pork, cooked	1 (3 oz)	268	8	21
italian pork, cooked	1 (2.4 oz)	216	6	17
kielbasa pork	1 oz	88	3	8
knockwurst pork & beef	1 oz	87	3	8
knockwurst pork & beef	1 (2.4 oz)	209	7	19
mettwurst, uncooked	3.5 oz	483	—	45
plockwurst, uncooked	3.5 oz	312	—	45
polish pork	1 oz	92	3	8
polish pork	1 (8 oz)	739	23	65
pork & beef, cooked	1 link (½ oz)	52	2	5
pork & beef, cooked	1 patty (1 oz)	107	4	10
pork, cooked	1 link (½ oz)	48	1	4
pork, cooked	1 patty (1 oz)	100	3	8
regensburger, uncooked	3.5 oz	354	—	31
smoked beef, cooked	1 (1.4 oz)	134	—	12
smoked pork	1 sm link(½ oz)	62	2	5
smoked pork	1 link (2.4 oz)	265	8	22
smoked pork & beef	1 sm link (½ oz)	54	2	5
smoked pork & beef	1 link (2.4 oz)	229	7	21
vienna, canned	1 (½ oz)	45	1	4
vienna, canned	7 (4 oz)	315	10	28
weisswurst, uncooked	3.5 oz	305	—	27
TAKE-OUT				
Tyson Country Pork	3.5 oz	320	—	29
pork	1 link (½ oz)	48	1	4
pork	1 patty (1 oz)	100	3	8

SAUSAGE DISHES
FROZEN

FOOD	PORTION	CALS.	SAT. FAT	FAT
Jimmy Dean Sausage Biscuits Microwave	1	210	—	14
Ovenstuffs French Roll Italian Sausage	1 (4.75 oz)	390	—	22
Ovenstuffs French Roll Pepperoni	1 (4.75 oz)	370	—	20
TAKE-OUT				
sausage roll	1 (2.3 oz)	311	—	24

SAUSAGE SUBSTITUTES

FOOD	PORTION	CALS.	SAT. FAT	FAT
Knox Mountain Farm Not-So-Sausage	1 serv (⅒ pkg)	120	—	1
LaLoma Linketts	2 (71 g)	140	—	8
LaLoma Little Links	2 (46 g)	90	—	5

FOOD	PORTION	CALS.	SAT. FAT	FAT
Lightlife Lean Links Breakfast	1.25 oz	69	tr	3
Lightlife Lean Links Italian	1.5 oz	83	tr	3
Morningstar Farms				
Breakfast Patties	2 (76 g)	190	—	12
Breakfast Links	2 (45 g)	90	—	5
Country Crisp Patties	1 (71 g)	220	—	15
Grillers	1 (64 g)	180	—	12
White Wave Meatless Healthy Links	2 (1.6 oz)	140	2	10
Worthington				
Leanies	1 link (40 g)	100	—	6
Prosage Links	2 (45 g)	130	—	9
Saucettes	2 links (67 g)	150	—	11
Super-Links	1 (48 g)	100	—	7
Veja-Links	2 (62 g)	140	—	10

SAVORY

ground	1 tsp	4	—	tr

SCALLOP

fresh, raw	3 oz	75	tr	1
FROZEN				
Fried (Mrs. Paul's)	2 oz	160	—	7
Lightly Breaded (King & Prince)	3.5 oz	120	—	tr
HOME RECIPE				
breaded & fried	2 lg	67	1	3
TAKE-OUT				
breaded & fried	6 (5 oz)	386	5	19

SCONE

HOME RECIPE				
apricot scone	1	232	—	7
TAKE-OUT				
cheese	1 (1.75 oz)	182	—	9
fruit	1 (1.75 oz)	158	—	5
plain	1 (1.75 oz)	181	—	7

SCROD

FROZEN				
Microwave Entree Baked (Gorton's)	1 pkg	320	4	18
Ready-to-Bake (King & Prince)	5 oz	252	—	16

FOOD	PORTION	CALS.	SAT. FAT	FAT
SCUP				
fresh, baked	3 oz	115	—	3
SEA BASS				
(*see* BASS)				
SEA TROUT				
(*see* TROUT)				
SEAWEED				
DRIED				
agar	1 oz	87	tr	tr
spirulina	1 oz	83	1	2
FRESH				
agar	1 oz	tr	tr	tr
irishmoss	1 oz	14	tr	tr
kelp	1 oz	12	tr	tr
kombu	1 oz	12	tr	tr
laver	1 oz	10	tr	tr
nori	1 oz	10	tr	tr
spirulina	1 oz	7	tr	tr
tangle	1 oz	12	tr	tr
wakame	1 oz	13	tr	tr
SEITAN				
(*see* WHEAT)				
SEMOLINA				
dry	½ cup	303	tr	tr
SESAME				
Sesame Butter (Erewhon)	2 tbsp (32 g)	190	—	17
Sesame Tahini (Arrowhead)	1 oz	170	—	17
Sesame Tahini (Erewhon)	2 tbsp	200	—	18
seeds	1 tsp	16	—	2
seeds, dried	1 tbsp	52	1	5
seeds, dried	1 cup	825	10	72
seeds, roasted & toasted	1 oz	161	2	14
sesame butter	1 tbsp	95	1	8
tahini from roasted & toasted kernels	1 tbsp	89	1	8
tahini from stone ground kernels	1 tbsp	86	1	7
tahini from unroasted kernels	1 tbsp	85	1	8

FOOD	PORTION	CALS.	SAT. FAT	FAT
SESBANIA				
flowers	1	1	0	0
flowers	1 cup	5	—	tr
flowers, cooked	1 cup	23	—	tr
SHAD				
american, baked	3 oz	214	—	15
roe, raw	3.5 oz	130	—	2
roe, baked w/ butter & lemon	3.5 oz	126	—	3
SHALLOTS				
dried	1 tbsp	3	0	0
fresh, raw, chopped	1 tbsp	7	tr	tr
SHARK				
batter-dipped & fried	3 oz	194	3	12
raw	3 oz	111	1	4
SHEEPSHEAD FISH				
cooked	3 oz	107	1	1
cooked	1 fillet (6.5 oz)	234	1	3
raw	3 oz	92	1	2
SHELLFISH				
(see individual names, SHELLFISH SUBSTITUTES)				
SHELLFISH SUBSTITUTES				
Kibun Sea Pasta w/ dressing	½ pkg	220	—	7
Kibun Sea Pasta w/o dressing	½ pkg	110	—	1
Kibun Sea Pasta & Shrimp w/ dressing	½ pkg	210	—	9
Kibun Sea Pasta & Shrimp w/o dressing	½ pkg	140	—	1
Kibun Sea Stix Salad Style	4 oz	110	—	tr
Kibun Sea Stix Whole Leg	4 oz	110	—	tr
Kibun Sea Tails	4 oz	110	—	tr
Louis Kemp Crab Delights Chunk Style	2 oz	60	—	tr
Louis Kemp Lobster Delights	2 oz	60	—	tr
Louis Kemp Maryland Style Cakes	2.5 oz	154	—	9
crab, imitation	3 oz	87	—	1

FOOD	PORTION	CALS.	SAT. FAT	FAT
scallop, imitation	3 oz	84	—	tr
shrimp, imitation	3 oz	86	—	1
surimi	1 oz	28	—	tr
surimi	3 oz	84	—	1

SHELLIE BEANS

canned shellie beans	½ cup	37	tr	tr

SHERBET
(see also ICES AND ICE POPS)

All Flavors (Bresler's)	3.5 oz	140	—	2
Borden Orange	½ cup	110	—	1
Sealtest Lime	½ cup (3 oz)	130	0	1
Sealtest Orange	½ cup (3 oz)	130	1	1
Sealtest Rainbow Orange, Red Raspberry, Lime	½ cup (3 oz)	130	1	1
Sealtest Red Raspberry	½ cup (3 oz)	130	1	1
orange	1 cup	270	2	4
orange	½ gal	2158	19	31
orange home recipe	½ cup	120	—	2

SHRIMP

canned	3 oz	102	tr	2
FRESH				
cooked	4 large	22	tr	tr
cooked	3 oz	84	tr	1
raw	4 large	30	tr	tr
raw	3 oz	90	tr	1
FROZEN				
Butterfly Shrimp (Gorton's)	4 oz	160	—	tr
Cooked in the Shell (King & Prince)	4 oz	70	—	tr
Gourmet Hand Breaded Shrimp Butterfly (King & Prince)	3.5 oz	150	—	tr
Gourmet Hand Breaded Shrimp Round (King & Prince)	3.5 oz	150	—	tr
Light Seafood Entrees Shrimp & Clams w/ Linguini (Mrs. Paul's)	10 oz	240	2	5
Microwave Crunchy Shrimp (Gorton's)	5 oz	380	3	20

FOOD	PORTION	CALS.	SAT. FAT	FAT
Microwave Entree Shrimp Scampi (Gorton's)	1 pkg	390	—	30
Shrimp Creole (Cajun Cookin')	12 oz	390	—	11
Shrimp Crisps (Gorton's)	4 oz	280	—	15
Shrimp Del Ray (King & Prince)	3 oz	85	—	6
Western Style Breaded Shrimp (King & Prince)	3.5 oz	115	—	tr
READY-TO-USE				
Fried Shrimp (American Original Foods)	4 oz	253	2	12
TAKE-OUT				
breaded & fried	4 large	73	1	4
breaded & fried	3 oz	206	2	10
breaded & fried	6–8 (6 oz)	454	5	25
jambalaya	¾ cup	188	2	5

SMELT

FOOD	PORTION	CALS.	SAT. FAT	FAT
rainbow, cooked	3 oz	106	tr	3
rainbow, raw	3 oz	83	tr	2

SNACKS

(*see also* CHIPS, FRUIT SNACKS, NUTS MIXED, POPCORN, PRETZELS)

FOOD	PORTION	CALS.	SAT. FAT	FAT
Apple Chips (Weight Watchers)	¾ oz	70	0	0
Bakem-ets	21 pieces (1 oz)	160	—	10
Bakem-ets Hot'N Spicy	21 pieces (1 oz)	150	—	9
Bugles	1 oz	150	—	8
Bugles Nacho Cheese	1 oz	160	—	9
Bugles Ranch	1 oz	150	—	9
Carrot Lites (Health Valley)	½ oz	75	—	4
Cheese Balls (Lance)	1 pkg (32 g)	190	3	13
Cheese Curls (Weight Watchers)	½ oz	70	1	2
Cheetos Cheddar Valley	26 pieces (1 oz)	160	—	9
Cheetos Crunchy	26 pieces (1 oz)	150	—	9
Cheetos Curls	15 pieces (1 oz)	150	—	9
Cheetos Flamin' Hot	26 pieces (1 oz)	150	—	9
Cheetos Light	38 pieces (1 oz)	140	—	6
Cheetos Paws	16 pieces (1 oz)	160	—	10
Cheetos Puffed Ball	38 pieces (1 oz)	160	—	10
Cheetos Puffs	33 pieces (1 oz)	160	—	10
Cheez Doodles Crunchy	1 oz	160	—	10

FOOD	PORTION	CALS.	SAT. FAT	FAT
Cheez Doodles Puffed	1 oz	150	—	9
Cheez Waffles	1 oz	140	—	8
Chex Snack Mix Barbeque Flavor (Ralston)	½ cup (1.1 oz)	130	1	5
Chex Snack Mix Cool Sour Cream & Onion (Ralston)	½ cup (1 oz)	130	1	4
Chex Snack Mix Golden Cheddar (Ralston)	½ cup (1 oz)	130	1	4
Chex Snack Mix Traditional (Ralston)	⅔ cup (1.2 oz)	150	1	5
Combos Cheddar	1 pkg (1.7 oz)	250	3	13
Combos Cheddar Cheese Cracker	1 oz	140	2	8
Combos Cheddar Cheese Pretzel	1 oz	130	1	5
Combos Cheddar Cheese Pretzel	1 pkg (1.8 oz)	240	2	9
Combos Chili Cheese w/ Corn Shell	1 oz	140	1	6
Combos Chili Cheese w/ Corn Shell	1 pkg (1.7 oz)	230	2	11
Combos Mustard Pretzel	1 oz	130	1	5
Combos Mustard Pretzel	1 pkg (1.8 oz)	230	1	8
Combos Nacho	1 pkg (1.8 oz)	230	2	8
Combos Nacho Cheese Pretzel	1 oz	130	1	5
Combos Nacho Cheese w/ Tortilla Shell	1 oz	140	1	6
Combos Nacho Cheese w/ Tortilla Shell	1 pkg (1.7 oz)	230	2	11
Combos Pepperoni And Cheese Pizza	1 oz	140	1	7
Combos Pepperoni And Cheese Pizza	1 pkg (1.7 oz)	240	2	11
Combos Pizzeria Pretzel	1 oz	130	1	5
Combos Pizzeria Pretzel	1 pkg (1.8 oz)	230	2	8
Combos Tortilla Ranch	1 bag (1.7 oz)	240	3	12
Combos Tortilla Ranch	1 oz	140	2	7
Cornnuts Barbecue	1 oz	120	tr	4
Cornnuts Nacho Cheese	1 oz	120	tr	4
Cornnuts Original	1 oz	120	tr	4
Cornnuts Original	1 pkg (2 oz)	260	2	8
Cornnuts Picante	1 oz	120	tr	4
Cornnuts Ranch	1 oz	120	tr	4

FOOD	PORTION	CALS.	SAT. FAT	FAT
Crunchy Cheese Twists (Lance)	1 pkg (42 g)	260	4	16
Doo Dads	1 oz	130	1	6
Eagle Cheese Crunch	1 oz	160	—	10
Easy Cheddar Nacho (Nabisco)	1 oz	80	4	6
Easy Cheese American (Nabisco)	1 oz	80	4	6
Easy Cheese Cheddar (Nabisco)	1 oz	80	4	6
Easy Cheese Cheese 'N Bacon (Nabisco)	1 oz	80	4	6
Easy Cheese Sharp Cheddar (Nabisco)	1 oz	80	4	6
Estee Snack Crisps				
Apple Cinnamon	1 pkg (0.66 oz)	90	0	2
Apple Cinnamon	27 crips (1 oz)	130	0	3
Chocolate	1 pkg (0.66 oz)	90	0	2
Chocolate	30 crips (1 oz)	130	1	3
Lemon	1 pkg (0.66 oz)	90	0	2
Lemon	30 (1 oz)	130	1	3
Ranch	1 pkg (0.6 oz)	90	0	2
Ranch	30 (1 oz)	130	1	3
White Cheddar	1 pkg (0.6 oz)	90	1	2
White Cheddar	27 crisps (1 oz)	130	1	3
Frito Lay Corn Nuggets Toasted	1.38 oz	170	—	5
Funyums Onions Rings	11 pieces (1 oz)	140	—	7
Gold-N-Chees Lance	1 pkg (39 g)	180	2	9
Hain Carrot Chips	1 oz	150	—	9
Hain Carrot Chips Barbecue	1 oz	140	—	8
Hain Carrot Chips No Salt Added	1 oz	150	—	7
Health Valley Cheddar Lites	0.75 oz	40	—	2
Health Valley Cheddar Lites With Green Onion	0.75 oz	40	—	2
Lance Pork Skins	1 pkg (14 g)	80	2	5
Lance Pork Skins BBQ	1 pkg (14 g)	80	2	5
Munchos	16 pieces (1 oz)	160	—	10
Ritz Snack Mix Cheese (Nabisco)	1 oz	130	1	6
Ritz Snack Mix Traditional (Nabisco)	1 oz	130	1	6

FOOD	PORTION	CALS.	SAT. FAT	FAT
Snyder's				
Cheddar Cheese Twists	1 oz	150	—	8
Kruncheez	1 oz	160	—	10
Onion Toasters Snyder's	1 oz	150	—	8
Snack Mix	1 oz	170	1	8
Sopaipillas Apple & Cinnamon	1 oz	150	1	8
Ultra Slim-Fast Lite N' Tasty Cheese Curls	1 oz	110	—	3
SNAIL				
fresh, cooked	3 oz	233	tr	1
raw	3 oz	117	tr	tr
SNAP BEANS				
CANNED				
green	½ cup	13	tr	tr
green low sodium	½ cup	13	tr	tr
italian	½ cup	13	tr	tr
italian low sodium	½ cup	13	tr	tr
yellow	½ cup	13	tr	tr
yellow low sodium	½ cup	13	tr	tr
FRESH				
green, cooked	½ cup	22	tr	tr
green, raw	½ cup	17	tr	tr
yellow, cooked	½ cup	22	tr	tr
yellow, raw	½ cup	17	tr	tr
FROZEN				
green, cooked	½ cup	18	tr	tr
italian, cooked	½ cup	18	tr	tr
yellow, cooked	½ cup	18	tr	tr
SNAPPER				
fresh, cooked	3 oz	109	tr	1
fresh, cooked	1 fillet (6 oz)	217	1	3
raw	3 oz	85	tr	1
SODA				
(*see also* DRINK MIXERS, MINERAL/BOTTLED WATER)				
7Up	1 oz	12	—	0
7Up Cherry	1 oz	13	—	0
7Up Cherry Diet	1 oz	tr	—	0
7Up Diet	1 oz	tr	—	0
7Up Gold	1 oz	13	—	0
7Up Gold Diet	1 oz	tr	—	0

FOOD	PORTION	CALS.	SAT. FAT	FAT
Caffeine Free Diet Pepsi (Pepsi-Cola)	8 fl oz	1	0	0
Caffeine Free Pepsi (Pepsi-Cola)	8 fl oz	105	0	0
Canada Dry				
Barrelhead Root Beer	8 fl oz	110	0	0
Birch Beer Brown	8 fl oz	110	0	0
Birch Beer Clear	8 fl oz	110	0	0
Black Cherry Wishniak	8 fl oz	130	0	0
Cactus Cooler	8 fl oz	110	0	0
California Strawberry	8 fl oz	110	0	0
Club	8 fl oz	0	0	0
Club Sodium Free	8 fl oz	0	0	0
Concord Grape	8 fl oz	120	0	0
Ginger Ale	8 fl oz	100	0	0
Ginger Ale Cherry	8 fl oz	110	0	0
Ginger Ale Cranberry	8 fl oz	100	0	0
Ginger Ale Golden	8 fl oz	100	0	0
Ginger Ale Lemon	8 fl oz	100	0	0
Ginger Ale Diet	8 fl oz	0	0	0
Ginger Ale Diet Cherry	8 fl oz	0	0	0
Ginger Ale Diet Cranberry	8 fl oz	0	0	0
Ginger Ale Diet Lemon	8 fl oz	5	0	0
Half and Half	8 fl oz	110	0	0
Hi-Spot	8 fl oz	110	0	0
Island Lime	8 fl oz	140	0	0
Jamaica Cola	8 fl oz	110	0	0
Lemon Sour	8 fl oz	100	0	0
Peach	8 fl oz	120	0	0
Pina Pineapple	8 fl oz	110	0	0
Seltzer	8 fl oz	0	0	0
Seltzer Cherry	8 fl oz	0	0	0
Seltzer Cranberry Lime	8 fl oz	0	0	0
Seltzer Grapefruit	8 fl oz	0	0	0
Seltzer Lemon Lime	8 fl oz	0	0	0
Seltzer Mandarin Orange	8 fl oz	0	0	0
Seltzer Peach	8 fl oz	0	0	0
Seltzer Raspberry	8 fl oz	0	0	0
Seltzer Strawberry	8 fl oz	0	0	0
Seltzer Tropical	8 fl oz	0	0	0
Sunripe Orange	8 fl oz	140	0	0
Tahitian Treat	8 fl oz	150	0	0

FOOD	PORTION	CALS.	SAT. FAT	FAT
Tonic Water	8 fl oz	100	0	0
Tonic Water Twist Of Lime	8 fl oz	100	0	0
Tonic Water Diet	8 fl oz	0	0	0
Tonic Water Diet Twist Of Lime	8 fl oz	0	0	0
Vanilla Cream	8 fl oz	120	0	0
Vichy Water	8 fl oz	0	0	0
Wild Cherry	8 fl oz	110	0	0
Clearly 2				
Black Cherry (Clearly Canadian)	8 fl oz	2	—	0
Boysenberry Mist (Clearly Canadian)	8 fl oz	2	—	0
Key Lime (Clearly Canadian)	8 fl oz	2	—	0
Clearly Canadian	8 fl oz	0	0	0
Alpine Fruit & Berries	8 fl oz	90	—	0
Costal Cranberry	8 fl oz	90	—	0
Country Raspberry	8 fl oz	80	—	0
Green Apple	8 fl oz	80	—	0
Mountain Blackberry	8 fl oz	100	—	0
Orchard Peach Strawberry	8 fl oz	90	—	0
Summer Strawberry	8 fl oz	80	—	0
Western Loganberry	8 fl oz	80	—	0
Wild Cherry	8 fl oz	90	—	0
Coca-Cola				
Cherry	8 fl oz	104	0	0
Classic	8 fl oz	97	0	0
Classic Caffeine-free	8 fl oz	97	0	0
Diet Cherry	8 fl oz	1	0	0
Coke II	8 fl oz	105	0	0
Cott				
Cola	8 fl oz	110	0	0
Ginger Ale	8 fl oz	90	0	0
Grape	8 fl oz	130	0	0
Orange	8 fl oz	140	0	0
Pineapple	8 fl oz	130	0	0
Punch	8 fl oz	130	0	0
Seltzer	8 fl oz	0	0	0
Crush Cherry	6 oz	100	0	0
Crush Grape	6 oz	100	0	0
Crush Orange	6 oz	100	0	0

FOOD	PORTION	CALS.	SAT. FAT	FAT
Crush Orange Diet	6 oz	12	0	0
Crush Pineapple	6 oz	100	0	0
Crush Strawberry	6 oz	90	0	0
Crush Tropical Fruit Punch	1 bottle (10 fl oz)	180	0	0
Crush Tropical Fruit Punch	1 can (11.5 fl oz)	200	0	0
Diet Coke (Coca-Cola)	8 fl oz	1	0	0
Diet Coke Caffeine-Free (Coca-Cola)	8 fl oz	1	0	0
Diet Cranberry Apple Salt/ Sodium Free (Royal Crown)	8 fl oz	2	0	0
Diet Cranberry Salt/ Sodium Free (Royal Crown)	8 fl oz	2	0	0
Diet Mountain Dew	8 fl oz	2	0	0
Diet Mug Cream	8 fl oz	2	0	0
Diet Mug Root Beer	8 fl oz	1	0	0
Diet Pepsi	8 fl oz	1	0	0
Diet Rite (Royal Crown)				
Black Cherry Salt/ Sodium Free	8 fl oz	2	0	0
Cola Caffeine/Sugar Free	8 fl oz	1	0	0
Cola Salt/Sodium Free	8 fl oz	1	0	0
Fruit Punch Salt/Sodium Free	8 fl oz	2	0	0
Golden Peach Salt/ Sodium Free	8 fl oz	2	0	0
Key Lime Salt/Sodium Free	8 fl oz	7	0	0
Pink Grapefruit Salt/ Sodium Free	8 fl oz	2	0	0
Red Raspberry Salt/ Sodium Free	8 fl oz	3	0	0
Tangerine Salt/Sodium Free	8 fl oz	2	0	0
White Grape Salt/ Sodium Free	8 fl oz	1	0	0
Diet Royal Crown	8 fl oz	1	0	0
Diet Royal Crown Caffeine Free	8 fl oz	1	0	0
Diet Tropical Chill Soda (Pepsi-Cola)	8 fl oz	1	0	0
Diet Upper 10 (Royal Crown)	8 fl oz	3	0	0
Diet Upper 10 Salt/Sodium Free (Royal Crown)	8 fl oz	3	0	0

FOOD	PORTION	CALS.	SAT. FAT	FAT
Dr Pepper	1 oz	13	—	0
Dr Pepper Diet	1 oz	tr	tr	0
Fanta Ginger Ale	8 oz	86	0	0
Fanta Grape	8 oz	117	0	0
Fanta Orange	8 oz	118	0	0
Fanta Root Beer	8 oz	111	0	0
Fresca	8 oz	3	0	0
Health Valley Ginger Ale	12 oz	153	—	1
Health Valley Rootbeer Old Fashioned	12 oz	120	—	1
Health Valley Sarsaparilla Rootbeer	12 oz	153	—	1
Health Valley Wild Berry	12 oz	142	—	1
Hires				
Cream	8 fl oz	130	0	0
Cream Soda Diet	8 fl oz	0	0	0
Original Mocha	8 fl oz	100	0	0
Original Mocha Diet	8 fl oz	5	0	0
Root Beer	8 oz	130	0	0
Root Beer Diet	8 oz	0	0	0
Kick (Royal Crown)	8 fl oz	120	0	0
Like Cola	1 oz	13	—	0
Like Cola Sugar Free	1 oz	tr	—	0
Lucozade	7 oz	136	0	0
Manischewitz Seltzer No Salt Added No Calories	8 oz	0	0	0
Mello Yellow	8 oz	119	0	0
Mello Yellow Diet	8 fl oz	4	0	0
Minute Maid	8 fl oz	110	0	0
Berry	8 fl oz	111	0	0
Diet Orange	8 fl oz	2	0	0
Fruit Punch	8 fl oz	117	0	0
Grape	8 fl oz	121	0	0
Grapefruit	8 fl oz	108	0	0
Orange	8 fl oz	118	0	0
Peach	8 fl oz	110	0	0
Pineapple	8 fl oz	109	0	0
Raspberry	8 fl oz	111	0	0
Strawberry	8 fl oz	122	0	0
Mountain Dew	8 fl oz	118	0	0
Mr. PiBB	6 oz	97	0	0
Mr. PiBB Diet	8 fl oz	1	0	0
Mug Cream (Pepsi-Cola)	8 fl oz	122	0	0
Mug Root Beer (Pepsi-Cola)	8 fl oz	141	0	0

FOOD	PORTION	CALS.	SAT. FAT	FAT
Nehi (Royal Crown)				
Cream	8 fl oz	120	0	0
Fruit Punch	8 fl oz	120	0	0
Ginger Ale	8 fl oz	90	0	0
Grape	8 fl oz	120	0	0
Orange	8 fl oz	130	0	0
Peach	8 fl oz	130	0	0
Pineapple	8 fl oz	130	0	0
Quinine Water	8 fl oz	90	0	0
Root Beer	8 fl oz	120	0	0
Strawberry	8 fl oz	120	0	0
Wild Red	8 fl oz	120	0	0
Old Colony Grape	8 fl oz	140	0	0
Orangina	6 fl oz	80	0	0
Pepper Free	1 oz	12	—	0
Pepper Free Diet	1 oz	tr	—	0
Pepsi-Cola	8 fl oz	105	0	0
Raging Razzberry Cola (Pepsi-Cola)	8 fl oz	117	0	0
Ramblin' Root Beer	8 fl oz	120	0	0
Royal Crown Caffeine Free Cola	8 fl oz	110	0	0
Royal Crown Cherry	8 fl oz	110	0	0
Royal Crown Cola	8 fl oz	100	0	0
Royal Mistic				
'N Juice Black Cherry	12 fl oz	146	0	0
'N Juice Peach Vanilla	12 fl oz	146	0	0
'N Juice Tangerine Orange	12 fl oz	146	0	0
'N Juice Tropical Supreme	12 fl oz	152	0	0
'N Juice Wild Berry	12 fl oz	156	0	0
Caribbean Fruit Punch	16 fl oz	230	0	0
Grape Strawberry	16 fl oz	230	0	0
Sparkling Diet With Lime Kiwi	11.1 fl oz	0	0	0
Sparkling Diet With Raspberry Boysenberry	11.1 fl oz	0	0	0
Sparkling Diet With Royal Peach	11.1 fl oz	0	0	0
Sparkling Diet With Wild Cherry	11.1 fl oz	0	0	0
Sparkling With Lime Kiwi	11.1 fl oz	112	0	0

FOOD	PORTION	CALS.	SAT. FAT	FAT
Sparkling With Mandarin Orange Pineapple	11.1 fl oz	120	0	0
Sparkling With Mango Passion	11.1 fl oz	112	0	0
Sparkling With Raspberry Boysenberry	11.1 fl oz	112	0	0
Sparkling With Royal Peach	11.1 fl oz	112	0	0
Sparkling With Wild Cherry	11.1 fl oz	112	0	0
Schweppes				
Bitter Lemon	8 fl oz	110	0	0
Club	8 fl oz	0	0	0
Club Sodium Free	8 fl oz	0	0	0
Ginger Ale	8 fl oz	90	0	0
Ginger Ale Diet	8 fl oz	0	0	0
Ginger Ale Dry Grape	8 fl oz	100	0	0
Ginger Ale Dry Grape Diet	8 fl oz	2	0	0
Ginger Ale Raspberry	8 fl oz	100	0	0
Ginger Ale Raspberry Diet	8 fl oz	0	0	0
Ginger Beer	8 fl oz	100	0	0
Grape	8 fl oz	130	0	0
Grapefruit	8 fl oz	110	0	0
Lemon Lime	8 fl oz	100	0	0
Lemon Sour	8 fl oz	110	0	0
Seltzer Water Black Berry	8 fl oz	0	0	0
Seltzer Water Lemon	8 fl oz	0	0	0
Seltzer Water Lemon Lime	8 fl oz	0	0	0
Seltzer Water Lime	8 fl oz	0	0	0
Seltzer Water Orange	8 fl oz	0	0	0
Seltzer Water Peaches & Cream	8 fl oz	0	0	0
Seltzer Water Raspberry	8 fl oz	0	0	0
Tonic Citrus	8 fl oz	90	0	0
Tonic Cranberry	8 fl oz	90	0	0
Tonic Raspberry	8 fl oz	90	0	0
Tonic Water Diet	8 fl oz	0	0	0
Shasta				
Birch Beer Diet	12 oz	4	—	0
Black Cherry	12 oz	162	—	0

FOOD	PORTION	CALS.	SAT. FAT	FAT
Shasta *(cont.)*				
Cherry Cola	12 oz	140	—	0
Citrus Mist	12 oz	170	—	0
Club	12 oz	0	—	0
Cola	8 oz	98	—	0
Cola	12 oz	147	—	0
Cola Diet	8 oz	0	—	0
Collins	12 oz	118	—	0
Creme	12 oz	154	—	0
Dr. Diablo	12 oz	140	—	0
Free Cola	12 oz	151	—	0
Fruit Punch	12 oz	173	—	0
Ginger Ale	8 oz	80	—	0
Ginger Ale	12 oz	120	—	0
Ginger Ale Diet	8 oz	0	—	0
Grape	12 oz	177	—	0
Lemon Lime	8 oz	97	—	0
Lemon Lime	12 oz	146	—	0
Lemon Lime Diet	8 oz	0	—	0
Orange	12 oz	177	—	0
Red Berry	12 oz	158	—	0
Red Pop	12 oz	158	—	0
Root Beer	12 oz	154	—	0
Strawberry	12 oz	147	—	0
Tonic Water	12 oz	0	—	0
Slice				
Diet Lemon Lime	8 fl oz	5	0	0
Diet Mandarin	8 fl oz	5	0	0
Lemon Lime	8 fl oz	100	0	0
Mandarin Orange	8 fl oz	128	0	0
Red	8 fl oz	128	0	0
Sprite	8 fl oz	100	0	0
Sprite Diet	8 fl oz	3	0	0
Sundrop	8 fl oz	140	0	0
Sundrop Cherry	8 fl oz	130	0	0
Sundrop Diet	8 fl oz	5	0	0
Sunkist				
Cactus Cooler	8 fl oz	110	0	0
Cherry	8 fl oz	140	0	0
Fruit Punch	8 fl oz	130	0	0
Orange	8 fl oz	140	0	0
Peach	8 fl oz	120	0	0
Pineapple	8 fl oz	140	0	0
Strawberry	8 fl oz	140	0	0

FOOD	PORTION	CALS.	SAT. FAT	FAT
Sunkist Diet				
Citrus	8 fl oz	0	0	0
Orange	8 fl oz	5	0	0
TAB	8 fl oz	1	0	0
Tropical Chill Cola (Pepsi-Cola)	8 fl oz	117	0	0
Upper 10 (Royal Crown)	8 fl oz	100	0	0
Upper 10 Salt Free (Royal Crown)	8 fl oz	100	0	0
Welch's Sparkling Apple	12 oz	180	—	0
Welch's Sparkling Grape	12 oz	180	—	0
Welch's Sparkling Orange	12 oz	180	—	0
Welch's Strawberry Sparkling	12 oz	180	—	0
Wink	8 fl oz	130	0	0
Wink Diet (Wink)	8 fl oz	5	0	0
Yoo-Hoo	9 fl oz	150	tr	tr
club	12 oz	0	0	0
cola	12 oz	151	0	tr
cream	12 oz	191	0	0
diet cola	12 oz	2	0	0
diet cola w/ Nutrasweet	12 oz	2	0	0
diet cola w/ saccharin	12 oz	2	0	0
ginger ale	12 oz	124	—	0
grape	12 oz	161	0	0
lemon lime	12 oz	149	0	0
orange	12 oz	177	0	0
pepper type	12 oz	151	0	tr
quinine	12 oz	125	0	0
root beer	12 oz	152	0	0
tonic water	12 oz	125	0	0

SOLDIER BEANS
DRIED
Bean Cuisine	½ cup	115	—	1

SOLE
FRESH
raw	3.5 oz	90	—	1
w/ lemon, raw	3.5 oz	85	—	1
FROZEN				
A La Monterey (King & Prince)	6 oz	221	—	13
Fishmarket Fresh (Gorton's)	5 oz	110	—	1

FOOD	PORTION	CALS.	SAT. FAT	FAT
Light Fillets (Mrs. Paul's)	1 fillet	240	—	10
Light Fillets (Van De Kamp's)	1 piece	250	2	12
Microwave Entree in Lemon Butter (Gorton's)	1 pkg	380	11	24
Microwave Entree in Wine Sauce (Gorton's)	1 pkg	180	3	8
Natural Fillets (Van De Kamp's)	4 oz	100	1	2

SORBET
(see ICES AND ICE POPS)

SORGHUM

sorghum	½ cup	325	tr	3

SOUFFLE
HOME RECIPE

cheese	3.5 oz	253	—	20
grand marnier	1 cup	109	—	4
lemon, chilled	1 cup	176	—	tr
raspberry, chilled	1 cup	173	—	tr
spinach	1 cup	218	—	18

SOUP
CANNED

FOOD	PORTION	CALS.	SAT. FAT	FAT
Asparagus Cream of, as prep (Campbell's)	8 oz	80	—	4
Bean & Ham (Healthy Choice)	1 cup (8.7 oz)	180	1	3
Bean & Ham Home Cookin' (Campbell)	10.75 oz	210	1	4
Bean Homestyle, as prep (Campbell)	8 oz	130	—	1
Bean w/ Bacon, as prep (Campbell)	8 oz	140	—	4
Bean w/ Bacon Healthy Request, as prep (Campbell)	8 oz	140	—	4
Beef, as prep (Campbell)	8 oz	80	—	2
Beef (Progresso)	1 can (10.5 fl oz)	180	—	6
Beef Barley (Progresso)	1 can (10.5 fl oz)	150	—	5
Beef Broth (College Inn)	½ can (7 oz)	16	0	0
Beef Broth (Health Valley)	7.5 oz	10	—	tr
Beef Broth (Pritikin)	6.88 oz	20	—	tr
Beef Broth (Swanson)	7.25 oz	18	—	1

FOOD	PORTION	CALS.	SAT. FAT	FAT
Beef Broth, as prep (Campbell)	8 oz	16	—	0
Beef Broth No Salt Added (Health Valley)	7.5 oz	10	—	tr
Beef Chunky Ready-to-Serve (Campbell)	10.75 oz	200	—	5
Beef Minestrone (Progresso)	1 can (10.5 fl oz)	180	—	6
Beef Noodle (Progresso)	9.5 fl oz	170	—	4
Beef Noodle, as prep (Campbell)	8 oz	70	—	3
Beef Noodle Homestyle, as prep (Campbell)	8 oz	80	—	4
Beef Stroganoff Style Chunky Ready-to-Serve (Campbell)	10.75 oz	320	—	16
Beef Vegetable (Progresso)	1 can (10.5 fl oz)	170	—	3
Beef w/ Vegetables & Pasta Home Cookin' (Campbell)	10.75 oz	140	—	2
Beefy Mushroom, as prep (Campbell)	8 oz	60	—	3
Black Bean (Goya)	7.5 oz	160	—	4
Black Bean (Health Valley)	7.5 oz	150	—	2
Black Bean No Salt Added (Health Valley)	7.5 oz	150	—	2
Borscht (Gold's)	8 oz	100	0	0
Borscht Lo-Cal (Gold's)	8 oz	20	—	tr
Borscht Low Calorie (Manischewitz)	8 oz	20	0	0
Borscht w/ Beets (Manischewitz)	8 oz	80	0	0
Broccoli Cream Of, as prep (Campbell)	8 oz	80	—	5
Broccoli Cream Of, as prep w/ 2% milk (Campbell)	8 oz	140	—	7
Celery Cream Of, as prep (Campbell)	8 oz	100	—	7
Cheddar Cheese, as prep (Campbell)	8 oz	110	—	6
Chickarina (Progresso)	9 fl oz	130	—	5
Chicken Alphabet, as prep (Campbell)	8 oz	80	—	3
Chicken & Stars, as prep (Campbell)	8 oz	70	—	2

FOOD	PORTION	CALS.	SAT. FAT	FAT
Chicken Barley (Progresso)	9.25 fl oz	100	—	2
Chicken Barley, as prep (Campbell)	8 oz	70	—	2
Chicken Broth (College Inn)	½ can (7 oz)	35	1	3
Chicken Broth (Hain)	8.75 fl oz	70	—	6
Chicken Broth (Health Valley)	7.5 oz	35	—	2
Chicken Broth (Pritikin)	6.86 oz	14	—	0
Chicken Broth (Progresso)	4 fl oz	8	—	0
Chicken Broth (Swanson)	7.25 oz	30	—	2
Chicken Broth, as prep (Campbell)	8 oz	30	—	2
Chicken Broth & Noodles, as prep (Campbell)	8 oz	45	—	1
Chicken Broth Healthy Request Ready-to-Serve (Campbell)	8 oz	10	—	0
Chicken Broth Low Sodium Ready-to-Serve (Campbell)	10.5 oz	30	—	1
Chicken Broth Lower Salt (College Inn)	½ can (7 oz)	20	1	2
Chicken Broth No Salt Added (Hain)	8.75 fl oz	60	—	5
Chicken Broth No Salt Added (Health Valley)	7.5 oz	35	—	2
Chicken Corn Chowder Chunky Ready-to-Serve (Campbell)	10.75 oz	340	—	21
Chicken Cream Of, as prep (Campbell)	8 oz	110	—	7
Chicken Cream of (Progresso)	9.5 fl oz	190	—	11
Chicken Gumbo (Pritikin)	7.38 oz	60	—	1
Chicken Gumbo, as prep (Campbell)	8 oz	60	—	2
Chicken Gumbo w/ Sausage Home Cookin' (Campbell)	10.75 oz	140	—	4
Chicken Minestrone (Progresso)	1 can (10.5 fl oz)	140	—	4
Chicken Minestrone Home Cookin' (Campbell)	10.75 oz	180	—	6
Chicken Mushroom Creamy, as prep (Campbell)	8 oz	120	—	8

FOOD	PORTION	CALS.	SAT. FAT	FAT
Chicken 'N Dumplings, as prep (Campbell)	8 oz	80	—	3
Chicken Noodle (Hain)	9.5 fl oz	120	—	4
Chicken Noodle (Progresso)	1 can (10.5 fl oz)	120	—	4
Chicken Noodle (Weight Watchers)	10.5 oz	80	—	2
Chicken Noodle, as prep (Campbell)	8 oz	60	—	2
Chicken Noodle Chunky Ready-to-Serve (Campbell)	10.75 oz	200	—	7
Chicken Noodle Healthy Request (Campbell)	8 oz	60	—	2
Chicken Noodle Homestyle, as prep (Campbell)	8 oz	70	—	3
Chicken Noodle No Salt Added (Hain)	9.5 fl oz	120	—	4
Chicken Noodle-O's, as prep (Campbell)	8 oz	70	—	2
Chicken Nuggets w/ Vegetables & Noodles Chunky Ready-to-Serve (Campbell)	10.75 oz	190	—	6
Chicken Rice (Progresso)	1 can (10.5 fl oz)	120	—	4
Chicken Rice Home Cookin' (Campbell)	10.75 oz	150	—	6
Chicken Vegetable (Pritikin)	7.25 oz	70	—	tr
Chicken Vegetable (Progresso)	1 can (10.5 fl oz)	150	—	4
Chicken Vegetable, as prep (Campbell)	8 oz	70	—	3
Chicken Vegetable Beef Low Sodium Ready-to-Serve (Campbell)	10.75 oz	180	—	5
Chicken Vegetable Chunky Ready-to-Serve (Campbell)	9.5 oz	170	—	6
Chicken With Noodle (Healthy Choice)	1 cup (8.8 oz)	130	1	2
Chicken w/ Noodles Home Cookin' (Campbell)	10.75 oz	140	—	4
Chicken w/ Noodles Low Sodium Ready-to-Serve (Campbell)	10.75 oz	170	—	5

FOOD	PORTION	CALS.	SAT. FAT	FAT
Chicken w/ Pasta (Healthy Choice)	1 cup (8.6 oz)	120	2	3
Chicken w/ Ribbon Pasta (Pritikin)	7.25 oz	60	—	tr
Chicken w/ Rice (Healthy Choice)	1 cup (8.4 oz)	100	2	3
Chicken w/ Rice, as prep (Campbell)	8 oz	60	—	3
Chicken w/ Rice Chunky Ready-to-Serve (Campbell)	9.5 oz	140	—	4
Chicken w/ Rice Healthy Request (Campbell)	8 oz	60	—	3
Chili Beef, as prep (Campbell)	8 oz	140	—	5
Chili Beef Chunky Ready-to-Serve (Campbell)	11 oz	290	—	7
Chunky Chicken Vegetable (Health Valley)	7.5 oz	125	—	2
Chunky Five Bean Vegetable (Health Valley)	7.5 oz	110	—	2
Chunky Five Bean Vegetable No Salt Added (Health Valley)	7.5 oz	110	—	2
Chunky Vegetable Chicken No Salt Added (Health Valley)	7.5 oz	125	—	2
Clam Chowder Manhattan Style, as prep (Campbell)	8 oz	70	—	2
Clam Chowder Manhattan Style Chunky Ready-to-Serve (Campbell)	10.75 oz	160	—	4
Clam Chowder New England, as prep (Campbell)	8 oz	80	—	3
Clam Chowder New England, as prep w/ whole milk (Campbell)	8 oz	150	—	7
Clam Chowder New England Chunky Ready-to-Serve (Campbell)	10.75 oz	290	—	17
Consomme, as prep (Campbell)	8 oz	25	—	0

FOOD	PORTION	CALS.	SAT. FAT	FAT
Country Vegetable (Healthy Choice)	½ can (7.5 oz)	120	1	1
Country Vegetable Home Cookin' (Campbell)	10.75 oz	120	—	2
Cream of Chicken Healthy Request (Campbell)	8 oz	70	—	2
Cream of Mushroom Healthy Request, as prep (Campbell)	8 oz	60	—	2
Creamy Chicken Mushroom Chunky Ready-to-Serve (Campbell)	10.5 oz	270	—	19
Creole Style Chunky Ready-to-Serve (Campbell)	10.75 oz	240	—	8
Curly Noodle w/ Chicken, as prep (Campbell)	8 oz	80	—	3
Escarole in Chicken Broth (Progresso)	9.25 oz	30	—	1
French Onion, as prep (Campbell)	8 oz	60	—	2
Garden Vegetable (Healthy Choice)	1 cup (8.6 oz)	110	1	1
Green Pea, as prep (Campbell)	8 oz	160	—	3
Green Split Pea (Health Valley)	7.5 oz	180	—	tr
Green Split Pea No Salt Added (Health Valley)	7.5 oz	180	—	tr
Ham & Bean (Progresso)	9.5 oz	140	—	2
Ham 'N Butter Bean Chunky Ready-to-Serve (Campbell)	10.75 oz	280	—	10
Hearty Beef (Healthy Choice)	½ can (7.5 oz)	120	1	2
Hearty Chicken (Progresso)	1 can (10.5 oz)	130	—	4
Hearty Chicken Noodle Healthy Request Ready-to-Serve (Campbell)	8 oz	80	—	2
Hearty Chicken Rice Healthy Request Ready-to-Serve (Campbell)	8 oz	110	—	2

FOOD	PORTION	CALS.	SAT. FAT	FAT
Hearty Chicken Vegetable Healthy Request (Campbell)	8 oz	120	—	2
Hearty Lentil Home Cookin' (Campbell)	10.75 oz	170	—	2
Hearty Vegetable Beef Healthy Request Ready-to-Serve (Campbell)	8 oz	120	—	3
Hearty Vegetable Healthy Request Ready-to-Serve (Campbell)	8 oz	110	—	3
Homestyle Chicken (Progresso)	9.5 fl oz	110	—	3
Italian Vegetable Pasta (Hain)	9.5 fl oz	160	—	5
Italian Vegetable Pasta Low Sodium (Hain)	9.5 fl oz	140	—	6
Lentil (Health Valley)	7.5 oz	220	—	4
Lentil (Health Choice)	1 cup (8.7 oz)	140	0	1
Lentil (Pritikin)	7.38 oz	100	—	0
Lentil (Progresso)	1 can (10.5 fl oz)	140	—	4
Lentil With Sausage (Progresso)	9.5 fl oz	170	—	8
Macaroni & Bean (Progresso)	1 can (10.5 fl oz)	150	—	4
Manhattan Clam Chowder (Health Valley)	7.5 oz	110	—	2
Manhattan Clam Chowder (Pritikin)	7.38 oz	70	—	tr
Manhattan Clam Chowder (Progresso)	9.5 fl oz	120	—	2
Manhattan Clam Chowder, as prep w/ water (Snow's)	7.5 oz	70	—	2
Manhattan Clam Chowder No Salt Added (Health Valley)	7.5 oz	110	—	2
Mediterranean Vegetable Chunky Ready-to-Serve (Campbell)	9.5 oz	170	—	6
Micro Cup (Hormel)				
Bean & Ham	1 cup (7.5 oz)	190	2	4
Beef Vegetable	1 cup (7.5 oz)	90	0	1
Broccoli Cheese With Ham	1 cup (7.5 oz)	170	5	13
Chicken & Rice	1 cup (7.5)	110	1	3

FOOD	PORTION	CALS.	SAT. FAT	FAT
Chicken Noodle	1 cup (7.5 oz)	110	1	3
New England Clam Chowder	1 cup (7.5 oz)	130	3	5
Potato Cheese With Ham	1 cup (7.5 oz)	190	5	13
Minestrone (Hain)	9.5 fl oz	170	—	2
Minestrone (Health Valley)	7.5 oz	130	—	3
Minestrone (Healthy Choice)	½ can (7.5 oz)	160	—	2
Minestrone (Pritikin)	7.38 oz	110	—	tr
Minestrone (Progresso)	1 can (10.5 fl oz)	120	—	3
Minestrone, as prep (Campbell)	8 oz	80	—	2
Minestrone Chunky Ready-to-Serve (Campbell)	9.5 oz	160	—	4
Minestrone Home Cookin' (Campbell)	10.75 oz	140	—	3
Minestrone No Salt Added (Hain)	9.5 fl oz	160	—	4
Minestrone No Salt Added (Health Valley)	7.5 oz	130	—	3
Mushroom (Pritikin)	7.38 oz	60	—	tr
Mushroom Barley (Hain)	9.5 fl oz	100	—	2
Mushroom Barley (Health Valley)	7.5 oz	100	—	2
Mushroom Barley No Salt Added (Health Valley)	7.5 oz	100	—	2
Mushroom Cream Of (Progresso)	9.25 fl oz	160	—	10
Mushroom Cream Of (Weight Watchers)	10.5 oz	90	—	2
Mushroom Cream Of Low Sodium Ready-to-Serve (Campbell)	10½ oz	210	—	14
Mushroom Cream Of, as prep (Campbell)	8 oz	100	—	7
Mushroom Golden, as prep (Campbell)	8 oz	70	—	3
Nacho Cheese, as prep (Campbell)	8 oz	110	—	8
Nacho Cheese, as prep w/ milk (Campbell)	8 oz	180	—	12
Natural Goodness Clear Chicken Broth (Swanson)	7.5 oz	20	—	1

FOOD	PORTION	CALS.	SAT. FAT	FAT
Navy Bean (Pritikin)	7.38 oz	130	—	tr
New England Chowder (American Original Foods)	4 oz	64	tr	1
New England Chowder, as prep w/ milk (American Original Foods)	4 oz	145	tr	6
New England Clam Chowder (Hain)	9.25 fl oz	180	—	4
New England Clam Chowder (Pritikin)	7.38 oz	118	tr	tr
New England Clam Chowder, as prep w/ milk (Snow's)	7.5 oz	140	tr	6
New England Clam Chowder, as prep w/ whole milk (Gorton's)	¼ can	140	tr	5
New England Corn Chowder, as prep w/ milk (Snow's)	7.5 oz	150	tr	6
New England Fish Chowder, as prep w/ milk (Snow's)	7.5 oz	130	—	6
New England Seafood Chowder, as prep w/ milk (Snow's)	7.5 oz	130	—	6
New England Style Clam Chowder (Progresso)	1 can (10.5 fl oz)	220	—	12
Noodles & Ground Beef, as prep (Campbell)	8 oz	90	—	4
Old Fashioned Bean w/ Ham Chunky Ready-to-Serve (Campbell)	11 oz	290	—	9
Old Fashioned Chicken Chunky Ready-to-Serve (Campbell)	10.75 oz	180	—	5
Old Fashioned Vegetable Beef Chunky Ready-to-Serve (Campbell)	10.75 oz	190	—	6
Onion Cream Of, as prep (Campbell)	8 oz	100	—	5
Onion Cream Of, as prep w/ whole milk & water (Campbell)	8 oz	140	—	7
Oyster Stew, as prep (Campbell)	8 oz	70	—	5

FOOD	PORTION	CALS.	SAT. FAT	FAT
Oyster Stew, as prep w/ whole milk (Campbell)	8 oz	140	—	9
Pepper Pot, as prep (Campbell)	8 oz	90	—	4
Pepper Steak Chunky Ready-to-Serve (Campbell)	10.75 oz	180	—	3
Potato Cream Of, as prep (Campbell)	8 oz	80	—	3
Potato Cream Of, as prep w/ whole milk & water (Campbell)	8 oz	120	—	4
Potato Leek (Health Valley)	7.5 oz	130	—	2
Potato Leek No Salt Added (Health Valley)	7.5 oz	130	—	2
Schav (Gold's)	8 oz	25	—	0
Schav (Manischewitz)	1 cup	11	—	tr
Scotch Broth, as prep (Campbell)	8 oz	80	—	3
Season Beef Broth (Progresso)	4 fl oz	40	—	tr
Shrimp Cream Of, as prep (Campbell)	8 oz	90	—	6
Shrimp Cream Of, as prep w/ whole milk (Campbell)	8 oz	160	—	10
Sirloin Burger Chunky Ready-to-Serve (Campbell)	10.75 oz	220	—	9
Split Pea (Hain)	9.5 fl oz	170	—	1
Split Pea (Pritikin)	7.5 oz	130	—	tr
Split Pea & Ham (Healthy Choice)	1 cup (8.8 oz)	160	1	2
Split Pea Low Sodium Ready-to-Serve (Campbell)	10.75 oz	230	—	4
Split Pea No Salt Added (Hain)	9.5 fl oz	170	—	1
Split Pea w/ Bacon, as prep (Campbell)	8 oz	160	—	4
Split Pea w/ Ham (Progresso)	1 can (10.5 fl oz)	160	—	5
Split Pea w/ Ham Chunky Ready-to-Serve (Campbell)	10.75 oz	230	—	6

FOOD	PORTION	CALS.	SAT. FAT	FAT
Split Pea w/ Ham Home Cookin' (Campbell)	10.75 oz	230	—	1
Steak & Potato Chunky Ready-to-Serve (Campbell)	10.75 oz	200	—	5
Teddy Bear, as prep (Campbell)	8 oz	70	—	2
Tomato (Health Valley)	7.5 oz	130	—	3
Tomato (Progresso)	9.5 fl oz	120	—	3
Tomato, as prep (Campbell)	8 oz	90	—	2
Tomato, as prep w/ 2% milk (Campbell)	8 oz	150	—	4
Tomato Beef with Rotini (Progresso)	9.5 fl oz	170	—	6
Tomato Bisque, as prep (Campbell)	8 oz	120	—	3
Tomato Garden (Healthy Choice)	1 cup (8.6 oz)	110	1	2
Tomato Garden Home Cookin' (Campbell)	10.75 oz	150	—	3
Tomato Healthy Request, as prep (Campbell)	8 oz	90	—	2
Tomato Healthy Request, as prep w/ Skim Milk (Campbell)	8 oz	130	—	2
Tomato Homestyle Cream Of, as prep (Campbell)	8 oz	110	—	3
Tomato Homestyle Cream Of, as prep w/ whole milk (Campbell)	8 oz	180	—	7
Tomato No Salt Added (Health Valley)	7.5 oz	130	—	3
Tomato Rice Old Fashioned, as prep (Campbell)	8 oz	110	—	2
Tomato Tortellini (Progresso)	9.5 fl oz	130	—	5
Tomato w/ Tomato Pieces (Pritikin)	7.5 oz	70	—	0
Tomato w/ Tomato Pieces Low Sodium Ready-to-Serve (Campbell)	10.5 oz	190	—	6
Tomato Zesty, as prep (Campbell)	8 oz	100	—	2

FOOD	PORTION	CALS.	SAT. FAT	FAT
Tortellini (Progresso)	9.5 fl oz	90	—	3
Tortellini Creamy (Progresso)	9.25 fl oz	240	—	16
Turkey Noodle, as prep (Campbell)	8 oz	70	—	2
Turkey Rice (Hain)	9½ fl oz	100	—	3
Turkey Rice No Salt Added (Hain)	9½ fl oz	120	—	4
Turkey Vegetable (Healthy Choice)	1 cup (8.5 oz)	120	1	3
Turkey Vegetable, as prep (Campbell)	8 oz	70	—	3
Turkey Vegetable Chunky Ready-to-Serve (Campbell)	9.38 oz	150	—	6
Turkey Vegetable w/ Ribbon Pasta (Pritikin)	7.38 oz	50	—	tr
Turkey w/ White and Wild Rice (Healthy Choice)	1 cup (8.4 oz)	110	1	3
Vegetable (Health Valley)	7.5 oz	110	—	1
Vegetable (Pritikin)	7.38 oz	70	—	0
Vegetable (Progresso)	1 can (10.5 fl oz)	80	—	2
Vegetable, as prep (Campbell)	8 oz	90	—	2
Vegetable Beef, as prep (Campbell)	8 oz	70	—	2
Vegetable Beef Healthy Request, as prep (Campbell)	8 oz	70	—	2
Vegetable Broth (Hain)	9.5 fl oz	45	—	0
Vegetable Broth (Swanson)	7.25 fl oz	20	—	1
Vegetable Broth Low Sodium (Hain)	9.5 fl oz	40	—	tr
Vegetable Chicken (Hain)	9.5 fl oz	120	—	4
Vegetable Chicken No Salt Added (Hain)	9.5 fl oz	130	—	4
Vegetable Chunky Ready-to-Serve (Campbell)	10.75 oz	160	—	4
Vegetable Healthy Request, as prep (Campbell)	8 oz	90	—	2
Vegetable Homestyle, as prep (Campbell)	8 oz	60	—	2
Vegetable No Salt Added (Health Valley)	7.5 oz	110	—	1
Vegetable Beef Home Cookin' (Campbell)	10.75 oz	140	—	3

FOOD	PORTION	CALS.	SAT. FAT	FAT
Vegetable Old Fashioned, as prep (Campbell)	8 oz	60	—	2
Vegetable Split Pea (Hain)	9.5 fl oz	170	—	1
Vegetable Split Pea No Salt Added (Hain)	9.5 fl oz	170	—	1
Vegetarian Lentil (Hain)	9.5 fl oz	160	—	3
Vegetarian Lentil No Salt Added (Hain)	9.5 fl oz	160	—	3
Vegetarian Vegetable (Hain)	9.5 fl oz	140	—	4
Vegetarian Vegetable No Salt Added (Hain)	9.5 fl oz	150	—	5
Vegetarian Vegetable, as prep (Campbell)	8 oz	80	—	2
Won Ton, as prep (Campbell)	8 oz	40	—	1
Zesty Minestrone (Progresso)	9.5 fl oz	150	—	8
asparagus, cream of, as prep w/ milk	1 cup	161	3	8
asparagus, cream of, as prep w/ water	1 cup	87	1	4
beef broth, ready-to-serve	1 can (14 oz)	27	tr	1
beef broth, ready-to-serve	1 cup	16	tr	1
beef noodle, as prep w/ water	1 cup	84	1	3
black bean, as prep w/ water	1 cup	116	tr	2
black bean turtle soup	1 cup	218	tr	1
celery, cream of, as prep w/ milk	1 cup	165	4	10
celery, cream of, as prep w/ water	1 cup	90	1	6
cheese, as prep w/ milk	1 cup	230	9	15
cheese, as prep w/ water	1 cup	155	7	10
cheese, not prep	1 can (11 oz)	377	16	25
chicken broth, as prep w/ water	1 cup	39	tr	1
chicken, cream of, as prep w/ milk	1 cup	191	5	11
chicken, cream of, as prep w/ water	1 cup	116	2	7
chicken gumbo, as prep w/ water	1 cup	56	tr	1

FOOD	PORTION	CALS.	SAT. FAT	FAT
chicken noodle, as prep w/ water	1 cup	75	1	2
chicken rice, as prep w/ water	1 cup	251	tr	2
clam chowder, Manhattan, as prep w/ water	1 cup	77	tr	2
clam chowder, New England, as prep w/ milk	1 cup	163	3	7
clam chowder, New England, as prep w/ water	1 cup	95	tr	3
consomme w/ gelatin, as prep w/ water	1 cup	29	0	0
consomme w/ gelatin, not prep	1 can (10.5 oz)	71	0	0
escarole, ready-to-serve	1 cup	27	1	2
french onion, as prep w/ water	1 cup	57	tr	2
gazpacho, ready-to-serve	1 cup	57	tr	2
minestrone, as prep w/ water	1 cup	83	1	3
mushroom, cream of, as prep w/ milk	1 cup	203	5	14
mushroom, cream of, as prep w/ water	1 cup	129	2	9
oyster stew, as prep w/ milk	1 cup	134	5	8
oyster stew, as prep w/ water	1 cup	59	3	4
pepperpot, as prep w/ water	1 cup	103	2	5
potato, cream of, as prep w/ milk	1 cup	148	4	6
potato, cream of, as prep w/ water	1 cup	73	1	2
scotch broth, as prep w/ water	1 cup	80	1	3
split pea w/ ham, as prep w/ water	1 cup	189	2	4
tomato, as prep w/ milk	1 cup	160	3	6
tomato, as prep w/ water	1 cup	86	tr	2
vegetarian vegetable, as prep w/ water	1 cup	72	tr	2

FOOD	PORTION	CALS.	SAT. FAT	FAT
vichyssoise	1 cup	148	4	6
DRY				
13 Bean, uncooked (Hodgson Mill)	1.5 oz	100	0	1
15 Bean Soup Beef (Hurst)	1 serv (1.7 oz)	160	0	1
15 Bean Soup Cajun (Hurst)	1 serv (1.7 oz)	160	0	1
15 Bean Soup Chicken (Hurst)	1 serv (1.7 oz)	160	0	1
15 Bean Soup Chili (Hurst)	1 serv (1.7 oz)	160	0	1
15 Bean Soup Ham (Hurst)	1 serv (1.7 oz)	160	0	1
Bean Bouillabisse (Bean Cuisine)	1 cup (7.5 fl oz)	174	tr	tr
Bean & Barley (Arrowhead)	¼ cup (1.9 oz)	170	0	0
Bean With Bacon 'n Ham Microwave (Campbell)	7½ oz	230	—	5
Beef Cup Of Soup (Goodman's)	1 pkg (1½ cups)	180	1	3
Beef Base (Emes)	1 tsp	18	0	tr
Beef Bouillon (Herb-Ox)	1 cube (3.5 g)	10	0	0
Beef, as prep (Diamond Crystal)	6 oz	30	—	1
Beef, as prep (Ramen Noodle)	8 oz	190	—	8
Beef Bouillon Instant (Wylers)	1 tsp	6	—	tr
Beef Bouillon Instant Cube (Wylers)	1	6	—	tr
Beef Bouillon Instant Low Sodium (Lite Line)	1 tsp	12	—	tr
Beef Broth Instant (Weight Watchers)	1 pkg	8	—	tr
Beef Flavor Bouillon, as prep (Diamond Crystal)	6 oz	17	—	tr
Beef Instant Bouillon Powder (Herb-Ox)	1 tsp (4 g)	10	0	0
Beef Instant Broth & Seasoning Pack (Herb-Ox)	1 pkg (4.5 g)	10	0	0
Beef Instant Broth & Seasoning Pack Low Sodium (Herb-Ox)	1 pkg (4 g)	15	0	0
Beef Instant Oriental Noodle (Lipton)	8 oz	177	—	1

FOOD	PORTION	CALS.	SAT. FAT	FAT
Beef Low Fat, as prep (Ramen Noodle)	8 oz	160	—	1
Beef Mushroom (Lipton)	8 oz	38	—	1
Beef Noodle (Campbell's Cup)	1 (1.35 oz)	130	—	2
Beef Noodle (Ultra Slim-Fast)	6 oz	45	—	tr
Beef With Vegetables Low Fat, as prep (Cup-A-Ramen)	8 oz	220	—	2
Beef With Vegetables, as prep (Cup-A-Ramen)	8 oz	270	—	10
Beefy Onion (Lipton)	8 oz	27	tr	1
Black Bean Cup-A-Soup, as prep (Knorr)	1 pkg	200	0	1
Broccoli, as prep (Knorr)	8 fl oz	160	—	8
Broth & Brown Seasoning (George Washington)	1 serving	6	—	0
Broth & Golden Seasoning (George Washington)	1 serving	6	—	0
Broth & Onion Seasoning (George Washington)	1 serving	12	—	0
Broth & Vegetable Seasoning (George Washington)	1 serving	12	—	0
Cauliflower, as prep (Knorr)	8 oz	100	—	3
Cheese & Broccoli (Hain)	¾ cup	310	—	22
Cheese Savory (Hain)	¾ cup	250	—	16
Chef's Series Wild Mushroom as prep (Knorr)	8 fl oz	100	—	3
Chick 'N Pasta, as prep (Knorr)	8 oz	90	—	2
Chicken, as prep (Ramen Noodle)	8 oz	190	—	8
Chicken Base (Emes)	1 tsp	18	0	tr
Chicken Bouillon (Herb-Ox)	1 cube (4 g)	10	0	0
Chicken Bouillon, as prep w/ water (Knorr)	8 oz	16	—	1
Chicken Bouillon Instant (Wylers)	1 tsp	8	—	tr
Chicken Bouillon Instant Cube (Wylers)	1	8	—	tr
Chicken Bouillon Instant Low Sodium (Lite Line)	1 tsp	12	—	tr

FOOD	PORTION	CALS.	SAT. FAT	FAT
Chicken Broth (Cup-A-Soup)	6 oz	19	—	1
Chicken Broth Instant (Weight Watchers)	1 pkg	8	—	0
Chicken Low Fat Ramen Noodle, as prep	8 oz	160	—	1
Chicken Flavor Noodle (Campbell's Cup)	1 (1.35 oz)	140	—	3
Chicken Flavor Ramen Noodle, as prep	8 oz	190	—	8
Chicken Flavor w/ Vegetables, as prep (Cup-A-Ramen)	8 oz	270	—	10
Chicken Flavor w/ Vegetables Low Fat, as prep (Cup-A-Ramen)	8 oz	220	—	2
Chicken Flavored Noodle as prep (Knorr)	8 fl oz	100	—	2
Chicken Instant Bouillon Powder (Herb-Ox)	1 tsp (4 g)	10	0	0
Chicken Instant Broth & Seasoning Pack (Herb-Ox)	1 pkg (5 g)	10	0	0
Chicken Instant Broth & Seasoning Pack Low Sodium (Herb-Ox)	1 pkg (4 g)	15	0	0
Chicken Instant Oriental Noodle (Lipton)	8 oz	180	—	2
Chicken Leek (Ultra Slim-Fast)	6 oz	50	—	tr
Chicken Noodle (Lipton)	8 oz	82	—	2
Chicken Noodle (Ultra Slim-Fast)	6 oz	45	—	tr
Chicken Noodle (Weight Watchers)	7.5 oz	90	—	1
Chicken Noodle, as prep (Campbell)	8 oz	100	1	2
Chicken Noodle, as prep (Knorr)	8 oz	100	—	2
Chicken Noodle Cup of Soup (Goodman's)	1 pkg (1½ cups)	180	1	3
Chicken Noodle Hearty (Lipton)	8 oz	81	—	4
Chicken Noodle Microwave (Campbell)	7.5 oz	100	—	4

FOOD	PORTION	CALS.	SAT. FAT	FAT
Chicken Noodle w/ White Meat, as prep (Campbell's Cup)	6 oz	90	—	2
Chicken Vegetable (Cup-A-Soup)	6 oz	47	—	1
Chicken w/ Rice Microwave Soup (Campbell)	7.5 oz	100	—	4
Chili Beef Microwave Soup (Campbell)	7.5 oz	190	—	4
Chunky Beef Stew (Weight Watchers)	7.5 oz	120	—	2
Country Vegetable (Lipton)	8 oz	80	—	1
Couscous (Nile Spice)				
Almondine	1 pkg	200	0	3
Garbanzo	1 pkg	220	0	3
Lentil Curry	1 pkg	200	0	2
Minestrone	1 pkg	180	0	2
Parmesan	1 pkg	200	2	3
Cream, as prep (Diamond Crystal)	6 oz	90	—	3
Creamy Broccoli (Ultra Slim Fast)	6 oz	75	tr	—
Creamy Broccoli and Cheese (Cup-A-Soup)	6 oz	70	—	3
Creamy Chicken w/ White Meat, as prep (Campbell's Cup)	6 oz	90	—	4
Creamy Tomato (Ultra Slim-Fast)	6 oz	60	—	tr
Fines Herb, as prep (Knorr)	8 oz	130	—	6
Fish Bouillon, as prep w/ water (Knorr)	8 oz	10	—	tr
French Onion, as prep (Knorr)	8 oz	50	—	1
Giggle Noodle (Lipton)	8 oz	72	—	2
Hearty Chicken And Noodles (Cup-A-Soup)	6 oz	110	—	2
Hearty Creamy Chicken Lots-A-Noodles (Cup-A-Soup)	7 oz	179	—	8
Hearty Minestrone Cup-A-Soup, as prep (Knorr)	1 pkg	150	1	1
Hearty Noodle, as prep (Campbell)	8 oz	90	—	1

FOOD	PORTION	CALS.	SAT. FAT	FAT
Hearty Noodle w/ Vegetable (Lipton)	8 oz	75	—	2
Hearty Noodle w/ Vegetables (Campbell's Cup)	1 (1.7 oz)	180	—	2
Hearty Vegetable (Ultra Slim-Fast)	6 oz	50	—	tr
Homestyle (Nile Spice)				
Black Bean	1 pkg	190	0	2
Chicken Flavored Vegetable	1 pkg	120	1	2
Lentil	1 pkg	180	0	2
Minestrone	1 pkg	160	0	2
Red Beans & Rice	1 pkg	190	0	2
Split Pea	1 pkg	200	0	2
Sweet Corn Chowder	1 pkg	120	1	3
Instant Lunch(Maruchan)				
Oriental Noodles Beef	1 pkg (2.25 oz)	290	—	13
Oriental Noodles Chicken	1 pkg (2.25 oz)	290	7	13
Oriental Noodles Chicken Mushroom	1 pkg (2.25 oz)	280	—	13
Oriental Noodles Mushroom	1 pkg(2.25 oz)	290	—	13
Oriental Noodles Pork	1 pkg (2.25 oz)	290	—	13
Oriental Noodles Shrimp	1 pkg (2.25 oz)	290	—	13
Oriental Noodles Toasted Onion	1 pkg (2.25 oz)	270	—	12
Oriental Noodles Vegetable Beef	1 pkg (2.25 oz)	290	—	12
Instant Wonton (Maruchan)				
Chicken	1 pkg (1.49 oz)	200	—	12
Hot & Sour	1 pkg (1.49 oz)	200	—	11
Oriental	1 pkg (1.49 oz)	190	—	12
Pork	1 pkg (1.49 oz)	200	—	12
Shrimp	1 pkg (1.49 oz)	200	—	12
Island Black Bean (Bean Cuisine)	1 cup (8.6 fl oz)	202	tr	tr
Italian Tomato (Nile Spice)	1 pkg	140	3	4
Lentil Cup-A-Soup, as prep (Knorr)	1 pkg	220	0	0
Lentil Savory (Hain)	¾ cup	130	—	2
Lobster Bisque (Golden Dipt)	¼ pkg	30	—	1

FOOD	PORTION	CALS.	SAT. FAT	FAT
Lots of Lentil (Bean Cuisine)	1 cup (7.7 oz)	166	tr	tr
Manhattan Clam Chowder (Golden Dipt)	¼ pkg	80	—	2
Matzo Ball & Soup (Goodman's)	1 cup	40	0	1
Matzo Ball & Soup 50% Less Salt (Goodman's)	1 serv	50	0	1
Mesa Maize (Bean Cuisine)	1 cup (9.2 fl oz)	179	tr	tr
Minestrone Savory (Hain)	¾ cup	110	—	1
Minestrone as prep (Manischewitz)	6 fl oz	50	—	tr
Mushroom, as prep (Knorr)	8 oz	100	—	4
New England Clam Chowder (Golden Dipt)	¼ pkg	24	—	2
New England Clam Chowder (Weight Watchers)	7.5 oz	90	—	0
Noodle (4C)	8 oz	50	—	2
Noodle, as prep (Campbell)	8 oz	110	—	2
Noodle w/ Chicken Broth, as prep (Campbell's Cup)	6 oz	90	—	2
Noodleman (Goodman's)	1 cup	45	0	1
Noodleman Low Sodium (Goodman's)	1 cup	50	0	1
Onion (Cup-A-Soup)	6 oz	27	—	1
Onion (Goodman's)	1 cup	30	1	1
Onion (Lipton)	8 oz	20	—	tr
Onion (Ultra Slim-Fast)	6 oz	45	—	tr
Onion, as prep (Campbell)	8 oz	30	—	0
Onion Bouillon Instant (Wylers)	1 tsp	10	—	tr
Onion Golden (Lipton)	8 oz	62	—	2
Onion Low Sodium (Goodman's)	1 cup	30	0	1
Onion Mushroom (Lipton)	8 oz	41	—	1
Onion Reduced Salt (4C)	8 oz	30	—	1
Onion Savory (Hain)	¾ cup	50	—	2
Onion Savory No Salt Added (Hain)	¾ cup	50	—	1
Oriental Hot and Sour as prep (Knorr)	8 fl oz	50	—	1

FOOD	PORTION	CALS.	SAT. FAT	FAT
Oriental Low Fat, as prep (Ramen Noodle)	8 oz	150	—	1
Oriental Noodle Picante Style Beef (Maruchan)	1 pkg (2.25 oz)	290	—	15
Oriental Noodle Picante Style Chicken (Maruchan)	1 pkg (2.25 oz)	290	—	15
Oriental Noodle Picante Style Shrimp (Maruchan)	1 pkg (2.25 oz)	300	—	16
Oriental With Vegetables Low Fat, as prep (Cup-A-Ramen)	8 oz	220	—	2
Oriental With Vegetables, as prep (Cup-A-Ramen)	8 oz	270	—	10
Oriental, as prep (Ramen Noodle)	8 oz	190	—	8
Oxtail Hearty Beef, as prep (Knorr)	8 oz	70	—	2
Pork, as prep (Ramen Noodle)	8 oz	200	—	8
Pork Flavor Low Fat Ramen Noodle, as prep	8 oz	150	—	1
Pork Flavor Ramen Noodle, as prep	8 oz	200	—	8
Potato Leek (Nile Spice)	1 pkg	150	4	6
Potato Leek (Ultra Slim-Fast)	6 oz	80	—	tr
Potato Leek Cup-A-Soup as prep (Knorr)	1 pkg	120	0	0
Potato Leek Savory (Hain)	¾ cup	260	—	18
Potato Ramono (Nile Spice)	10 oz	140	4	5
Ramen (Maruchan)				
Beef	½ pkg (1.5 oz)	190	—	9
Chicken	½ pkg (1.5 oz)	190	—	8
Chicken Mushroom	½ pkg (1.5 oz)	190	—	8
Chili	½ pkg (1.5 oz)	190	—	9
Mushroom	½ pkg (1.5 oz)	190	—	9
Oriental	½ pkg (1.5 oz)	190	—	9
Pork	½ pkg (1.5 oz)	190	—	9
Shrimp	½ pkg (1.5 oz)	190	—	9
Ring-O-Noodle (Lipton)	8 oz	67	—	2
Rocky Mountain Red Bean (Bean Cuisine)	1 cup (8.6 oz)	202	tr	tr
Sante Fe Corn Chowder (Bean Cuisine)	1 cup (9.2 oz)	179	tr	tr

FOOD	PORTION	CALS.	SAT. FAT	FAT
Seafood Chowder (Golden Dipt)	¼ pkg	70	—	2
Shrimp Bisque (Golden Dipt)	¼ pkg	30	—	1
Shrimp Flavor w/ Vegetables Cup-A-Ramen, as prep	8 oz	280	—	10
Shrimp Flavor w/ Vegetables Low Fat Cup-A-Ramen, as prep	8 oz	230	—	2
Spanish-American Black Bean (Hurst)	1 serv (1.3 oz)	120	0	1
Spinach as prep (Knorr)	8 fl oz	100	—	5
Split Pea Savory (Hain)	¾ cup	310	—	10
Split Pea Soup Mix, as prep (Manischewitz)	6 oz	45	—	tr
Spring Vegetable w/ Herbs, as prep (Knorr)	8 oz	30	—	tr
Thick As Fog Split Pea (Bean Cuisine)	1 cup (8.6 oz)	189	tr	tr
Tomato (Cup-A-Soup)	6 oz	103	—	1
Tomato, as prep (Diamond Crystal)	6 oz	70	—	2
Tomato Basil, as prep (Knorr)	8 oz	90	—	3
Tomato Savory (Hain)	¾ cup	220	—	14
Tortellini in Brodo, as prep (Knorr)	8 oz	60	—	1
Ultima Pasta E Fagioli (Bean Cuisine)	1 cup (8.6 oz)	179	0	tr
Vegetable (Lipton)	8 oz	37	—	1
Vegetable, as prep (Campbell)	8 oz	40	—	0
Vegetable, as prep (Knorr)	8 oz	35	—	1
Vegetable Bouillon (Herb-Ox)	1 cube (4 g)	10	0	0
Vegetable Bouillon Instant (Wylers)	1 tsp	6	0	tr
Vegetable Beef (Weight Watchers)	7.5 oz	90	0	1
Vegetable Beef Microwave Soup (Campbell)	7.5 oz	100	0	2
Vegetable Cup Of Soup (Goodman's)	1 pkg (1½ cups)	180	1	3
Vegetable Cup-A-Soup as prep (Knorr)	1 pkg	100	0	0

FOOD	PORTION	CALS.	SAT. FAT	FAT
Vegetable Savory (Hain)	¾ cup	80	—	1
Vegetable Savory No Salt Added (Hain)	¾ cup	80	—	1
Vegetable Soup Mix, as prep (Manischewitz)	6 oz	50	0	tr
Vegetarian Vegetable Bouillon, as prep w/ water (Knorr)	8 oz	16	0	2
White Bean Provencal (Bean Cuisine)	1 cup (7.7 fl oz)	166	tr	tr
Wonton (Maruchan)				
Beef	⅓ pkg (0.68 oz)	90	—	5
Chicken	⅓ pkg (0.67 oz)	90	—	5
Pork	⅓ pkg (0.68 oz)	90	—	5
Vegetable	⅓ pkg (0.7 oz)	90	—	6
asparagus, cream of, as prep w/ water	1 cup	59	tr	2
beef broth, as prep w/ water	1 cup	19	tr	1
beef broth cube	1 cube (3.6 g)	6	tr	tr
beef broth cube, as prep w/ water	1 cup	8	tr	tr
celery, cream of, as prep w/ water	1 cup	63	tr	2
chicken broth, as prep w/ water	1 cup	21	tr	1
chicken broth cube	1 cube (4.8 g)	9	tr	tr
chicken broth cube, as prep w/ water	1 cup	13	tr	tr
chicken broth, not prep	1 pkg (0.2 oz)	16	tr	1
chicken, cream of, as prep w/ water	1 cup	107	3	5
chicken noodle, as prep w/ water	1 cup	53	tr	1
french onion, not prep	1 pkg (1.4 oz)	115	1	2
leek, as prep w/ water	1 cup	71	1	2
onion, as prep w/ water	1 cup	28	tr	1
tomato, as prep w/ water	1 cup	102	1	2
FROZEN				
Asparagus Cream of (Kettle Ready)	6 oz	62	2	5
Barley & Mushroom (Jaclyn's)	7.5 oz	90	—	1
Black Bean w/ Ham (Kettle Ready)	6 oz	154	1	6

FOOD	PORTION	CALS.	SAT. FAT	FAT
Boston Clam Chowder (Kettle Ready)	6 oz	131	2	7
Broccoli Cream Of (Kettle Ready)	6 oz	94	3	7
Cauliflower Cream Of (Kettle Ready)	6 oz	93	3	7
Cheedar Broccoli Cream Of (Kettle Ready)	6 oz	137	5	11
Chicken Cream Of (Kettle Ready)	6 oz	98	2	6
Chicken Gumbo (Kettle Ready)	6 oz	94	1	4
Chicken Noodle (Kettle Ready)	6 oz	94	1	3
Chili (Kettle Ready)	6 oz	161	2	7
Corn & Broccoli Chowder (Kettle Ready)	6 oz	102	2	5
Creamy Cheddar (Kettle Ready)	6 oz	158	6	13
French Onion (Kettle Ready)	6 oz	42	tr	2
Garden Vegetable (Kettle Ready)	6 oz	85	1	3
Hearty Minestrone (Kettle Ready)	6 oz	104	1	4
Hearty Beef Vegetable (Kettle Ready)	6 oz	85	1	3
Manhattan Clam Chowder (Kettle Ready)	6 oz	69	1	3
Mushroom Cream Of (Kettle Ready)	6 oz	85	2	6
New England Clam Chowder (Kettle Ready)	6 oz	116	2	7
Potato Cream Of (Kettle Ready)	6 oz	121	2	5
Savory Bean With Ham (Kettle Ready)	6 oz	113	1	4
Split Pea (Jaclyn's)	7.5 oz	180	—	2
Split Pea w/ Ham (Kettle Ready)	6 oz	155	1	4
Tomato Florentine (Kettle Ready)	6 oz	106	1	4
Tortellini In Tomato (Kettle Ready)	6 oz	122	1	5
Vegetable (Jaclyn's)	7.5 oz	90	—	1

FOOD	PORTION	CALS.	SAT. FAT	FAT
HOME RECIPE				
black bean turtle soup	1 cup	241	tr	1
corn & cheese chowder	¾ cup	215	7	12
greek	¾ cup	63	1	2
hot & sour	1 cup	74	—	2
TAKE-OUT				
gazpacho	1 cup	46	—	tr
oxtail	5 oz	64	—	3

SOUR CREAM

(*see also* SOUR CREAM SUBSTITUTES)

FOOD	PORTION	CALS.	SAT. FAT	FAT
Breakstone	1 tbsp	30	2	3
Breakstone Light Choice Cultured Half & Half	1 tbsp	25	1	2
Cabot	1 oz	60	4	6
Cabot Light	1 oz	33	—	2
Friendship	2 tbsp	60	4	5
Friendship Light	2 tbsp (1 oz)	35	2	3
Heluva Good Cheese	2 tbsp (1.1 oz)	60	4	5
Heluva Good Cheese Fat-Free	2 tbsp (1.1 oz)	20	0	0
Heluva Good Cheese Light	2 tbsp (1.1 oz)	40	2	3
Knudsen Hampshire	1 oz	60	3	6
Knudsen Light N'Lively Light	1 oz	40	2	3
Naturally Yours No Fat	2 tbsp (1 fl oz)	15	0	0
Sealtest	1 tbsp	30	2	3
Sealtest Light Cultured Half & Half	1 tbsp	25	1	2
Weight Watchers Light Sour	2 tbsp	35	—	2
sour cream	1 tbsp	26	2	3
sour cream	1 cup	493	30	48

SOUR CREAM SUBSTITUTES

FOOD	PORTION	CALS.	SAT. FAT	FAT
Better Than Sour Cream Sour Supreme Tofutti	1 oz	50	2	5
Pet Imitation	1 tbsp	25	—	2
nondairy	1 cup	479	41	45
nondairy	1 oz	59	5	6

SOURSOP

FOOD	PORTION	CALS.	SAT. FAT	FAT
fresh	1	416	—	2
fresh, cut up	1 cup	150	—	1

FOOD	PORTION	CALS.	SAT. FAT	FAT

SOY
(*see also* TOFU, MILK SUBSTITUTES, ICE CREAM AND FROZEN DESSERTS)

FOOD	PORTION	CALS.	SAT. FAT	FAT
Soy Sauce (Kikkoman)	1 tbsp	12	0	0
Soy Sauce (La Choy)	½ tsp	2	—	tr
Soy Sauce Chef Magic (Trappey)	1 tbsp (0.5 oz)	23	tr	tr
Soy Sauce Dark (House of Tsang)	1 tbsp (0.6 oz)	10	0	0
Soy Sauce Ginger Flavored Low Sodium (House Of Tsang)	1 tbsp (0.6 oz)	10	0	0
Soy Sauce Ginger Flavored (House Of Tsang)	1 tbsp (0.6 oz)	20	0	0
Soy Sauce Light (House of Tsang)	1 tbsp (0.6 oz)	5	0	0
Soy Sauce Lite (Kikkoman)	1 tbsp	13	—	0
Soy Sauce Lite (La Choy)	½ tsp	1	—	tr
Soy Sauce Low Sodium (House of Tsang)	1 tbsp (0.6 oz)	10	0	0
Soy Sauce Mix (Diamond Crystal)	1 tsp	5	—	tr
Soy Sauce Mushroom Flavored Low Sodium (House of Tsang)	1 tbsp (0.6 oz)	10	0	0
Soyagen All Purpose (LaLoma)	¼ cup	130	—	6
Soyagen Carob (LaLoma)	¼ cup	140	—	6
Soyagen No Sucrose (LaLoma)	¼ cup	130	—	6
Soyamel (Worthington)	1 oz	130	—	7
Tempeh (Lightlife)	4 oz	182	1	6
lecithin	1 tbsp	104	2	14
soy milk	1 cup	79	1	5
soy sauce	1 tbsp	7	tr	tr
soy sauce, shoyu	1 tbsp	9	tr	tr
soy sauce, tamari	1 tbsp	11	tr	tr
soya cheese	1.4 oz	128	tr	11
soybean sprouts, raw	½ cup	43	tr	2
soybean sprouts, steamed	½ cup	38	tr	2
soybean sprouts, stir-fried	1 cup	125	1	7
soybeans, dry-roasted	½ cup	387	3	19
soybeans, roasted	½ cup	405	3	22
soybeans, roasted & toasted	1 oz	129	1	7

FOOD	PORTION	CALS.	SAT. FAT	FAT
soybeans, roasted & toasted	1 cup	490	3	26
soybeans, salted, roasted & toasted	1 oz	129	1	7
soybeans, salted, roasted & toasted	1 cup	490	3	26
soybeans, cooked	1 cup	298	2	15

SPAGHETTI
(*see* PASTA, PASTA DINNERS, PASTA SALAD, SPAGHETTI SAUCE)

SPAGHETTI SAUCE
(*see also* PIZZA, TOMATO)

JARRED
Classico

FOOD	PORTION	CALS.	SAT. FAT	FAT
Beef & Pork	4 fl oz	80	—	4
Four Cheese	4 fl oz	70	—	4
Ripe Olives & Mushrooms	4 fl oz	50	—	2
Spicy Red Pepper	4 fl oz	50	—	2
Sweet Peppers & Onions	4 fl oz	50	—	4
Tomato & Basil	4 fl oz	60	—	3
Contadina	¼ cup	20	0	0
Contadina Italian	¼ cup	15	0	0
Contadina Thick & Zesty	¼ cup	15	0	0
Healthy Choice				
Extra Chunky Garlic & Onions	½ cup (4.4 oz)	50	0	1
Extra Chunky Italian Style Vegetable	½ cup (4.4 oz)	50	0	1
Extra Chunky Mushrooms	½ cup (4.4 oz)	50	0	1
Original Garlic & Herbs	½ cup (4.4 oz)	50	0	1
Original Mushrooms	½ cup (4.4 oz)	50	0	1
Original Traditional	½ cup (4.4 oz)	50	0	1
Original With Meat	½ cup (4.4 oz)	50	0	1
Hunt's				
Chunky	¼ cup (2.2 fl oz)	30	0	1
Classic Italian With Parmesan	½ cup (4.4 fl oz)	50	0	2
Homestyle Traditional No Sugar Added	½ cup (4.4 fl oz)	60	0	3
Traditional	4 oz	70	tr	2
Traditional Light	½ cup (4 oz)	40	0	1
w/ Meat	4 oz	70	tr	2

FOOD	PORTION	CALS.	SAT. FAT	FAT
w/ Mushrooms	4 oz	70	tr	2
Newman's Own Marinara	4 oz	70	—	2
Newman's Own Sockaroooni	4 oz	70	—	2
Newman's Own w/ Mushrooms	4 oz	70	—	2
Prego Chunky Sausage & Green Peppers	4 oz	160	—	8
Extra Chunky Garden Combination	4 oz	80	—	2
Extra Chunky Mushroom & Green Pepper	4 oz	100	—	4
Extra Chunky Mushroom & Onion	4 oz	100	—	4
Extra Chunky Mushroom & Tomato	4 oz	110	—	5
Extra Chunky Mushroom w/ Extra Spice	4 oz	100	—	3
Extra Chunky Tomato & Onion	4 oz	110	—	5
Marinara	4 oz	100	—	6
Meat Flavored	4 oz	140	—	6
Mushroom	4 oz	130	—	5
Onion & Garlic	4 oz	110	—	4
Regular	4 oz	130	—	5
Three Cheese	4 oz	100	—	2
Tomato & Basil	4 oz	100	—	2
Pritikin	4 oz	60	—	0
Pritikin w/ Mushrooms	4 oz	60	—	0
Progresso	½ cup	110	1	5
Bolognese	½ cup	150	2	12
Marinara	½ cup	90	1	5
Meat Flavored	½ cup	110	1	5
Mushroom	½ cup	110	1	5
Sicilian	½ cup	30	tr	3
Ragu				
Fino Italian Garden Medley	½ cup (4.5 oz)	90	0	3
Fino Italian Garlic & Basil	½ cup (4.5 oz)	90	0	3
Fino Italian Parmesan	½ cup (4.5 oz)	100	1	3
Fino Italian Sliced Mushroom	½ cup (4.5 oz)	90	0	3

FOOD	PORTION	CALS.	SAT. FAT	FAT
Ragu *(cont.)*				
Fino Italian Tomato & Herb	½ cup (4.5 oz)	90	0	3
Fino Italian Zesty Tomato	½ cup (4.5 oz)	90	0	3
Gardenstyle Chunky Garden Combination	½ cup (4.5 oz)	120	1	4
Gardenstyle Chunky Green & Red Pepper	½ cup (4.5 oz)	120	1	4
Gardenstyle Chunky Mushroom & Green Pepper	½ cup (4.5 oz)	120	1	4
Gardenstyle Chunky Mushroom & Onion	½ cup (4.5 oz)	120	1	4
Gardenstyle Chunky Tomato, Garlic & Onion	½ cup (4.5 oz)	120	1	4
Gardenstyle Super Mushroom	½ cup (4.5 oz)	120	1	4
Gardenstyle Super Vegetable Primavera	½ cup (4.5 oz)	110	1	4
Homestyle Mushroom	½ cup (4.5 oz)	120	1	4
Homestyle Tomato & Herb	½ cup (4.5 oz)	120	1	4
Homestyle With Meat	½ cup (4.5 oz)	130	1	4
Light Chunky Mushroom	½ cup (4.4 oz)	50	0	0
Light Garden Harvest	½ cup (4.4 oz)	50	0	0
Light No Sugar Added	½ cup (4.4 oz)	60	0	0
Light Tomato & Herb	½ cup (4.4 oz)	50	0	0
Old World Style Marinara	½ cup (4.4 oz)	90	1	5
Old World Style Mushrooms	½ cup (4.4 oz)	80	1	3
Old World Style Traditional	½ cup (4.4 oz)	80	1	3
Old World Style With Meat	½ cup (4.4 oz)	90	1	5
Spaghetti Sauce	4 fl oz	80	—	4
Thick & Hearty Mushroom	½ cup (4.5 oz)	120	1	3
Thick & Hearty Spaghetti Sauce	4 oz	100	—	3
Thick & Hearty Tomato & Herb	½ cup (4.5 oz)	120	1	3

FOOD	PORTION	CALS.	SAT. FAT	FAT
Thick & Hearty With Meat	1.2 cup (4.5 oz)	130	1	5
Weight Watchers Flavored w/ Meat	⅓ cup	45	0	1
Weight Watchers Flavored w/ Mushrooms	⅓ cup	35	0	0
marinara sauce	1 cup	171	tr	8
spaghetti sauce	1 cup	272	2	12
REFRIGERATED				
Contadina				
Alfredo	½ cup (4.2 fl oz)	400	21	38
Four Cheese Sauce With White Wine & Shallots	½ cup (4.2 fl oz)	320	14	25
Light Alfredo	½ cup (4.2 fl oz)	190	7	13
Light Chunky Tomato	½ cup (4.4 fl oz)	45	0	0
Light Garden Vegetable	½ cup (4.4 fl oz)	45	0	1
Marinara	½ cup (4.4 fl oz)	80	1	4
Pesto With Basil	¼ cup (2 oz)	310	5	30
Pesto With Sun Dried Tomatoes	¼ cup (2 oz)	250	4	24
Plum Tomato With Basil	½ cup (4.4 fl oz)	70	1	3
Spicy Italian Sausage & Bell Pepper	½ cup (4.4 fl oz)	100	1	5
TAKE-OUT				
bolognese	5 oz	195	—	15

SPANISH FOOD

(see also BEANS, CHIPS, DINNER, PEPPERS, SALSA, SNACKS, SAUCE, TORTILLA)

FOOD	PORTION	CALS.	SAT. FAT	FAT
CANNED				
Enchilada Sauce Hot (El Molino)	2 tbsp	16	—	1
Enchilada Sauce Mild (Rosarita)	2.5 oz	25	tr	1
Enchiladas (Gebhardt)	2	310	9	24
Fajita Marinade (Old El Paso)	⅛ jar	14	0	0
Green Chili Sauce Mild (El Molino)	2 tbsp	10	0	0
Menudo (Old El Paso)	½ can	476	21	52
Mexican Sauce (Pritikin)	4 oz	50	—	1
Picante Chunky Hot (Rosarita)	3 tbsp (2 fl oz)	18	—	tr
Picante Chunky Medium (Rosarita)	3 tbsp (2 fl oz)	16	—	tr

FOOD	PORTION	CALS.	SAT. FAT	FAT
Picante Chunky Mild (Rosarita)	3 tbsp (2 oz)	25	—	tr
Picante Hot (Chi-Chi's)	2 tbsp (1 oz)	10	0	0
Picante Medium (Chi-Chi's)	2 tbsp (1 oz)	10	0	0
Picante Mild (Casa Fiesta)	1 oz	9	—	tr
Picante Mild (Chi-Chi's)	2 tbsp (1 oz)	10	0	0
Picante Mild (Guiltless Gourmet)	1 oz	6	0	0
Pico De Gallo (Chi-Chi's)	2 tbsp (1.2 oz)	10	0	0
Queso Mild Cheddar (Guiltless Gourmet)	1 oz	22	—	tr
Taco Sauce Thick & Chunky (Chi-Chi's)	1 tbsp (0.5 oz)	10	0	0
Taco Sauce Western Style (Ortego)	1 oz	8	—	0
Taco Sauce Mild (Casa Fiesta)	1 oz	9	—	tr
Taco Sauce Red Mild (El Molino)	2 tbsp	10	0	0
Taco Sauce Thick and Smooth Hot (Ortego)	1 tbsp	8	0	0
Taco Sauce Thick And Smooth Mild (Ortega)	1 tbsp	8	0	0
Tamales (Derby)	2	160	3	7
Tamales (Gebhardt)	2	290	8	22
Tamales (Old El Paso)	2	190	—	12
Tamales (Van Camp's)	2 (5.1 oz)	210	5	13
Tamales (Wolf Brand)	7.5 oz	328	—	25
Tamales (Beef Hormel)	3 (7.5 oz)	280	8	21
Tamales Beef (Hormel)	1 can (7.5 oz)	290	8	21
Tamales Chicken (Hormel)	3 (7.5 oz)	210	4	10
Tamales Hot Spicy Beef (Hormel)	3 (7.5 oz)	280	8	21
Tamales Jumbo Gebhardt	2	400	11	30
Tamales Jumbo Beef (Hormel)	2 (6.9 oz)	270	8	20
FROZEN				
Banquet				
Beef & Bean Burrito	9.5 oz	390	—	12
Beef Echilada & Tamale w/ Chili Gravy	10 oz	300	—	10
Chimichanga	9.5 oz	480	—	21
Enchilada Chicken	11 oz	340	—	9
Enchilada Beef	11 oz	370	—	12

FOOD	PORTION	CALS.	SAT. FAT	FAT
Enchilada Cheese	11 oz	340	—	9
Enchiladas Beef w/ Chili Sauce	7 oz	270	—	13
Tamale Beef	11 oz	420	—	18
El Charrito				
Burrito Grande B&B	1 pkg (6 oz)	430	—	16
Burrito Grande Green Chili B&B	1 pkg (6 oz)	410	—	14
Burrito Grande Jalapeno	1 pkg (6 oz)	410	—	15
Burrito Grande Red Chili B&B	1 pkg (6 oz)	410	—	15
Burrito Green Chili B&B	1 pkg (5 oz)	370	—	16
Burrito Red Chili B&B	1 pkg (5 oz)	380	—	18
Burrito Red Hot B&B	1 pkg (5 oz)	540	—	18
Burrito Red Hot Beef	1 pkg (5 oz)	340	—	17
Enchilada Chicken Dinner	1 pkg (13.75 oz)	510	—	17
Enchilada Beef Dinner	1 pkg (13.75 oz)	620	—	31
Enchilada Cheese Dinner	1 pkg (13.75 oz)	570	—	24
Enchilada Grande Beef Dinner	1 pkg (21 oz)	950	—	49
Enchiladas 3 Beef	1 pkg (11 oz)	560	—	31
Enchiladas 3 Cheese	1 pkg (11 oz)	470	—	20
Enchiladas 3 Chicken	1 pkg (11 oz)	440	—	13
Enchiladas 4 Grande Beef	1 pkg (16.5 oz)	890	—	47
Enchiladas 6 Beef	1 pkg (16.25 oz)	880	—	49
Enchiladas 6 Beef & Cheese	1 pkg (16.25 oz)	880	—	42
Enchiladas 6 Cheese	1 pkg (16.25 oz)	780	—	30
Grande Mexican Dinner	1 pkg (20 oz)	850	—	47
Mexican Dinner	1 pkg (14.25 oz)	690	—	35
Queso Dinner	1 pkg (13.25 oz)	490	—	16
Satillo Dinner	1 pkg (13.5 oz)	570	—	24
Satillo Grande Dinner	1 pkg (20.75 oz)	820	—	34
Tortillas Corn	2	95	—	1
Tortillas Flour	2	170	—	4
Healthy Choice				
Burrito Con Queso Chicken	1 (5.4 oz)	280	2	6
Burrito Ranchero Beef Medium	1 (5.4 oz)	290	3	7
Burrito Ranchero Beef Mild	1 (5.4 oz)	300	3	7

FOOD	PORTION	CALS.	SAT. FAT	FAT
Healthy Choice *(cont.)*				
Enchilada Suprema Chicken	1 meal (13.4 oz)	390	5	9
Enchilada Beef Rio Grande	1 meal (13.4 oz)	410	3	8
Enchiladas Suiza Chicken	1 meal (10 oz)	270	2	4
Feista Fajitas Chicken	1 meal (7 oz)	260	1	4
Le Menu Entree LightStyle Enchiladaa Chicken	8 oz	280	—	8
Lean Cuisine Chicken Enchanadas	1 pkg (9.9 oz)	220	2	6
Lean Cuisine Chicken Enchilada Suiza	1 pkg (9 oz)	290	2	5
Lightlife Vegetarian Taco	2 oz	51	tr	1
Old El Paso				
Beef and Bean Burrito	11 oz	470	—	9
Beef and Cheese Chimichanga	11 oz	510	—	23
Burrito Bean And Cheese	1	330	—	11
Burrito Beef and Bean Hot	1	310	—	11
Burrito Beef and Bean Medium	1	330	—	13
Burrito Beef and Bean Mild	1	320	—	11
Chimichangas Beef	1 pkg (11 oz)	540	—	21
Chimichanges Bean & Cheese	1	380	—	19
Chimichanges Beef & Pork	1	340	—	16
Chimichanges Chicken	1	370	—	21
Enchilada Beef	1 pkg (11 oz)	390	—	8
Enchilada Cheese	1 pkg (11 oz)	590	—	31
Enchilada Chicken	1 pkg (11 oz)	460	—	18
Enchiladas w/ Sour Cream Sauce	1	280	—	19
Patio Britos				
Beef & Bean	1 (3 oz)	210	—	9
Nacho Beef	1 (3 oz)	220	—	11
Nacho Cheese	1 (3.63 oz)	250	—	10
Spicy Chicken & Cheese	1 (3 oz)	210	—	9
Patio Burritos Hot Beef & Bean Red Chili	1 (5 oz)	340	—	13

FOOD	PORTION	CALS.	SAT. FAT	FAT
Patio Burritos Medium Beef & Bean	1 (5 oz)	370	—	16
Patio Burritos Mild Beef & Bean Green Chili	1 (5 oz)	330	—	12
Patio Enchilada Beef Dinner	13.25 oz	520	—	24
Patio Enchilada Cheese Dinner	12 oz	370	—	10
Patio Fiesta Dinner	12 oz	460	—	20
Patio Mexican Dinner	13.25 oz	540	—	25
Patio Tamale Dinner	13 oz	470	—	21
Stouffer's Cheese Enchilada	1 pkg (9.75 oz)	370	5	14
Stouffer's Chicken Enchilada	1 pkg (10 oz)	370	4	14
Swanson Enchiladas Beef	13¾ oz	480	—	21
Swanson Mexican Style Combination	14¼ oz	490	—	18
Swanson Mexican Style Hungry Man	20¼ oz	820	—	41
Tyson Fajita Kit Beef	3.84 oz	160	—	4
Tyson Fajita Kit Chicken	4 oz	80	—	2
Van De Kamp's Mexican Holiday Enchilada Dinner Beef	12 oz	390	—	15
Van De Kamp's Mexican Holiday Enchilada Dinner Cheese	12 oz	450	—	20
Weight Watchers				
Enchiladas Ranchero Beef	9.12 oz	190	2	5
Enchiladas Ranchero Cheese	8.87 oz	260	2	10
Enchiladas Suiza Chicken	9 oz	230	2	7
Fajitas Chicken	6.75 oz	210	2	5
MIX				
Burrito Seasoning Mix (Old El Paso)	⅙ pkg	17	0	0
Enchilada Seasoning Mix (Old El Paso)	⅛ pkg	6	0	0
Guacamole Seasoning Mix (Old El Paso)	½ pkg	7	0	0
Masa Harina De Maiz (Quaker)	2 tortillas	137	2	2

FOOD	PORTION	CALS.	SAT. FAT	FAT
Masa Trigo (Quaker)	2 tortillas	149	1	4
Menudo Mix (Gebhardt)	1 tsp	5	—	tr
Taco Seasoning Mix (Old El Paso)	½ pkg	8	—	tr
Taco Meat Seasoning Mix Mild (Ortega)	1 filled taco	90	0	1
Taco Seasoning Mix (Hain)	⅒ pkg	10	0	0
READY-TO-USE				
Taco Shells (Casa Fiesta)	3.5 oz	480	—	23
Taco Shells (Gebhardt)	1	50	2	2
Taco Shells (Old El Paso)	1	55	—	3
Taco Shells (Rosarita)	1 shell (11 g)	50	2	2
Taco Shells Super (Old El Paso)	1	100	—	6
Taco Shells White Corned (Chi-Chi's)	2 (1 oz)	130	1	6
Tastaco Shells (Old El Paso)	1	100	—	5
Toco Shells Mini (Old El Paso)	3	70	—	4
Tostada Shells (Old El Paso)	1	65	—	3
Tostada Shells (Rosarita)	1 shell (14 g)	60	2	3
taco shell baked	1 med (½ oz)	61	tr	3
taco shell baked w/o salt	1 med (½ oz)	61	tr	3
TAKE-OUT				
burrito w/ apple	1 lg (5.4 oz)	484	7	20
burrito w/ apple	1 sm (2.6 oz)	231	5	10
burrito w/ beans	2 (7.6 oz)	448	7	14
burrito w/ beans & cheese	2 (6.5 oz)	377	7	12
burrito w/ beans & chili peppers	2 (7.2 oz)	413	8	15
burrito w/ beans & meat	2 (8.1 oz)	508	8	18
burrito w/ beans, cheese & beef	2 (7.1 oz)	331	7	13
burrito w/ beans, cheese & chili peppers	2 (11.8 oz)	663	11	23
burrito w/ beef	2 (7.7 oz)	523	10	21
burrito w/ beef & chili peppers	2 (7.1 oz)	426	8	17
burrito w/ beef, cheese & chili peppers	2 (10.7 oz)	634	10	25
burrito w/ cherry	1 lg (5.4 oz)	484	7	20
burrito w/ cherry	1 sm (2.6 oz)	231	5	10

FOOD	PORTION	CALS.	SAT. FAT	FAT
chimichanga w/ beef	1 (6.1 oz)	425	9	20
chimichanga w/ beef & cheese	1 (6.4 oz)	443	11	23
chimichanga w/ beef & red chili peppers	1 (6.7 oz)	424	8	19
chimichanga w/ beef, cheese & red chili peppers	1 (6.3 oz)	364	8	18
enchilada w/ cheese	1 (5.7 oz)	320	11	19
enchilada w/ cheese & beef	1 (6.7 oz)	324	9	18
enchiladas eggplant	1	142	—	5
enchirito w/ cheese, beef & beans	1 (6.8 oz)	344	8	16
frijoles w/ cheese	1 cup (5.9 oz)	226	4	8
nachos w/ cheese	6 to 8 (4 oz)	345	8	19
nachos w/ cheese & jalapeno peppers	6 to 8 (7.2 oz)	607	14	34
nachos w/ cheese, beans, ground beef & peppers	6 to 8 (8.9 oz)	568	12	31
nachos w/ cinnamon & sugar	6 to 8 (3.8 oz)	592	18	36
taco	1 sm (6 oz)	370	11	21
taco salad	1½ cups	279	7	15
taco salad w/ chili con carne	1½ cups	288	6	13
tostada w/ beans & cheese	1 (5.1 oz)	223	5	10
tostada w/ beans, beef & cheese	1 (7.9 oz)	334	11	17
tostada w/ beef & cheese	1 (5.7 oz)	315	10	16
tostada w/ guacamole	2 (9.2 oz)	360	10	23

SPARE RIBS
(*see* PORK)

SPELT
Arrowhead	1 oz	83	tr	1

SPICES
(*see* HERBS/SPICES, INDIVIDUAL NAMES)

SPINACH
CANNED
Popeye Chopped	½ cup (4.1 oz)	40	0	1
Popeye Leaf	½ cup (4.2 oz)	45	0	1
Popeye Low Sodium	½ cup (4.2 oz)	35	0	1

FOOD	PORTION	CALS.	SAT. FAT	FAT
S&W Northwest Premium	½ cup	25	0	0
Sunshine Chopped	½ cup (4.1 oz)	40	0	1
spinach	½ cup	25	tr	1
FRESH				
Dole	3 oz	9	—	tr
cooked	½ cup	21	tr	tr
mustard, chopped, cooked	½ cup	14	—	tr
mustard, raw, chopped	½ cup	17	—	tr
new zealand, chopped, cooked	½ cup	11	tr	tr
new zealand, raw	½ cup	4	tr	tr
raw, chopped	½ cup	6	tr	tr
raw, copped	1 pkg (10 oz)	46	tr	1
FROZEN				
Birds Eye Chopped	½ cup	20	0	0
Birds Eye Creamed	½ cup	90	2	5
Birds Eye Leaf	½ cup	20	0	0
Budget Gourmet Au Gratin	1 pkg (5.5 oz)	160	—	11
Fresh Like Cut Leaf	3.5 oz	21	—	tr
Green Giant	½ cup	25	0	0
Green Giant Creamed	½ cup	70	tr	3
Green Giant Cut Leaf in Butter Sauce	½ cup	40	tr	2
Green Giant Harvest Fresh	½ cup	25	0	0
Stouffer's Creamed	½ cup (2.25 oz)	150	4	12
Stouffer's Souffle	½ cup (4 oz)	150	2	10
cooked	½ cup	27	tr	tr
JUICE				
spinach juice	3.5 oz	7	0	0

SPORTS DRINKS

FOOD	PORTION	CALS.	SAT. FAT	FAT
All Sport Diet Lemon Lime (Slice)	8 fl oz	1	0	0
All Sport Lemon Lime (Slice)	8 fl oz	72	0	0
All Sport Orange (Slice)	8 fl oz	74	0	0
All Sport Punch (Slice)	8 fl oz	81	0	0
PowerAde				
Fruit Punch	8 fl oz	72	0	0
Grape	8 fl oz	73	0	0
Lemon-Lime	8 fl oz	72	0	0
Orange	8 fl oz	72	0	0

SPOT

FOOD	PORTION	CALS.	SAT. FAT	FAT
fresh, baked	3 oz	134	2	5

FOOD	PORTION	CALS.	SAT. FAT	FAT
SQUAB				
breast w/o skin, raw	1 (3.5 oz)	135	1	5
w/ skin, raw	1 squab (6.9 oz)	584	17	47
w/o skin, raw	1 squab (5.9 oz)	239	3	13
SQUASH				
(*see also* ZUCCHINI)				
CANNED				
Yellow (Allen)	½ cup (4.2 oz)	25	0	0
Yellow (Sunshine)	½ cup (4.2 oz)	25	0	0
crookneck, sliced	½ cup	14	tr	tr
FRESH				
Spaghetti Squash (Nature's Pasta)	1 cup (5.5 oz)	20	0	0
acorn, cooked, mashed	½ cup	41	tr	tr
acorn, cubed, baked	½ cup	57	tr	tr
butternut, baked	½ cup	41	tr	tr
crookneck, sliced, cooked	½ cup	18	tr	tr
crookneck, raw, sliced	½ cup	12	tr	tr
hubbard, baked	½ cup	51	tr	tr
hubbard, cooked, mashed	½ cup	35	tr	tr
scallop, raw, sliced	½ cup	12	tr	tr
scallop, sliced, cooked	½ cup	14	tr	tr
spaghetti, cooked	½ cup	23	tr	tr
FROZEN				
Butternut (Southland)	4 oz	45	—	0
Prepared Squash (Southland)	3.6 oz	80	—	2
Winter Cooked (Birds Eye)	½ cup	45	0	tr
butternut, cooked, mashed	½ cup	47	tr	tr
crookneck, sliced, cooked	½ cup	24	tr	tr
SEEDS				
dried	1 oz	154	2	13
dried	1 cup	747	12	63
roasted	1 oz	148	2	12
roasted	1 cup	1184	18	96
salted & roasted	1 oz	148	2	12
salted & roasted	1 cup	1184	18	96
whole, roasted	1 oz	127	1	6
whole, roasted	1 cup	285	2	12
whole, salted & roasted	1 oz	127	1	6
whole, salted & roasted	1 cup	285	2	12
SQUID				
fresh, fried	3 oz	149	2	6
raw	3 oz	78	tr	1

FOOD	PORTION	CALS.	SAT. FAT	FAT

SQUIRREL

FOOD	PORTION	CALS.	SAT. FAT	FAT
roasted	3 oz	147	tr	4

STRAWBERRIES

CANNED

FOOD	PORTION	CALS.	SAT. FAT	FAT
in heavy syrup	½ cup	117	tr	tr
FRESH				
Dole	8	50	—	0
strawberries	1 cup	45	tr	1
strawberries	1 pint	97	tr	1
FROZEN				
Halved in Delicious Syrup (Birds Eye)	½ cup	120	0	0
Halved in Lite Syrup (Birds Eye)	½ cup	90	0	0
Whole in Lite Syrup (Birds Eye)	½ cup	80	0	0
sweetened, sliced	1 cup	245	tr	tr
sweetened, sliced	1 pkg (10 oz)	273	tr	tr
unsweetened	1 cup	52	tr	tr
whole, sweetened	1 cup	200	tr	tr
whole, sweetened	1 pkg (10 oz)	223	tr	tr
JUICE				
Juice Works	6 oz	100	—	0
Kern's Nectar	6 oz	110	0	0
Kool-Aid Koolers	1 (8.45 oz)	136	0	0
Libby's Nectar	1 can (11.5 fl oz)	210	0	0
Smucker's Juice	8 oz	130	0	0
Tang Strawberry	8.45 fl oz	121	0	0
Wylers Drink Mix Unsweetened Strawberry Split	8 oz	2	0	0

STUFFING/DRESSING

HOME RECIPE

FOOD	PORTION	CALS.	SAT. FAT	FAT
bread, as prep w/ water & fat	½ cup	251	6	15
bread, as prep w/ water, egg & fat	½ cup	107	4	7
plain, as prep	½ cup (3.5 oz)	195	2	8
sausage	½ cup	292	2	11
MIX				
Arnold				
All Purpose Seasoned	½ oz	50	0	0

FOOD	PORTION	CALS.	SAT. FAT	FAT
Corn	½ oz	50	0	1
Herb Seasoned	½ oz	50	—	tr
Sage & Onion	½ oz	50	0	tr
Betty Crocker Chicken	½ cup	180	—	9
Betty Crocker Traditional Herb	½ cup	180	—	8
Brownberry Corn	1 oz	103	—	2
Brownberry Herb	1 oz	100	—	1
Brownberry Sage & Onion	1 oz	97	—	1
Golden Grain Bread Stuffing				
Chicken	½ cup	180	—	9
Corn Bread	½ cup	180	—	9
Herb & Butter	½ cup	180	—	9
With Wild Rice	½ cup	180	—	9
Pepperidge Farm				
Corn Bread	1 oz	110	—	1
Country Style	1 oz	100	—	1
Cube	1 oz	110	—	1
Distinctive Apple Raisin	1 oz	110	—	1
Distinctive Classic Chicken	1 oz	110	—	1
Distinctive Country Garden Herb	1 oz	120	—	4
Distinctive Vegetable & Almond	1 oz	110	—	3
Distinctive Wild Rice & Mushroom	1 oz	130	—	5
Herb Seasoned	1 oz	110	—	1
Stove Top				
Beef, as prep	½ cup	178	—	9
Chicken, as prep	½ cup	181	tr	8
Chicken w/ Rice, as prep	½ cup	182	tr	9
Cornbread, as prep	½ cup	175	tr	8
Flexible Serve Chicken, as prep	½ cup	173	tr	9
Flexible Serve Cornbread, as prep	½ cup	181	tr	9
Flexible Serve Herb Homestyle, as prep	½ cup	173	tr	9
Long Grain & Wild Rice, as prep	½ cup	182	tr	9
bread, dry, as prep	½ cup	178	2	9
cornbread, as prep	½ cup	179	2	9

FOOD	PORTION	CALS.	SAT. FAT	FAT
STURGEON				
FRESH				
roe, raw	3.5 oz	207	—	10
cooked	3 oz	115	1	4
raw	3 oz	90	1	3
SMOKED				
sturgeon	1 oz	48	tr	1
sturgeon	3 oz	147	1	4
SUCKER				
white, baked	3 oz	101	tr	3
SUGAR				
(see also FRUCTOSE, SUGAR SUBSTITUTES, SYRUP)				
C&H White	1 tsp	16	0	0
Domino White	1 tsp	16	0	0
Hain Turbinado	1 tbsp	50	0	0
Hollywood Turbinado	1 tbsp	50	0	0
brown	1 cup	820	0	0
powdered, sifted	1 cup	385	0	0
white	1 pkt (6 g)	25	0	0
white	1 tbsp	45	0	0
white	1 cup	770	0	0
SUGAR SUBSTITUTES				
(see also FRUCTOSE)				
Equal	1 pkt	4	0	0
S&W Liquid Table Sweetener	⅛ tsp	0	0	0
Sprinkle Sweet	1 tsp	2	0	0
SugarTwin	1 tsp (0.4 g)	2	—	0
SugarTwin	1 pkt (0.8 g)	3	—	0
SugarTwin Brown	1 tsp (0.4 g)	2	—	0
Sweet 'N Low Granulated	1 pkt (1 g)	4	—	0
Sweet One	1 pkg (1 g)	4	0	0
Sweet* 10	⅛ tsp	0	0	0
Weight Watchers Sweet'ner	1 pkt	4	0	0
SUGAR-APPLE				
fresh	1	146	—	tr
fresh, cut up	1 cup	236	—	1
SUNDAE TOPPINGS				
(see ICE CREAM TOPPINGS)				

FOOD	PORTION	CALS.	SAT. FAT	FAT
SUNFISH				
pumpkinseed, baked	3 oz	97	tr	1
SUNFLOWER SEEDS				
Frito Lay	1 oz	160	—	14
Oil Roasted (Fisher)	1 oz	170	2	15
Salted In Shell, shelled (Fisher)	1 oz	160	1	14
Salted In Shell, unshelled (Fisher)	1 oz	170	2	15
Sunflower Butter (Erewhon)	2 tbsp (32 g)	200	—	18
Sunflower Nuts Dry Roasted (Planters)	1 oz	170	2	15
Sunflower Seeds (Planters)	1 oz	160	0	14
dried	1 oz	162	7	14
dried	1 cup	821	7	71
dry roasted	1 oz	165	1	14
dry roasted	1 cup	745	7	64
dry roasted, salted	1 oz	165	1	14
dry roasted, salted	1 cup	745	7	64
oil roasted	1 cup	830	8	78
oil roasted, salted	1 oz	175	2	16
oil roasted, salted	1 cup	830	8	78
sunflower butter	1 tbsp	93	1	8
sunflower butter w/o salt	1 tbsp	93	1	8
toasted	1 oz	176	2	16
toasted	1 cup	826	8	76
toasted, salted	1 oz	176	2	16
toasted, salted	1 cup	826	8	76
SURF				
CANNED				
American Original Foods	4 oz	100	1	tr
FRESH				
American Original Foods	4 oz	90	tr	tr
SUSHI				
TAKE-OUT				
california roll	1 piece (0.8 oz)	28	tr	1
kim chi	⅓ cup (5.8 oz)	18	tr	tr
sashimi	1 serving (6 oz)	198	1	7
tuna roll	1 piece (0.7 oz)	23	tr	tr
vegetable roll	1 piece (1.2 oz)	27	tr	1
vinegared ginger	⅓ cup (1.6 oz)	48	tr	tr

FOOD	PORTION	CALS.	SAT. FAT	FAT
wasabi	2 tsp (0.3 oz)	5	0	tr
yellowtail roll	1 piece (0.6 oz)	25	tr	1

SWAMP CABBAGE
chopped, cooked	½ cup	10	—	tr
raw, chopped	1 cup	11	—	tr

SWEET POTATO
(see also YAM)
CANNED
Candied (Royal Prince)	½ cup (4.9 oz)	210	0	1
Halves (Royal Prince)	3 pieces (5.7 oz)	190	0	1
Mashed (Princella)	⅔ cup (5.1 oz)	120	0	1
Mashed (Sugary Sam)	⅔ cup (5.1 oz)	120	0	1
Orange Pineapple (Royal Prince)	½ cup (4.8 oz)	210	0	1
in syrup	½ cup	106	tr	tr
pieces	1 cup	183	tr	tr

FRESH
baked w/ skin	1 (3.5 oz)	118	tr	tr
leaves, cooked	½ cup	11	tr	tr
mashed	½ cup	172	tr	tr

FROZEN
Candied Sweet Potatoes (Mrs. Paul's)	4 oz	170	—	0
Candied Sweets 'N Apples (Mrs. Paul's)	4 oz	160	—	0
cooked	½ cup	88	tr	tr

HOME RECIPE
candied	3.5 oz	144	1	3

SWEETBREADS
beef, braised	3 oz	230	—	15
lamb, braised	3 oz	199	6	13
veal, braised	3 oz	218	—	12

SWISS CHARD
fresh, cooked	½ cup	18	—	tr
fresh, raw, chopped	½ cup	3	—	tr

SWORDFISH
cooked	3 oz	132	1	4
raw	3 oz	103	1	3

FOOD	PORTION	CALS.	SAT. FAT	FAT

SYRUP
(see also ICE CREAM TOPPINGS, PANCAKE/WAFFLE SYRUP)

FOOD	PORTION	CALS.	SAT. FAT	FAT
Blueberry	1 oz	45	—	tr
(Whistling Wings)				
Blueberry Diet (S&W)	1 tbsp	4	0	0
Blueberry Lite (Estee)	¼ cup (2.4 g)	80	0	0
Cane (McIlhenny)	2 tbsp (1.4 oz)	130	0	0
Corn Syrup Dark (Karo)	1 tbsp	60	0	0
Corn Syrup Dark (Karo)	1 cup	975	0	0
Corn Syrup Light (Karo)	1 tbsp	60	0	0
Corn Syrup Light (Karo)	1 cup	960	0	0
Fruit Syrup, All Flavors	2 tbsp	100	0	0
(Smuckers)				
Maple Flavored Diet	1 tbsp	4	0	0
(S&W)				
Maple Rich (Home Brands)	1 oz	110	0	0
Quik Strawberry (Nestle)	1⅔ tbsp	100	—	0
Raspberry	1 oz	60	—	tr
(Whistling Wings)				
Strawberry Diet (S&W)	1 tbsp	4	0	0
corn	2 tbsp	122	0	0
raspberry	3.5 oz	267	0	0

TACO
(see SPANISH FOOD)

TAHINI
(see SESAME)

TAMARIND
FRESH

FOOD	PORTION	CALS.	SAT. FAT	FAT
cut up	1 cup	287	tr	1
tamarind	1	5	tr	tr

TANGERINE
CANNED

FOOD	PORTION	CALS.	SAT. FAT	FAT
in light syrup	½ cup	76	tr	tr
juice pack	½ cup	46	tr	tr
FRESH				
Dole	2	70	—	1
sections	1 cup	86	tr	tr
tangerine	1	37	tr	tr
JUICE				
Dole Mandarin frzn as	8 fl oz	140	0	0
prep				

FOOD	PORTION	CALS.	SAT. FAT	FAT
Minute Maid Frozen	8 fl oz	120	0	0
canned, sweetened	1 cup	125	tr	1
fresh	1 cup	106	tr	tr
frzn, sweetened, as prep	1 cup	110	tr	tr
frzn, sweetened, not prep	6 oz	344	tr	1

TAPIOCA

Minute Tapioca (General Foods)	1 tbsp	35	—	tr
pearl dry	⅓ cup	174	0	0
starch	3.5 oz	344	—	tr

TARO

chips	10 (0.8 oz)	115	1	6
chips	1 oz	141	2	7
leaves, cooked	½ cup	18	tr	tr
raw, sliced	½ cup	56	tr	tr
shoots, sliced, cooked	½ cup	10	tr	tr
sliced, cooked	½ cup	94	tr	tr
tahitian, sliced, cooked	½ cup	30	tr	tr

TARRAGON

ground	1 tsp	5	—	tr

TEA/HERBAL TEA
HERBAL

Almond Orange (Bigelow)	5 oz	tr	—	tr
Almond Sunset (Celestial Seasonings)	1 cup	3	—	tr
Apple Orchard (Bigelow)	1 cup	5	—	tr
Apple Spice (Bigelow)	5 oz	tr	—	tr
Bengal Spice (Celestial Seasonings)	8 fl oz	5	—	tr
Caffeine Free (Celestial Seasonings)	8 fl oz	2	—	tr
Chamomile (Bigelow)	5 oz	tr	—	tr
Chamomile (Celestial Seasonings)	1 cup	2	—	tr
Chamomile Mint (Bigelow)	5 oz	tr	—	tr
Cinnamon Apple Spice (Celestial Seasonings)	1 cup	3	—	tr
Cinnamon Orange (Bigelow)	5 oz	tr	—	tr
Cinnamon Rose (Celestial Seasonings)	1 cup	2	—	tr

FOOD	PORTION	CALS.	SAT. FAT	FAT
Country Peach Spice (Celestial Seasonings)	1 cup	3	—	tr
Cranberry Cove (Celestial Seasonings)	1 cup	3	—	tr
Early Riser (Bigelow)	1 cup	3	—	3
Emperor's Choice (Celestial Seasonings)	1 cup	4	—	tr
Feeling Free (Bigelow)	1 cup	1	—	1
Fruit & Almond (Bigelow)	1 cup	1	—	tr
Ginseng Plus (Celestial Seasonings)	1 cup	3	—	tr
Grandma's Tummy Mints (Celestial Seasonings)	1 cup	2	—	tr
Hibiscus & Rose Hips (Bigelow)	5 oz	1	—	1
I Love Lemon (Bigelow)	1 cup	1	—	1
Lemon & C (Bigelow)	5 oz	tr	—	tr
Lemon Mist (Celestial Seasonings)	1 cup	2	—	tr
Lemon Zinger (Celestial Seasonings)	1 cup	4	—	tr
Looking Good (Bigelow)	1 cup	1	—	tr
Mama Bear's Cold Care (Celestial Seasonings)	8 fl oz	6	—	tr
Mandarin Orange Spice (Celestial Seasonings)	1 cup	5	—	tr
Mellow Mint (Celestial Seasonings)	1 cup	2	—	tr
Mint Blend (Bigelow)	5 oz	tr	—	1
Mint Magic (Celestial Seasonings)	1 cup	1	—	tr
Mint Medley (Bigelow)	1 cup	1	—	1
Orange & C (Bigelow)	5 oz	tr	—	tr
Orange & Spice (Bigelow)	1 cup	1	—	tr
Orange Zinger (Celestial Seasonings)	1 cup	5	—	tr
Peppermint (Bigelow)	5 oz	tr	—	tr
Peppermint (Celestial Seasonings)	1 cup	2	—	tr
Raspberry Patch (Celestial Seasonings)	1 cup	4	—	tr
Red Zinger (Celestial Seasonings)	1 cup	4	—	tr
Roastaroma (Celestial Seasonings)	1 cup	11	—	tr

FOOD	PORTION	CALS.	SAT. FAT	FAT
Roasted Grain & Carob (Bigelow)	5 oz	3	—	2
Sleepytime (Celestial Seasonings)	1 cup	5	—	tr
Spearmint (Bigelow)	5 oz	tr	—	tr
Spearmint (Celestial Seasonings)	1 cup	5	—	tr
Strawberry Fields (Celestial Seasonings)	1 cup	4	—	tr
Sunburst C (Celestial Seasonings)	1 cup	3	—	tr
Sweets Dreams (Bigelow)	1 cup	1	—	2
Take-a-Break (Bigelow)	1 cup	3	—	2
Tropical Escape (Celestial Seasonings)	8 fl oz	1	—	tr
Wild Forest Blueberry (Celestial Seasonings)	1 cup	2	—	tr
ICED				
4C Instant (4C)	8 oz	90	—	0
Arizona Raspberry	8 fl oz	95	0	0
Bigelow Nice Over Ice	5 fl oz	1	—	tr
Celestial Seasonings Iced Delight (Celestial Seasonings)	8 fl oz	4	—	tr
Crystal Light Decaffeinated Sugar Free	8 oz	2	0	0
Crystal Light Sugar Free	8 oz	3	0	0
Lipton				
Instant	6 oz	0	0	0
Instant Decaffeinated	6 oz	0	0	0
Instant Raspberry	8 oz	3	0	0
Instant Lemon	8 oz	3	—	0
Lemon	6 oz	55	—	0
Lemon w/ Vitamin C	6 oz	58	0	0
Sugar Free	8 oz	1	—	0
Sugar Free Peach	8 oz	5	—	0
Sugar Free Raspberry	8 oz	5	—	0
With Nutrasweet	8 oz	3	—	0
With Nutrasweet Decaffeinated	8 oz	3	—	0
Nestea				
Lemon	8 oz	6	0	0
Mix With Sugar And Lemon, as prep	8 oz	70	0	0
Peach	8 fl oz	88	—	tr

FOOD	PORTION	CALS.	SAT. FAT	FAT
Raspberry	8 fl oz	88	—	tr
With Sugar & Lemon	1 bottle (16 fl oz)	176	0	0
With Sugar And Lemon	1 can (11.5 fl oz)	127	0	0
Nestea 100% Instant Tea, as prep	8 oz	2	0	0
Nestea Ice Teasers				
Citrus	8 oz	6	0	0
Lemon	8 oz	6	0	0
Orange	8 oz	6	0	0
Tropical	8 oz	6	0	0
Wild Cherry	8 oz	6	0	0
Nestea Sugarfree Iced Tea Mix	8 oz	4	0	0
Royal Mistic				
Diet	12 fl oz	8	0	0
Lemon	12 fl oz	144	0	0
Orange	12 fl oz	144	0	0
Wild Berry	12 fl oz	144	0	0
Schweppes	8 fl oz	90	0	0
Shasta	12 oz	124	—	0
Sipps	8.45 oz	100	—	0
Tropicana				
Diet Lemon Fruit	8 fl oz	15	0	0
Lemon Fruit	8 fl oz	100	0	0
Peach Fruit	1 bottle (10 fl oz)	140	0	0
Peach Fruit	1 can (11.5 fl oz)	160	0	0
Peach Fruit	8 fl oz	120	0	0
Rasperry Fruit	1 bottle (10 fl oz)	140	0	0
Raspberry Fruit	1 can (11.5 fl oz)	160	0	0
Raspberry Fruit	8 fl oz	120	0	0
Tangerine Fruit	1 bottle (10 fl oz)	140	0	0
Tangerine Fruit	1 can (11.5 fl oz)	170	0	0
Tangerine Fruit	8 fl oz	110	0	0
Twister Apple Berry	8 fl oz	100	0	0
Twister Lemon Citrus	8 fl oz	110	0	0
Veryfine With Lemon	8 oz	80	0	0
instant artificially sweetened lemon flavored, as prep w/ water	8 oz	5	0	0
instant sweetened lemon flavor, as prep w/ water	9 oz	87	tr	tr
instant unsweetened lemon flavor, as prep w/ water	8 oz	4	0	0

FOOD	PORTION	CALS.	SAT. FAT	FAT
REGULAR				
Chinese Fortune (Bigelow)	5 fl oz	1	—	tr
Cinnamon Stick (Bigelow)	5 fl oz	1	—	tr
Cinnamon Vienna (Celestial Seasonings)	8 fl oz	2	—	tr
Constant Comment (Bigelow)	5 fl oz	1	—	1
Darjeeling Blend (Bigelow)	5 fl oz	1	—	tr
Earl Gray (Bigelow)	5 fl oz	1	—	tr
Earl Grey Extraordinary (Celestial Seasonings)	8 fl oz	3	—	tr
English Breakfast Classic (Celestial Seasonings)	8 fl oz	3	—	tr
English Teatime (Bigelow)	5 fl oz	1	—	tr
Kaffree (Natural Touch)	8 fl oz	0	0	0
Lemon (Celestial Seasonings)	8 fl oz	7	—	tr
Lemon Lift (Bigelow)	5 fl oz	1	—	tr
Mint (Celestial Seasonings)	8 fl oz	4	—	tr
Morning Thunder (Celestial Seasonings)	8 fl oz	3	—	tr
Naturally Decaffeinated (Celestial Seasonings)	8 fl oz	10	—	1
Nestea Tea Bag, as prep	6 oz	0	0	0
Orange Pekoe (Bigelow)	5 fl oz	1	—	tr
Orange Spice (Celestial Seasonings)	8 fl oz	7	—	tr
Orange Spice Decaff (Celestial Seasonings)	8 fl oz	7	—	tr
Organically Grown (Celestial Seasonings)	8 fl oz	12	—	tr
Peppermint Stick (Bigelow)	5 fl oz	1	—	tr
Plantation Mint (Bigelow)	5 fl oz	1	—	tr
Raspberry (Celestial Seasonings)	8 fl oz	7	—	tr
Raspberry Royale (Bigelow)	5 fl oz	1	—	tr
brewed tea	6 oz	2	0	0
instant unsweetened, as prep w/ water	8 oz	2	0	0
TEFF				
Whole Grain (Arrowhead)	¼ cup (1.6 oz)	160	0	1

FOOD	PORTION	CALS.	SAT. FAT	FAT
TEMPEH				
White Wave				
Burger	1 patty (3 oz)	110	0	3
Lemon Broil	1 patty (2 oz)	130	1	6
Organic Wild Rice	⅓ block (2.7 oz)	140	1	4
Teriyaki Burger	1 patty (3 oz)	110	0	2
tempeh	½ cup	165	1	6
THYME				
ground	1 tsp	4	tr	tr
TILEFISH				
fresh, cooked	3 oz	125	1	4
fresh, cooked	½ fillet (5.3 oz)	220	1	7
raw	3 oz	81	tr	2
TOFU				
Azumaya Blue Label	3.5 oz	46	—	1
Azumaya Green Label	3.5 oz	68	—	2
Azumaya Name Age Fried	3.5 oz	144	—	4
Azumaya Red Label	3.5 oz	68	—	1
Jaclyn's Grilled In Black Bean Sauce	10.75 oz	270	—	8
Jaclyn's Grilled In Peanut Sauce	10.75 oz	260	—	9
Mori-Nu Extra Firm	1 in slice (3 oz)	55	0	2
Mori-Nu Firm	1 in slice (3 oz)	50	0	3
Mori-Nu Soft	1 in slice (3 oz)	45	0	3
Mori-Nu Lite Extra Firm Mori-Nu	1 in slice (3 oz)	35	0	1
Mori-Nu Lite Firm Mori-Nu	1 in slice (3 oz)	35	0	1
Nasoya				
Extra Firm	⅕ block (3 oz)	90	1	5
Firm	⅕ block (3 oz)	80	1	4
Silken	⅙ block (3 oz)	50	0	2
Soft	⅕ block (3 oz)	60	0	3
Spring Creek				
Baked Barbeque	2 oz	88	—	4
Baked Cajun	2 oz	87	—	4
Baked Teriyaki	2 oz	84	—	4
Great Balls Of Tofu!	2 (3 oz)	107	—	5
Nigari Firm	4 oz	140	1	8
Tofu Salads !Onion Dip	2 oz	46	—	14
Tufo Salads !Taco Dip	2 oz	46	—	14
Tofu Salads Missing Egg	2 oz	49	—	14

FOOD	PORTION	CALS.	SAT. FAT	FAT
White Wave				
Baked Tofu Teriyaki Oriental Style	¼ block (2 oz)	120	1	6
Hard	4 oz	120	—	7
International Baked Italian Garlic Herb	¼ pkg (2 oz)	120	1	6
International Baked Mexican Jalapeno	¼ pkg (2 oz)	120	1	6
International Baked Oriental Teriyaki	¼ pkg (2 oz)	120	1	6
International Baked Thai Sesame Peanut	¼ pkg (2 oz)	120	1	6
Soft	4 oz	120	—	7
firm	¼ block (3 oz)	118	1	7
firm	½ cup	183	2	11
fresh, fried	1 piece (½ oz)	35	tr	3
fuyu, salted & fermented	1 block (⅓ oz)	13	tr	1
koyadofu, dried, frozen	1 piece (½ oz)	82	1	5
okara	½ cup	47	tr	1
regular	¼ block (4 oz)	88	1	6
regular	½ cup	94	1	6
YOGURT				
Stir Fruity				
Black Cherry	6 oz	141	—	2
Blueberry	6 oz	140	—	1
Lemon Chiffon	6 oz	152	—	3
Mixed Berry	6 oz	149	—	2
Orange	6 oz	143	—	2
Peach	6 oz	160	—	3
Pina Colada	6 oz	162	—	3
Raspberry	6 oz	155	—	2
Spiced Apple	6 oz	167	—	2
Strawberry	6 oz	140	—	2
Tropical Fruit	6 oz	170	—	2

TOFUTTI
(*see* CREAM AND FROZEN DESSERTS)

TOMATILLO

FOOD	PORTION	CALS.	SAT. FAT	FAT
fresh	1 (1.2 oz)	11	—	tr
fresh, chopped	½ cup	21	—	1

FOOD	PORTION	CALS.	SAT. FAT	FAT

TOMATO
(*see also* PIZZA, SPAGHETTI SAUCE)

CANNED

FOOD	PORTION	CALS.	SAT. FAT	FAT
Claussen Kosher	1	9	—	tr
Contadina California Sliced	½ cup	40	—	tr
Contadina Crushed	¼ cup	20	0	0
Contadina Italian Paste	2 tbsp	40	—	1
Contadina Italian Style Pear	½ cup	25	0	0
Contadina Italian Style Stewed	½ cup	40	0	0
Contadina Mexican Style Stewed	½ cup	40	0	0
Contadina Pasta Ready Primavera	½ cup	50	1	2
Contadina Pasta Ready Tomatoes	½ cup	50	0	2
Contadina Pasta Ready With Crushed Red Pepper	½ cup	60	1	3
Contadina Pasta Ready With Mushrooms	½ cup	50	1	2
Contadina Pasta Ready With Olives	½ cup	60	1	3
Contadina Pasta Ready With Three Cheeses	½ cup	70	0	4
Contadina Paste	2 tbsp	30	0	0
Contadina Peeled Whole	½ cup	25	0	0
Contadina Puree	¼ cup	20	0	0
Contadina Recipe Ready	½ cup	25	0	0
Contadina Stewed	½ cup	40	0	0
Health Valley Sauce	1 cup	70	0	1
Health Valley Sauce Low Sodium	1 cup	70	—	1
Hebrew National Pickled	⅓ tomato (1 oz)	4	0	0
Hunt's All Natural Sauce	¼ cup (2.2 fl oz)	15	0	0
Hunt's Paste	1 oz	25	0	0
Hunt's Crushed Angela Mia	4 oz	35	—	tr
Hunt's Crushed Italian	4 oz	40	—	tr
Hunt's Italian Pear Shaped	4 oz	20	—	tr
Hunt's Paste Italian Style	2 oz	50	—	tr
Hunt's Paste No Salt Added	2 oz	45	—	tr
Hunt's Paste w/ Garlic	2 oz	50	—	tr

FOOD	PORTION	CALS.	SAT. FAT	FAT
Hunt's Peeled Choice-Cut	4 oz	20	—	tr
Hunt's Puree	4 oz	45	—	tr
Hunt's Sauce Herb	4 oz	70	1	2
Hunt's Sauce Italian	4 oz	60	1	2
Hunt's Sauce Meatloaf Fixin's	4 oz	20	—	tr
Hunt's Sauce No Salt Added	4 oz	35	—	tr
Hunt's Sauce Special	4 oz	35	—	tr
Hunt's Sauce w/ Bits	4 oz	30	—	tr
Hunt's Sauce w/ Garlic	4 oz	70	—	2
Hunt's Sauce w/ Mushrooms	4 oz	25	—	tr
Hunt's Stewed	4 oz	35	—	tr
Hunt's Stewed Italian	4 oz	40	—	tr
Hunt's Stewed No Salt Added	4 oz	35	—	tr
Hunt's Whole	4 oz	20	—	tr
Hunt's Whole Italian	4 oz	25	—	tr
Hunt's Whole No Salt Added	4 oz	20	—	tr
Rosoff's Pickled	⅓ tomato (1 oz)	5	0	0
S&W Aspic Supreme	½ cup	60	0	0
S&W Diced in Rich Puree	½ cup	35	0	0
S&W Italian Stewed Sliced	½ cup	35	0	0
S&W Italian Style w/ Basil	½ cup	25	0	0
S&W Mexican Style Stewed	½ cup	40	0	0
S&W Paste	6 oz	150	0	0
S&W Peeled Ready Cut	½ cup	25	0	0
S&W Puree	½ cup	60	0	0
S&W Sauce	½ cup	40	0	0
S&W Sauce Chunky	½ cup	45	0	0
S&W Stewed 50% Salt Reduced	½ cup	35	0	0
S&W Stewed Sliced	½ cup	35	0	0
S&W Whole Diet	½ cup	25	0	0
S&W Whole Peeled	½ cup	25	0	0
Schorr's Pickled	⅓ tomato (1 oz)	4	0	0
paste	½ cup	110	tr	1
puree	1 cup	102	tr	tr
puree w/o salt	1 cup	102	tr	tr
red whole	½ cup	24	tr	tr
sauce	½ cup	37	tr	tr
sauce spanish style	½ cup	40	tr	tr

FOOD	PORTION	CALS.	SAT. FAT	FAT
sauce w/ mushrooms	½ cup	42	tr	tr
sauce w/ onion	½ cup	52	tr	tr
stewed	½ cup	34	tr	tr
tomato w/ green chiles	½ cup	18	tr	tr
wedges in tomato juice	½ cup	34	tr	tr
DRIED				
sun dried	1 piece	5	tr	tr
sun dried	1 cup	140	tr	2
sun dried in oil	1 piece	6	tr	tr
sundried in oil	1 cup	235	2	15
FRESH				
cooked	½ cup	32	tr	1
green	1	30	tr	tr
red	1 (4.5 oz)	26	tr	tr
red, chopped	1 cup	35	tr	tr
JUICE				
Campbell	6 oz	40	—	0
Hunt's	6 oz	30	—	tr
Hunt's No Salt Added	6 oz	35	—	tr
Libby's	6 oz	35	0	0
Mott's Beefamato	6 oz	80	0	0
Mott's Clamato	6 oz	96	0	0
Mott's Clamato Ceasar	8 fl oz	100	0	0
S&W California	6 oz	35	0	0
S&W Diet	½ cup	35	0	0
beef broth & tomato	5.5 oz	61	tr	tr
clam & tomato	1 can (5.5 oz)	77	tr	tr
juice	6 oz	32	tr	tr
juice	½ cup	21	tr	tr
TAKE-OUT				
stewed	1 cup	80	1	3

TONGUE

beef, simmered	3 oz	241	8	18
lamb, braised	3 oz	234	7	17
pork, braised	3 oz	230	5	16

TOPPINGS
(*see* ICE CREAM TOPPINGS)

TORTILLA
(*see also* SPANISH FOOD)

Mariachi	1	112	—	3
Old El Paso	1	150	—	3

FOOD	PORTION	CALS.	SAT. FAT	FAT
Tyson				
Burrito Style Flour	1	170	—	4
Burrito Style Flour	1	182	—	4
Large Heat Pressed				
Burrito Style Flour	1	106	—	2
Small Hand Stretched				
Enchilada Style Corn	1	54	—	tr
Fajito Style Flour	1	89	—	2
Soft Taco Flour	1	121	—	3
Whole Wheat	1	120	—	3
Wonder Wheat Low Fat	1 (1.4 oz)	120	1	2
Wonder White Low Fat	1 (1.4 oz)	110	1	2
corn	1 (6 in diam)	56	tr	1
corn w/o salt	1 (6 in diam) (0.9 oz)	56	tr	1
flour w/o salt	1-8 in diam (1.2 oz)	114	tr	3

TORTILLA CHIPS
(*see* CHIPS)

TREE FERN

chopped, cooked	½ cup	28	—	tr

TRITICALE
(*see also* FLOUR)

dry	½ cup	323	tr	2

TROUT
FRESH

Rainbow (Clear Springs)	3.5 oz	140	—	7
baked	3 oz	162	1	7
rainbow, cooked	3 oz	129	1	4
sea trout, baked	3 oz	113	1	4

TRUFFLES

fresh	3.5 oz	25	—	1

TUNA
(*see also* TUNA DISHES)
CANNED

Bumble Bee Chunk Light in Oil	2 oz	160	3	12
Bumble Bee Chunk Light in Water	2 oz	60	1	1
Bumble Bee Chunk White in Oil	2 oz	160	3	12

FOOD	PORTION	CALS.	SAT. FAT	FAT
Bumble Bee Chunk White in Water	2 oz	70	1	2
Bumble Bee Diet Chunk White in Water	2 oz	60	—	1
Bumble Bee Solid White in Oil	2 oz	130	2	8
Bumble Bee Solid White in Water	2 oz	70	1	2
Empress Chunk Light	2 oz	60	—	1
Empress Chunk Light Tongol	2 oz	50	—	1
Empress Solid White	2 oz	70	—	2
Progresso	⅓ cup	150	—	13
S&W Chunk Light Fancy in Oil	2 oz	140	—	10
S&W Chunk Light Fancy in Water	2 oz	60	—	1
S&W Fancy White Albacore in Oil	2 oz	160	—	12
light in oil	3 oz	169	1	7
light in oil	1 can (6 oz)	399	3	14
light in water	3 oz	99	tr	1
light in water	1 can (5.8 oz)	192	tr	1
white in oil	3 oz	158	—	7
white in oil	1 can (6.2 oz)	331	—	14
white in water	3 oz	116	1	2
white in water	1 can (6 oz)	234	1	4
FRESH				
bluefin, cooked	3 oz	157	1	5
bluefin, raw	3 oz	122	1	4
skipjack, baked	3 oz	112	tr	1
yellowfin, baked	3 oz	118	tr	1

TUNA DISHES

FROZEN				
Microwave Tuna Sandwich (Mrs. Paul's)	1	200	—	6
Tuna Melt (Chefwich)	5 oz	360	—	14
MIX				
Bumble Bee Tuna Mix-ins Garden Herb	⅙ pkg (0.17 oz)	25	—	0
Bumble Bee Tuna Mix-ins Lemon Herb	⅙ pkg (0.17 oz)	25	0	0
Bumble Bee Tuna Mix-ins Zesty Tomato	⅙ pkg (0.17 oz)	25	0	0

FOOD	PORTION	CALS.	SAT. FAT	FAT
Tuna Helper				
Au Gratin, as prep	⅕ pkg (6 oz)	280	—	11
Buttery Rice, as prep	⅕ pkg (6 oz)	280	—	11
Cheesy Noodles, as prep	⅕ pkg (7.75 oz)	240	—	8
Creamy Mushroom, as prep	⅕ pkg (7 oz)	220	—	6
Creamy Noodles, as prep	⅕ pkg (8 oz)	300	—	14
Fettucine Alfredo, as prep	⅕ pkg (7 oz)	300	—	13
Romanoff, as prep	⅕ pkg (8 oz)	290	—	8
Tetrazzini, as prep	⅕ pkg (6 oz)	240	—	8
Tuna Pot Pie, as prep	⅙ pkg (5.1 oz)	420	—	27
Tuna Salad, as prep	⅕ pkg (5.5 oz)	420	—	27
READY-TO-USE				
The Spreadables Tuna Salad	¼ can	90	—	6
Wampler Longacre Tuna Salad	1 oz	61	—	13
TAKE-OUT				
tuna salad	3 oz	159	1	8
tuna salad	1 cup	383	3	19
tuna salad submarine sandwich w/ lettuce & oil	1	584	5	28

TURBOT
fresh european, baked	3 oz	104	—	3

TURKEY
(*see also* DINNER, HOT DOG, TURKEY DISHES, TURKEY SUBSTITUTES)

FOOD	PORTION	CALS.	SAT. FAT	FAT
CANNED				
Chunk (Hormel)	2 oz	70	1	3
Chunk Turkey Ham (Hormel)	2 oz	70	2	4
Chunk White (Hormel)	2 oz	60	1	1
Chunky Light (Underwood)	2.08 oz	75	tr	2
White (Swanson)	2.5 oz	80	—	1
w/ broth	1 can (5 oz)	231	3	10
w/ broth	½ can (2.5 oz)	116	1	5
FRESH				
Bil Mar Foods Ground	3 oz	163	—	12
Breast Cutlets Thin-Sliced Skinless & Boneless (Perdue)	1 oz	28	tr	tr

FOOD	PORTION	CALS.	SAT. FAT	FAT
Breast Fillets Skinless & Boneless, Fit 'N Easy (Perdue)	1 oz	28	tr	tr
Breast Hotel Style Prime w/ skin (Perdue)	1 oz	43	1	2
Breast Prime Young (Shady Brook)	3 oz	140	—	7
Breast Skinless & Boneless, Fit 'N Easy (Purdue)	1 oz	28	tr	tr
Breast Tenderloins Skinless & Boneless (Perdue)	1 oz	29	tr	tr
Breast Fresh Young w/ skin (Perdue)	1 oz	44	—	2
Drumsticks Fresh Young w/ skin, cooked (Perdue)	1 oz	36	1	2
Ground (Louis Rich)	3 oz	140	3	9
Ground (Perdue)	1 oz	35	2	1
Ground All White Meat (Butterball)	3 oz	100	—	3
Ground All White (Swift-Eckrich)	3 oz	100	—	3
Ground Breast Meat (Perdue)	1 oz	28	tr	tr
Thighs Fresh Young w/ skin (Perdue)	1 oz	48	1	3
Thighs Skinless & Boneless, Fit 'N Fresh (Perdue)	1 oz	36	1	2
Whole Dark Meat w/ skin (Perdue)	1 oz	48	1	3
Whole White Meat Fresh Young w/ skin (Perdue)	1 oz	44	1	2
Wing Drummettes Fresh Young w/ skin (Perdue)	1 oz	43	1	2
Wing Portions Fresh Young w/ skin (Perdue)	1 oz	51	1	3
Wings (Shady Brook)	3 oz	130	—	6
Wings Fresh Young w/ skin (Perdue)	1 oz	45	tr	2
back w/ skin, roasted	½ back (9 oz)	637	11	38
breast w/ skin, roasted	4 oz	212	2	8
dark meat w/ skin, roasted	3.6 oz	230	4	12

FOOD	PORTION	CALS.	SAT. FAT	FAT
dark meat w/o skin, roasted	3 oz	170	2	7
dark meat w/o skin, roasted	1 cup (5 oz)	262	3	10
ground, cooked	3 oz	188	3	11
leg w/ skin, roasted	2.5 oz	147	2	7
leg w/ skin, roasted	1 (1.2 lbs)	1133	17	54
light meat w/ skin, roasted	4.7 oz	268	3	11
light meat w/ skin, roasted	from ½ turkey (2.8 lbs)	2069	25	87
light meat w/o skin, roasted	4 oz	183	1	4
neck, simmered	1 (5.3 oz)	274	4	11
skin, roasted	1 oz	141	3	13
skin, roasted	from ½ turkey (9 oz)	1096	26	98
w/ skin, neck & giblets, roasted	½ turkey 8.8 lbs)	4123	56	190
w/ skin, roasted	8.4 oz	498	7	23
w/ skin, roasted	½ turkey (4 lbs)	3857	53	181
w/o skin, roasted	1 cup (5 oz)	238	2	7
w/o skin, roasted	7.3 oz	354	3	10
wing w/ skin, roasted	1 (6.5 oz)	426	6	23
FROZEN				
Tyson Breast Boneless Skinless	3.5 oz	160	—	3
Empire Patties	1 (3.1 oz)	200	2	10
roast boneless seasoned light & dark meat, roasted	1 pkg (1.7 lbs)	1213	—	45
READY-TO-USE				
Bil Mar Foods				
Breast	1 slice (1 oz)	31	—	tr
Buffet Style Smoked Ham	1 oz	32	—	1
Cheese Patties	3 oz	213	—	13
Ham Smoked	1 oz	32	—	1
Ham Square Chopped	1 slice (1 oz)	37	—	2
Luncheon Loaf Square Spiced	1 slice (1 oz)	51	—	4
Smoked Breast	1 oz	31	—	tr
Smoked Sliced Breast	1 oz	31	—	tr
Carl Buddig	1 oz	50	1	3
Carl Buddig Honey Turkey	1 oz	40	1	2

FOOD	PORTION	CALS.	SAT. FAT	FAT
Carl Buddig Turkey Ham	1 oz	40	1	2
Deli Chef Breast & White	1 oz	39	—	6
Empire				
Bologna	3 slices (1.8 oz)	90	2	6
Breast Slices Oven Prepared	3 slices (1.8 oz)	50	0	1
Breast Slices Smoked	3 slices (1.8 oz)	40	0	0
Pastrami	3 slices (1.8 oz)	60	5	2
Salami	3 slices (1.8 oz)	70	1	4
Whole Barbecue	5 oz	250	4	12
Falls BBQ	3 oz	140	—	8
Falls Gourmet Breast	3 oz	80	—	1
Falls Premium Breast Cooked	3 oz	100	—	2
Hansel 'N Gretel				
Doubledecker Turkey-Corned Beef	1 oz	30	—	1
Doubledecker Turkey Ham	1 oz	30	—	1
Gourmet Breast	1 oz	28	—	1
Gourmet Smoked Breast	1 oz	31	—	1
Honey Breast	1 oz	28	—	1
Lessalt Cooked Breast	1 oz	25	—	1
Oven Cooked Breast	1 oz	26	—	tr
Healthy Choice				
Breast Oven Roasted	1 slice (1 oz)	35	0	1
Breast Smoked	1.9 oz	60	1	2
Deli-Thin Variety Pack Breast	2.2 oz	70	1	2
Deli-Thin Variety Pack Honey Roast & Smoked	1.9 oz	60	1	2
Honey Roasted & Smoked	1 slice (1 oz)	35	0	1
Hebrew National Deli Thin Hickory Smoked National	1.8 oz	55	—	1
Hebrew National Deli Thin Lemon Garlic National	1.8 oz	50	—	1
Hebrew National Deli Thin Oven Roasted	1.8 oz	80	—	1
Hillshire				
Breast Honey Cured	1 oz	35	—	1
Breast Smoked	1 oz	35	—	1

FOOD	PORTION	CALS.	SAT. FAT	FAT
Hillshire *(cont.)*				
Deli Select Breast Honey Roasted	1 slice	10	—	tr
Deli Select Breast Oven Roasted	1 slice	10	—	tr
Deli Select Breast Smoked	1 slice	10	—	tr
Deli Select Turkey Ham	1 slice	10	—	tr
Flavor Pack 90–99% Fat Free Breast Honey Roasted	1 slice (0.75 oz)	20	—	tr
Flavor Pack 90–99% Fat Free Breast Oven Roasted	1 slice (0.75 oz)	20	—	tr
Flavor Pack 90–99% Fat Free Breast Smoked	1 slice (0.75 oz)	20	—	tr
Lunch 'N Munch Smoked Turkey/ Cheddar	1 pkg (4.5 oz)	350	—	21
Lunch 'N Munch Smoked Turkey/ Cheddar/ Brownie	1 pkg (4.5 oz)	400	—	22
Lunch 'N Munch Turkey/ Cheddar/ Brownie/Hi-C	1 pkg (4.5 oz + 6 fl oz)	500	—	22
Hormel Light & Lean 97				
Breast Sliced	1 slice (1 oz)	30	0	1
Breast Smoked	3 oz	80	1	1
Cuts	16 pieces (1 oz)	30	0	1
Cuts Smoked	16 pieces (1 oz)	30	0	1
Louis Rich				
Bologna	1 slice (28 g)	50	1	4
Breaded Nuggets	4 (3.2 oz)	260	3	15
Breaded Patties	1 (3 oz)	220	3	13
Breaded Sticks	3 (3 oz)	230	3	15
Breast Honey Roasted	1 slice (1 oz)	30	0	1
Breast Oven Roasted	1 slice (1 oz)	30	0	1
Breast Oven Roasted	2 oz	60	1	2
Breast Smoked	1 slice (1 oz)	25	0	1
Carving Board Breast Oven Roasted	2 slices (1.6 oz)	40	0	1
Carving Board Breast Oven Roasted Thin Carved	6 slices (2.1 oz)	60	0	1

FOOD	PORTION	CALS.	SAT. FAT	FAT
Carving Board Breast Smoked	2 slices (1.6 oz)	40	0	1
Chopped Ham	1 slice (1 oz)	46	1	3
Cotto Salami	1 slice (28 g)	40	1	3
Deli-Thin Breast Oven Roasted	4 slices (1.8 oz)	50	0	1
Deli-Thin Breast Smoked	4 slices (1.8 oz)	50	0	1
Dinner Slices Breast Hickory Smoked	1 slice (2.8 oz)	80	0	1
Dinner Slices Breast Honey Roasted	1 slice (2.8 oz)	80	1	1
Dinner Slices Breast Oven Roasted	1 slice (2.8 oz)	70	0	1
Fat Free Breast Hickory Smoked	1 slice (1 oz)	25	0	0
Fat Free Breast Oven Roasted	1 slice (28 g)	25	0	0
Ham	4 slices (1.8 oz)	60	1	2
Ham Round	1 slice (28 g)	34	0	1
Ham Square	3 slices (2.2 oz)	70	1	3
Honey Cured Ham	3 slices (2.2 oz)	70	1	2
Pastrami	2 slices (1.6 oz)	45	0	2
Salami	1 slice (28 g)	45	1	3
Skinless Breast Barbecued	2 oz	60	0	1
Skinless Breast Hickory Smoked	2 oz	60	0	1
Skinless Breast Honey Roasted	2 oz	60	0	1
Skinless Breast Oven Roasted	2 oz	50	0	1
White Smoked	1 slice (1 oz)	30	0	1
Mr. Turkey				
BBQ Breast Quarter	1 oz	34	—	1
Bologna	1 oz	63	—	5
Bologna Red Rind	1 oz	63	—	5
Breakfast Smoked Ham	1 oz	33	—	1
Cotto Salami	1 oz	45	—	3
Diced White Meat	2 oz	84	—	2
Nuggets	1 nugget	33	—	2
Oven Roasted Quarter Breast	1 oz	34	—	1
Patties	3 oz	195	—	11

FOOD	PORTION	CALS.	SAT. FAT	FAT
Mr. Turkey *(cont.)*				
Smoked Breast Quarter	1 oz	35	—	1
Sticks	1 stick	65	—	4
Oscar Mayer				
Deli-Thin Roast	4 slices (1.8 oz)	50	0	1
Deli-Thin Smoked, Honey Roasted	4 slices (1.8 oz)	60	0	1
Healthy Favorites Breast Oven Roasted	4 slices (1.8 oz)	40	0	0
Healthy Favorites Breast Smoked	4 slices (1.8 oz)	40	0	0
Lunchables Fun Pack Turkey/Pacific Cooler	1 pkg (11.2 oz)	460	10	21
Lunchables Fun Pack Turkey/Surfer Cooler	1 pkg (11.2 oz)	440	8	16
Lunchables Turkey Oven Roasted/Green Onion Cheese	1 pkg (4.5 oz)	380	9	20
Lunchables Turkey Smoked/Ranch & Herb Cheese	1 pkg (4.5 oz)	380	9	20
Lunchables Turkey/ Cheddar	1 pkg (4.5 oz)	360	11	22
Perdue Done It! Nuggets	1 (.67 oz)	54	3	1
Tyson Breast	1 slice	20	tr	—
Tyson Ham	1 slice	23	tr	—
Wampler Longacre				
Baked Ham	1 oz	38	—	6
Baked Ham w/ 12% Water	1 oz	33	—	5
Baked Ham w/ 20% Water	1 oz	39	—	6
Bologna	1 oz	56	—	16
Breaded Nuggets	1 oz	87	—	20
Chunk Ham w/ 12% Water	1 oz	36	—	6
Chunk Ham w/ 20% Water	1 oz	39	—	6
Chunk Pastrami	1 oz	35	—	5
Combination Roll	1 oz	43	—	10
Dark Smoked Cured	1 oz	45	—	10
Diced Combination Roll	1 oz	43	—	10
Diced Ham w/ 20% Water	1 oz	39	—	6
Diced White Roll	1 oz	43	—	10

FOOD	PORTION	CALS.	SAT. FAT	FAT
Gourmet Breast	1 oz	31	—	2
Gourmet Brown & Glazed Breast	1 oz	28	—	2
Gourmet Brown & Roasted Breast	1 oz	35	—	3
Gourmet High Yield Skinless Breast	1 oz	28	—	tr
Gourmet Mini Breast	1 oz	35	—	4
Gourmet Skinless Brown & Roasted Breast	1 oz	31	—	1
Gourmet Smoked Breast	1 oz	37	—	3
Ham w/ 20% Water	1 oz	39	—	6
Lean-Lite Ham	1 oz	36	—	5
Lean-Lite Smoked Ham	1 oz	38	—	4
Mini Gourmet Smoked Breast	1 oz	37	—	3
Oven Roasted Oven Lite Breast	1 oz	35	—	3
Pastrami	1 oz	35	—	5
Premium Breast	1 oz	29	—	2
Premium Brown & Glazed Breast	1 oz	29	—	2
Premium Skinless Breast	1 oz	26	—	1
Premium Skinless Brown & Roasted Breast	1 oz	26	—	1
Roasted Thighs	1 oz	38	—	6
Roll Sliced Breast	1 oz	37	—	5
Roll White	1 oz	43	—	10
Salami	1 oz	45	—	8
Salt Watchers Breast	1 oz	35	—	tr
Sliced Bologna	1 oz	57	—	16
Sliced Ham	1 oz	37	—	5
Sliced Pastrami	1 oz	34	—	5
Sliced Salami	1 oz	46	—	9
Smoked Sliced Breast	1 oz	27	—	tr
Smoked Whole	1 oz	40	—	4
Turkey Deli Chef Breast & White	1 oz	35	—	5
Turkey No Skin Breast & White	1 oz	39	—	5
Weight Watchers				
Oven Roasted Breast	2 slices (¾ oz)	25	—	1

FOOD	PORTION	CALS.	SAT. FAT	FAT
Weight Watchers *(cont.)*				
Oven Roasted Turkey Ham	2 slices (¾ oz)	25	—	1
Roasted & Smoked Breast	2 slices (¾ oz)	25	—	1
Smoked Deli Thin Breast	5 slices (½ oz)	10	—	tr
bologna	1 oz	57	—	4
breast	1 slice (¾ oz)	23	tr	tr
diced light & dark, seasoned	1 oz	39	1	2
diced light & dark, seasoned	½ lb	313	4	14
ham thigh meat	2 oz	73	1	3
ham thigh meat	1 pkg (8 oz)	291	4	12
pastrami	2 oz	80	1	4
pastrami	1 pkg (8 oz)	320	4	14
patties, battered & fried	1 (2.3 oz)	181	—	12
patties, battered & fried	1 (3.3 oz)	266	—	17
poultry salad sandwich spread	1 tbsp	109	tr	2
poultry salad sandwich spread	1 oz	238	1	4
prebasted breast w/ skin, roasted	½ breast (1.9 lbs)	1087	8	30
prebasted breast w/ skin, roasted	1 breast (3.8 lbs)	2175	17	60
prebasted thigh w/ skin, roasted	1 thigh (11 oz)	494	8	27
roll, light & dark meat	1 oz	42	1	2
roll, light meat	1 oz	42	1	2
salami, cooked	2 oz	111	—	8
salami, cooked	1 pkg (8 oz)	446	—	31
turkey loaf breast meat	2 slices (1.5 oz)	47	tr	1
turkey loaf breast meat	1 pkg (6 oz)	187	1	3
turkey sticks, battered & fried	1 stick (2.3 oz)	178	—	11
turkey sticks, breaded & fried	1 stick (2.3 oz)	178	—	11

TURKEY DISHES
(*see also* DINNER, TURKEY SUBSTITUTES)

CANNED

American Classics Chicken With Mashed Potatoes (Dinty Moore)	1 bowl (10 oz)	250	3	7

FOOD	PORTION	CALS.	SAT. FAT	FAT
American Classics Turkey & Dressing With Gravy (Dinty Moore)	1 bowl (10 oz)	280	2	7
FROZEN				
Kibun Turkey Pasta Salad w/ Dressing	½ pkg	250	—	12
Kibun Turkey Pasta Salad w/o Dressing	½ pkg	140	—	2
Ovenstuffs Turkey Turnover	1 (4.75 oz)	350	—	16
gravy & turkey	1 pkg (5 oz)	95	1	4
gravy & turkey	1 cup (8.4 oz)	160	2	6
READY-TO-USE				
Turkey Salad (The Spreadables)	¼ can	100	—	6
Turkey Salad (Wampler Longacre)	1 oz	71	—	17

TURKEY SUBSTITUTES

Harvest Direct TVP Poultry Chunks	3.5 oz	280	tr	1
Harvest Direct TVP Poultry Ground	3.5 oz	280	tr	1
White Wave Meatless Sandwich Slices	2 slices (1.6 oz)	80	0	0
Worthington Smoked Turkey Slices	4 slices (76 g)	180	—	12
Worthington Turkee Slices	2 slices (63 g)	130	—	9

TURMERIC

ground	1 tsp	8	—	tr

TURNIPS

CANNED				
Chopped Greens And Diced Turnip (Allen)	½ cup (4.2 oz)	30	0	1
Chopped Greens And Diced Turnip (Sunshine)	½ cup (4.2 oz)	30	0	1
Greens (Allen)	½ cup (4.2 oz)	25	0	1
Greens (Sunshine)	½ cup (4.2 oz)	25	0	1
Turnip Greens w/ Diced Turnips Seasoned w/ Pork (Luck's)	7.5 oz	90	—	6
greens	½ cup	17	tr	tr
FRESH				
cooked, mashed	½ cup (4.2 oz)	47	tr	tr
cubed, cooked	½ cup (3 oz)	33	tr	tr

FOOD	PORTION	CALS.	SAT. FAT	FAT
greens, chopped, cooked	½ cup	15	tr	tr
greens, raw, chopped	½ cup	7	tr	tr
raw, cubed	½ cup (2.4 oz)	25	tr	tr
FROZEN				
Mashed (Southland)	3.6 oz	90	—	6
Rutabaga Yellow Turnips (Southland)	4 oz	50	—	0
greens, cooked	½ cup	24	tr	tr

TURTLE

FOOD	PORTION	CALS.	SAT. FAT	FAT
raw	3.5 oz	85	—	tr

TUSK FISH

FOOD	PORTION	CALS.	SAT. FAT	FAT
raw	3.5 oz	79	—	tr

VANILLA

FOOD	PORTION	CALS.	SAT. FAT	FAT
Vanilla Milk Chips (Hershey)	¼ cup	240	—	14
Virginia Dare Vanilla Extract	1 tsp	10	—	0

VEAL
(see also BEEF, VEAL DISHES)

FOOD	PORTION	CALS.	SAT. FAT	FAT
FRESH				
cutlet, lean only, braised	3 oz	172	2	4
cutlet, lean only, fried	3 oz	156	1	4
ground, broiled	3 oz	146	3	6
loin chop w/ bone, lean & fat, braised	1 (2.8 oz)	227	5	14
loin chop w/ bone, lean only, braised	1 (2.4 oz)	155	2	6
shoulder w/ bone, lean only, braised	3 oz	169	1	5
sirloin w/ bone, lean & fat, roasted	3 oz	171	4	9
sirloin w/ bone, lean only, roasted	3 oz	143	2	5

VEAL DISHES
TAKE-OUT

FOOD	PORTION	CALS.	SAT. FAT	FAT
parmigiana	4.2 oz	279	10	18

VEGETABLE JUICE

FOOD	PORTION	CALS.	SAT. FAT	FAT
Mott's Vegetable Juice, as prep	8 fl oz	60	0	0
Odwalla Vegetable Cocktail	8 fl oz	70	0	0

FOOD	PORTION	CALS.	SAT. FAT	FAT
Smucker's Vegetable Juice Hearty	8 fl oz	58	—	tr
Smucker's Vegetable Juice Hot & Spicy	8 fl oz	58	—	tr
V8	6 fl oz	35	—	0
V8 No Salt Added V8	6 fl oz	35	—	0
V8 Spicy Hot V8	6 fl oz	35	—	0
vegetable juice cocktail	½ cup	22	tr	tr
vegetable juice cocktail	6 fl oz	34	tr	tr

VEGETABLES, MIXED

(*see also* INDIVIDUAL VEGETABLES, VEGETABLE JUICES)

CANNED

FOOD	PORTION	CALS.	SAT. FAT	FAT
Chop Suey Vegetables (La Choy)	½ cup	10	tr	tr
Diced Tomatoes & Green Chilies (Chi-Chi's)	¼ cup (2.5 oz)	20	0	0
Garden Medley (Green Giant)	½ cup	40	0	tr
Garden Salad Marinated (S&W)	½ cup	60	0	0
Green Beans and Potatoes (Allen)	½ cup (4.2 oz)	35	0	0
Green Beans And Potatoes (Sunshine)	½ cup (4.2 oz)	35	0	0
Mixed (Hanover)	½ cup	110	—	0
Mixed Vegetables Old Fashion Harvest Time (S&W)	½ cup	35	0	0
Okra & Tomatoes (Allen)	½ cup (4 oz)	25	0	0
Okra & Tomatoes (Trappey)	½ cup (4 oz)	25	0	0
Okra, Tomatoes & Corn (Allen)	½ cup (4.1 oz)	30	0	0
Okra, Tomatoes & Corn (Trappey)	½ cup (4.1 oz)	30	0	0
Peas & Carrots (Seneca)	½ cup	60	0	0
Peas & Carrots Water Pack (S&W)	½ cup	35	0	0
Succotash Country Style (S&W)	½ cup	80	—	1
Succotash (Seneca)	½ cup	90	0	0
Sweet Peas & Diced Carrots (S&W)	½ cup	50	0	0

FOOD	PORTION	CALS.	SAT. FAT	FAT
Sweet Peas w/ Tiny Pearl Onions (S&W)	½ cup	60	—	1
Vegetable Salad (Hanover)	½ cup	90	—	0
Vegetables & Sauce (House of Tsang)				
Cantonese Classic	½ cup (4.2 oz)	70	0	1
Hong Kong Sweet & Sour	½ cup (4.5 oz)	160	0	0
Szechuan Hot & Spicy	½ cup (4.2 oz)	70	0	1
Tokyo Teriyaki	½ cup (4.4 oz)	100	0	0
mixed vegetables	½ cup	39	tr	tr
peas & carrots	½ cup	48	tr	tr
peas & carrots, low sodium	½ cup	48	tr	tr
peas & onions	½ cup	30	tr	tr
succotash	½ cup	102	tr	1
FROZEN				
American Mixtures (Green Giant)				
Califoria	½ cup	25	0	0
Heartland	½ cup	25	0	0
New England	½ cup	70	—	1
San Francisco	½ cup	25	0	0
Santa Fe	½ cup	70	—	1
Seattle	½ cup	25	0	0
Broccoli & Cauliflower, Cut (Hanover)	½ cup	20	—	0
Broccoli, Cauliflower & Carrots in Butter Sauce (Green Giant)	½ cup	30	tr	1
Broccoli, Cauliflower & Carrots in Cheese Sauce (Green Giant)	½ cup	60	tr	2
Broccoli, Cauliflower & Carrots w/ Cheese Sauce (Birds Eye)	½ pkg	80	2	4
California Blend (Big Valley)	¾ cup (3 oz)	25	0	0
California Blend (Fresh Like)	3.5 oz	31	—	tr
Caribbean Blend (Hanover)	½ cup	20	—	0
Chuckwagon Blend (Fresh Like)	3.5 oz	71	—	1
Country Wisconsin Blend (Veg-All)	3.5 oz	52	—	tr

FOOD	PORTION	CALS.	SAT. FAT	FAT
Farm Fresh (Birds Eye)				
Broccoli Cauliflower And Carrots	¾ cup	35	0	0
Broccoli and Cauliflower	¾ cup	30	0	0
Broccoli, Carrots And Water Chestnuts	¾ cup	40	0	0
Broccoli, Cauliflower And Red Peppers	¾ cup	30	0	0
Broccoli, Corn And Red Peppers	⅔ cup	60	tr	1
Broccoli, Green Beans, Pearl Onions and Red Peppers	¾ cup	35	0	0
Broccoli, Red Peppers, Onions And Mushrooms	¾ cup	30	0	0
Brussels Sprouts Cauliflower and Carrots	¾ cup	40	0	0
Cauliflower, Carrots And Snow Peas	⅔ cup	35	0	0
Garden Medley (Hanover)	½ cup	20	—	0
Harvest Fresh Mixed Vegetables (Green Giant)	½ cup	40	0	0
In Butter Sauce Broccoli, Cauliflower And Carrots (Birds Eye)	½ cup	40	1	2
In Sauce Peas And Pearl Onions With Seasonings (Birds Eye)	½ cup	70	0	0
Internationals (Birds Eye)				
Austrian	3.3 oz	70	2	3
Bavarian	3.3 oz	90	2	5
California	3.3 oz	90	3	4
French Country	3.3 oz	70	3	4
Japanese	3.3 oz	60	2	3
New England	3.3 oz	100	3	5
Italian	3.3 oz	80	3	5
Italian Blend (Fresh Like)	3.5 oz	33	—	tr
Italian Blend (Big Valley)	¾ cup (3 oz)	30	0	0
Mandarin Vegetables (Budget Gourmet)	1 pkg (5.25 oz)	160	—	11
Midwestern Blend (Fresh Like)	3.5 oz	42	—	tr
Mixed Fancy (La Choy)	½ cup	12	tr	tr

FOOD	PORTION	CALS.	SAT. FAT	FAT
Mixed Vegetables (Birds Eye)	½ cup	60	0	0
Mixed Vegetables (Green Giant)	½ cup	40	0	0
Mixed Vegetables (Hanover)	½ cup	50	—	0
Mixed Vegetables in Butter Sauce (Green Giant)	½ cup	60	tr	2
New England Recipe Vegetables (Budget Gourmet)	1 pkg. (5.5 oz)	230	—	13
One Serve Broccoli, Carrots & Rotini in Cheese Sauce (Green Giant)	1 pkg	120	tr	3
One Serve Broccoli, Cauliflower & Carrots (Green Giant)	1 pkg	25	0	0
Oriental Blend (Big Valley)	¾ cup (3 oz)	25	0	0
Oriental Blend (Fresh Like)	3.5 oz	26	—	tr
Oriental Blend (Hanover)	½ cup	25	0	0
Peas & Carrots (Fresh Like)	3.5 oz	63	—	tr
Peas & Potatoes w/ Cream Sauce (Birds Eye)	½ cup	100	1	3
Peppers & Onions (Southland)	2 oz	15	—	0
Polybag (Birds Eye)	½ cup	60	0	0
Scandinavian Blend (Veg-All)	3.5 oz	48	—	tr
Soup Mix Vegetables (Southland)	3.2 oz	50	—	0
Spring Vegetables in Cheese Sauce (Budget Gourmet)	1 pkg (5 g)	120	—	8
Stew Vegetables (Big Valley)	⅔ cup (3 oz)	40	0	0
Stew Vegetables (Ore Ida)	3 oz	50	0	tr
Stew Vegetables (Southland)	4 oz	60	0	0
Succotash (Hanover)	½ cup	80	0	0
Summer Vegetables (Hanover)	½ cup	35	—	0

FOOD	PORTION	CALS.	SAT. FAT	FAT
Valley Combinations Broccoli & Cauliflower (Green Giant)	½ cup	60	—	2
Vegetables for Soup (Hanover)	½ cup	60	—	0
Vegetables For Soup (Eight) (Veg-All)	3.5 oz	34	—	tr
Vegetables For Soup (Potatoes) (Veg-All)	3.5 oz	53	—	tr
Vegetables For Stew 4-Way (Veg-All)	3.5 oz	51	—	tr
Vegetables For Stew 5-Way (Veg-All)	3.5 oz	54	—	tr
Winter Blend (Big Valley)	¾ cup (3 oz)	25	0	0
Winter Blend (Fresh Like)	3.5 oz	26	—	tr
mixed vegetables, cooked	½ cup	54	tr	tr
peas & carrots, cooked	½ cup	38	tr	tr
peas & onions, cooked	½ cup	40	tr	tr
succotash, cooked	½ cup	79	tr	1
HOME RECIPE				
succotash	½ cup	111	tr	1
SHELF STABLE				
Corn, Green Beans, Carrots & Pasta in Tomato Sauce (Pantry Express)	½ cup	80	0	2
Green Beans, Potatoes & Mushrooms in a Seasoned Sauce (Pantry Express)	½ cup	50	tr	2
Mixed Vegetables (Pantry Express)	½ cup	35	0	tr
TAKE-OUT				
caponata	¼ cup	28	—	1
curry	7.7 oz	398	—	33
pakoras	1 (2 oz)	108	—	5
ratatouille	8.8 oz	190	—	16
samosa	2 (4 oz)	519	—	46

VENISON

FOOD	PORTION	CALS.	SAT. FAT	FAT
Antelope Chili Meat (Broken Arrow Ranch)	3.5 oz	115	1	2

FOOD	PORTION	CALS.	SAT. FAT	FAT
Antelope Ground Venison (Broken Arrow Ranch)	3.5 oz	110	1	2
Antelope Stew Meat (Broken Arrow Ranch)	3.5 oz	110	1	2
Nilgai Chili Meat (Broken Arrow Ranch)	3.5 oz	115	1	2
Nilgai Leg (Broken Arrow Ranch)	3.5 oz	100	tr	1
Nilgai Stew Meat (Broken Arrow Ranch)	3.5 oz	110	1	2
Venison & Beef Smoked Sausage (Broken Arrow Ranch)	6 oz	432	—	30
Venison Meat Chunks (Broken Arrow Ranch)	6 oz	175	—	2
Venison Salami (Broken Arrow Ranch)	6 oz	252	—	8
roasted	3 oz	134	1	3

VINEGAR

FOOD	PORTION	CALS.	SAT. FAT	FAT
Apple Cider (White House)	2 tbsp	2	0	0
Cider (Hain)	1 tbsp	2	0	0
Red Wine (Regina)	1 oz	4	0	0
Red Wine (White House)	2 tbsp	4	0	0
Rice (Nakano)	1 tbsp	tr	0	0
cider	1 tbsp	tr	0	0

WAFFLES

FROZEN

FOOD	PORTION	CALS.	SAT. FAT	FAT
Apple Cinnamon (Aunt Jemima)	2.5 oz	176	1	6
Apple Cinnamon (Eggo)	1	130	1	5
Belgian (Weight Watchers)	1 (1.5 oz)	120	2	4
Belgian Chef	1	90	—	2
Belgian Waffles & Sausage (Great Starts)	2.85 oz	280	—	19
Belgian Waffles w/ Strawberries & Sausage (Great Starts)	3.5 oz	210	—	8
Blueberry (Aunt Jemima)	2.5 oz	175	1	5
Blueberry (Downyflake)	2	180	—	4
Blueberry (Eggo)	1	130	1	5
Blueberry Batter, as prep (Aunt Jemima)	3.6 oz	204	1	4
Buttermilk (Aunt Jemima)	2.5 oz	179	1	6

FOOD	PORTION	CALS.	SAT. FAT	FAT
Buttermilk (Downyflake)	1	130	1	5
Buttermilk (Eggo)	1	130	1	5
Homestyle (Eggo)	1	130	1	5
Hot-N-Buttery (Downyflake)	2	180	—	6
Minis (Eggo)	4	90	1	3
Multi-Bran (Nutri-Grain)	1	120	1	5
Multi-Grain Belgian (Weight Watchers)	1 (1.5 oz)	120	1	4
Multi-Grain (Downyflake)	2	250	—	14
Nut & Honey (Eggo)	1	130	1	5
Oat Bran (Common Sense)	1	110	1	4
Oat Bran (Downyflake)	2	260	—	13
Oat Bran w/ Fruit & Nut (Common Sense)	1	120	1	5
Original (Aunt Jemima)	2.5 oz	173	1	6
Plain (Nutri-Grain)	1	120	1	5
Raisin & Bran (Nutri-Grain)	1	120	1	5
Regular (Downyflake)	2	120	—	3
Regular Jumbo (Downyflake)	2	170	—	4
Rice Bran (Downyflake)	2	210	—	11
Roman Meal (Downyflake)	2	280	—	14
Special K (Kellogg's)	1	80	0	0
Strawberry (Eggo)	1	130	1	5
Waffle (Kid Cuisine)	3.6 oz	160	—	3
Waffle w/ Bacon (Great Starts)	2.2 oz	230	—	14
Wholegrain Wheat/Oat Bran (Aunt Jemima)	2.5 oz	154	tr	3
buttermilk	1–4 in sq (1.2 oz)	88	tr	3
plain	1–4 in sq (1.2 oz)	88	tr	3
HOME RECIPE				
plain	1 (7 in diam)	218	2	11
MIX				
plain as prep	1–7 in diam (2.6 oz)	218	2	10

WALNUTS

FOOD	PORTION	CALS.	SAT. FAT	FAT
Black (Planters)	1 oz	180	1	17
English Halves (Planters)	1 oz	190	2	20
black, dried	1 oz	172	1	16
black, dried, chopped	1 cup	759	5	71
english, dried	1 oz	182	2	18

FOOD	PORTION	CALS.	SAT. FAT	FAT
english, dried, chopped	1 cup	770	7	74

WATER
(see MINERAL/BOTTLED WATER)

WATER CHESTNUTS
CANNED

Empress Sliced	2 oz	14	0	0
Empress Whole	2 oz	14	0	0
La Choy Sliced	¼ cup	18	tr	tr
La Choy Whole	4	14	tr	tr
chinese sliced	½ cup	35	tr	tr

FRESH

sliced	½ cup	66	tr	tr

WATERCRESS
(see also CRESS)

raw, chopped	½ cup	2	tr	tr

WATERMELON
FRESH

cut up	1 cup	50	—	1
wedge	1⁄16	152	—	2

SEEDS

dried	1 oz	158	3	13
dried	1 cup	602	3	51

WAX BEANS
CANNED

Cut (Owatonna)	½ cup	20	—	0
Cuts Natural Pack (Seneca)	½ cup	25	0	0
Golden Cut Premium (S&W)	½ cup	20	0	0
Wax Beans (Seneca)	½ cup	20	0	0

WHALE

raw	3.5 oz	134	—	3

WHEAT
(see also BULGUR, BRAN, CEREAL, COUSCOUS, FLOUR, WHEAT GERM)

Kamut Grain (Arrowhead)	¼ cup (1.7 oz)	140	0	1
Seitan (White Wave)	½ pkg (4 oz)	140	0	0
Seitan Fajita Strips (White Wave)	⅓ cup (1.8 oz)	60	0	0

FOOD	PORTION	CALS.	SAT. FAT	FAT
Seitan Marinated Slices (White Wave)	3 slices (1.8 oz)	60	0	0
Seitan Quick Mix (Arrowhead)	⅓ cup (1.4 oz)	150	0	1
Vital Wheat Gluten Plus Ascorbic Acid (Hodgson Mill)	1 tbsp (0.3 oz)	30	0	0
sprouted	⅓ cup	71	tr	tr
starch	3.5 oz	348	—	tr

WHEAT GERM

Arrowhead	3 tbsp (0.5 oz)	50	0	1
Hodgson Mill	2 tbsp (0.5 oz)	55	0	1
Kretschmer	¼ cup	103	1	3
Kretschmer Honey Crunch	¼ cup	105	tr	3
plain, toasted	¼ cup	108	tr	3
plain, toasted	1 cup	431	2	12
plain, untoasted	¼ cup	104	tr	3
w/ brown sugar & honey, toasted	1 oz	107	tr	2
w/ brown sugar & honey, toasted	1 cup	426	2	9

WHIPPED TOPPINGS
(see also CREAM)

Cool Whip Extra Creamy	1 tbsp	13	—	1
Cool Whip Non Dairy	1 tbsp	11	—	1
Diamond Crystal	1 tbsp	7	—	tr
Dream Whip	1 tbsp	9	—	tr
D-Zerta, as prep	1 tbsp	7	—	tr
Estee Whipped Topping	1 tbsp	4	—	tr
Kraft Real Cream Topping	¼ cup	30	2	2
Kraft Whipped Topping	¼ cup	35	3	3
La Creme	1 tbsp	16	—	1
Pet Whip	1 tbsp	14	—	1
cream, pressurized	1 tbsp	8	tr	tr
cream, pressurized	1 cup	154	8	13
nondairy, powdered, as prep w/ whole milk	1 tbsp	8	tr	tr
nondairy, powdered, as prep w/ whole milk	1 cup	151	9	10
nondairy, pressurized	1 tbsp	11	1	1
nondairy, pressurized	1 cup	184	13	16
nondairy, frzn	1 tbsp	13	1	1

FOOD	PORTION	CALS.	SAT. FAT	FAT

WHITE BEANS

CANNED

FOOD	PORTION	CALS.	SAT. FAT	FAT
Goya Spanish Style	7.5 oz	130	—	1
Progresso Cannellini	½ cup	80	—	tr
white beans	1 cup	306	tr	1

DRIED

FOOD	PORTION	CALS.	SAT. FAT	FAT
regular, cooked	1 cup	249	tr	1
small, cooked	1 cup	253	tr	1

WHITEFISH

FOOD	PORTION	CALS.	SAT. FAT	FAT
fresh, baked	3 oz	146	1	6
smoked whitefish	1 oz	39	tr	tr
smoked whitefish	3 oz	92	tr	1

WHITING

FOOD	PORTION	CALS.	SAT. FAT	FAT
fresh, cooked	3 oz	98	tr	1
raw	3 oz	77	tr	1

WILD RICE

(*see also* RICE)

FOOD	PORTION	CALS.	SAT. FAT	FAT
cooked	½ cup	83	tr	tr

WINE

(*see also* CHAMPAGNE, WINE COOLERS)

FOOD	PORTION	CALS.	SAT. FAT	FAT
Boone's				
Country Kwencher	1 fl oz	24	0	0
Delicious Apple	1 fl oz	21	0	0
Sangria	1 fl oz	22	0	0
Snow Creek Berry	1 fl oz	18	0	0
Strawberry Hill	1 fl oz	22	0	0
Sun Peak Peach	1 fl oz	18	0	0
Wild Island	1 fl oz	18	0	0
Carlo Rossi				
Blush	1 fl oz	21	0	0
Burgundy	1 fl oz	22	0	0
Chablis	1 fl oz	21	0	0
Paisano	1 fl oz	23	0	0
Red Sangria	1 fl oz	24	0	0
Rhine	1 fl oz	21	0	0
Vin Rosé	1 fl oz	21	0	0
White Grenache	1 fl oz	20	0	0
Fairbanks				
Cream Sherry	1 fl oz	42	0	0
Port	1 fl oz	44	0	0
Sherry	1 fl oz	34	0	0

FOOD	PORTION	CALS.	SAT. FAT	FAT
White Port	1 fl oz	44	0	0
Gallo				
Blush Chablis	1 fl oz	22	0	0
Burgundy	1 fl oz	22	0	0
Cabernet Sauvignon	1 fl oz	22	0	0
Chablis Blanc	1 fl oz	20	0	0
Chardonnay	1 fl oz	23	0	0
Classic Burgundy	1 fl oz	21	0	0
French Colombard	1 fl oz	21	0	0
Hearty Burgundy	1 fl oz	22	0	0
Johannisberg Riesling '88	1 fl oz	20	0	0
Pink Chablis	1 fl oz	20	0	0
Red Rosé	1 fl oz	23	0	0
Rhine	1 fl oz	22	0	0
Sauvignon Blanc '90	1 fl oz	20	0	0
White Grenache '92	1 fl oz	20	0	0
White Grenache New Vintage	1 fl oz	20	0	0
White Zinfandel '91	1 fl oz	18	0	0
White Zinfandel New Vintage	1 fl oz	18	0	0
Zinfandel '87	1 fl oz	23	0	0
Sheffield Cellars				
Sherry	1 fl oz	44	0	0
Tawny Port	1 fl oz	45	0	0
Vermouth Extra Dry	1 fl oz	28	0	0
Vermouth Sweet	1 fl oz	43	0	0
Very Dry Sherry	1 fl oz	32	0	0
red	3.5 oz	74	0	0
rose	3.5 oz	73	0	0
sherry	2 oz	84	0	0
sweet dessert	2 oz	90	0	0
vermouth, dry	3.5 oz	105	0	0
vermouth, sweet	3.5 oz	167	0	0
white	3.5 oz	70	0	0

WINE COOLERS

Bartles & Jaymes				
Berry	12 fl oz	210	0	0
Margarita	12 fl oz	260	0	0
Original	12 fl oz	190	0	0
Peach	12 fl oz	210	0	0
Pina Colada	12 fl oz	280	0	0

FOOD	PORTION	CALS.	SAT. FAT	FAT
Bartles & Jaymes *(cont.)*				
Planter's Punch	12 fl oz	230	0	0
Strawberry	12 fl oz	210	0	0
Strawberry Daquiri	12 fl oz	230	0	0
Tropical	12 fl oz	230	0	0
WINGED BEANS				
dried, cooked	1 cup	252	1	10
WOLFFISH				
fresh atlantic, baked	3 oz	105	tr	3
YAM				
(see also SWEET POTATO)				
CANNED				
Allen Cut	⅔ cup (5.8 oz)	160	—	1
Bruce				
Cut	½ cup	139	—	1
Mashed	½ cup	130	—	1
Vacuum Pack	½ cup	122	—	1
Whole	½ cup	139	—	1
Princella Cut	⅔ cup (5.8 oz)	160	0	1
Royal Prince Whole	4 pieces (5.9 oz)	200	0	1
S&W Candied	½ cup	180	0	0
S&W Southern Whole In Extra Heavy Syrup	½ cup	139	—	1
Sugary Sam Cut	⅔ cup (5.8 oz)	160	0	1
Trappey Whole	4 pieces (5.9 oz)	200	0	1
FRESH				
mountain yam, hawaiian, cooked	½ cup	59	tr	tr
yam, cubed, cooked	½ cup	79	tr	tr
YAM BEAN				
cooked	¾ cup	38	—	tr
YARDLONG BEANS				
dried, cooked	1 cup	202	tr	1
YEAST				
Fleischmann's				
Active Dry	1 pkg (¼ oz)	20	0	0
Fresh Active	1 pkg (0.6 oz)	15	0	0
Household Yeast	½ oz	15	0	0
RapidRise	1 pkg (¼ oz)	20	0	0
Red Star	4 tbsp (0.5 oz)	47	0	tr

FOOD	PORTION	CALS.	SAT. FAT	FAT
Red Star Small Flakes	3 tbsp (0.5 oz)	47	0	tr
Red Star Yeast Flakes	3 tbsp (0.5 oz)	47	0	tr
baker's compressed	1 cake (0.6 oz)	18	tr	tr
baker's dry	1 pkg (¼ oz)	21	tr	tr
baker's, dry	1 tbsp	35	1	tr
brewer's, dry	1 tbsp	25	tr	tr

YELLOW BEANS
CANNED

B&M Baked Beans	8 oz	326	—	7

DRIED

Bean Cuisine Yellow Eye	½ cup	115	—	1
dried, cooked	1 cup	254	tr	2

YELLOW-EYE BEANS
CANNED

B&M Yellow Eye Baked Beans	⅞ cup	290	—	7

YELLOWTAIL

fresh, baked	3 oz	159	—	6

YOGURT
(*see also* YOGURT FROZEN)

All Flavors (Cabot)	8 oz	220	2	3
All Flavors Ultimate 90 (Weight Watchers)	1 cup	90	—	0
Amaretto Almond Yo Creme (Yoplait)	5 oz	240	—	10
Apple (La Yogurt)	6 oz	190	—	4
Apple Crisp Lowfat (New Country)	6 oz	150	—	2
Apple Original (Yoplait)	6 oz	190	—	3
Apples 'N Spice Fat Free (Colombo)	8 oz	190	0	0
Apricot Fat Free (Colombo)	8 oz	190	0	0
Banana Custard Style	6 oz	190	—	4
Banana Fruit on Bottom (Dannon)	8 oz	240	—	3
Banana Strawberry Fat Free (Colombo)	8 oz	200	0	0
Banana Strawberry Low Fat (Colombo)	8 oz	210	2	4
Bavarian Chocolate Yo Creme	5 oz	270	—	11

FOOD	PORTION	CALS.	SAT. FAT	FAT
Black Cherry 100 Calorie w/ Aspartame (Light N'Lively)	8 oz	100	0	0
Black Cherry Lowfat (Breyers)	8 oz	260	1	3
Black Cherry Lowfat (Colombo)	8 oz	200	2	4
Black Cherry Lowfat (Light N'Lively)	8 oz	230	1	2
Black Cherry w/ Aspartame (Knudsen Cal 70)	8 oz	70	0	0
Blueberry (Dannon)	8 oz	200	—	4
Blueberry (La Yogurt)	6 oz	190	—	4
Blueberry (La Yogurt 25)	8 oz	200	—	0
Blueberry (Mountain High)	1 cup	220	—	6
Blueberry 100 Calorie w/ Aspartame (Light N'Lively)	8 oz	90	0	0
Blueberry Custard Style (Yoplait)	6 oz	190	—	4
Blueberry Fat Free (Colombo)	8 oz	190	0	0
Blueberry Fat Free (Yoplait)	6 oz	150	—	0
Blueberry Fruit Crunch (Friendship)	6 oz	190	2	4
Blueberry Fruit on Bottom (Dannon)	4.4 oz	130	—	2
Blueberry Fruit on Bottom (Dannon)	8 oz	240	—	3
Blueberry Light (Yoplait)	4 oz	60	—	0
Blueberry Light (Yoplait)	6 oz	80	—	0
Blueberry Light 100 (Colombo)	8 oz	100	0	0
Blueberry Lowfat (Breyers)	8 oz	250	1	2
Blueberry Lowfat (Colombo)	8 oz	200	2	4
Blueberry Lowfat (Light N'Lively)	4.4 oz	130	1	1
Blueberry Lowfat (Light N'Lively)	8 oz	240	1	2
Blueberry Nonfat (Dannon)	6 oz	140	—	0
Blueberry Nonfat Light (Dannon)	4.4 oz	60	—	0

FOOD	PORTION	CALS.	SAT. FAT	FAT
Blueberry Nonfat Light (Dannon)	8 oz	100	—	0
Blueberry Nonfat Lite (Colombo)	8 oz	190	—	tr
Blueberry Original (Yoplait)	4 oz	120	—	2
Blueberry Original (Yoplait)	6 oz	190	—	3
Blueberry Supreme Lowfat (New Country)	6 oz	150	—	2
Blueberry w/ Aspartame (Knudsen Cal 70)	8 oz	70	0	0
Blueberry w/ Aspartame (Light N'Lively Free)	8 oz	50	0	0
Boysenberry Fruit on Bottom (Dannon)	8 oz	240	—	3
Boysenberry Lowfat (Knudsen)	8 oz	240	1	4
Boysenberry Original (Yoplait)	4 oz	120	—	2
Cappuccino Fat Free (Colombo)	8 oz	180	0	0
Cherries Jubilee (Yoplait)	5 oz	220	—	8
Cherry (La Yogurt)	6 oz	190	—	4
Cherry (La Yogurt 25)	8 oz	200	—	0
Cherry Custard Style (Yoplait)	6 oz	180	—	4
Cherry Fat Free (Colombo)	8 oz	190	0	0
Cherry Fruit on Bottom (Dannon)	4.4 oz	130	—	2
Cherry Fruit on Bottom (Dannon)	8 oz	240	—	3
Cherry Light (Yoplait)	4 oz	60	—	0
Cherry Light (Yoplait)	6 oz	80	—	0
Cherry Lowfat (Knudsen)	8 oz	240	2	4
Cherry Lowfat (Light N'Lively)	4.4 oz	140	1	1
Cherry Original (Yoplait)	6 oz	190	—	3
Cherry Supreme Lowfat (New Country)	6 oz	150	—	2
Cherry Vanilla (La Yogurt)	6 oz	190	—	4
Cherry Vanilla Lowfat Swiss Style (Lite Line)	1 cup	240	—	2
Cherry Vanilla Nonfat Light (Dannon)	8 oz	100	0	0
Cherry Vanilla Light 100 (Colombo)	8 oz	100	0	0

FOOD	PORTION	CALS.	SAT. FAT	FAT
Coffee (Friendship)	8 oz	210	2	3
Coffee Lowfat (Dannon)	8 oz	200	—	3
Creamy Vanilla Light 100 (Colombo)	8 oz	100	0	0
Dutch Apple Fruit on Bottom (Dannon)	8 oz	240	—	3
Exotic Fruit Fruit on Bottom (Dannon)	8 oz	240	—	3
French Roast Fat Free (Colombo)	8 oz	180	0	0
French Vanilla Lowfat (New Country)	6 oz	150	—	2
Fruit Cocktail Fat Free (Colombo)	8 oz	190	0	0
Fruit Crunch Lowfat (New Country)	6 oz	150	—	2
Fruit Medley Light 100 (Colombo)	8 oz	100	0	0
Grape Lowfat (Light N'Lively)	4.4 oz	130	1	1
Hawaiian Salad Lowfat (New Country)	6 oz	150	—	2
Juicy Peach Light 100 (Colombo)	8 oz	100	0	0
Key Lime (La Yogurt)	6 oz	190	—	4
Lemon 100 Calorie w/ Aspartame (Light N'Lively)	8 oz	100	0	0
Lemon Creme Light 100 (Colombo)	8 oz	100	0	0
Lemon Custard Style (Yoplait)	6 oz	190	—	4
Lemon Fat Free (Colombo)	8 oz	170	0	0
Lemon Lowfat (Dannon)	8 oz	200	—	3
Lemon Lowfat (Knudsen)	8 oz	240	2	4
Lemon Original (Yoplait)	6 oz	190	—	3
Lemon Supreme Lowfat (New Country)	6 oz	150	—	2
Lemon w/ Aspartame (Knudsen Cal 70)	8 oz	70	0	0
Lime Lowfat (Knudsen)	8 oz	240	2	4
Mandarin Orange Light 100 (Colombo)	8 oz	100	0	0
Mixed Berries Fruit on Bottom (Dannon)	4.4 oz	130	—	2

FOOD	PORTION	CALS.	SAT. FAT	FAT
Mixed Berries Fruit on Bottom (Dannon)	8 oz	240	—	3
Mixed Berries Light 100 (Colombo)	8 oz	100	0	0
Mixed Berries Lowfat (New Country)	6 oz	150	tr	2
Mixed Berries Lowfat (Dannon)	8 oz	240	—	3
Mixed Berry (La Yogurt)	6 oz	190	—	4
Mixed Berry Custard Style (Yoplait)	6 oz	180	—	4
Mixed Berry Fat Free (Yoplait)	6 oz	150	—	0
Mixed Berry Lowfat (Breyers)	8 oz	250	1	2
Mixed Berry Original (Yoplait)	4 oz	120	—	2
Orange Original (Yoplait)	6 oz	190	—	3
Orange Supreme Lowfat (New Country)	6 oz	150	—	2
Peach (La Yogurt)	6 oz	190	—	4
Peach Fat Free (Yoplait)	6 oz	150	—	0
Peach 100 Calorie w/ Aspartame (Light N'Lively)	8 oz	100	0	0
Peach Fruit on Bottom (Dannon)	8 oz	240	—	3
Peach Light (Yoplait)	4 oz	60	—	0
Peach Light (Yoplait)	6 oz	80	—	0
Peach Lowfat (Breyers)	8 oz	250	1	2
Peach Lowfat (Knudsen)	8 oz	240	2	4
Peach Lowfat (Light N'Lively)	4.4 oz	130	1	1
Peach Lowfat (Light N'Lively)	8 oz	240	1	2
Peach Lowfat Blended w/ Fruit (Dannon)	4 oz	110	—	2
Peach Melba Low Fat (Colombo)	8 oz	200	2	4
Peach Nonfat (Dannon)	6 oz	140	—	0
Peach Nonfat Light (Dannon)	8 oz	100	—	0
Peach Original (Yoplait)	4 oz	120	—	2
Peach Original (Yoplait)	6 oz	190	—	3

FOOD	PORTION	CALS.	SAT. FAT	FAT
Peach w/ Aspartame (Knudsen Cal 70)	8 oz	70	0	0
Peaches 'N Cream Lowfat (New Country)	6 oz	150	—	2
Pina Colada (La Yogurt)	6 oz	190	—	4
Pina Colada Fruit on Bottom (Dannon)	8 oz	240	—	3
Pina Colada Original (Yoplait)	4 oz	120	—	2
Pineapple Lowfat (Breyers)	8 oz	250	1	2
Pineapple Lowfat (Light N'Lively)	4.4 oz	130	1	1
Pineapple Lowfat (Light N'Lively)	8 oz	230	1	2
Pineapple Original (Yoplait)	6 oz	190	—	3
Pineapple w/ Aspartame (Knudsen Cal 70)	8 oz	70	0	0
Plain (Cabot)	8 oz	140	2	4
Plain (Friendship)	8 oz	150	2	3
Plain (Knudsen)	8 oz	200	5	9
Plain (La Yogurt)	6 oz	140	—	6
Plain (Mountain High)	1 cup	200	—	9
Plain Fat Free (Colombo)	8 oz	110	0	0
Plain Low Fat (Colombo)	8 oz	120	3	5
Plain Lowfat (Breyers)	8 oz	140	2	3
Plain Lowfat (Dannon)	8 oz	140	—	4
Plain Lowfat (Knudsen)	8 oz	160	1	5
Plain Lowfat (Meadow Gold)	1 cup	160	—	5
Plain Lowfat Swiss Style (Lite Line)	1 cup	140	—	2
Plain Nonfat (Dannon)	8 oz	110	—	0
Plain Nonfat (Weight Watchers)	1 cup	90	—	0
Plain Nonfat (Yoplait)	8 oz	120	—	0
Plain Original (Yoplait)	6 oz	130	—	3
Raspberries & Cream (Yoplait)	5 oz	230	—	9
Raspberry (La Yogurt 25)	8 oz	200	—	0
Raspberry Custard Style (Yoplait)	6 oz	190	—	4
Raspberry Fat Free (Colombo)	8 oz	190	0	0
Raspberry Fat Free (Yoplait)	6 oz	150	—	0

FOOD	PORTION	CALS.	SAT. FAT	FAT
Raspberry Fruit on Bottom (Dannon)	4.4 oz	120	—	1
Raspberry Fruit on Bottom (Dannon)	8 oz	240	—	3
Raspberry Light (Yoplait)	4 oz	60	—	0
Raspberry Light (Yoplait)	6 oz	80	—	0
Raspberry Lowfat (Knudsen)	8 oz	240	2	4
Raspberry Lowfat Blended w/ Fruit (Dannon)	4.4 oz	130	—	2
Raspberry Nonfat (Dannon)	6 oz	140	—	0
Raspberry Nonfat (Dannon)	8 oz	200	—	4
Raspberry Nonfat Light (Dannon)	8 oz	100	—	0
Raspberry Original (Yoplait)	4 oz	120	—	2
Raspberry Sundae Style (Meadow Gold)	1 cup	250	—	4
Raspberry Supreme Lowfat (New Country)	6 oz	150	—	2
Red Raspberry 100 Calorie w/ Aspartame (Light N'Lively)	8 oz	90	0	0
Red Raspberry Light 100 (Colombo)	8 oz	100	0	0
Red Raspberry Lowfat (Breyers)	8 oz	250	1	2
Red Raspberry Lowfat (Light N'Lively)	4.4 oz	130	1	1
Red Raspberry Lowfat (Light N'Lively)	8 oz	230	1	2
Red Raspberry w/ Aspartame (Knudsen Cal 70)	8 oz	70	0	0
Red Raspberry w/ Aspartame (Light N'Lively)	8 oz	50	0	0
Sprinkl'ns All Flavors (average) (Dannon)	1 pkg (4.1 oz)	145	1	2
Strawberries Romanoff (Yoplait)	5 oz	220	—	8
Strawberry (Colombo)	8 oz	200	2	4
Strawberry (La Yogurt)	6 oz	190	—	4

FOOD	PORTION	CALS.	SAT. FAT	FAT
Strawberry (La Yogurt 25)	8 oz	200	—	0
Strawberry Banana (La Yogurt)	6 oz	190	—	4
Strawberry Banana (La Yogurt 25)	8 oz	200	—	0
Strawberry Banana 100 Calorie w/ Aspartame (Light N'Lively)	8 oz	90	0	0
Strawberry Banana Custard Style (Yoplait)	4 oz	130	—	3
Strawberry Banana Custard Style (Yoplait)	6 oz	190	—	4
Strawberry Banana Fat Free (Yoplait)	6 oz	150	—	0
Strawberry Banana Fruit Crunch (Friendship)	6 oz	190	2	4
Strawberry Banana Fruit on Bottom (Dannon)	4.4 oz	130	—	2
Strawberry Banana Light (Yoplait)	4 oz	60	—	0
Strawberry Banana Light (Yoplait)	6 oz	80	—	0
Strawberry Banana Lowfat (Breyers)	8 oz	250	1	2
Strawberry Banana Lowfat (Dannon)	8 oz	200	—	4
Strawberry Banana Lowfat (Knudsen)	8 oz	250	2	4
Strawberry Banana Lowfat (Light N'Lively)	4.4 oz	140	1	1
Strawberry Banana Lowfat (Light N'Lively)	8 oz	260	1	2
Strawberry Banana Lowfat (New Country)	6 oz	150	—	2
Strawberry Banana Lowfat Blended w/ Fruit (Dannon)	4.4 oz	130	—	2
Strawberry Banana Nonfat Light (Dannon)	8 oz	100	—	0
Strawberry Banana Original (Yoplait)	6 oz	190	—	3
Strawberry Banana w/ Aspartame (Knudsen Cal 70)	8 oz	70	0	0

FOOD	PORTION	CALS.	SAT. FAT	FAT
Strawberry Banana w/ Aspartame (Light N'Lively Free)	8 oz	50	0	0
Strawberry Custard Style (Yoplait)	4 oz	130	—	3
Strawberry Custard Style (Yoplait)	6 oz	190	—	4
Strawberry Fat Free (Colombo)	8 oz	190	0	0
Strawberry Fruit Crunch (Friendship)	6 oz	190	2	5
Strawberry Fruit Basket w/ Aspartame (Knudsen Cal 70)	8 oz	70	0	0
Strawberry Fruit Cup (La Yogurt)	6 oz	190	—	4
Strawberry Fruit Cup Lowfat (Light N'Lively)	4.4 oz	130	1	1
Strawberry Fruit Cup Lowfat (Light N'Lively)	8 oz	240	1	2
Strawberry Fruit Cup Lowfat (New Country)	6 oz	150	—	2
Strawberry Fruit Cup Nonfat Light (Dannon)	8 oz	100	—	0
Strawberry Fruit Cup w/ Aspartame (Light N'Lively Free)	8 oz	50	0	0
Strawberry Fruit on Bottom (Dannon)	4.4 oz	130	—	2
Strawberry Fruit on Bottom (Dannon)	8 oz	240	—	3
Strawberry Light 100 (Colombo)	8 oz	100	0	0
Strawberry Lowfat (Breyers)	8 oz	250	1	2
Strawberry Lowfat (Dannon)	8 oz	200	—	4
Strawberry Lowfat (Knudsen)	8 oz	250	2	4
Strawberry Lowfat (Light N'Lively)	4.4 oz	130	1	1
Strawberry Lowfat (Light N'Lively)	8 oz	240	2	2
Strawberry Lowfat Blended w/ Fruit (Dannon)	4 oz	110	2	2

FOOD	PORTION	CALS.	SAT. FAT	FAT
Strawberry Lowfat Swiss Style (Lite Line)	1 cup	240	—	2
Strawberry Nonfat (Dannon)	6 oz	140	—	0
Strawberry Nonfat Light (Dannon)	4.4 oz	60	—	0
Strawberry Nonfat Light (Dannon)	8 oz	100	—	0
Strawberry Original (Yoplait)	4 oz	120	—	2
Strawberry Original (Yoplait)	6 oz	190	—	3
Strawberry Rhubarb Original (Yoplait)	4 oz	120	—	2
Strawberry Supreme Lowfat (New Country)	6 oz	150	—	2
Strawberry w/ Aspartame (Knudsen Cal 70)	8 oz	70	0	0
Strawberry w/ Aspartame (Light N'Lively Free)	8 oz	50	0	0
Tropical Orange (La Yogurt)	6 oz	190	—	4
Vanilla (La Yogurt)	6 oz	160	—	4
Vanilla Bean Lowfat (Breyers)	8 oz	230	2	3
Vanilla Custard Style (Yoplait)	4 oz	130	—	3
Vanilla Custard Style (Yoplait)	6 oz	180	—	4
Vanilla Fat Free (Colombo)	8 oz	170	0	0
Vanilla Lowfat (Dannon)	8 oz	200	—	3
Vanilla Lowfat (Knudsen)	8 oz	240	2	4
Vanilla Nonfat Light (Dannon)	8 oz	100	—	0
Vanilla Nonfat Lite (Yoplait)	8 oz	180	—	0
Vanilla w/ Aspartame (Knudsen Cal 70)	8 oz	70	0	0
coffee lowfat	8 oz	194	2	3
fruit lowfat	4 oz	113	1	1
fruit lowfat	8 oz	225	2	3
plain	8 oz	139	5	7
plain lowfat	8 oz	144	2	4
plain nonfat	8 oz	127	tr	tr
vanilla lowfat	8 oz	194	2	3

FOOD	PORTION	CALS.	SAT. FAT	FAT
YOGURT, FROZEN				
(*see also* TOFU YOGURT)				
All Flavors Gourmet Yogurt (Bresler's)	5 oz	145	—	2
All Flavors Just 10	1 oz	10	0	0
All Flavors Lite Yogurt (Bresler's)	5 oz	135	0	0
Apple Pie (Ben & Jerry's)	½ cup (4 fl oz)	140	2	3
Banana Strawberry (Ben & Jerry's)	½ cup (4 fl oz)	130	1	2
Banana Strawberry (Edy's)	3 oz	80	—	1
Better Than Yogurt (Tofutti)				
Chocolate Fudge	4 fl oz	120	1	2
Coffee Marshmallow Swirl	4 fl oz	100	0	1
Passion Island Fruit	4 fl oz	100	0	1
Peach Mango	4 fl oz	100	0	1
Strawberry Banana	4 fl oz	100	0	1
Vanilla Fudge	4 fl oz	120	0	2
Black Cherry (Breyers)	½ cup (2.7 oz)	140	3	3
Blueberry (Edy's)	3 oz	80	—	1
Blueberry (Elan)	4 oz	130	—	3
Blueberry Cheesecake (Ben & Jerry's)	½ cup (4 fl oz)	130	1	2
Blueberry Softy (Dannon)	4 oz	110	—	2
Butter Pecan Softy (Dannon)	4 oz	110	—	2
Cappuccino Softy (Dannon)	4 oz	110	—	2
Caramel Almond Praline (Elan)	4 oz	150	—	4
Cheesecake Softy (Dannon)	4 oz	110	—	2
Cherry (Edy's)	3 oz	80	—	1
Cherry Garcia (Ben & Jerry's)	½ cup (4 fl oz)	150	2	3
Chocolate (Ben & Jerry's)	½ cup (4 fl oz)	140	2	3
Chocolate (Ben & Jerry's)	1 pop (2.5 fl oz)	150	5	9
Chocolate (Breyers)	½ cup (2.7 oz)	150	3	4
Chocolate (Edy's)	3 oz	80	—	1
Chocolate (Elan)	4 oz	130	—	3
Chocolate (Haagen-Dazs)	3 oz	130	2	3
Chocolate (Sealtest Free)	½ cup (2.7 oz)	110	1	0

FOOD	PORTION	CALS.	SAT. FAT	FAT
Chocolate Almond (Elan)	4 oz	160	—	6
Chocolate Bee-Lite	4 oz	100	—	tr
Chocolate Chip (Edy's)	3 oz	100	—	1
Chocolate Fi-Bar	1	190	—	7
Chocolate Fudge Brownie (Ben & Jerry's)	½ cup (4 fl oz)	170	2	4
Chocolate Kissed w/ Honey	3.5 oz	100	—	3
Chocolate Kissed w/ Honey Nonfat	3.5 oz	85	—	tr
Chocolate Nonfat Softy (Dannon)	4 oz	110	—	0
Chocolate Softy (Dannon)	4 oz	140	—	2
Citrus Heights (Edy's)	3 oz	80	—	1
Coffee (Elan)	4 oz	130	—	3
Coffee Almond Fudge (Ben & Jerry's)	½ cup (4 fl oz)	180	2	7
Cookies 'N' Cream (Edy's)	3 oz	100	—	1
Decaffeinated Coffee (Elan)	4 oz	130	—	3
Dutch Chocolate Desserve	4 oz	80	0	0
Frista Cup (Good Humor)	1 (6.2 oz)	220	4	5
Golden Vanilla Nonfat Softy (Dannon)	4 oz	100	—	0
Heath Bar Crunch (Ben & Jerry's)	½ cup (4 fl oz)	170	4	6
Lemon Meringue Softy (Dannon)	4 oz	110	—	2
Marble Fudge (Edy's)	3 oz	100	—	1
Mocha Fudge (Sealtest)	½ cup (2.6 oz)	130	2	2
Peach (Breyer's)	½ cup (2.7 oz)	140	2	3
Peach (Elan)	4 oz	130	—	3
Peach (Haagen-Dazs)	3 oz	120	2	3
Peach Softy (Dannon)	4 oz	110	—	2
Peanut Butter Softy (Dannon)	4 oz	130	—	3
Perfectly Peach (Edy's)	3 oz	80	—	1
Pina Colada Softy (Dannon)	4 oz	110	—	2
Plain Softy (Dannon)	4 oz	90	—	1
Pure Indulgence All Flavors (average) (Dannon)	½ cup	160	2	6
Raspberry (Ben & Jerry's)	4 oz	133	1	2
Raspberry (Edy's)	3 oz	80	—	1
Raspberry & Vanilla Bar (Haagen-Dazs)	1 bar (2.5 oz)	90	0	1

FOOD	PORTION	CALS.	SAT. FAT	FAT
Raspberry Softy (Dannon)	4 oz	110	—	2
Raspberry Vanilla Swirl (Edy's)	3 oz	80	—	1
Red Raspberry (Breyer's)	½ cup (2.7 oz)	140	3	4
Red Raspberry Nonfat Softy (Dannon)	4 oz	100	—	0
Rum Raisin (Elan)	4 oz	135	—	3
Rum Raisin Nonfat Softy (Dannon)	4 oz	100	—	0
Strawberry (Borden)	½ cup	100	—	2
Strawberry (Breyers)	½ cup (2.7 oz)	130	2	3
Strawberry (Edy's)	3 oz	80	—	1
Strawberry (Elan)	4 oz	125	—	3
Strawberry (Haagen-Dazs)	3 oz	120	2	3
Strawberry (Meadow Gold)	½ cup	100	—	2
Strawberry Banana (Breyers)	½ cup (2.7 oz)	140	2	3
Strawberry Banana Softy (Dannon)	4 oz	110	—	2
Strawberry Cheesecake (Breyers)	½ cup (2.7 oz)	160	3	5
Strawberry Fi-Bar	1	190	—	7
Strawberry Nonfat (Dannon)	6 oz	140	—	0
Strawberry Nonfat Softy (Dannon)	4 oz	100	—	0
Strawberry Softy (Dannon)	4 oz	110	—	2
Toffee Bar Crunch (Breyers)	½ cup (2.7 oz)	160	3	5
Vanilla (Breyers)	½ cup (2.7 oz)	140	3	4
Vanilla (Edy's)	3 oz	80	—	1
Vanilla (Elan)	4 oz	130	—	3
Vanilla (Haagen-Dazs)	3 oz	130	2	3
Vanilla (Sealtest)	½ cup (2.6 oz)	120	1	2
Vanilla Almond Crunch (Haagen-Dazs)	3 oz	150	2	5
Vanilla Bee-Lite	4 oz	110	—	tr
Vanilla Desserve	4 oz	70	0	0
Vanilla Fi-Bar	1	190	—	7
Vanilla Kissed w/ Honey	3.5 oz	100	—	3
Vanilla Kissed w/ Honey Nonfat	3.5 oz	85	—	tr
Vanilla Raspberry Swirl (Breyers)	½ cup (2.7 oz)	140	3	4

FOOD	PORTION	CALS.	SAT. FAT	FAT
Vanilla Fudge Twirl (Breyers)	½ cup (2.7 oz)	150	3	4
Vanilla Softy (Dannon)	4 oz	110	—	2

ZABAGLIONE
(*see* CUSTARD)

ZUCCHINI
CANNED
Italian Style (Progresso)	½ cup	50	tr	2
Italian Style (S&W)	½ cup	45	—	1
italian style	½ cup	33	tr	tr

FRESH
baby, raw	1 (.5 oz)	3	tr	tr
raw, sliced	½ cup	9	tr	tr
sliced, cooked	½ cup	14	tr	tr

FROZEN
Big Valley	¾ cup (3 oz)	10	0	0
Breaded (Empire)	1 (2.9 oz)	100	0	0
Zucchini Sliced (Southland)	3.2 oz	15	—	0
cooked	½ cup	19	tr	tr

PART II

Restaurant, Take-Out and Fast-Food Chains

FOOD	PORTION	CALS.	SAT. FAT	FAT
ARBY'S				
Cheese Cake	1 serving	306	7	23
Chocolate Chip Cookie	1	130	2	4
Turnover Blueberry	1	320	6	19
Turnover Apple	1	303	7	18
Turnover Cherry	1	280	5	18
BEVERAGES				
7UP	12 oz	144	0	0
Chocolate Shake	12 fl oz	451	3	12
Coca-Cola Classic	12 oz	141	0	0
Coffee	8 oz	3	0	0
Diet 7UP	12 oz	4	0	0
Diet Coke	12 oz	1	0	0
Hot Chocolate	8 oz	110	1	1
Iced Tea	16 oz	6	0	0
Jamocha Shake	11.5 fl oz	368	3	11
Milk, 2%	8 oz	121	3	4
Nehi Orange	12 oz	190	0	0
Orange Juice	6 oz	82	0	0
Pepsi-Cola	12 oz	159	0	0
R.C. Cola	12 oz	173	0	0
R.C. Diet Rite	12 oz	1	0	0
R.C. Root Beer	12 oz	173	0	0
Sugar Substitute	1 pkg (0.8 g)	4	0	0
Upper Ten	12 oz	169	0	0
Vanilla Shake	11 fl oz	330	4	12
BREAKFAST SELECTIONS				
Biscuit, Bacon	1	318	4	18
Biscuit, Ham	1	323	4	17
Biscuit, Plain	1	280	3	14
Biscuit, Sausage	1	460	9	32
Blueberry Muffin	1	200	2	6
Cinnamon Nut Danish	1	340	2	10
Croissant, Bacon & Egg	1	389	14	26
Croissant, Ham & Cheese	1	345	12	21
Croissant, Mushroom & Cheese	1	493	15	38
Croissant, Plain	1	260	10	16
Croissant, Sausage & Egg	1	519	19	39
Maple Syrup	1.5 oz	120	0	tr
Platter, Bacon	1	860	10	32
Platter, Egg	1	460	7	24
Platter, Ham	1	518	26	89
Platter, Sausage	1	640	13	41

FOOD	PORTION	CALS.	SAT. FAT	FAT
Toastix	1 serving	420	5	25
ICE CREAM				
Polar Swirl				
Butterfinger	1	457	8	18
Heath	1	543	5	22
Oreo	1	482	10	20
P'nut Butter Cup	1	517	8	24
Snickers	1	511	7	19
MAIN MENU SELECTIONS				
Arby's Sauce	0.5 oz	15	0	tr
Au Jus	4 oz	7	0	0
Bac N'Cheddar Deluxe Sandwich	1	532	8	33
Baked Potato, Broccoli 'N Cheddar	1	417	7	18
Baked Potato, Deluxe	1	621	18	36
Baked Potato, Mushroom & Cheese	1	515	6	27
Baked Potato, Plain	1	240	0	2
Baked Potato w/ Butter/ Margarine & Sour Cream	1	463	12	25
Beef N'Cheddar Sandwich	1	451	7	20
Cheddar Fries	1 serving (5 oz)	399	9	22
Chicken Breast Sandwich	1	489	4	46
Chicken Cordon Bleu Sandwich	1	658	9	37
Chicken Fajita Pita	1	272	—	9
Curly Fries	1 serving (3.5 oz)	337	8	18
Fish Fillet Sandwich	1	537	6	29
French Dip	1	345	6	12
French Dip 'N Swiss	1	425	8	18
French Fries	1 serving	246	3	13
Grilled Chicken Barbeque Sandwich	1	378	4	14
Grilled Chicken Deluxe Sandwich	1	426	5	21
Ham 'N Cheese Sandwich	1	330	4	15
Horsey Sauce	0.5 oz	55	1	5
Ketchup	0.5 oz	16	0	0
Light Ham Deluxe	1	255	—	6
Light Roast Beef Deluxe	1	294	—	10
Light Roast Chicken Deluxe	1	263	—	6

FOOD	PORTION	CALS.	SAT. FAT	FAT
Light Roast Turkey Deluxe	1	260	—	5
Mayonnaise, Cholesterol Free	0.5 oz	90	1	10
Mustard	0.5 oz	11	0	1
Philly Beef N' Swiss Sandwich	1	498	6	26
Potato Cakes	1 serving	204	2	12
Roast Beef Sandwich, Giant	1	530	11	27
Roast Beef Sandwich, Junior	1	218	4	11
Roast Beef Sandwich, Regular	1	353	7	15
Roast Beef Sandwich, Super	1	529	8	28
Roast Chicken Club	1	513	5	29
Roast Chicken Deluxe Sandwich	1	373	3	20
Roast Chicken Salad	1	184	—	7
Sub Deluxe	1	482	5	26
Turkey Deluxe Sandwich	1	399	4	20
SALAD DRESSINGS				
Blue Cheese	2 oz	295	6	31
Buttermilk Ranch	2 oz	349	6	39
Honey French	2 oz	322	4	27
Italian Light	2 oz	23	tr	1
Thousand Island	2 oz	298	4	29
Weight Watchers Creamy French	1 oz	48	1	3
Weight Watchers Creamy Italian	1 oz	29	1	3
SALADS AND SALAD BARS				
Cashew Chicken Salad	1	590	9	37
Chef Salad	1	210	5	11
Croutons	0.5 oz	59	tr	2
Garden Salad	1	149	4	9
SOUPS				
Beef w/ Vegetables & Barley	8 oz	96	1	3
Boston Clam Chowder	8 oz	207	4	11
Cream of Broccoli	8 oz	180	5	8
French Onion	8 oz	67	1	3
Lumberjack Mixed Vegetable	8 oz	89	2	4

FOOD	PORTION	CALS.	SAT. FAT	FAT
Old Fashioned Chicken Noodle	8 oz	99	1	2
Pilgrim's Corn Chowder	5 oz	193	4	11
Split Pea w/ Ham	8 oz	200	5	10
Tomato Florentine	8 oz	244	1	2
Wisconsin Cheese	8 oz	287	8	19

AU BON PAIN

BAGELS

Cinnamon Raisin	1	280	—	1
Onion	1	270	—	1
Plain	1	270	—	1
Sesame	1	270	—	1

BREAD AND ROLLS

3-Seed Raisin	1	250	tr	4
Alpine Roll	1	220	tr	3
Baguette Loaf	1	810	tr	2
Braided Roll	1	387	3	11
Cheese Loaf	1	1670	4	29
Country Seed Roll	1	220	tr	4
Four Grain Loaf	1	1420	tr	11
French Roll	1	320	tr	9
Hearth Roll	1	250	tr	2
Hearth Sandwich Roll	1	370	tr	3
Multigrain	2 slices	391	1	3
Onion Herb Loaf	1	1430	tr	13
Parisienne Loaf	1	1490	tr	4
Petit Pain Roll	1	220	tr	tr
Pita Pocket	1	80	—	tr
Pumpernickel Roll	1	210	tr	2
Rye	2 slices	374	1	4
Rye Roll	1	230	tr	2
Sandwich Croissant	1	300	8	14
Vegetable Roll	1 roll	230	tr	5

COOKIES

Chocolate Chip	1	280	9	15
Chocolate Chunk Pecan	1	290	6	17
Oatmeal Raisin	1	250	3	9
Peanut Butter	1	290	6	15
White Chocolate Chunk Pecan	1	300	6	17

CROISSANTS

Almond	1	420	12	25
Apple	1	250	6	10

FOOD	PORTION	CALS.	SAT. FAT	FAT
Blueberry Cheese	1	380	12	20
Chocolate	1	400	14	24
Chocolate Hazelnut	1	480	14	28
Cinnamon Raisin	1	390	8	13
Coconut Pecan	1	440	12	23
Ham & Cheese	1	370	12	20
Plain	1	220	6	10
Raspberry Cheese	1	400	12	20
Spinach & Cheese	1	290	10	16
Strawberry Cheese	1	400	12	20
Sweet Cheese	1	420	14	23
Turkey & Cheddar	1	410	13	22
Turkey & Havariti	1	410	13	21
MUFFINS				
Blueberry	1	390	4	11
Bran	1	390	3	11
Carrot	1	450	5	22
Corn	1	460	3	17
Cranberry Walnut	1	350	2	13
Oat Bran Apple	1	400	2	10
Pumpkin	1	410	2	16
Whole Grain	1	440	2	16
SALAD DRESSINGS				
Balsamic Vinaigrette	1 serving (2.25 fl oz)	311	5	33
Champagne Vinaigrette	1 serving (2.25 fl oz)	251	4	26
County Blue Cheese	1 serving (2.25 fl oz)	325	6	31
Honey With Poppy Seed	1 serving (2.25 fl oz)	354	—	35
Italian Low Cal	1 serving (2.25 fl oz)	68	tr	6
Olive Oil Ceasar	1 serving (2.25 fl oz)	255	—	16
Parmesan & Pepper	1 serving (2.25 fl oz)	235	5	21
Sesame French	1 serving (2.25 fl oz)	339	4	27
Tomato Basil	1 serving (2.25 fl oz)	66	0	tr
SALADS AND SALAD BARS				
Chicken Cracked Pepper Garden	1	100	tr	2

FOOD	PORTION	CALS.	SAT. FAT	FAT
Chicken Grilled Garden	1	110	tr	2
Chicken Tarragon Garden	1	310	2	15
Garden, Large	1	40	tr	tr
Garden, Small	1	20	tr	tr
Shrimp Garden	1	102	tr	2
Tuna Garden	1	350	4	25
SANDWICHES AND FILLINGS				
Bacon	1 serving	140	4	12
Brie	1 serving	300	15	24
Cheddar Cheese	1 serving	110	5	9
Chicken Cracked Pepper	1 serving	120	tr	2
Chicken Grilled	1 serving	130	tr	4
Chicken Tarragon	1 serving	270	2	15
Country Ham	1 serving	150	3	7
Herb Cheese	1 serving	290	18	29
Provolone Cheese	1 serving	155	7	13
Roast Beef	1 serving	180	4	8
Smoked Turkey	1 serving	100	tr	1
Swiss	1 serving	330	15	24
Tuna Salad	1 serving	310	4	24
SOUPS				
Beef Barley	1 cup	75	tr	2
Beef Barley	1 bowl	112	1	3
Chicken Noodle	1 cup	79	tr	1
Chicken Noodle	1 bowl	119	tr	2
Clam Chowder	1 cup	289	9	18
Clam Chowder	1 bowl	302	12	26
Cream of Broccoli	1 cup	201	8	17
Cream of Broccoli	1 bowl	302	12	26
Garden Vegetarian	1 cup	29	tr	tr
Garden Vegetarian	1 bowl	44	tr	tr
Minestrone	1 cup	105	tr	1
Minestrone	1 bowl	158	tr	2
Split Pea	1 cup	176	tr	1
Split Pea	1 bowl	264	tr	2
Tomato Florentine	1 cup	61	tr	1
Tomato Florentine	1 bowl	92	tr	2
Vegetarian Chili	1 cup	139	tr	3
Vegetarian Chili	1 bowl	208	tr	4

BASKIN-ROBBINS

Sugar Cone	1	60	—	1
Waffle Cone	1	140	—	2

FOOD	PORTION	CALS.	SAT. FAT	FAT
FROZEN YOGURT				
Cafe Mocha	½ cup (4 fl oz)	70	0	0
Chocolate Nonfat	½ cup	110	0	0
Chocolate Vanilla	½ cup	110	0	0
Dutch Chocolate Chip Bar	1	260	—	14
Pralines Vanilla Bar	1	250	—	14
Strawberry Low-Fat	½ cup (4 fl oz)	120	—	1
Strawberry Nonfat	½ cup	110	0	0
Wild Cherry	½ cup (4 fl oz)	70	0	0
ICE CREAM				
Almond Butter Crunch Light	½ cup	130	4	6
Butter Pecan	½ cup	160	7	10
Butterfinger	½ cup	170	6	8
Caramel Banana Fat Free	½ cup	100	0	0
Cherry Cordial Sugar Free	½ cup	100	1	1
Chewy Babyruth	½ cup	190	6	10
Chilly Burgers Vanilla	1	240	—	11
Chocolate	½ cup	150	5	8
Chocolate Raspberry Truffle	½ cup	180	7	10
Chocolate Vanilla Fat Free	½ cup	100	0	0
Chocolate Almond	½ cup	170	7	10
Chocolate Chip	½ cup	150	6	9
Chocolate Chip Sugar Free	½ cup	100	1	2
Chocolate Fudge	½ cup	170	6	9
Chocolate Mousse Royale	½ cup	180	6	9
Chocolate Wonder Fat Free	½ cup	120	0	0
Chunky Banana Sugar Free	½ cup	80	1	1
Coconut Caramel Nut Light	½ cup	130	3	5
Cookies N Cream	½ cup	160	6	10
Double Raspberry Light	½ cup	120	3	4
Espresso N Cream Light	½ cup	120	3	5
French Vanilla	½ cup	170	7	11
Fudge Brownie	½ cup	180	7	10
Gold Medal Ribbon	½ cup	150	5	7
Jamoca Swirl Fat Free	½ cup	100	0	0
Jamoca Swiss Almond Sugar Free	½ cup	90	1	2
Jamoca Almond Fudge	½ cup	150	5	8
Just Peachy Fat Free	½ cup	100	0	0
Kahula N Cream	½ cup	160	6	8
Mint Chocolate Chip	½ cup	150	6	9
Peanut Butter Chocolate	½ cup	190	8	12

FOOD	PORTION	CALS.	SAT. FAT	FAT
Pineapple Cheesecake Fat Free	½ cup	110	0	0
Pineapple Coconut Sugar Free	½ cup	90	1	1
Pistachio Almond	½ cup	160	7	10
Praline Dream Light	½ cup	130	4	6
Pralines N Cream	½ cup	160	5	8
Reeses Peanut Butter Cup	½ cup	170	7	10
Rocky Road	½ cup	170	5	8
Strawberry Sugar Free	½ cup	80	1	1
Strawberry Royal Light	½ cup	110	2	3
Thin Mint Chip Sugar Free	½ cup	90	1	2
Tiny Toon Adventures Toonwiches Chocolate	1	330	—	14
Tiny Toon Adventures Toonwiches Vanilla	1	340	—	16
Tiny Toon Adventures Bar Mint Chocolate Chip	1	230	—	15
Tiny Toon Adventures Bar Vanilla	1	210	—	14
Vanilla	½ cup	140	5	8
Vanilla Fudge Light	½ cup	110	3	4
Very Berry Strawberry	½ cup	120	4	6
World Class Chocolate	½ cup	160	5	8
ICES AND ICE POPS				
Daiquiri Ice	1 scoop	140	0	0
Rainbow Sherbet	1 scoop	160	—	2
Sorbet Strawberry	½ cup (4 fl oz)	100	0	0

BEN & JERRY'S
FROZEN YOGURT

FOOD	PORTION	CALS.	SAT. FAT	FAT
Apple Pie	½ cup (4 fl oz)	140	2	3
Banana Strawberry	½ cup (4 fl oz)	130	1	2
Blueberry Cheesecake	½ cup (4 fl oz)	130	1	2
Cherry Garcia	½ cup (4 fl oz)	150	2	3
Chocolate	½ cup (4 fl oz)	140	2	3
Chocolate Fudge Brownie	½ cup (4 fl oz)	170	2	4
Coffee Almond Fudge	½ cup (4 fl oz)	180	2	7
Heath Bar Crunch	½ cup (4 fl oz)	170	4	6
Pop Chocolate	1 (2.5 fl oz)	150	5	9
Raspberry	½ cup (4 fl oz)	120	1	2
ICE CREAM				
Cherry Garcia	½ cup (4 fl oz)	230	9	16
Chocolate	½ cup (4 fl oz)	230	8	14

FOOD	PORTION	CALS.	SAT. FAT	FAT
Chocolate Chip Cookie Dough	½ cup (4 fl oz)	260	10	17
Chocolate Fudge Brownie	½ cup (4 fl oz)	250	8	14
Chocolate Peanut Butter Chocolate Chip Cookie Dough	½ cup (4 fl oz)	280	9	18
Chunky Monkey	½ cup (4 fl oz)	270	10	19
Coffee Heath Bar Crunch	½ cup (4 fl oz)	270	11	19
Heath Bar Crunch	½ cup (4 fl oz)	270	12	19
Mint Cookie	½ cup (4 fl oz)	250	9	17
New York Super Fudge	½ cup (4 fl oz)	290	10	20
Pop Cherry Garcia	1 (3.7 fl oz)	250	10	18
Pop Chocolate Chip Cookie Dough	1 (2.5 fl oz)	240	9	16
Pop Heath Bar Crunch	1 (2.5 fl oz)	260	10	18
Pop Heath Bar Crunch	1 (3.7 fl oz)	340	13	23
Pop Milk Chocolate Almond	1 (2.5 fl oz)	250	10	19
Pop New York Super Fudge	1 (3.7 fl oz)	330	11	26
Pop Rain Forest Crunch	1 (3.7 fl oz)	350	14	27
Rain Forest Crunch	½ cup (4 fl oz)	270	10	21
Vanilla	½ cup (4 fl oz)	215	9	16
Vanilla Brownie Bar	1 (4 fl oz)	260	6	14
Vanilla Chocolate Chunk	½ cup (4 fl oz)	250	11	18

BIG BOY
ICE CREAM

FOOD	PORTION	CALS.	SAT. FAT	FAT
Frozen Yogurt	1 serving	72	—	0
Frozen Yogurt Shake	1 serving	184	—	tr
No-No Frozen Dessert	1 serving	75	—	0

MAIN MENU SELECTIONS

FOOD	PORTION	CALS.	SAT. FAT	FAT
Baked Cod Dinner	1 serving	392	—	13
Baked Cod Dijon Dinner	1 serving	455	—	19
Baked Potato	1	163	—	tr
Bran Muffin	1	367	—	10
Breast of Chicken Dinner	1 serving	358	—	13
Breast of Chicken w/ Mozzarella Dinner	1 serving	379	—	12
Breast of Chicken w/ Mozzarella Sandwich	1	390	—	13
Broiled Cod Dijon Dinner	1 serving	455	—	19
Broiled Cod Dinner	1 serving	392	—	13
Cajun Chicken Dinner	1 serving	358	—	13

FOOD	PORTION	CALS.	SAT. FAT	FAT
Cajun Cod Dinner	1 serving	392	—	13
Carrots	1 serving	35	—	tr
Chicken Breast Salad w/ Dijon And Pita Bread	1 serving	377	—	11
Corn	1 serving	90	—	1
Dijon Sauce	1 serving	63	—	6
Dinner Salad	1	19	—	tr
Green Beans	1 serving	28	—	tr
Mixed Vegetables	1 serving	27	—	tr
Peas	1 serving	77	—	tr
Promise Margarine	1 pat (5 g)	35	—	4
Rice	1 serving	114	—	tr
Roll	1	139	—	tr
Spaghetti Marinara Dinner	1 serving	450	—	6
Stir Fry Vegetable	1 serving	408	—	10
Stir Fry Dinner Chicken 'n Vegetable	1 serving	562	—	14
Turkey Pita	1	224	—	5
Vegetable Pita	1	144	—	3
SALAD DRESSINGS				
Buttermilk	1 serving	36	—	2
SOUPS				
Cabbage	1 bowl	43	—	1
Cabbage	1 cup	37	—	tr

BOSTON CHICKEN

DESSERTS

FOOD	PORTION	CALS.	SAT. FAT	FAT
Brownie	1 (3.36 oz)	452	8	27
Cookie Chocolate Chip	1 (2.79 oz)	369	6	16
Cookie Oatmeal Raisin	1 (2.79 oz)	341	3	13
MAIN MENU SELECTIONS				
½ Chicken With Skin	1 serving (10.05 oz)	642	14	39
¼ Dark Meat With Skin	1 serving (4.67 oz)	330	7	22
¼ Dark Meat Without Skin	1 serving (3.65 oz)	218	3	12
¼ White Meat With Skin	1 serving (5.39 oz)	332	5	18
¼ White Meat Without Skin & Wing	1 serving (3.68 oz)	164	2	4
BBQ Baked Beans	1 serving (7.1 oz)	290	3	7
Buttered Corn	1 serving (5. 14 oz)	181	1	6

FOOD	PORTION	CALS.	SAT. FAT	FAT
Butternut Squash	1 serving (6.79 oz)	247	7	11
Chicken Pot Pie	1 serving (15.01 oz)	703	9	34
Chicken Soup	1 serving (6.8 oz)	87	1	3
Chunky Chicken Salad	1 serving (5.57 oz)	460	5	39
Cole Slaw	1 serving (6.49 oz)	289	3	17
Corn Bread	1 serving (2.4 oz)	253	2	8
Cranberry Relish	1 serving (7.95 oz)	371	tr	6
Creamed Spinach	1 serving (6.37 oz)	298	15	24
Cucumber Salad	1 serving (4.79 oz)	79	tr	7
Fruit Salad	1 serving (4.4 oz)	49	tr	tr
Homestyle Mashed Potatoes & Gravy	1 serving (6.69 oz)	205	6	10
Macaroni & Cheese	1 serving (6.76 oz)	290	5	11
Mediterranean Pasta Salad	1 serving (4.54 oz)	160	2	9
New Potatoes	1 serving (4.61 oz)	129	1	4
Rice Pilaf	1 serving (5.13 oz)	188	1	5
Sandwich Chicken Breast	1 (9.13 oz)	422	1	4
Sandwich Chunky Chicken Salad	1 (12.11 oz)	763	7	43
Steamed Vegetables	1 serving (3.69 oz)	32	tr	tr
Stuffing	1 serving (6.14 oz)	282	2	11
Tortellini Salad	1 serving (5.62 oz)	430	5	25
Zucchini Marinara	1 serving (6.68 oz)	80	1	4

BURGER KING
BEVERAGES

FOOD	PORTION	CALS.	SAT. FAT	FAT
Cocoa Cola Classic	1 med (22 fl oz)	264	0	0
Coffee, Black	1 (8.6 fl oz)	2	0	0
Diet Coke	1 med (22 fl oz)	1	0	0
Milk, 2%	8.6 fl oz	121	3	5

FOOD	PORTION	CALS.	SAT. FAT	FAT
Orange Juice	6.4 fl oz	82	0	0
Shake Chocolate	1 med (10 fl oz)	320	5	7
Shake Chocolate Syrup Added	1 med (11 fl oz)	400	5	9
Shake Strawberry Syrup Added	1 med (10.9 fl oz)	370	4	6
Shake Vanilla	1 med (10 fl oz)	310	4	6
Sprite	1 med (22 fl oz)	264	0	0
BREAKFAST SELECTIONS				
A.M. Express Dip	1 oz	84	0	0
Breakfast Buddy With Sausage, Egg And Cheese	1 (2.9 oz)	255	6	16
Cream Cheese	1 serving (1 oz)	98	5	7
Croissan'wich Bacon, Egg And Cheese	1 (4.1 oz)	353	8	23
Croissan'wich Ham, Egg And Cheese	1 (5.1 oz)	351	7	22
Croissan'wich Sausage, Egg And Cheese	1 (5.6 oz)	534	14	40
French Toast Sticks	1 serving (4.9 oz)	440	7	27
Hash Browns	1 serving (2.5 oz)	213	3	12
Mini Muffins Blueberry	1 serving (3.3 oz)	292	3	14
DESSERTS				
Dutch Apple Pie	1 serving (4 oz)	308	3	15
Popcorn	1 serving (1 oz)	130	3	6
Snickers Ice Cream Bar	1 (2 oz)	220	7	14
MAIN MENU SELECTIONS				
American Cheese	1 slice (1 oz)	92	5	7
BK Big Fish Sandwich	1 (8.9 oz)	710	8	43
BK Broiler	1 (5.4 oz)	280	2	10
BK Broiler Sauce	1 serving (0.4 fl oz)	37	1	4
Bacon Bits	½ tsp (3 g)	16	tr	1
Bacon Double Cheeseburger	1 (5.2 oz)	470	13	28
Bacon Double Cheeseburger Deluxe	1 (6.5 oz)	570	15	38
Baked Potato	1 (7 oz)	210	0	0
Bull's Eye Barbecue Sauce	0.5 fl oz	22	0	0
Butterfly Shrimp	1 serving (4.1 oz)	300	5	17
Cheeseburger	1 (4 oz)	300	6	14
Chicken Sandwich	1 (8 oz)	700	8	42
Chicken Tenders	6 pieces (3.2 oz)	236	3	13

FOOD	PORTION	CALS.	SAT. FAT	FAT
Cocktail Sauce	1 serving (0.7 oz)	20	0	0
Croutons	1 serving (0.2 oz)	31	—	1
Dinner Roll	1 (0.9 oz)	80	0	2
Dipping Sauce Barbecue	1 oz	36	0	0
Dipping Sauce Honey	1 oz	91	0	0
Dipping Sauce Ranch	1 oz	171	3	18
Dipping Sauce Sweet & Sour	1 oz	45	0	0
Double Cheeseburger	1 (5.6 oz)	450	12	25
Double Whopper	1 (12.3 oz)	860	19	55
French Fries Salted	1 med (4.1 oz)	372	5	20
Hamburger	1 (3.6 oz)	260	4	10
Ketchup	0.5 fl oz	17	0	0
Lettuce	1 leaf (0.7 oz)	3	0	0
Mayonnaise	1 oz	210	3	23
Mustard	½ tsp (3 g)	2	0	0
Onion	0.5 oz	5	0	0
Onion Rings	1 serving (3.4 oz)	339	5	19
Pickles	0.5 oz	1	0	0
Sour Cream	1 oz	60	4	6
Tartar Sauce	1 oz	175	3	19
Tomato	1 oz	6	0	0
Whipped Classic Blend	1 serving (0.4 oz)	65	—	7
Whopper	1 (9.5 oz)	630	11	38
Whopper Double With Cheese	1 (13.2 oz)	950	23	63
Whopper Jr.	1 (4.6 oz)	330	5	19
Whopper Jr. With Cheese	1 (5.1 oz)	380	7	22
Whopper With Cheese	1 (10.3 oz)	720	16	46
SALAD DRESSINGS				
Bleu Cheese	1 serving (1.1 fl oz)	150	3	16
French	1 serving (1.1 fl oz)	145	2	11
Italian Reduced Calorie Light	1 serving (1.1 fl oz)	15	0	1
Ranch	1 serving (1.1 fl oz)	175	3	18
Thousand Island	1 serving (1.1 fl oz)	145	3	13
SALADS AND SALAD BARS				
Chef Salad w/o Dressing	1 (9.6 oz)	178	4	9
Chunky Chicken Salad w/o Dressing	1 (9.1 oz)	142	1	4

FOOD	PORTION	CALS.	SAT. FAT	FAT
Dinner Side Salad	1 (3.5 oz)	20	0	0
Garden Salad w/o Dressing	1 (7.8 oz)	95	3	5

CAPTAIN D'S
DESSERTS

FOOD	PORTION	CALS.	SAT. FAT	FAT
Carrot Cake	1 piece (4 oz)	434	—	23
Cheesecake	1 piece (4 oz)	420	—	31
Chocolate Cake	1 piece (4 oz)	303	—	10
Lemon Pie	1 piece (4 oz)	351	—	10
Pecan Pie	1 piece (4 oz)	458	—	20

MAIN MENU SELECTIONS

FOOD	PORTION	CALS.	SAT. FAT	FAT
Baked Fish Dinner w/ Slaw	1 dinner	451	—	19
Baked Potato	1 (9 oz)	277	—	tr
Breadstick	1 (1.3 oz)	91	—	1
Breadsticks	6 (7.5 oz)	545	—	7
Broiled Chicken Sandwich	1 (8.2 oz)	451	—	19
Cheese	1 slice (0.5 oz)	54	—	5
Chicken Dinner w/ Salad	1 dinner	414	—	8
Cob Corn	1 serving (9.5 oz)	251	—	2
Cocktail Sauce	1 lg serving (4 fl oz)	137	—	tr
Cole Slaw	1 pt (16 oz)	633	—	47
Cole Slaw	1 serving (4 oz)	158	—	12
Crackers	4	50	—	1
Cracklins	1 serving (1 oz)	218	—	17
Creamer	1 serving (0.4 fl oz)	14	—	1
Dinner Salad w/o Dressing	1 (2.5 oz)	27	—	1
French Fried Potatoes	1 serving (3.5 oz)	302	—	10
Fried Okra	1 serving (4 oz)	300	—	16
Green Beans Seasoned	1 serving (4 oz)	46	—	2
Hushpuppies	6 (6.7 oz)	756	—	25
Hushpuppy	1 (1.1 oz)	126	—	4
Orange Roughy Dinner w/ Salad	1 dinner	537	—	19
Rice	1 serving (4 oz)	124	0	0
Shrimp Dinner w/ Salad	1 dinner	457	—	10
Stuffed Crab	1 serving	91	—	7
Sugar	1 pkg	18	0	0
Sweet & Sour Sauce	1 lg serving (4 fl oz)	206	0	0
Sweet & Sour Sauce	1 serving (1 fl oz)	52	0	0
Tartar Sauce	1 lg serving (4 fl oz)	298	—	27
Tartar Sauce	1 serving (1 fl oz)	75	—	7

FOOD	PORTION	CALS.	SAT. FAT	FAT
White Beans	1 serving (4 oz)	126	—	1
SALAD DRESSINGS				
Blue Cheese	1 pkg (1 fl oz)	105	—	12
French	1 pkg (1 fl oz)	111	—	11
Italian Lo Cal	1 pkg (1 fl oz)	9	0	0
Ranch	1 pkg (1 fl oz)	92	—	10

CARL'S JR.

BAKED SELECTIONS

FOOD	PORTION	CALS.	SAT. FAT	FAT
Cheese Danish	1 (4 oz)	520	4	22
Cheesecake	1 serving (3.5 oz)	310	8	17
Chocolate Cake	1 serving (3 oz)	300	3	11
Chocolate Chip Cookies	2.5 oz	330	—	17
Cinnamon Roll	1 (4 oz)	460	—	18
Fudge Moussecake	1 slice (4 oz)	400	—	23
Muffin, Blueberry	1 (4.2 oz)	340	0	9
Muffin, Bran	1 (4.7 oz)	310	0	6
BEVERAGES				
Iced Tea	1 reg (21 fl oz)	2	0	0
Milk, 1%	1 (11 fl oz)	150	2	3
Orange Juice	1 sm (3.2 fl oz)	90	—	tr
Shake	1 reg (11.6 fl oz)	350	4	7
Soda	1 reg (21 fl oz)	240	0	0
Soda, Diet	1 reg (21 fl oz)	2	0	0
BREAKFAST SELECTIONS				
Bacon	2 strips (0.3 oz)	45	—	4
Breakfast Burrito	1 (5.3 oz)	430	12	26
English Muffin w/ Margarine	1 (2.2 oz)	190	1	5
French Toast Dips w/o Syrup	1 serving (5.4 oz)	490	6	20
Hash Brown Nuggets	1 serving (3.3 oz)	270	4	17
Hot Cakes w/ Margarine w/o Syrup	1 serving (6.6 oz)	510	5	24
Sausage	1 patty (1.6 oz)	190	1	18
Scrambled Eggs	1 serving (2.4 oz)	120	4	9
Sunrise Sandwich	1 (4.1 oz)	300	6	13
MAIN MENU SELECTIONS				
American Cheese	1 (0.6 oz)	60	—	5
Carl's Catch Fish Sandwich	1 (7.4 oz)	560	—	30
Carl's Original Hamburger	1 (6.8 oz)	460	9	20
Charbroiled Chicken Club Sandwich	1 (8.8 oz)	570	8	29
Charbroiled BBQ Chicken Sandwich	1 (6.7 oz)	310	2	6

FOOD	PORTION	CALS.	SAT. FAT	FAT
Chicken Strips	6 pieces (3.7 oz)	260	5	19
CrissCut Fries	1 reg (3.2 oz)	330	3	22
Cheeseburger, Double Western Bacon	1 (11.5 oz)	1030	32	63
Famous Star Hamburger	1 (8.6 oz)	610	13	38
French Fries	1 reg (4.4 oz)	420	5	20
Great Stuff Potato Broccoli & Cheese	1 (15 oz)	590	11	31
Great Stuffs Potato Bacon & Cheese	1 (14.9 oz)	730	15	43
Great Stuffs Potato Cheese	1 (14.6 oz)	690	15	36
Great Stuffs Potato Chili	1 (14.3 oz)	500	11	26
Great Stuffs Potato Lite	1 (10 oz)	290	0	1
Great Stuffs Potato Sour Cream & Chives	1 (12.3 oz)	470	7	19
Hamburger	1 (4.2 oz)	320	5	14
Onion Rings	1 serving (5.3 oz)	520	6	26
Roast Beef Deluxe Sandwich	1 (9.3 oz)	540	—	26
Salsa	1 oz	8	—	0
Sante Fe Chicken Sandwich	1 (7.9 oz)	530	7	29
Super Star Hamburger	1 (11.2 oz)	820	24	53
Swiss Cheese	1 serving (0.6 oz)	60	—	4
Turkey Club Sandwich	1 (9.3 oz)	530	6	23
Western Bacon Cheeseburger	1 (8.1 oz)	730	20	39
Zucchini	1 serving (5.9 oz)	390	6	23
SALADS AND DRESSINGS				
1000 Island	1 fl oz	110	3	11
Blue Cheese	1 fl oz	150	3	15
French Reduced Calorie	1 fl oz	40	0	2
House	1 fl oz	110	3	11
Italian Reduced Calorie	1 fl oz	40	0	2
Salad-to-Go Chicken	1 (12 oz)	200	4	8
Salad-to-Go Garden	1 (4.8 oz)	50	2	3

CARVEL

FROZEN YOGURT

Lo-Yo	4 fl oz	140	—	4
Low Fat Frozen Yogurt	4 fl oz	110	—	2
ICE CREAM				
Carvella	4 fl oz	180	—	10
Chocolate	4 fl oz	180	—	10
Thinny-Thin	4 fl oz	90	—	1

FOOD	PORTION	CALS.	SAT. FAT	FAT
CHICK-FIL-A				
BEVERAGES				
Iced Tea, Unsweetened	9 fl oz	3	—	tr
Lemonade	10 fl oz	124	—	tr
Lemonade Diet	10 fl oz	32	—	tr
DESSERTS				
Cheesecake	1 slice (3.2 oz)	299	—	19
Cheesecake w/ Blueberry Topping	1 slice (4.3 oz)	350	—	19
Cheesecake w/ Strawberry Topping	1 slice (4.3 oz)	343	—	19
Fudge Brownie w/ Nuts	1 (2.78 oz)	369	—	19
Icedream	4.5 oz	134	—	5
Lemon Pie	1 slice (4.1 oz)	329	—	5
MAIN MENU SELECTIONS				
Carrot-Raisin Salad	1 serving (2.67 oz)	116	—	5
Chargrilled Chicken Deluxe Sandwich	1 (7.15 oz)	266	—	5
Chargrilled Chicken Garden Salad	10.4 oz	126	—	2
Chargrilled Chicken Sandwich	1 (5.46 oz)	258	—	5
Chargrilled Chicken w/o Bun	1 piece (3.6 oz)	128	—	2
Chick-N-Q Sandwich	1 (6.8 oz)	409	—	15
Chicken Sandwich	1 (5.76 oz)	360	—	9
Chicken Deluxe Sandwich	1 (7.45 oz)	368	—	9
Chicken Salad Plate	1 (12.6 oz)	291	—	19
Chicken Salad Sandwich w/ Wheat Bread	1 (5.7 oz)	365	—	26
Chicken w/o Bun	1 piece (3.6 oz)	219	—	7
Cole Slaw	1 serving (3.72 oz)	175	—	14
Grilled 'n Lites	2 skewers (2.7 oz)	97	—	2
Hearty Breast of Chicken Soup	8.5 oz	152	—	3
Nuggets	8 pack (4 oz)	287	—	15
Potato Salad	1 serving (3.84 oz)	198	—	15
Waffle Potato Fries	1 sm (3 oz)	270	—	14
SALADS AND SALAD BARS				
Tossed Salad	4.5 oz	21	—	tr

FOOD	PORTION	CALS.	SAT. FAT	FAT
Tossed Salad w/ Blue Cheese Dressing	6 oz	243	—	24
Tossed Salad w/ Honey French	6 oz	246	—	24
Tossed Salad w/ Lite Italian	6 oz	46	—	2
Tossed Salad w/ Ranch	6 oz	177	—	16
Tossed Salad w/ Ranch Lite	6 oz	114	—	6
Tossed Salad w/ Thousand Island	6 oz	231	—	22

CHURCH'S FRIED CHICKEN

FOOD	PORTION	CALS.	SAT. FAT	FAT
Apple Pie	1 serving (3.1 oz)	280	—	12
Biscuit	1 serving (2.1 oz)	250	—	16
Breast	1 serving (2.8 oz)	200	—	12
Cajun Rice	1 serving (3.1 oz)	130	—	7
Cole Slaw	1 serving (3 oz)	92	—	6
Corn On The Cob	1 serving (5.7 oz)	190	—	5
French Fries	1 serving (2.7 oz)	210	—	11
Leg	1 serving (2 oz)	140	—	9
Okra	1 serving (2.8 oz)	210	—	16
Potatoes & Gravy	1 serving (3.7 oz)	90	—	3
Thigh	1 serving (2.8 oz)	230	—	16
Wing	1 serving (3.1 oz)	250	—	16

COLOMBO FROZEN YOGURT

FOOD	PORTION	CALS.	SAT. FAT	FAT
Alpine Strawberry Nonfat	4 fl oz	100	0	0
Banana Strawberry Nonfat	4 fl oz	50	0	0
Brazilian Banana Nonfat	4 fl oz	100	0	0
Butter Pecan Nonfat	4 fl oz	100	0	0
Cappuccino Nonfat	4 fl oz	100	0	0
Cherry Amaretto Nonfat	4 fl oz	50	0	0
Cherry Vanilla Nonfat	4 fl oz	100	0	0
Chocolate Nonfat	4 fl oz	50	0	0
Coconut Cooler Nonfat	4 fl oz	100	0	0
Cool Berry Blue Nonfat	4 fl oz	100	0	0
Country Pumpkin Nonfat	4 fl oz	100	0	0
Double Dutch Chocolate Nonfat	4 fl oz	100	0	0
Egg Nog Nonfat	4 fl oz	100	0	0
French Vanilla Lowfat	4 fl oz	110	1	2
French Vanilla Nonfat	4 fl oz	100	0	0
Georgia Peach Nonfat	4 fl oz	100	0	0

FOOD	PORTION	CALS.	SAT. FAT	FAT
German Fudge Chocolate Nonfat	4 fl oz	100	0	0
Hawaiian Pineapple Nonfat	4 fl oz	100	0	0
Hazelnut Amaretto Nonfat	4 fl oz	100	0	0
Honey Almond Nonfat	4 fl oz	100	0	0
Irish Cream Nonfat	4 fl oz	100	0	0
New York Cheesecake Nonfat	4 fl oz	100	0	0
Old World Chocolate Lowfat	4 fl oz	110	1	2
Orange Bavarian Creme Nonfat	4 fl oz	100	0	0
Peanut Butter Lowfat	4 fl oz	110	1	2
Pecan Praline Nonfat	4 fl oz	100	0	0
Pina Colada Nonfat	4 fl oz	100	0	0
Raspberry Nonfat	4 fl oz	50	0	0
Rockin' Raspberry Nonfat	4 fl oz	100	0	0
Simply Vanilla Lowfat	4 fl oz	110	1	2
Simply Vanilla Nonfat	4 fl oz	100	0	0
Strawberry Nonfat	4 fl oz	50	0	0
Tropical Tango Nonfat	4 fl oz	100	0	0
Vanilla Nonfat	4 fl oz	50	0	0
White Chocolate Almond Nonfat	4 fl oz	100	0	0
Wild Strawberry Lowfat	4 fl oz	110	1	2

D'ANGELO SANDWICH SHOPS

ICE CREAM

Frozen Banana Yogurt	5 oz	125	—	3
Frozen Banana Yogurt w/ Cone	5 oz	215	—	4
Frozen Peach Yogurt	5 oz	130	—	3
Frozen Peach Yogurt w/ Cone	5 oz	220	—	3

SALADS AND SALAD BARS

Beef	1 serving	350	—	5
Chicken	1 serving	325	—	4
Tuna	1 serving	305	—	2
Turkey	1 serving	375	—	4

SANDWICHES

D'Lite Pocket, Chicken Stir Fry	1	340	—	4
D'Lite Pocket, Roast Beef	1	325	—	5
D'Lite Pocket, Steak	1	415	—	11

FOOD	PORTION	CALS.	SAT. FAT	FAT
D'Lite Pocket, Steak & Mushroom	1	420	—	11
D'Lite Pocket, Steak & Pepper	1	420	—	11
D'Lite Pocket, Turkey	1	350	—	4
D'Lite Pocket, Vegetarian	1	350	—	11
D'Lite Small Sub, Roast Beef	1	365	—	7
D'Lite Small Sub, Turkey	1	390	—	6

DAIRY QUEEN/BRAZIER
FOOD SELECTION

FOOD	PORTION	CALS.	SAT. FAT	FAT
¼-lb Super Dog	1	590	16	38
BBQ Beef Sandwich	1	225	1	4
Breaded Chicken Fillet Sandwich	1	430	4	20
Breaded Chicken Fillet Sandwich w/ Cheese	1	480	7	25
Double Hamburger	1	460	12	25
Double Hamburger w/ Cheese	1	570	18	34
DQ Homestyle Ultimate Burger	1	700	21	47
Fish Fillet Sandwich	1	370	3	16
Fish Fillet Sandwich w/ Cheese	1	420	6	21
French Dressing, Reduced Calorie	2 oz	90	1	5
French Fries	1 sm	210	2	10
French Fries	1 reg	300	3	14
French Fries	1 lg	390	4	18
Garden Salad	1	200	7	13
Grilled Chicken Fillet Sandwich	1	300	2	8
Hot Dog	1	280	6	16
Hot Dog w/ Cheese	1	330	9	21
Hot Dog w/ Chili	1	320	7	19
Lettuce	0.5 oz	2	0	0
Onion Rings	1 reg	240	3	12
Side Salad	1	25	0	0
Single Hamburger	1	310	6	13
Single Hamburger w/ Cheese	1	365	9	18
Thousand Island Dressing	2 oz	225	3	21
Tomato	0.5 oz	3	0	0

FOOD	PORTION	CALS.	SAT. FAT	FAT
ICE CREAM				
Banana Split	1	510	8	11
Blizzard, Strawberry	1 sm	500	8	12
Blizzard, Strawberry	1 reg	740	11	16
Breeze, Strawberry	1 sm	400	tr	tr
Breeze, Strawberry	1 reg	590	tr	1
Buster Bar	1	450	9	29
Cone, Chocolate	1 reg	230	5	7
Cone, Chocolate	1 lg	350	8	11
Cone, Dipped Chocolate	1 reg	330	8	16
Cone, Vanilla	1 sm	140	3	4
Cone, Vanilla	1 reg	230	5	7
Cone, Vanilla	1 lg	340	7	10
Cone, Yogurt	1 reg	180	tr	tr
Cone, Yogurt	1 lg	260	tr	tr
Cup, Yogurt	1 reg	170	tr	tr
Cup, Yogurt	1 lg	230	tr	tr
Dilly Bar	1	210	6	13
DQ Frozen Cake Slice Undecorated	1	380	8	18
DQ Sandwich	1	140	2	4
Heath Blizzard	1 sm	560	11	23
Heath Blizzard	1 reg	820	17	36
Heath Breeze	1 sm	450	3	12
Heath Breeze	1 reg	680	6	21
Hot Fudge Brownie Delight	1	710	14	29
Malt, Vanilla	1 reg	610	8	14
Mr. Misty	1 reg	250	0	0
Nutty Double Fudge	1	580	10	22
Peanut Buster Parfait	1	710	10	32
QC Big Scoop, Chocolate	1	310	10	14
QC Big Scoop, Vanilla	1	300	9	14
Shake, Chocolate	1 reg	540	8	14
Shake, Vanilla	1 reg	520	8	14
Shake, Vanilla	1 lg	600	10	16
Sundae, Chocolate	1 reg	300	5	7
Sundae, Strawberry Yogurt	1 reg	200	tr	tr
Sundae, Strawberry Waffle Cone	1	350	5	12
DELTACO				
BEVERAGES				
Coffee	1 serving	6	tr	tr
Coke Classic	1 lg	287	0	0
Coke Classic	1 med	198	0	0

FOOD	PORTION	CALS.	SAT. FAT	FAT
Coke Classic	1 sm	144	0	0
Coke Classic Best Value	1 serving	395	0	0
Diet Coke	1 lg	2	0	0
Diet Coke	1 med	1	0	0
Diet Coke	1 sm	1	0	0
Diet Coke Best Value	1 serving	2	0	0
Iced Tea	1 lg	6	0	tr
Iced Tea	1 med	4	0	tr
Iced Tea	1 sm	3	0	tr
Iced Tea Best Value	1 serving	8	0	tr
Milk	1	126	2	3
Mr Pibb	1 lg	283	0	0
Mr Pibb	1 med	195	0	0
Mr Pibb	1 sm	142	0	0
Mr Pibb Best Value	1 serving	390	0	0
Orange Juice	1	83	0	tr
Shake				
Chocolate	1 med	755	14	22
Chocolate	1 sm	549	10	16
Orange	1 med	837	14	22
Orange	1 sm	609	10	16
Strawberry	1 med	668	14	22
Strawberry	1 sm	486	10	16
Vanilla	1 med	707	17	25
Vanilla	1 sm	514	12	18
Sprite	1 lg	287	0	0
Sprite	1 med	198	0	0
Sprite	1 sm	144	0	0
Sprite Best Value	1 serving	395	0	0
BREAKFAST SELECTIONS				
Burrito				
Beef And Egg	1	529	10	27
Breakfast	1	256	4	11
Egg And Cheese	1	443	8	22
Egg and Bean	1	470	8	22
Steak And Egg	1	500	9	25
CHILDREN'S MENU SELECTIONS				
Kid's Meal Hamburger	1	617	7	20
Kid's Meal Taco	1	532	6	17
ICE CREAM				
M&M's Toppers	1	256	4	8
Oreos Toppers	1	257	4	10
Snickers Toppers	1	254	5	10

FOOD	PORTION	CALS.	SAT. FAT	FAT
MAIN MENU SELECTIONS				
American Cheese	1 slice	53	3	4
Beans And Cheese	1	122	2	3
BURRITO				
Chicken	1	264	4	10
Combination	1	413	7	17
Del Beef	1	440	9	20
Deluxe Chicken	1	549	10	34
Deluxe Combo	1	453	9	20
Deluxe Del Beef	1	479	10	23
Green	1	229	3	8
Green Regular	1	330	5	11
Macho Beef	1	893	18	41
Macho Combo	1	774	15	31
Red	1	235	4	8
Red Regular	1	324	5	12
Cheeseburger	1	284	6	13
Chicken Salad	1	254	6	19
Chicken Salad Deluxe	1	716	15	47
Del Burger	1	385	6	20
Del Cheeseburger	1	439	9	25
Double Del Cheeseburger	1	618	16	39
French Fries	1 lg	566	9	26
French Fries	1 reg	404	6	19
French Fries	1 sm	242	4	11
Fries Chili Cheese	1 serving	562	13	30
Fries Deluxe Chili Cheese	1 serving	600	15	33
Fries Nacho	1 serving	669	11	34
Guacamole	1 oz	60	4	6
Hamburger	1	231	3	8
Hot Sauce	1 pkg	2	0	tr
Nacho Cheese Sauce Side Order	1 serving	100	2	8
Nachos	1	390	4	32
Nachos Super Deluxe	1	684	10	45
Quesadilla	1	257	6	12
Quesadilla Chicken	1	544	16	31
Quesadilla Regular	1	483	16	27
Salsa	2 oz	14	0	tr
Salsa Dressing	1 oz	33	2	3
Sour Cream	1 oz	60	4	6
Taco	1	140	3	8
Taco Chicken	1	186	3	13
Taco Deluxe Double Beef	1	205	5	13

FOOD	PORTION	CALS.	SAT. FAT	FAT
Taco Double Beef	1	172	3	10
Taco Soft	1	146	3	6
Taco Salad	1	235	6	19
Taco Salad Deluxe	1	741	16	49
Taco Soft Chicken	1	197	3	11
Taco Soft Deluxe Double Beef	1	211	5	11
Taco Soft Double Beef	1	178	3	8
Tostada	1	140	3	8

DENNY'S
BREAKFAST SELECTIONS

FOOD	PORTION	CALS.	SAT. FAT	FAT
Harvest Slam	1 serving	1050	14	55
Harvest Slam w/ Eggbeaters	1 serving	960	11	46
Omelette				
Chili Cheese	1 serving	490	2	33
Denver	1 serving	720	18	62
Ham 'N' Cheddar	1 serving	480	2	33
Mexican	1 serving	540	6	40
Senior	1 serving	640	11	57
Ultimate	1 serving	850	25	75
Vegetable	1 serving	590	16	48
Vegetable w/ Eggbeaters	1 serving	450	12	34
Pancakes	3	410	—	6
Senior				
Belgian Waffle Slam	1 serving	370	—	25
Grand Slam Breakfast	1 serving	380	—	22
Starter w/ Sausage	1 serving	440	—	24
Starter w/ Bacon	1 serving	370	—	18

DESSERTS

FOOD	PORTION	CALS.	SAT. FAT	FAT
Apple Pie Regular	1 slice	480	8	26
Apple Pie w/ Equal	1 slice	460	8	30

MAIN MENU SELECTIONS

FOOD	PORTION	CALS.	SAT. FAT	FAT
BLT	1	620	8	38
Bacon Swiss w/o Lettuce And Tomato	1	750	18	45
Baked Potato	1 med	90	0	0
Carrots	1 serving (3 oz)	20	—	tr
Catfish	2 pieces (8 oz)	640	13	58
Chicken Fried Steak w/o Gravy	2 pieces	500	21	41
Chicken Stir Fry w/ Rice	1 serving	420	6	20
Club Sandwich	1	590	6	34

FOOD	PORTION	CALS.	SAT. FAT	FAT
Cole Slaw	1 cup	120	—	10
Corn	1 serving (3 oz)	60	—	1
Denny Burger	1	490	7	24
French Fries	1 serving (4 oz)	300	—	16
Fried Chicken	4 pieces	460	—	30
Green Beans	1 serving (3 oz)	15	—	tr
Grilled Cheese	1	710	22	48
Grilled Chicken	1	520	2	26
Grilled Chicken Breast	1 serving	125	1	3
Ham & Swiss Sandwich	1	500	5	28
Liver w/ Bacon & Onions	2 pieces	370	8	22
Mashed Potatoes	1 serving (4 oz)	70	—	tr
Onion Rings	1 ring	90	—	5
Patty Melt	1	775	12	57
Peas	1 serving (3 oz)	40	—	tr
Quesadila Beef	1	730	10	48
Quesadila Chicken	1	620	5	36
Quesadila Denny's	1	510	4	33
Rice Pilaf	⅓ cup	90	—	2
Senior				
Fried Shrimp w/o Vegetable or Bread	1 serving	330	—	13
Grilled Catfish Dinner	1 serving	320	—	29
Grilled Chicken Breast Entree	1 serving	100	—	3
Roast Beef Dinner w/o Vegetable	1 serving	280	3	9
Roast Turkey & Stuffing Entree	1 serving	440	—	16
Sirloin Tips & Noodles	1 serving	220	—	5
Spaghetti Dinner	1 serving	580	10	25
Turkey Sandwich	1 serving	340	—	27
Stuffing	½ cup	180	—	9
Super Bird	1	750	3	37
Top Sirloin Steak	1 serving	270	5	10
Tuna Sandwich	1	400	4	23
Turkey Sandwich	1	340	2	16
Turkey w/o Gravy	6 slices	200	1	6
Veggie Cheese	1	560	5	40
Veggie Cheese Melt	1	560	5	39
Works Burger w/o Lettuce And Tomato	1	950	20	66
SALADS AND SALAD BARS				
Chef Salad	1	370	10	26

FOOD	PORTION	CALS.	SAT. FAT	FAT
Garden Salad	1	110	1	4
Grilled Chicken Salad	1	290	1	12
Taco Salad	1	910	25	55
SOUPS				
Cheese	1 serving	406	15	30
Chicken Noodle	1 serving	120	—	4
Cream of Potato	1 serving	250	—	9
Vegetable Beef	1 serving	159	1	27

DOMINO'S PIZZA
(*see also* GODFATHER'S, PIZZA, PIZZA HUT, SHAKEY'S)

FOOD	PORTION	CALS.	SAT. FAT	FAT
12 INCH PIZZA				
Pepperoni	1 slice	219	4	7
Veggie	1 slice	204	3	5
15 INCH PIZZA				
Deluxe	2 slices	498	9	20
16 INCH PIZZA				
Cheese	2 slices	376	5	10
Double Cheese Pepperoni	2 slices	545	13	25
Ham	2 slices	417	6	11
Pepperoni	2 slices	460	8	18
Sausage Mushroom	2 slices	430	8	16
Veggie	2 slices	498	10	19

DUNKIN' DONUTS
(*see also* DOUGHNUT, WINCHELL'S)

FOOD	PORTION	CALS.	SAT. FAT	FAT
COOKIES				
Chocolate Chunk	1 (1.6 oz)	200	5	10
Chocolate Chunk w/ Nuts	1 (1.5 oz)	210	5	11
Oatmeal Pecan Raisin	1 (1.6 oz)	200	4	9
CROISSANTS				
Almond	1 (3.7 oz)	420	5	26
Chocolate	1 (3.3 oz)	440	10	29
Plain	1 (2.5 oz)	310	4	19
DOUGHNUTS				
Apple Crumb	1 (3 oz)	250	3	10
Apple-Filled w/ Cinnamon Sugar	1 (2.8 oz)	250	2	11
Blueberry-Filled	1 (2.4 oz)	210	2	8
Boston Kreme	1 (2.8 oz)	240	2	11
Butternut Cake Ring	1 (3.5 oz)	410	6	20
Chocolate Frosted Yeast Ring	1 (1.9 oz)	200	2	10
Chocolate Frosted Cake Ring	1 (2.3 oz)	280	3	16

FOOD	PORTION	CALS.	SAT. FAT	FAT
Chocolate Glazed Ring	1 (3.4 oz)	420	8	24
Chocolate Kreme	1 (2.4 oz)	250	3	14
Cinnamon Cake Ring	1 (2.2 oz)	260	3	15
Coconut Coated Cake Ring	1 (3.1 oz)	360	8	21
Dunkin Donut	1 (2.1 oz)	240	3	14
Glazed Buttermilk Ring	1 (2.6 oz)	290	3	14
Glazed Chocolate Ring	1 (2.7 oz)	320	4	18
Glazed Coffee Roll	1 (2.8 oz)	280	—	12
Glazed Cruller	1 (2.4 oz)	260	2	11
Glazed French Cruller	1 (1.4 oz)	140	2	8
Glazed Whole Wheat Ring	1 (2.5 oz)	280	3	15
Glazed Yeast Ring	1 (1.9 oz)	200	2	9
Jelly-Filled	1 (2.4 oz)	220	2	9
Lemon-Filled	1 (2.8 oz)	260	2	12
Mini				
Cake	1 (0.9 oz)	100	1	6
Chocolate Glazed	1 (1.1 oz)	122	1	7
Cinnamon Cake	1 (1 oz)	116	2	7
Coconut	1 (1.2 oz)	140	3	8
Coffee Roll	1 (0.8 oz)	78	1	3
Eclairs	1 (1.3 oz)	114	1	5
Munchkin				
Butternut Cake	1 (0.6 oz)	70	1	3
Coconut Cake	1 (0.6 oz)	70	2	4
Glazed Cake	1 (0.6 oz)	60	1	3
Glazed Chocolate	1 (0.7 oz)	70	1	3
Glazed Yeast	1 (0.5 oz)	50	tr	2
Jelly Filled Yeast	1 (0.5 oz)	50	tr	2
Plain Cake	1 (0.5 oz)	50	1	3
Powdered Cake	1 (0.5 oz)	50	1	3
Peanut	1 (3.7 oz)	480	5	29
Plain Cake Ring	1 (2 oz)	262	4	18
Powdered Cake Ring	1 (2.2 oz)	270	3	16
Sugared Cake Ring	1 (2.1 oz)	270	4	18
Sugared Jelly Stick	1 (3 oz)	310	2	12
Vanilla Frosted Yeast Ring	1 (2 oz)	200	2	9
Vanilla Kreme	1 (2.4 oz)	250	3	12
MUFFINS				
Apple N'Spice	1 (3.4 oz)	300	2	8
Banana Nut	1 (3.3 oz)	310	2	10
Blueberry	1 (3.6 oz)	280	2	8
Bran w/ Raisins	1 (3.68 oz)	310	1	9
Corn	1 (3.4 oz)	340	2	12
Cranberry Nut	1 (3.4 oz)	290	2	9
Oat Bran	1 (3.3 oz)	330	2	11

FOOD	PORTION	CALS.	SAT. FAT	FAT
EL POLLO LOCO				
DESSERTS				
Cheesecake	1 serving (3.5 oz)	160	9	18
Churros	1 serving (1.5 oz)	140	2	9
Orange Bang	1 serving (7 oz)	110	0	0
Pina Colada Bang	1 serving (7 oz)	110	0	0
MAIN MENU SELECTIONS				
Beans	1 serving (4 oz)	100	1	3
Burrito Chicken	1 (7 oz)	310	2	11
Burrito Steak	1 (6 oz)	450	9	22
Burrito Vegetarian	1 (6 oz)	340	2	7
Cheddar Cheese	1 serving (1 oz)	90	3	5
Chicken Breast	1 piece (3 oz)	160	2	6
Chicken Leg	1 piece (1.75 oz)	90	2	5
Chicken Thigh	1 piece (2 oz)	180	4	12
Chicken Wing	1 (1.5 oz)	110	2	6
Chicken Fajita Meal	1 (17.5 oz)	780	3	18
Coleslaw	1 serving (3 oz)	70	0	8
Corn	1 serving (3 oz)	110	1	2
Guacamole	1 serving (1 oz)	60	0	6
Potato Salad	1 serving (4 oz)	180	2	10
Rice	1 serving (2 oz)	110	0	2
Salsa	2 oz	10	0	0
Sour Cream	1 serving (1 oz)	60	4	6
Steak Fajita Meal	1 (17.5 oz)	1040	14	38
Taco Chicken	1 (5 oz)	180	1	7
Taco Steak	1 (4.5 oz)	250	4	12
Tortillas Corn	1 (1 oz)	60	0	1
Tortillas Flour	1 (1 oz)	90	2	3
SALAD DRESSINGS				
Blue Cheese	1 fl oz	80	1	6
Deluxe French	1 fl oz	60	0	4
Honey Dijon Mustard	1 fl oz	50	0	1
Italian Reduced Calorie	1 fl oz	25	0	2
Ranch	1 fl oz	75	0	6
Thousand Island	1 fl oz	110	0	10
SALADS AND SALAD BARS				
Chicken Salad	1 (12 oz)	160	1	4
Side Salad	1 (9 oz)	50	0	1
FRIENDLY'S				
Heath English Toffee	½ cup (2.7 oz)	190	6	10

FOOD	PORTION	CALS.	SAT. FAT	FAT
GODFATHER'S PIZZA				
Golden Crust Cheese	⅙ sm (3 oz)	213	—	8
Golden Crust Cheese	⅛ med (3.1)	229	—	9
Golden Crust Cheese	⅒ lg (3.5 oz)	261	—	11
Golden Crust Combo	⅙ sm (4.5 oz)	273	—	12
Golden Crust Combo	⅛ med (4.5 oz)	283	—	13
Golden Crust Combo	⅒ lg (5.1 oz)	322	—	15
Original Crust Cheese	¼ mini (2 oz)	138	—	4
Original Crust Cheese	⅙ sm (3. 5 oz)	239	—	7
Original Crust Cheese	⅛ med (3.5 oz)	242	—	7
Original Crust Cheese	⅒ lg (4 oz)	271	—	8
Original Crust Combo	¼ mini (2.8 oz)	164	—	5
Original Crust Combo	⅙ sm (5 oz)	299	—	11
Original Crust Combo	⅛ med (5.2 oz)	318	—	12
Original Crust Combo	⅒ lg (5.5 oz)	332	—	12
GODIVA				
Almond Butter Dome	3 pieces (1.5 oz)	240	6	17
Bouchee Au Chocolat	1 piece (1.5 oz)	210	6	11
Bouchee Ivory Raspberry	1 piece (1 oz)	160	3	9
Gold Ballotin	3 pieces (1.5 oz)	210	4	10
Truffle Amaretto Di Saronno	2 pieces (1.5 oz)	210	6	12
Truffle Deluxe Liqueur	2 pieces (1.5 oz)	210	6	13
H-SALT SEAFOOD				
Chicken	3 oz	108	—	6
Cod	3 oz	62	—	2
Hamburger	3 oz	228	—	18
Pork Loin	3 oz	254	—	21
Sirloin Steak	3 oz	239	—	20
HAAGEN-DAZS				
FROZEN YOGURT				
Banana Nonfat Soft	1 oz	25	0	0
Chocolate	3 oz	130	2	3
Chocolate Nonfat Soft	1 oz	30	0	0
Chocolate Soft	1 oz	30	—	1
Coffee Soft	1 oz	28	—	1
Peach	3 oz	120	2	3
Raspberry Soft	1 oz	30	—	1
Strawberry	3 oz	120	2	3
Strawberry Nonfat Soft	1 oz	25	0	0
Vanilla	3 oz	130	2	3
Vanilla Soft	1 oz	28	—	1

FOOD	PORTION	CALS.	SAT. FAT	FAT
Vanilla Almond Crunch	3 oz	150	2	5
ICE CREAM				
Butter Pecan	4 oz	390	9	24
Caramel Almond Crunch Bar	1	240	7	18
Caramel Nut Sundae	4 oz	310	—	21
Chocolate	4 oz	270	8	17
Chocolate Chocolate Chip	4 oz	290	10	20
Chocolate Chocolate Mint	4 oz	300	—	20
Chocolate Dark Chocolate Bar	1	390	—	27
Coffee	4 oz	270	8	17
Deep Chocolate	4 oz	290	—	14
Deep Chocolate Fudge	4 oz	290	—	14
Honey Vanilla	4 oz	250	8	16
Macadamia Brittle	4 oz	280	—	18
Orange & Cream Pop	1	130	—	6
Peanut Butter Crunch Bar	1 (6.3 fl oz)	270	7	21
Rum Raisin	4 oz	250	8	17
Strawberry	4 oz	250	8	15
Vanilla	4 oz	260	8	17
Vanilla Crunch Bar	1	220	6	16
Vanilla Fudge	4 oz	270	—	17
Vanilla Milk Chocolate Almond Bar	1	370	—	27
Vanilla Milk Chocolate Bar	1	360	—	27
Vanilla Milk Chocolate Brittle Bar	1	370	—	25
Vanilla Peanut Butter Swirl	4 oz	280	8	21
Vanilla Swiss Almond	4 oz	290	—	19
ICES AND ICE POPS				
Blueberry Sorbet & Cream	4 oz	190	—	8
Fudge Pop Bar	1	210	—	14
Keylime Sorbet & Cream	4 oz	190	—	7
Lemon Sorbet	4 oz	140	—	0
Orange Sorbet	4 oz	113	—	0
Orange Sorbet & Cream	4 oz	190	—	8
Raspberry Sorbet	4 oz	93	—	0
Raspberry Sorbet & Cream	4 oz	180	—	8

HARDEE'S

BAKED SELECTIONS

FOOD	PORTION	CALS.	SAT. FAT	FAT
Big Cookie	1 (2.0 oz)	280	4	12
Blueberry Muffin	1 (4 oz)	400	4	17

FOOD	PORTION	CALS.	SAT. FAT	FAT
BEVERAGES				
Orange Juice	1 serving (11 oz)	140	tr	tr
Shake Chocolate	1 (11.4 fl oz)	390	6	10
Shake Peach	1 (11.4 fl oz)	530	7	11
Shake Strawberry	1 (11.4 fl oz)	390	5	8
Shake Vanilla	1 (11.4 fl oz)	370	6	9
BREAKFAST SELECTIONS				
Bacon & Egg Biscuit	1 (4.4 oz)	490	9	27
Bacon, Egg & Cheese Biscuit	1 (4.8 oz)	530	11	31
Big Country Breakfast, Bacon	1 (7.6 oz)	740	13	43
Big Country Breakfast, Sausage	1 (9.6 oz)	930	19	61
Biscuit 'N' Gravy	1 (7.8 oz)	510	9	28
Canadian Rise 'N' Shine Biscuit	1 (5.8 oz)	570	11	32
Chicken Biscuit	1 (5.1 oz)	510	7	25
Cinnamon 'N' Raisin Danish	1 (2.8 oz)	370	5	18
Country Ham Biscuit	1 (3.8 oz)	430	6	22
Frisco Breakfast Sandwich Ham	1 (6.5 oz)	460	8	22
Ham Biscuit	1 (4 oz)	400	6	20
Ham, Egg & Cheese Biscuit	1 (5.6 oz)	500	10	27
Hash Rounds	1 serving (2.8 oz)	230	3	14
Rise 'N' Shine Biscuit	1 (2.9 oz)	390	6	21
Sausage & Egg Biscuit	1 (5.2 oz)	560	11	35
Sausage Biscuit	1 (4.1 oz)	510	10	31
Steak Biscuit	1 (5.2 oz)	580	10	32
Three Pancakes	1 serving (4.8 oz)	280	1	2
Three Pancakes w/ 1 Sausage Pattie	1 serving (6.2 oz)	430	6	16
Three Pancakes w/ 2 Bacon Strips	1 serving (5.3 oz)	350	3	9
ICE CREAM				
Cool Twist Sundae, Hot Fudge	1 (5.9 oz)	320	5	10
Cool Twist Sundae, Strawberry	1 (5.8 oz)	260	3	6
Cool Twist Cone, Chocolate	1 (4.1 oz)	180	3	4
Cool Twist Cone, Vanilla	1 (4.1 oz)	180	3	4

FOOD	PORTION	CALS.	SAT. FAT	FAT
Cool Twist Cone, Vanilla/ Chocolate	1 (4.1 oz)	170	3	4
MAIN MENU SELECTIONS				
Bacon Cheeseburger	1 (7.9 oz)	600	15	36
Big Deluxe Burger	1 (8.5 oz)	530	13	30
Big Roast Beef Sandwich	1 (5.9 oz)	370	7	16
Cheeseburger	1 (4.2 oz)	300	7	13
Chef Salad	1 (9.4 oz)	200	8	13
Chicken Fillet Sandwich	1 (6.6 oz)	400	3	14
Cole Slaw	1 serving (4 oz)	240	3	20
Crispy Curls	1 serving (3.0 oz)	300	3	16
Fisherman's Fillet Sandwich	1 (7.6 oz)	500	6	22
French Fries	1 sm (3.4 oz)	240	3	10
French Fries	1 med (5.0 oz)	350	4	15
French Fries	1 lg (6.1 oz)	430	5	18
Fried Chicken Breast	1 piece (5.2 oz)	370	4	15
Fried Chicken Leg	1 piece (2.4 oz)	170	2	7
Fried Chicken Thigh	1 piece (4.2 oz)	330	4	15
Fried Chicken Wing	1 piece (2.3 oz)	200	2	8
Frisco Burger	1 (8.5 oz)	760	18	50
Frisco Grilled Chicken Sandwich	1 (8.6 oz)	620	10	34
Garden Salad	1 (9.3 oz)	190	9	14
Grilled Chicken Sandwich	1 (9.8 oz)	120	1	4
Hamburger	1 (3.6 oz)	260	4	9
Hot Dog	1 (6.8 oz)	450	6	20
Hot Ham 'N' Cheese	1 (7.1 oz)	530	9	30
Mashed Potatoes	1 serving (4 oz)	70	tr	tr
Mushroom 'N' Swiss Burger	1 (7.1 oz)	520	13	27
Quarter-Pound Cheeseburger	1 (6.5 oz)	490	12	25
Regular Roast Beef	1 (4.4 oz)	270	5	11
Side Salad	1 (4.9 oz)	20	tr	tr
IHOP				
Pancake Buckwheat	1 (2.5 oz)	134	1	5
Pancake Buttermilk	1 (2 oz)	108	1	3
Pancake Egg	1 (2 oz)	102	1	5
Pancake Harvest Grain 'N Nut	1 (2.25 oz)	160	1	8
Waffle	1 (4 oz)	305	3	15
Waffle Belgian	1 (6 oz)	408	11	20

FOOD	PORTION	CALS.	SAT. FAT	FAT
Waffle Belgian Harvest Grain 'N Nut	1 (6 oz)	445	12	28

JACK IN THE BOX
BEVERAGES

Coca-Cola Classic	1 sm (16 fl oz)	190	0	0
Coffee, Black	8 oz	0	0	0
Diet Coke	1 sm (16 oz)	0	0	0
Dr. Pepper	1 sm (16 oz)	190	0	0
Iced Tea	1 sm (16 oz)	5	0	0
Milk, 2%	8 oz	120	3	5
Milk Shake, Chocolate	11 oz	330	4	7
Milk Shake, Strawberry	11 oz	320	4	7
Milk Shake, Vanilla	11 oz	320	4	6
Orange Juice	6 oz	80	0	0
Ramblin' Root Beer	1 sm (16 oz)	240	0	0
Sprite	1 sm (16 oz)	190	0	0

BREAKFAST SELECTIONS

Breakfast Jack	1 (4.4 oz)	310	5	13
Country Crock Spread	1 pat (5 g)	25	tr	3
Grape Jelly	1 serving (0.5 oz)	40	0	0
Hash Browns	1 serving (2 oz)	160	3	11
Pancake Platter	1 (8.1 oz)	612	9	22
Pancake Syrup	1 serving (1.5 fl oz)	121	0	0
Sausage Crescent	1 (5.5 oz)	584	16	43
Scrambled Egg Platter	1 (7.5 oz)	559	9	32
Scrambled Egg Pocket	1 (6.4 oz)	431	8	21
Sourdough Breakfast Sandwich	1 (5.2 oz)	381	7	20
Supreme Crescent	1 (5.1 oz)	547	13	40

DESSERTS

Cheesecake	1 serving (3.5 oz)	310	9	18
Cinnamon Churritos	1 serving (2.6 oz)	330	5	21
Double Fudge Cake	1 slice (3 oz)	290	2	9
Hot Apple Turnover	1 (3.9 oz)	350	4	19

MAIN MENU SELECTIONS

¼ lb Burger	1 (6 oz)	510	10	27
Bacon Cheeseburger	1 (8.5 oz)	710	15	45
BBQ Sauce	1 oz	45	tr	tr
Beef Gyro	1 (9.1 oz)	620	12	32
Buttermilk House Sauce	1 serving (0.9 fl oz)	130	2	13
Cheeseburger	1 (3.9 oz)	320	6	14

FOOD	PORTION	CALS.	SAT. FAT	FAT
Chicken & Mushroom Sandwich	1 (7.8 oz)	440	5	18
Chicken Fajita Pita	1 (6.6 oz)	290	3	8
Chicken Sandwich	1 (5.6 oz)	400	4	18
Chicken Strips	4 pieces (3.9 oz)	290	3	13
Chicken Strips	6 pieces (6.2 oz)	450	5	20
Chicken Supreme	1 (8.6 oz)	670	11	42
Chimichangas Mini	4 pieces (7.3 oz)	570	9	28
Chimichangas Mini	6 pieces (10.9 oz)	860	13	42
Country Fried Steak	1 (5.4 oz)	450	7	25
Double Cheeseburger	1 (5.2 oz)	470	12	27
Egg Rolls	3 (5.5 oz)	440	7	24
Egg Rolls	5 (10 oz)	750	12	41
Fish Supreme	1 (8.6 oz)	590	8	32
French Fries	1 sm (2.4 oz)	220	3	11
French Fries	1 reg (3.8 oz)	350	4	17
French Fries	1 jumbo (4.3 oz)	400	5	19
Grilled Chicken Fillet	1 (7.4 oz)	430	5	19
Grilled Sourdough Burger	1 (7.8 oz)	710	16	50
Guacamole	1 serving (0.9 oz)	30	tr	3
Hamburger	1 (3.4 oz)	270	4	11
Hot Sauce	1 serving (0.5 fl oz)	5	0	0
Jumbo Jack	1 (7.8 oz)	580	11	34
Jumbo Jack w/ Cheese	1 (8.9 oz)	680	14	40
Onion Rings	1 serving (3.6 oz)	380	6	23
Salsa	1 oz	10	tr	tr
Seasoned Curly French Fries	1 serving (3.8 oz)	360	5	20
Sesame Breadsticks	1 (0.6 oz)	70	—	2
Sirloin Steak Sandwich	1 (8.3 oz)	520	5	23
Smoked Chicken Cheddar & Bacon Sandwich	1 (7.8 oz)	540	11	30
Spicy Crispy Chicken Sandwich	1 (7.8 oz)	560	5	27
Super Taco	1 (4.4 oz)	280	6	17
Sweet & Sour Sauce	1 oz	40	tr	tr
Taco	1 (2.7 oz)	190	4	11
Teriyaki Bowl Beef	1 serving (15.4 oz)	640	1	3
Teriyaki Bowl Chicken	1 serving (15.4 oz)	580	tr	2
Tortilla Chips	1 oz	140	—	6
Ultimate Cheeseburger	1 (9.8 oz)	940	26	69

FOOD	PORTION	CALS.	SAT. FAT	FAT
SALAD DRESSINGS				
Bleu Cheese	1 serving (2.5 fl oz)	260	4	22
Buttermilk House	1 serving (2.5 fl oz)	360	6	36
Italian Low Calorie	1 serving (2.5 fl oz)	25	tr	2
SALADS AND SALAD BARS				
Chef Salad	1 (11.4 oz)	320	11	19
Side Salad	1 (4 oz)	50	2	3
Taco Salad	1	503	13	31

KENTUCKY FRIED CHICKEN

FOOD	PORTION	CALS.	SAT. FAT	FAT
BAKED SELECTIONS				
Biscuit	1 (2.2 oz)	220	3	12
Breadstick	1 (1.2 oz)	110	0	3
Cornbread	1 (2 oz)	228	2	13
Sourdough Roll	1 (1.7 oz)	128	0	2
MAIN MENU SELECTIONS				
BBQ Baked Beans	1 serving (3.9 oz)	132	1	2
Chicken Littles Sandwich	1 (1.7 oz)	169	2	10
Cole Slaw	1 serving (3.2 oz)	114	1	6
Colonel's				
Chicken Sandwich	1 (5.9 oz)	482	6	27
Rotisserie Gold Dark Quarter	1 serving (5.1 oz)	333	7	24
Rotisserie Gold Dark Quarter Skin Removed	1 serving (4.1 oz)	217	4	12
Rotisserie Gold White Quarter	1 serving (6.2 oz)	335	5	19
Rotisserie Gold White Quarter Skin Removed	1 serving (4.1 oz)	199	2	6
Corn On The Cob	1 ear (5.3 oz)	222	2	12
Crispy Fries	1 serving (2.5 oz)	210	3	11
Extra Crispy Tasty Side Breast	1 (4.1 oz)	400	6	27
Extra Tasty Crispy				
Center Breast	1 (4.1 oz)	330	4	19
Drumstick	1 (2.3 oz)	190	3	12
Thigh	1 (3.8 oz)	380	7	29
Whole Wing	1 (2.1 oz)	240	4	17
Garden Rice	1 serving (3.8 oz)	75	0	1

FOOD	PORTION	CALS.	SAT. FAT	FAT
Green Beans	1 serving (3.6 oz)	36	0	1
Hot & Spicy				
Center Breast	1 (4.3 oz)	360	5	22
Drumstick	1 (2.4 oz)	180	3	12
Side Breast	1 (4.2 oz)	400	6	28
Thigh	1 (4.2 oz)	370	6	27
Whole Wing	1 (2.1 oz)	220	4	16
Hot Wings	6 (4.8 oz)	471	8	33
Kentucky Nuggets	6 (3.4 oz)	284	4	18
Macaroni & Cheese	1 serving (4 oz)	162	3	8
Mashed Potatoes With Gravy	1 serving (4.2 oz)	70	tr	1
Mean Greens	1 serving (3.9 oz)	52	1	2
Original				
Center Breast	1 (3.6 oz)	260	4	14
Drumstick	1 (2 oz)	152	2	9
Side Breast	1 (2.9 oz)	245	4	15
Thigh	1 (3.4 oz)	287	5	21
Whole Wing	1 (1.9 oz)	172	3	11
Potato Wedges	1 serving (3.3 oz)	192	3	9
Red Beans & Rice	1 serving (3.9 oz)	114	1	3
Vegetable Medley Salad	1 serving (4 oz)	126	1	4
SALAD DRESSINGS				
Italian	1 serving (1 fl oz)	15	0	1
Ranch	1 serving (1 fl oz)	170	3	18
SALADS AND SALAD BARS				
Garden Salad	1 (3.1 oz)	16	0	0
Macaroni	1 serving (3.8 oz)	248	3	17
Pasta Salad	1 serving (3.8 oz)	135	1	8
Potato	1 serving (4.4 oz)	180	2	11

KRYSTAL

BEVERAGES

Chocolate Shake	1 (12.8 fl oz)	271	5	10

BREAKFAST SELECTIONS

Biscuit	1 (3.2 oz)	289	3	14
Biscuit Bacon	1 (3.6 oz)	355	5	20
Biscuit Country Ham	1 (4.5 oz)	379	5	19
Biscuit Egg	1 (4.8 oz)	372	5	21
Biscuit Gravy	1 (8.2 oz)	445	5	26
Biscuit Sausage	1 (4.3 oz)	429	7	27
Sunriser	1 (3.6 oz)	264	6	17

DESSERTS

Apple Pie	1 serving (4.5 oz)	320	4	14

FOOD	PORTION	CALS.	SAT. FAT	FAT
Donut	1 (1.3 oz)	100	2	9
Donut w/ Chocolate Icing	1 (1.8 oz)	162	3	11
Donut w/ Vanilla Icing	1 (1.8 oz)	148	2	9
Lemon Meringue Pie	1 serving (4 oz)	340	3	9
Pecan Pie	1 serving (4 oz)	450	6	24
MAIN MENU SELECTIONS				
Bacon Cheeseburger	1 (6.4 oz)	583	14	35
Big K	1 (7.3 oz)	608	14	36
Burger Plus	1 (6.4 oz)	488	9	27
Burger Plus w/ Cheese	1 (7 oz)	545	12	31
Cheese Krystal	1 (2.6 oz)	189	4	10
Chicken Sandwich	1 (6.4 oz)	392	1	16
Chili	1 lg (12 oz)	322	4	11
Chili	1 reg (8 oz)	214	2	8
Chili Cheese Pup	1 (2.6 oz)	203	5	13
Chili Pup	1 (2.5 oz)	184	4	12
Corn Pup	1 (2.3 oz)	214	6	14
Double Cheese Krystal	1 (4.6 oz)	341	8	19
Double Krystal	1 (4 oz)	276	5	14
Fries	1 lg (5 oz)	615	8	17
Fries	1 med (3.9 oz)	474	6	13
Fries	1 sm (2.8 oz)	338	4	9
Krys Kross Fries	1 serving (2.6 oz)	242	5	11
Krys Kross Fries w/ Cheese	1 serving (3.6 oz)	292	6	15
Krystal	1 (2.2 oz)	157	3	7
Plain Pup	1 (1.9 oz)	164	4	10
LITTLE CAESARS PIZZA				
Antipasto Salad	1 sm	96	—	5
Crazy Bread	1 piece	98	—	1
Crazy Sauce	1 serving	63	—	1
Greek Salad	1 sm	85	—	5
Ham & Cheese Sandwich	1	552	—	27
Italian Sandwich	1	615	—	35
Tossed Salad	1 sm	37	—	1
Tuna Sandwich	1	610	—	31
Turkey Sandwich	1	450	—	17
Veggie Sandwich	1	784	—	47
PIZZA				
Baby Pan!Pan!	1 order	525	—	22
Cheese & Pepperoni Round Large	1 slice	185	—	7
Cheese & Pepperoni Round Medium	1 slice	168	—	7

FOOD	PORTION	CALS.	SAT. FAT	FAT
Cheese & Pepperoni Round Small	1 slice	151	—	6
Cheese & Pepperoni Square Large	1 slice	204	—	8
Cheese & Pepperoni Square Medium	1 slice	201	—	8
Cheese & Pepperoni Square Small	1 slice	204	—	8
Cheese Round Large	1 slice	169	—	6
Cheese Round Medium	1 slice	154	—	5
Cheese Round Small	1 slice	138	—	5
Cheese Square Large	1 slice	188	—	6
Cheese Square Medium	1 slice	185	—	6
Cheese Square Small	1 slice	188	—	6
Slice!Slice!	1 order	756	—	31

LONG JOHN SILVER'S

CHILDREN'S MENU SELECTIONS

Chicken Planks, 2 pieces & Fryes	7.8 oz	560	6	29
Fish & Fryes, 1 piece	7 oz	500	6	28
Fish, Chicken & Fryes	8.9 oz	620	7	34

DESSERTS

Apple Pie	1 slice (4.5 oz)	320	5	13
Cherry Pie	1 slice (4.5 oz)	360	4	13
Chocolate Chip Cookie	1 (1.8 oz)	230	6	9
Lemon Pie	1 slice (4 oz)	340	3	9
Oatmeal Raisin Cookie	1 (1.8 oz)	160	2	10
Pineapple Cream Cheese Cake	1 slice (3.2 oz)	310	9	18
Walnut Brownie	1 (3.4 oz)	440	5	22

MAIN MENU SELECTIONS

1 Fish & 2 Chicken w/ Fries & Slaw	1 serving (15.2 oz)	950	11	49
1 Fish, 1 Chicken & Fries	1 serving (8.1 oz)	550	7	32
2 Fish, 4 Shrimp Clams w/ Fries & Slaw	1 serving (18.1 oz)	1240	15	70
2 Fish, 5 Shrimp 1 Chicken w/ Fries & Slaw	1 serving (18.1 oz)	1160	14	65
2 Fish, 8 Shrimp w/ Fries & Slaw	1 serving (17.2 oz)	1140	14	65
Baked Chicken Entree	1 dinner (15.9 oz)	590	3	15
Baked Chicken Light Herb	1 piece (3.5 oz)	120	1	4

FOOD	PORTION	CALS.	SAT. FAT	FAT
Baked Fish w/ Lemon Crumb	3 pieces (5 oz)	150	tr	1
Baked Fish w/ Lemon Crumb Entree 3 pieces	1 dinner (17.4 oz)	610	2	13
Baked Light Fish w/ Lemon Crumb Entree 2 pieces	1 dinner (11.8 oz)	330	1	5
Batter Dipped Fish	1 piece (3.1 oz)	180	3	11
Batter Dipped Shrimp	1 piece (0.4 oz)	30	1	2
Catsup	1 serving (0.32 oz)	12	0	0
Chicken Plank	1 piece (2 oz)	120	2	6
Chicken Planks	2 pieces (4 oz)	240	3	12
Chicken Planks 2 Pieces & Fries	1 serving (6.9 oz)	490	6	26
Chicken Planks 3 Pieces w/ Fries & Slaw	1 serving (14.1 oz)	890	10	44
Clams w/ Fries & Slaw	1 serving (12.7 oz)	990	11	52
Cole Slaw	1 serving (3.4 oz)	140	1	6
Corn Cobbette	1 piece (3.3 oz)	140	—	8
Crispy Fish	1 piece (1.8 oz)	150	2	8
Crispy Fish & More 3 Pieces w/ Fries & Slaw	1 serving (13.5 oz)	980	11	50
Fish & Fries 2 Pieces	1 serving (9.2 oz)	610	8	37
Fish & More 2 Pieces w/ Fries & Slaw	1 serving (14.4 oz)	890	10	48
Fries	1 serving (3 oz)	250	3	15
Green Beans	1 serving (3.5 oz)	20	tr	tr
Honey Mustard Sauce	1 serving (0.42 fl oz)	20	tr	tr
Hushpuppies	1 (0.8 oz)	70	tr	2
Rice	1 serving (4 oz)	190	1	4
Roll	1 (1.5 oz)	110	tr	tr
Saltine Crackers	1 pkg (0.2 oz)	25	—	1
Sandwich Batter Dipped Chicken 1 Piece	1 (4.5 oz)	280	2	8
Sandwich Batter Dipped Fish 1 Piece	1 (5.6 oz)	340	3	13
Seafood Sauce	1 serving (0.42 fl oz)	14	tr	tr
Shrimp w/ Fries & Slaw	1 serving (11.7 oz)	840	10	47
Sweet 'N Sour Sauce	1 serving (0.42 oz)	20	tr	tr

FOOD	PORTION	CALS.	SAT. FAT	FAT
Tartar Sauce	1 serving (0.42 fl oz)	50	1	5
SALAD DRESSINGS				
Creamy Italian Dressing	1 fl oz	30	—	3
Malt Vinegar	0.28 fl oz	1	—	tr
Ranch Dressing	1 fl oz	180	4	19
Sea Salad Dressing	1 fl oz	140	6	15

MACHEEZMO MOUSE

CHILDREN'S MENU SELECTIONS

FOOD	PORTION	CALS.	SAT. FAT	FAT
Kid's Plate	7 oz	279	—	5
Kid's Plate w/ Chicken	9 oz	349	—	7
MAIN MENU SELECTIONS				
Bean/Cheese Enchilada	12 oz	405	—	8
Bean/Cheese Enchilada Dinner	22 oz	670	—	8
Beans	6 oz	214	—	0
Boss Sauce	1 oz	30	—	0
Cheese	1 oz	81	—	5
Cheese Quesadilla	5 oz	337	—	13
Chicken	3 oz	105	—	3
Chicken Burrito	13 oz	543	—	10
Chicken Burrito Dinner	23 oz	808	—	10
Chicken Enchilada	10 oz	332	—	10
Chicken Enchilada Dinner	20 oz	597	—	10
Chicken Quesadilla	9 oz	407	—	15
Chicken Majita	18 oz	704	—	9
Chicken Salad Small	10 oz	324	—	75
Chicken Salad Large	17 oz	612	—	15
Chicken Tacos	6 oz	294	—	8
Chicken Tacos Dinner	16 oz	559	—	8
Chicken w/ Green Salad	13 oz	377	—	6
Chili	3 oz	135	—	3
Chili Tacos	6 oz	314	—	8
Chili Tacos Dinner	16 oz	579	—	8
Chips	3 oz	394	—	17
Combo Burrito	14 oz	598	—	11
Combo Burrito Dinner	24 oz	863	—	11
Enchilada Sauce	1 oz	6	—	0
Famouse #5	14 oz	583	—	5
Guacamole	2 oz	201	—	5
Mex Cheese	1 oz	100	—	8
Mixed Greens	4 oz	tr	—	0
Nacho Grande	8 oz	704	—	38
Rice	6 oz	274	—	0

FOOD	PORTION	CALS.	SAT. FAT	FAT
Salad w/ Marinated, Small Veggies	5 oz	32	—	1
Salad w/ Marinated Veggies, Large	8 oz	54	—	1
Sour Cream Blend	1 oz	27	—	3
Tortilla Corn	2 oz	128	—	0
Tortilla Flour	2 oz	180	—	2
Tortilla Mini Corn	3 oz	160	—	0
Tortilla Whole Wheat	2 oz	160	—	2
Vegetables	4 oz	43	—	0
Vegetarian Burrito	14 oz	601	—	7
Vegetarian Burrito Dinner	24 oz	866	—	7
Vegetarian Plate	15 oz	531	—	5
Vegetarian Tacos	6 oz	295	—	6
Vegetarian Tacos Dinner	16 oz	560	—	6
Veggie Taco Salad, Small	10 oz	379	—	8
Veggie Taco Salad, Large	17 oz	647	—	13

McDONALD'S

BAKED SELECTIONS

FOOD	PORTION	CALS.	SAT. FAT	FAT
Apple Pie	1 (3 oz)	260	4	15
Cookies Chocolaty Chip	1 pkg (2 oz)	330	4	15
Cookies McDonaldland	1 pkg (2 oz)	290	1	9
Danish Apple	1	390	4	17
Danish Cinnamon Raisin	1	440	5	13
Danish Iced Cheese	1	390	6	21
Danish Raspberry	1	410	3	16

BEVERAGES

FOOD	PORTION	CALS.	SAT. FAT	FAT
Apple Juice	6 oz	90	0	0
Coca-Cola Classic	16 oz	145	0	0
Diet Coke	16 oz	1	0	0
Grapefruit Juice	6 oz	80	0	0
Milk, 1%	8 oz	110	2	2
Milk Shake, Lowfat Chocolate	10.4 oz	320	1	1
Milk Shake, Lowfat Strawberry	10.4 oz	320	1	1
Milk Shake, Lowfat Vanilla	10.4 oz	290	1	1
Orange Drink	16 oz	130	0	0
Orange Juice	6 oz	80	0	0
Sprite	16 oz	145	0	0

BREAKFAST SELECTIONS

FOOD	PORTION	CALS.	SAT. FAT	FAT
Biscuit w/ Bacon, Egg & Cheese	1	440	8	26
Biscuit w/ Sausage	1	420	8	28

FOOD	PORTION	CALS.	SAT. FAT	FAT
Biscuit w/ Sausage & Egg	1	505	10	33
Biscuit w/ Spread	1	260	3	13
Breakfast Burrito	1	280	6	17
Cheerios	¾ cup	80	tr	1
Egg McMuffin	1	280	4	11
English Muffin w/ Spread	1	170	1	4
Fat-Free Apple Bran Muffin	1	180	0	0
Hash Brown Potatoes	1 serving	130	1	7
Hotcakes w/ Margarine & Syrup	1 portion	440	2	12
Sausage	1	160	5	15
Sausage McMuffin	1	345	7	20
Sausage McMuffin w/ Egg	1	430	8	25
Scrambled Eggs	1 portion	140	3	10
Wheaties	¾ cup	90	1	1
ICE CREAM				
Cone, Vanilla Lowfat Frozen Yogurt	1 (3 oz)	105	1	1
Sundae, Lowfat Frozen Yogurt, Hot Caramel	1 (6 oz)	270	1	3
Sundae, Lowfat Frozen Yogurt, Hot Fudge	1 (6 oz)	240	3	3
Sundae, Lowfat Frozen Yogurt, Strawberry	1 (6 oz)	210	1	1
MAIN MENU SELECTIONS				
Big Mac	1	500	9	26
Cheeseburger	1	305	5	13
Chicken Fajita	1 (2.9 oz)	190	2	8
Chicken McNuggets	4 pieces (2.6 oz)	180	2	10
Chicken McNuggets	6	270	4	15
Chicken McNuggets	9 pieces (5.6 oz)	405	5	22
Filet-O-Fish	1	370	4	18
French Fries	1 sm	220	3	12
French Fries	1 med	320	4	17
French Fries	1 lg	400	5	22
Hamburger	1	255	3	9
McChicken	1	415	4	19
McLean Deluxe	1	320	4	10
McLean Deluxe w/ Cheese	1	370	5	14
Quarter Pounder	1	410	8	20
Quarter Pounder w/ Cheese	1	510	11	28
SALAD DRESSINGS				
1000 Island Dressing	1 pkg	225	5	20
Bleu Cheese Dressing	1 pkg	250	5	20

FOOD	PORTION	CALS.	SAT. FAT	FAT
Lite Vinaigrette Dressing	1 pkg	48	tr	2
Ranch Dressing	1 pkg	220	4	20
Red French Reduced Calorie Dressing	1 pkg	160	1	8
SALADS AND SALAD BARS				
Bacon Bits	0.1 oz	15	1	1
Chef Salad	1 serving	170	4	9
Chunky Chicken Salad	1 serving	150	1	4
Croutons	0.3 oz	50	1	2
Garden Salad	1	50	1	2
Side Salad	1 serving	30	tr	4

MORRISON'S

DESSERTS

FOOD	PORTION	CALS.	SAT. FAT	FAT
Boston Cream Cake	1 slice	218	—	4
MAIN MENU SELECTIONS				
Baked Potato	1	220	—	tr
Broccoli	1 serving (4 oz)	37	—	2
Cabbage	1 serving (4 oz)	36	—	tr
Cantaloupe Compote	1 serving (4 oz)	130	—	1
Cauliflower	1 serving (4 oz)	68	—	5
Chicken Stew & Dumplings	1 serving (7 oz)	362	—	14
Chicken Teriyaki	1 serving (5.5 oz)	232	—	10
French Bread	1 slice	207	—	2
Grilled Chicken Pecan Salad	1 serving (6 oz)	298	—	8
Lima Beans	1 serving (4 oz)	170	—	4
Okra & Tomatoes	1 serving (5 oz)	40	—	2
Pinto Beans	1 serving (4 oz)	105	—	4
Plain Jello	1 serving (3 oz)	131	—	tr
Rutabagas	1 serving (4 oz)	33	—	1
Sliced Tomato	4 slices	40	—	1
Soft Roll	1 (2 oz)	170	—	4
Strawberries Peaches & Bananas	1 serving (6 oz)	203	—	1
Strawberries & Banana Bowl	1 serving (6 oz)	203	—	1
Turnip Greens	1 serving (4 oz)	30	—	2
Watermelon	1 serving (6 oz)	102	—	1
Yellow Squash	1 serving (4 oz)	22	—	1
SALADS AND SALAD BARS				
Garden Salad	1 serving (2.5 oz)	75	—	2
Tossed Salad	1 serving (3 oz)	30	—	tr

FOOD	PORTION	CALS.	SAT. FAT	FAT
NATHAN'S				
BEVERAGES				
Lemonade	16 fl oz	189	—	0
Lemonade	22 fl oz	260	—	0
Lemonade	32 fl oz	378	—	0
MAIN MENU SELECTIONS				
Breaded Chicken Sandwich	1 (7.2 oz)	510	4	25
Charbroiled Chicken Sandwich	1 (4.5 oz)	288	1	5
Cheese Steak Sandwich	1 (6.1 oz)	485	10	26
Chicken 2 Pieces	1 serving (7.1 oz)	693	9	44
Chicken 4 Pieces	1 serving (14.2 oz)	1382	18	88
Chicken Platter 2 Pieces	1 serving (14.8 oz)	1096	14	66
Chicken Platter 4 Pieces	1 serving (21.9 oz)	1788	23	109
Chicken Salad	1 serving (12.7 oz)	154	1	4
Double Burger	1 (7.3 oz)	671	18	41
Filet of Fish Platter	1 serving (22 oz)	1455	10	74
Filet of Fish Sandwich	1 (5.2 oz)	403	2	15
Frank Nuggets	11 pieces (5.1 oz)	563	10	38
Frank Nuggets	15 pieces (6.9 oz)	764	13	52
Frank Nuggets	7 pieces (3.2 oz)	357	6	24
Frankfurter	1 (3.2 oz)	310	8	19
French Fries	1 serving (8.6 oz)	514	4	26
Fried Clam Platter	1 serving (13.1 oz)	1024	7	51
Fried Clam Sandwich	1 (5.4 oz)	620	4	29
Fried Shrimp	1 serving (4.4 oz)	348	2	11
Fried Shrimp Platter	1 serving (12.6 oz)	796	5	34
Hamburger	1 (4.7 oz)	434	10	23
Knish	1 (5.9 oz)	318	2	7
Pastrami Sandwich	1 (4.1 oz)	325	4	12
Sauteed Onions	1 serving (3.5 oz)	39	0	1
Super Burger	1 (7.6 oz)	533	9	32
Turkey Sandwich	1 (4.9 oz)	270	0	2
SALADS AND SALAD BARS				
Garden Salad	1 serving (10.9 oz)	193	7	13
OLIVE GARDEN				
Baked Lasagna	1 lunch serving	330	—	18
Breadstick	1	70	—	2
Breadstick w/o margarine	1	30	—	0
Breadstick w/o margarine & garlic salt	1	30	—	0
Eggplant Parmigiana	1 lunch serving	220	—	14
Fettuccine Alfredo	1 lunch serving	790	—	50

FOOD	PORTION	CALS.	SAT. FAT	FAT
Garden Salad	1 serving	230	—	15
Minestrone Soup	6 fl oz	45	—	tr
Pasta e Fagioli	6 fl oz	140	—	5
Salad Dressing	1 tbsp	60	—	7
Spaghetti w/ Marinara Sauce	1 lunch serving	315	—	8
Spaghetti w/ Tomato Sauce	1 lunch serving	400	—	9
Veal Marsala	1 dinner serving	330	—	29
Veal Parmigiana	1 dinner serving	590	—	40
Veal Piccata	1 dinner serving	230	—	16
Venetian Grilled Chicken w/o pasta or vegetable	1 dinner serving	320	—	12

PIZZA HUT

FOOD	PORTION	CALS.	SAT. FAT	FAT
Beef Medium Hand Tossed	1 slice	261	3	10
Beef Medium Pan	1 slice	288	3	18
Beef Medium Thin 'N Crispy	1 slice	231	3	11
Cheese Big Foot	1 slice	179	3	5
Cheese Medium Hand Tossed	1 slice	253	4	9
Cheese Medium Pan	1 slice	279	5	13
Cheese Medium Thin 'N Crispy	1 slice	223	5	10
Chunky Combo Hand Tossed	1 slice	280	5	12
Chunky Combo Pan	1 slice	306	5	16
Chunky Combo Thin 'N Crispy	1 slice	250	5	13
Chunky Meat Hand Tossed	1 slice	325	6	16
Chunky Meat Pan	1 slice	352	7	20
Chunky Meat Thin 'N Crispy	1 slice	295	6	17
Chunky Veggie Hand Tossed	1 slice	224	2	6
Chunky Veggie Pan	1 slice	251	3	10
Chunky Veggie Thin 'N Crispy	1 slice	193	3	8
Italian Sausage Medium Hand Tossed	1 slice	313	6	15
Italian Sausage Medium Pan	1 slice	399	6	24
Italian Sausage Medium Thin 'N Crispy	1 slice	282	6	17

FOOD	PORTION	CALS.	SAT. FAT	FAT
Meat Lovers Medium Hand Tossed	1 slice	321	4	15
Meat Lovers Medium Pan	1 slice	347	5	23
Meat Lovers Medium Thin 'N Crispy	1 slice	297	4	16
Pepperoni Big Foot	1 slice	195	3	7
Pepperoni Medium Hand Tossed	1 slice	253	3	10
Pepperoni Medium Pan	1 slice	280	3	18
Pepperoni Medium Thin 'N Crispy	1 slice	230	3	11
Pepperoni Personal Pan	1 pie	675	—	29
Pepperoni Lovers Medium Hand Tossed	1 slice	335	4	16
Pepperoni Lovers Medium Pan	1 slice	362	5	25
Pepperoni Lovers Medium Thin 'N Crispy	1 slice	320	4	19
Pepperoni, Italian Sausage And Mushroom Big Foot	1 slice	213	4	8
Pork Medium Hand Tossed	1 slice	270	3	11
Pork Medium Pan	1 slice	296	3	19
Pork Medium Thin 'N Crispy	1 slice	240	3	12
Super Supreme Medium Hand Tossed	1 slice	276	3	10
Super Supreme Medium Pan	1 slice	302	4	19
Super Supreme Medium Thin 'N Crispy	1 slice	253	3	12
Supreme Medium Hand Tossed	1 slice	289	3	12
Supreme Medium Pan	1 slice	315	3	16
Supreme Medium Thin 'N Crispy	1 slice	262	3	14
Supreme Personal Pan	1 pie	647	—	28
Veggie Lovers Medium Hand Tossed	1 slice	222	3	7
Veggie Lovers Medium Pan	1 slice	249	3	15
Veggie Lovers Medium Thin 'N Crispy	1 slice	192	3	8

FOOD	PORTION	CALS.	SAT. FAT	FAT
PONDEROSA				
BEVERAGES				
Cherry Coke	6 oz	77	—	0
Chocolate Milk	8 oz	208	—	9
Coca-Cola	6 oz	72	—	0
Coffee, Black	6 oz	2	—	0
Diet Coke	6 oz	tr	—	0
Diet Coke, Caffeine-Free	6 oz	tr	—	0
Diet Sprite	6 oz	2	—	0
Dr. Pepper	6 oz	72	—	0
Lemonade	6 oz	68	—	0
Milk	8 oz	159	—	9
Mr. Pibb	6 oz	71	—	0
Orange Soda	6 oz	82	—	0
Root Beer	6 oz	80	—	0
Sprite	6 oz	72	—	0
Tea	6 oz	2	—	0
DESSERTS				
Ice Milk, Chocolate	3.5 oz	152	—	3
Ice Milk, Vanilla	3.5 oz	150	—	3
Topping, Caramel	1 oz	100	—	1
Topping, Chocolate	1 oz	89	—	tr
Topping, Strawberry	1 oz	71	—	tr
Topping, Whipped	1 oz	80	—	6
MAIN MENU SELECTIONS				
Bake 'R Broil Fish	1 serving (5.2 oz)	230	—	13
BBQ Sauce	1 tbsp	25	—	0
Beans, Baked	1 serving (4 oz)	170	—	6
Beans, Green	1 serving (3.5 oz)	20	—	0
Breaded Cauliflower	1 serving (4 oz)	115	—	1
Breaded Okra	1 serving (4 oz)	124	—	1
Breaded Onion Rings	1 serving (4 oz)	213	—	9
Breaded Zucchini	1 serving (4 oz)	102	—	1
Carrots	1 serving (3.5 oz)	31	—	tr
Cheese Sauce	2 oz	52	—	2
Cheese, Herb & Garlic Spread	1 tbsp	100	—	10
Chicken Breast	1 serving (5.5 oz)	90	—	2
Chicken Wings	2	213	—	9
Chopped Steak	4 oz	225	—	16
Chopped Steak	5.3 oz	296	—	22
Corn	1 serving (3.5 oz)	90	—	tr
Fish Fried	1 serving (3.2 oz)	190	—	9

FOOD	PORTION	CALS.	SAT. FAT	FAT
Fish Nuggets	1	31	—	2
Gravy, Brown	2 oz	25	—	1
Gravy, Turkey	2 oz	25	—	tr
Halibut, Broiled	1 serving (6 oz)	170	—	2
Hot Dog	1	144	—	13
Italian Breadsticks	1	100	—	1
Kansas City Strip	5 oz	138	—	6
Macaroni & Cheese	4 oz	67	—	2
Margarine, Liquid	1 tbsp	100	—	11
Meatballs	1	58	—	2
Mini Shrimp	6	47	—	tr
New York Strip, Choice	8 oz	314	—	11
New York Strip, Choice	10 oz	384	—	15
Pasta Shells, Plain	2 oz	78	—	tr
Peas	1 serving (3.5 oz)	67	—	tr
Porterhouse	13 oz	441	—	30
Porterhouse, Choice	16 oz	640	—	31
Potato, Baked	1	145	—	tr
Potato Wedges	1 serving (3.5 oz)	130	—	6
Potatoes, French Fried	1 serving	120	—	4
Potatoes, Mashed	1 serving (4 oz)	62	—	tr
Ribeye	5 oz	219	—	13
Ribeye, Choice	6 oz	281	—	14
Rice Pilaf	1 serving (4 oz)	160	—	4
Roll, Dinner	1	184	—	3
Roll, Sourdough	1	110	—	1
Roughy, Broiled	1 serving (5 oz)	139	—	5
Salmon, Broiled	1 serving (6 oz)	192	—	3
Sandwich Steak	4 oz	408	—	11
Scrod, Baked	1 serving (7 oz)	120	—	1
Shrimp, Fried	7 pieces	231	—	tr
Sirloin, Choice	7 oz	241	—	11
Sirloin Tips, Choice	5 oz	473	—	8
Spaghetti, Plain	2 oz	78	—	tr
Spaghetti Sauce	4 oz	110	—	4
Steak Kabobs (Meat only)	3 oz	153	—	5
Stuffing	4 oz	230	—	11
Sweet & Sour Sauce	1 oz	37	—	1
Swordfish, Broiled	1 serving (6 oz)	271	—	9
T-Bone	8 oz	176	—	9
T-Bone, Choice	10 oz	444	—	18
Teriyaki Steak	5 oz	174	—	3
Tortilla Chips	1 oz	150	—	8
Trout, Broiled	1 serving (5 oz)	228	—	4
Winter Mix	1 serving (3.5 oz)	25	—	0

FOOD	PORTION	CALS.	SAT. FAT	FAT
SALADS AND SALAD BAR				
Alfalfa Sprouts	1 oz	10	—	0
Apple	1	80	—	1
Apples, Canned	4 oz	90	—	0
Applesauce	4 oz	80	—	0
Banana	1	87	—	tr
Banana Chips	0.2 oz	25	—	1
Banana Pudding	1 oz	52	—	2
Bean Sprouts	1 oz	10	—	tr
Beets, Diced	4 oz	55	—	tr
Breadsticks Sesame	2	35	—	0
Broccoli	1 oz	9	—	1
Cabbage, Green	1 oz	9	—	0
Cabbage, Red	1 oz	1	—	0
Cantaloupe	1 wedge	13	—	0
Carrots	1 oz	12	—	tr
Cauliflower	1 oz	8	—	tr
Celery	1 oz	4	—	0
Cheese, Imitation, Shredded	1 oz	90	—	7
Cheese Spread	1 oz	98	—	7
Cherry Peppers	2 pieces	7	—	tr
Chicken Salad	3.5 oz	212	—	15
Chow Mein Noodles	0.2 oz	25	—	1
Cocktail Sauce	1 oz	34	—	1
Coconut, Shredded	0.2 oz	25	—	2
Cottage Cheese	4 oz	120	—	5
Croutons	1 oz	115	—	4
Cucumber	1 oz	4	—	0
Eggs, Diced	2 oz	94	—	7
Fruit Cocktail	4 oz	97	—	tr
Garbanzo Beans	1 oz	102	—	0
Gelatin, Plain	4 oz	71	—	0
Granola	.2 oz	24	—	1
Grapes	10	34	—	tr
Green Onion	1	7	—	tr
Green Pepper	1 oz	6	—	tr
Ham, Diced	2 oz	120	—	10
Honeydew	1 wedge	24	—	tr
Lemon	1 wedge	3	—	tr
Lettuce	1 oz	5	—	0
Macaroni Salad	3.5 oz	335	—	12
Margarine, Whipped	1 tbsp	34	—	1
Meal Mates Sesame Crackers	2	45	—	2

FOOD	PORTION	CALS.	SAT. FAT	FAT
Melba Snacks	2	18	—	0
Mousse, Chocolate	1 oz	78	—	4
Mousse, Strawberry	1 oz	74	—	5
Mushrooms	1 oz	8	—	tr
Olives, Black	1	4	—	tr
Olives, Green	1	3	—	tr
Onions, Red & Yellow	1 oz	11	—	0
Orange	1	45	—	tr
Pasta Salad	3.5 oz	269	—	12
Peaches, Canned	4 oz	70	—	0
Peanuts, Chopped	0.2 oz	30	—	2
Pears, Canned	4 oz	98	—	tr
Pickles, Dill Spears	0.14 oz	tr	—	0
Pickles, Sweet Chips	0.14 oz	4	—	0
Pineapple, Fresh	1 wedge	11	—	tr
Pineapple Tidbits	4 oz	95	—	tr
Potato Salad	3.5 oz	126	—	6
Radishes	1 oz	4	—	0
Ritz Crackers	2	40	—	2
Saltine Crackers	2	25	—	tr
Spiced Apple Rings	4 oz	100	—	0
Spinach	1 oz	7	—	tr
Strawberries	2 oz	14	—	tr
Strawberry Glaze	1 oz	37	—	0
Tartar Sauce	1 oz	85	—	11
Tomatoes	1 oz	6	—	tr
Turkey & Ham Salad	3.5 oz	186	—	13
Turkey Julienne	1 oz	29	—	tr
Watermelon	1 wedge	111	—	1
Yogurt, Fruit	4 oz	115	—	1
Yogurt, Vanilla	4 oz	110	—	2
Zucchini	1 oz	5	—	0
SALAD DRESSINGS				
Blue Cheese	1 oz	130	—	13
Cole Slaw	1 oz	150	—	14
Creamy Italian	1 oz	103	—	10
Cucumber Reduced Calorie	1 oz	69	—	6
Italian Reduced Calorie	1 oz	31	—	3
Parmesan Pepper	1 oz	150	—	15
Ranch	1 oz	147	—	15
Salad Oil	1 tbsp	120	—	14
Sour Cream	1 tbsp	26	—	3
Sweet-N-Tangy	1 oz	122	—	9
Thousand Island	1 oz	113	—	10

FOOD	PORTION	CALS.	SAT. FAT	FAT
POPEYE'S				
Apple Pie	1 serving (3.1 oz)	290	—	16
Biscuit	1 serving (2.3 oz)	250	—	15
Cajun Rice	1 serving (3.9 oz)	150	—	5
Chicken Breast Mild	1 (3.7 oz)	270	—	16
Chicken Breast Spicy	1 (3.7 oz)	270	—	16
Chicken Leg Mild	1 (1.7 oz)	120	—	7
Chicken Leg Spicy	1 (1.7 oz)	120	—	7
Chicken Thigh Mild	1 (3.1 oz)	300	—	23
Chicken Thigh Spicy	1 (3.1 oz)	300	—	23
Chicken Wing Mild	1 (1.6 oz)	160	—	11
Chicken Wing Spicy	1 (1.6 oz)	160	—	11
Cole Slaw	1 serving (4 oz)	149	—	11
Corn On The Cob	1 serving (5.2 oz)	90	—	3
French Fries	1 serving (3 oz)	240	—	12
Nuggets	1 serving (4.2 oz)	410	—	32
Onion Rings	1 serving (3.1 oz)	310	—	19
Potatoes & Gravy	1 serving (3.8 fl oz)	100	—	6
Red Beans & Rice	1 serving (5.9)	270	—	17
Shrimp	1 serving (2.8 oz)	250	—	16
PUDGIE'S FAMOUS CHICKEN				
Fried Chicken	3.5 oz	233	3	13
QUINCY'S FAMILY STEAKHOUSE				
MAIN MENU SELECTIONS				
Baked Potato	1 (12 oz)	370	—	1
Broccoli Spears	1 serving (10 oz)	110	—	1
Chicken Breast Grilled	5 oz	120	—	2
Filet Mignon	7 oz	330	—	12
Peppers & Onions	1 serving (4.5 oz)	90	—	5
Rainbow Trout Grilled	6 oz	240	—	10
Ribeye	10 oz	670	—	60
Ribeye Thick	13 oz	870	—	78
Rice Pilaf	1 serving (4 oz)	180	1	3
Sirloin Club	6 oz	280	—	10
Sirloin Large	10 oz	850	—	70
Sirloin Petite	5.5 oz	450	—	37
Sirloin Regular	8 oz	650	—	54
Stir Fry Beef	1 serving (16 oz)	950	14	77
Stir Fry Chicken	1 serving (16 oz)	790	11	67
T-Bone	14 oz	1610	—	159
Yeast Roll	1 (1.5 oz)	160	—	4

FOOD	PORTION	CALS.	SAT. FAT	FAT
SOUPS				
Clam Chowder	9 oz	198	—	14
RAX				
BEVERAGES				
Chocolate Shake	11 oz	445	8	12
Coke	16 oz	205	0	0
Diet Coke	16 oz	1	0	0
DESSERTS				
Chocolate Chip Cookie	1 (2 oz)	262	4	12
MAIN MENU SELECTIONS				
Bacon	1 slice (0.1 oz)	14	tr	1
Baked Potato	1 (10 oz)	264	0	0
Baked Potato w/ 1 tbsp Margarine	1 (10.5 oz)	364	2	11
Barbecue Sauce	1 pkg (0.4 oz)	11	0	0
Beef, Bacon 'N Cheddar	1 (6.7 oz)	523	8	32
Cheddar Cheese Sauce	1 oz	29	0	tr
Country Fried Chicken Breast Sandwich	1 (7.4 oz)	618	15	29
Deluxe Roast Beef	1 (7.9 oz)	498	7	30
French Fries	1 serving (3.25 oz)	282	4	14
Grilled Chicken Breast Sandwich	1 (6.9 oz)	402	4	23
Grilled Chicken Garden Salad w/ French Dressing	1 serving (12.7 oz)	477	6	31
Grilled Chicken Garden Salad w/ Lite Italian Dressing	1 serving (12.7 oz)	264	3	12
Mushroom Sauce	1 oz	16	0	tr
Philly Melt	1 (8.2 oz)	396	7	16
Regular Rax	1 (4.7 oz)	262	4	10
Swiss Slice	1 slice (0.4 oz)	42	3	3
SALAD DRESSINGS				
French Dressing	2 oz	275	3	22
Lite Italian Dressing	2 oz	63	0	3
SALADS AND SALAD BARS				
Gourmet Garden Salad w/ French Dressing	1 serving (10.7 oz)	409	5	29
Gourmet Garden Salad w/ Lite Italian Dressing	1 serving (10.7 oz)	305	2	10

FOOD	PORTION	CALS.	SAT. FAT	FAT
Gourmet Garden Salad w/o Dressing	1 serving (8.7 oz)	134	2	6
Grilled Chicken Salad w/o Dressing	1 serving (10.7 oz)	202	2	9

RED LOBSTER

All of the following are for a cooked portion unless otherwise noted.

FOOD	PORTION	CALS.	SAT. FAT	FAT
Atlantic Cod	1 lunch serving	100	tr	1
Atlantic Ocean Perch	1 lunch serving	130	—	4
Blacktip Shark	1 lunch serving	150	—	1
Calamari, Breaded & Fried	1 lunch serving	360	—	21
Calico Scallops	1 lunch serving	180	—	2
Catfish	1 lunch serving	170	3	10
Chicken Breast, Skinless	4 oz	140	1	3
Deep Sea Scallops	1 lunch serving	130	—	2
Filet Mignon	8 oz	350	6	16
Flounder	1 lunch serving	100	—	1
Grouper	1 lunch serving	110	—	1
Haddock	1 lunch serving	110	—	1
Halibut	1 lunch serving	110	—	1
Hamburger	5 oz	410	11	28
King Crab Legs	1 lb	170	—	2
Langostino	1 lunch serving	120	—	1
Lemon Sole	1 lunch serving	120	—	1
Mackerel	1 lunch serving	190	—	12
Maine Lobster	18 oz	240	—	8
Mako Shark	1 lunch serving	140	—	1
Monkfish	1 lunch serving	110	—	1
Norwegian Salmon	1 lunch serving	230	—	12
Pollack	1 lunch serving	120	—	1
Rainbow Trout	1 lunch serving	170	—	9
Red Rockfish	1 lunch serving	90	—	1
Red Snapper	1 lunch serving	110	—	1
Ribeye Steak	12 oz	980	35	82
Rock Lobster	1 tail (13 oz)	230	—	3
Shrimp	8–12 pieces (7 oz)	120	—	2
Sirloin Steak	8 oz	350	6	15
Snow Crab Legs	1 lb	150	—	2
Sockeye Salmon	1 lunch serving	160	—	4
Strip Steak	9 oz	560	17	40
Swordfish	1 lunch serving	100	—	4
Tilefish	1 lunch serving	100	—	2
Yellowfin Tuna	1 lunch serving	180	—	6

FOOD	PORTION	CALS.	SAT. FAT	FAT
ROY ROGERS				
BEVERAGES				
Orange Juice	11 oz	140	tr	tr
BREAKFAST SELECTIONS				
3 Pancakes	1 serving (4.8 oz)	280	1	2
3 Pancakes w/ 1 Sausage	1 serving (6.2 oz)	430	6	16
3 Pancakes w/ 2 Bacon	1 serving (5.3 oz)	350	3	9
Bagel Cinnamon Raisin	1 (4 oz)	300	tr	1
Bagel Plain	1 (4 oz)	300	tr	2
Big Country Platters w/ Bacon	1 serving (7.6 oz)	740	13	43
Big Country Platters w/ Ham	1 serving (9.4 oz)	710	11	39
Big Country Platters w/ Sausage	1 serving (9.6 oz)	920	19	60
Biscuit	1 (2.9 oz)	390	6	21
Biscuit Bacon	1 (3.1 oz)	420	7	23
Biscuit Bacon & Egg	1 (4.2 oz)	470	8	26
Biscuit Cinnamon 'N' Raisin	1 (2.8 oz)	370	5	18
Biscuit Ham & Cheese	1 (4.5 oz)	450	8	24
Biscuit Ham & Egg	1 (5.1 oz)	460	7	23
Biscuit Ham, Egg & Cheese	1 (5.6 oz)	500	10	27
Biscuit Sausage	1 (4.1 oz)	510	10	31
Biscuit Sausage & Egg	1 (5.2 oz)	560	11	35
Hashrounds	1 serving (2.8 oz)	230	3	14
Sourdough Ham, Egg & Cheese	1 (6.8 oz)	480	9	24
DESSERTS				
Strawberry Shortcake	1 serving (6.6 oz)	480	5	21
ICE CREAM				
Ice Cream Cone	1 (4.1 oz)	180	3	4
Sundae Hot Fudge	1 (6 oz)	320	5	10
Sundae Strawberry	1 (5.5 oz)	260	3	6
MAIN MENU SELECTIONS				
¼ Roaster Dark Meat	7.4 oz	490	10	34
¼ Roaster Dark Meat w/ Skin Off	4 oz	190	3	10
¼ Roaster White Meat	8.6 oz	500	9	29
¼ Roaster White Meat w/ Skin Off	4.7 oz	190	2	6
Bacon Cheeseburger	1 (5.9 oz)	520	—	31
Baked Beans	1 serving (5 oz)	160	1	2

FOOD	PORTION	CALS.	SAT. FAT	FAT
Baked Potato	1 (3.9 oz)	130	0	1
Baked Potato w/ Margarine	1 (4.4 oz)	240	2	13
Baked Potato w/ Margarine & Sour Cream	1 (5.4 oz)	300	6	19
Cheeseburger	1 (4.2 oz)	300	7	13
Chicken Fillet Sandwich	1 (8.3 oz)	500	5	24
Cole Slaw	1 serving (5 oz)	295	4	25
Cornbread	1 serving (2.7 oz)	310	3	17
Fisherman's Fillet	1 (6.5 oz)	490	5	21
Fried Chicken Breast	1 (5.2 oz)	370	4	15
Fried Chicken Leg	1 (2.4 oz)	170	2	7
Fried Chicken Thigh	1 (4.2 oz)	330	4	15
Fried Chicken Wing	1 (2.3 oz)	200	2	8
Fry	1 lg (6.1 oz)	430	5	18
Fry	1 reg (5 oz)	350	4	15
Gravy	1 serving (1.5 fl oz)	20	tr	tr
Grilled Chicken Sandwich	1 (8.3 oz)	340	2	11
Hamburger	1 (3.8 oz)	260	4	9
Mashed Potatoes	1 serving (5 oz)	92	tr	tr
Nuggets	6 (4 oz)	290	4	18
Nuggets	9 (6.2 oz)	460	6	29
Pizza	1 serving (4.75 oz)	282	3	6
Quarter Pound Cheeseburger	1 (6 oz)	510	—	26
Quarter Pound Hamburger	1 (5.5 oz)	460	—	22
Roast Beef Sandwich	1 (5.7 oz)	260	1	4
Sourdough Grilled Chicken	1 (10.1 oz)	500	6	21
Sourdough Bacon Cheeseburger	1 (9.1 oz)	770	—	50
SALADS AND SALAD BARS				
Garden Salad	1 (9.3 oz)	190	9	14
Grilled Chicken Salad	1 serving (9.8 oz)	120	1	4
Side Salad	1 (4.9 oz)	20	tr	tr

SCHLOTZSKY'S DELI

FOOD	PORTION	CALS.	SAT. FAT	FAT
Pizza				
Chicken & Pesto	1	634	—	18
Onion & Mushroom	1	577	—	20
Smoked Turkey & Jalapeno	1	589	—	13
Vegetarian	1	555	—	17
SALAD AND SALAD BARS				
Chicken Chef	1 serving	192	—	8
Turkey Club	1 serving	233	—	10

FOOD	PORTION	CALS.	SAT. FAT	FAT
SANDWICHES				
Chicken Breast	1 sm	514	—	22
Dijon Chicken Breast	1 sm	469	—	16
Smoked Turkey	1 sm	510	—	22
The Original	1 sm	598	—	33
SOUPS				
Creole Vegetable	1 serving (8 fl oz)	120	—	3
Red Bean	1 serving (8 fl oz)	110	—	2
Shrimp & Okra	1 serving (8 fl oz)	100	—	3
Spicy Chicken	1 serving (8 fl oz)	120	—	3

SHAKEY'S

(*see also* DOMINO'S PIZZA, GODFATHER'S PIZZA, PIZZA HUT)

FOOD	PORTION	CALS.	SAT. FAT	FAT
MAIN MENU SELECTIONS				
3 Piece Fried Chicken And Potatoes	1 serving	947	—	56
5 Piece Fried Chicken and Potatoes	1 serving	1700	—	90
Hot Ham And Cheese	1	550	—	21
Potatoes	15 pieces	950	—	36
Spaghetti With Meat Sauce And Garlic Bread	1 serving	940	—	33
Super Hot Hero	1	810	—	44
PIZZA				
Homestyle Crust Cheese	1 slice	303	—	14
Homestyle Crust Onion, Green Pepper, Black Olives, Mushrooms	1 slice	320	—	15
Homestyle Crust Pepperoni	1 slice	343	—	15
Homestyle Crust Sausage, Mushroom	1 slice	343	—	17
Homestyle Crust Sausage, Pepperoni	1 slice	374	—	20
Homestyle Crust Shakey's Special	1 slice	384	—	21
Thick Crust Cheese	1 slice	170	—	5
Thick Crust Green Pepper, Black Olives, Mushrooms	1 slice	162	—	4
Thick Crust Pepperoni	1 slice	185	—	6
Thick Crust Sausage, Mushrooms	1 slice	179	—	6
Thick Crust Sausage, Pepperoni	1 slice	177	—	8

OOD	PORTION	CALS.	SAT. FAT	FAT
Thick Crust Shakey's Special	1 slice	208	—	8
Thin Crust Cheese	1 slice	133	—	5
Thin Crust Onion, Green Pepper, Black Olives, Mushrooms	1 slice	125	—	5
Thin Crust Pepperoni	1 slice	148	—	7
Thin Crust Sausage, Mushroom	1 slice	141	—	6
Thin Crust Sausage, Pepperoni	1 slice	166	—	8
Thin Crust Shakey's Special	1 slice	171	—	9

SHONEY'S

BEVERAGES

Clear Soda	1 sm	52	—	0
Clear Soda	1 lg	105	—	0
Coffee, Regular & Decaf	1 cup	8	—	0
Cola	1 sm	69	—	0
Cola	1 lg	139	—	0
Creamer	0.38 oz	14	—	1
Hot Chocolate	1 cup	110	—	2
Hot Tea	1 cup	0	—	0
Milk, 2%	1 cup	121	—	5
Orange Juice	4 oz	54	—	tr
Sugar	1 pkg	13	—	0

BREAKFAST SELECTIONS

100% Natural	½ cup	244	—	11
Ambrosia Salad	¼ cup	75	—	3
Apple	1	81	—	1
Apple Butter	1 tbsp	37	—	tr
Apple Grape Surprise	¼ cup	19	0	0
Apple Ring	1	15	0	0
Apple, Sliced	1 slice	13	—	tr
Bacon	1 strip	36	—	3
Beef Stick	1	43	—	1
Biscuit	1	170	—	8
Blueberries	¼ cup	21	—	tr
Blueberry Muffin	1	107	—	4
Bread Pudding	1 sq	305	—	11
Breakfast Ham	1 slice	26	—	1
Brunch Cake, Apple	1 sq	160	—	8
Brunch Cake, Banana	1 sq	152	—	7

FOOD	PORTION	CALS.	SAT. FAT	FAT
Brunch Cake, Carrot	1 sq	150	—	7
Brunch Cake, Pineapple	1 sq	147	—	7
Brunch Cake, Sour Cream	1 sq	160	—	8
Buttered Toast	2 slices	163	—	5
Cantaloupe, Diced	½ cup	28	—	tr
Cantaloupe, Sliced	1 slice	8	—	tr
Captain Crunch Berry	½ cup	73	—	1
Cheese Sauce	1 ladle	26	—	2
Cinnamon Honey Bun	1	344	—	12
Cottage Cheese	1 tbsp	12	—	tr
Cottage Fries	¼ cup	62	—	2
Country Gravy	¼ cup	82	—	7
Croissant	1	260	—	16
Donut Mini Cinnamon	1 (14 g)	56	—	3
DoughNugget	1	157	—	10
Egg, Fried	1	159	—	15
Egg, Scrambled	¼ cup	95	—	7
English Muffin w/ Margarine	1	140	—	2
Fluff	¼ cup	16	0	0
French Toast	1 slice	69	—	3
Fruit Delight	¼ cup	54	—	2
Fruit Topping, All Flavors	1 tbsp	24	0	0
Glaced Fruit	¼ cup	51	—	tr
Golden Pound Cake	1 slice	134	—	5
Grape Jelly	1 tbsp	60	0	0
Grapefruit, Canned	¼ cup	24	—	tr
Grapes	25	57	—	1
Grits	¼ cup	57	—	3
Hash Brown	¼ cup	43	—	2
Home Fries	¼ cup	53	—	2
Honey Bun	1	265	—	14
Honeydew, Sliced	1 slice	13	0	0
Jelly Packet	1	40	0	0
Jr. Bun, Chocolate	1	141	—	5
Jr. Bun, Honey	1	141	—	5
Jr. Bun, Maple	1	141	—	5
Kiwi, Sliced	1 slice	11	—	tr
Marble Cake w/ Icing	1 slice	136	—	5
Mixed Fruit	¼ cup	37	—	tr
Mushroom Topping	1 oz	25	—	2
Oleo, Whipped	1 tbsp	70	—	8
Omelette Topping	1 spoonful	23	—	2
Orange	1 med	65	—	tr

FOOD	PORTION	CALS.	SAT. FAT	FAT
Orange Sections	1 section	7	0	0
Oriental Salad	¼ cup	79	—	3
Pancake	1	41	—	tr
Pear	1	98	—	1
Pineapple Bits	1 tbsp	9	0	0
Pineapple, Fresh, Sliced	1 slice	10	—	tr
Pistachio Pineapple Salad	¼ cup	98	—	0
Prunes	1 tbsp	19	0	0
Raisin Bran	½ cup	87	0	1
Raisin English Muffin w/ Margarine	1	158	0	4
Sausage Link	1	91	0	9
Sausage Patty	1	136	0	13
Sausage Rice	¼ cup	110	0	6
Shortcake	1	60	0	2
Sirloin Steak, Charbroiled	6 oz	357	0	25
Smoked Sausage	1	103	0	10
Snow Salad	¼ cup	72	0	4
Strawberries	5	23	0	tr
Syrup, Light	1 ladle	60	0	0
Syrup, Low-Cal	2.2 oz	98	0	0
Tangerine	1	37	—	tr
Trix	½ cup	54	—	tr
Waldorf Salad	¼ cup	81	—	5
Watermelon, Diced	½ cup	50	—	1
Watermelon, Sliced	1 slice	9	—	tr
Whipped Topping	1 scoop	10	—	1
CHILDREN'S MENU SELECTIONS				
Jr. Burger All-American	1 serving	234	—	11
Kid's Fried Chicken Dinner	1 serving	244	—	13
Kid's Fish N' Chips (includes fries)	1 serving	337	—	17
Kid's Fried Shrimp	1 serving	194	—	12
Kid's Spaghetti	1 serving	247	—	8
DESSERTS				
Apple Pie a la Mode	1 slice	492	—	23
Carrot Cake	1 slice	500	—	26
Chocolate Pudding	¼ cup	81	—	2
Strawberry Pie	1 slice	332	—	17
Walnut Brownie a la Mode	1	576	—	34
ICE CREAM				
Hot Fudge Cake	1 slice	522	—	20
Hot Fudge Sundae	1	451	—	22
Strawberry Sundae	1	380	—	19

FOOD	PORTION	CALS.	SAT. FAT	FAT
MAIN MENU SELECTIONS				
All-American Burger	1	501	—	33
Bacon Burger	1	591	—	40
Baked Fish	1 serving	170	—	1
Baked Fish Light	1 serving	170	—	1
Baked Ham Sandwich	1	290	—	10
Baked Potato	10 oz	264	—	tr
BBQ Sauce	1 souffle cup	41	—	1
Beef Patty Light	1 serving	289	—	23
Charbroiled Chicken	1 serving	239	—	7
Charbroiled Chicken Sandwich	1	451	—	17
Chicken Fillet Sandwich	1	464	—	21
Chicken Pieces	1 piece	40	0	2
Chicken Tenders	1 serving	388	—	20
Cocktail Sauce	1 souffle cup	36	—	tr
Country Fried Sandwich	1	588	—	29
Country Fried Steak	1 serving	449	—	27
Fish N' Chips (includes fries)	1 serving	639	—	35
Fish N' Shrimp	1 serving	487	—	26
Fish Sandwich	1	323	—	13
French Fries	3 oz	189	—	8
French Fries	4 oz	252	—	10
Fried Fish Light	1 serving	297	—	14
Grecian Bread	1 slice	80	—	2
Grilled Bacon & Cheese Sandwich	1	440	—	28
Grilled Cheese Sandwich	1	302	—	17
Half O'Pound	1 serving	435	—	34
Ham Club on Whole Wheat	1	642	—	36
Hawaiian Chicken	1 serving	262	—	7
Italian Feast	1 serving	500	—	20
Lasagna	1 serving	297	—	10
Liver N' Onions	1 serving	411	—	23
Mushroom Swiss Burger	1	616	—	42
Old-Fashioned Burger	1	470	—	28
Onion Rings	1	52	—	3
Patty Melt	1	640	—	42
Philly Steak Sandwich	1	673	—	44
Reuben Sandwich	1	596	—	35
Ribeye	6 oz	605	—	51
Rice	3.5 oz	137	—	4
Sautéed Mushrooms	3 oz	75	—	7

FOOD	PORTION	CALS.	SAT. FAT	FAT
Sautéed Onions	2.5 oz	37	—	2
Seafood Platter	1 serving	566	—	28
Shoney Burger	1	498	—	36
Shrimp Charbroiled	1 serving	138	—	3
Shrimp Bite-Size	1 serving	387	—	25
Shrimp Broiled	1 serving	93	—	18
Shrimp Sampler	1 serving	412	—	23
Shrimper's Feast	1 serving	383	—	22
Shrimper's Feast Large	1 serving	575	—	33
Sirloin	6 oz	357	—	25
Slim Jim Sandwich	1	484	—	24
Spaghetti	1 serving	496	—	16
Steak N' Shrimp (charbroiled shrimp)	1 serving	361	—	23
Steak N' Shrimp (fried shrimp)	1 serving	507	—	33
Sweet N' Sour Sauce	1 souffle cup	58	—	0
Tartar Sauce	1 souffle cup	84	—	8
Turkey Club on Whole Wheat	1	635	—	33
SALAD AND SALAD BARS				
Ambrosia Salad	¼ cup	75	—	3
Apple Grape Surprise	¼ cup	19	—	0
Apple Ring	1	15	—	0
Bacon Bits	1 spoonful	15	—	1
Beet Onion Salad	¼ cup	25	—	1
Black Olives	2	10	—	1
Broccoli	¼ cup	4	—	tr
Broccoli, Cauliflower, Carrot Salad	¼ cup	53	—	4
Broccoli & Cauliflower	¼ cup	98	—	9
Broccoli & Cauliflower Ranch	¼ cup	65	—	6
Carrot	¼ cup	10	—	tr
Carrot Apple Salad	¼ cup	99	—	9
Cauliflower	¼ cup	8	—	tr
Celery	1 tbsp	5	—	0
Chow Mein Noodles	1 spoonful	13	—	1
Cole Slaw	¼ cup	69	—	5
Cottage Cheese	1 tbsp	12	—	tr
Croutons	1 spoonful	13	—	tr
Cucumber	1 tbsp	1	—	0
Cucumber Lite	¼ cup	12	—	tr
Diced Egg	1 tbsp	15	—	1

FOOD	PORTION	CALS.	SAT. FAT	FAT
Don's Pasta	¼ cup	82	—	5
Fruit Delight	¼ cup	54	—	2
Fruit Topping, All Flavors	¼ cup	64	—	tr
Glaced Fruit	¼ cup	51	—	tr
Granola	1 spoonful	25	—	1
Grapefruit	¼ cup	24	—	tr
Green Pepper	1 tbsp	1	—	0
Italian Vegetable	¼ cup	11	—	tr
Jell-O	¼ cup	40	—	0
Jell-O Fluff	¼ cup	16	—	tr
Kidney Bean Salad	¼ cup	55	—	2
Lettuce	1.8 oz	7	—	tr
Macaroni Salad	¼ cup	207	—	14
Melba Toast	2	20	—	0
Mixed Fruit Salad	¼ cup	37	—	tr
Mixed Squash	¼ cup	49	—	4
Mushrooms	1 tbsp	1	—	0
Oil	1 tsp	45	—	5
Oriental Salad	¼ cup	79	—	3
Pea Salad	¼ cup	73	—	6
Pepperoni	1 tbsp	30	—	3
Pickle Chips	1 slice	5	—	0
Pickle Spear	1 spear	2	—	0
Pineapple Bits	1 tbsp	9	—	0
Pistachio Pineapple Salad	¼ cup	98	—	3
Prunes	1 tbsp	19	—	0
Radish	1 tbsp	1	—	0
Raisins	1 spoonful	26	—	0
Rotelli Pasta	¼ cup	78	—	4
Seign Salad	¼ cup	72	—	4
Shredded Cheese	1 tbsp	21	—	2
Snow Delight	¼ cup	72	—	4
Spaghetti Salad	¼ cup	81	—	5
Spinach	¼ cup	1	—	0
Spring Pasta	¼ cup	38	—	3
Summer Salad	¼ cup	114	—	12
Sunflower Seeds	1 spoonful	40	—	3
Three Bean Salad	¼ cup	96	—	5
Trail Mix	1 spoonful	30	—	1
Turkey Ham	1 tbsp	12	—	1
Waldorf	¼ cup	81	—	5
Wheat Bread	1 slice	71	—	1
Whipped Margarine	1 tsp	23	—	3
SALAD DRESSINGS				
Biscayne Lo-Cal	2 tbsp	62	—	1

FOOD	PORTION	CALS.	SAT. FAT	FAT
Blue Cheese	2 tbsp	113	—	13
Creamy Italian	2 tbsp	135	—	15
French	2 tbsp	124	—	12
Golden Italian	2 tbsp	141	—	15
Honey Mustard	2 tbsp	165	—	17
Ranch	2 tbsp	95	—	10
Rue French	2 tbsp	122	—	10
Thousand Island	2 tbsp	130	—	13
W. W. Italian	2 tbsp	10	—	0
SOUP				
Bean	6 oz	63	—	1
Beef Cabbage	6 oz	86	—	3
Broccoli Cauliflower	6 oz	124	—	9
Cheddar Chowder	6 oz	91	—	2
Cheese Florentine Ham	6 oz	110	—	8
Chicken Gumbo	6 oz	60	—	2
Chicken Noodle	6 oz	62	—	1
Chicken Rice	6 oz	72	—	1
Clam Chowder	6 oz	94	—	5
Corn Chowder	6 oz	148	—	5
Cream of Broccoli	6 oz	75	—	5
Cream of Chicken	6 oz	136	—	9
Cream of Chicken Vegetable	6 oz	79	—	1
Onion	6 oz	29	—	2
Potato	6 oz	102	—	3
Tomato Florentine	6 oz	63	—	1
Tomato Vegetable	6 oz	46	—	tr
Vegetable Beef	6 oz	82	—	2

SKIPPER'S

BEVERAGES

FOOD	PORTION	CALS.	SAT. FAT	FAT
Coke Classic	1 (12 fl oz)	144	0	0
Coke Diet	1 (12 fl oz)	2	0	0
Milk Lowfat	1 (12 fl oz)	181	—	10
Root Beer	1 (12 fl oz)	154	0	0
Root Beer Float	1 (12 fl oz)	302	—	10
Sprite	1 (12 fl oz)	142	0	0

DESSERTS

FOOD	PORTION	CALS.	SAT. FAT	FAT
Jell-O	1 serving (2.75 oz)	55	0	0

MAIN MENU SELECTIONS

FOOD	PORTION	CALS.	SAT. FAT	FAT
Baked Fish With Margarine & Seasoning	1 serving (4.4 oz)	147	—	3
Baked Potato	1 (6 oz)	145	0	0

FOOD	PORTION	CALS.	SAT. FAT	FAT
Captain's Cut	1 piece (2.6 oz)	160	—	7
Cocktail Sauce	1 tbsp	20	0	0
Coleslaw	1 serving (5 oz)	289	—	27
Corn Muffin	1 (2 oz)	91	—	5
English Style Fish	1 piece (2.4 oz)	187	—	12
French Fries	1 serving (3.5 oz)	239	—	12
Green Salad (no dressing)	1 serving (4 oz)	24	0	0
Ketchup	1 tbsp	17	0	0
Margarine	1 serving (0.5 oz)	50	—	6
Shrimp Fried Cajun	1 serving (4 oz)	342	—	21
Shrimp Fried Jumbo	1 piece (.65 oz)	51	—	2
Shrimp Fried Original	1 serving (4 oz)	266	—	13
Tartar Original	1 tbsp	65	—	7
SOUPS				
Clam Chowder	1 cup (6 fl oz)	100	—	4
Clam Chowder	1 pint (12 fl oz)	200	—	7

SONIC DRIVE-IN

FOOD	PORTION	CALS.	SAT. FAT	FAT
#1 Hamburger	1 (6.6 oz)	409	—	27
#2 Hamburger	1 (6.6 oz)	323	—	16
B-L-T Sandwich	1 (6.1 oz)	327	—	19
Bacon Cheeseburger	1 (7.2 oz)	548	—	39
Chicken Sandwich Breaded	1 (7.4 oz)	455	—	25
Chili Pie	1 (3.7 oz)	327	—	23
Corn Dog	1 (3 oz)	280	—	15
Extra Long Cheese Cony w/ Onions	1 (9.4 oz)	640	—	39
Extra Long Cheese Coney	1 (8.9 oz)	635	—	39
Fish Sandwich	1 (6.1 oz)	277	—	7
French Fries	1 lg (6.7 oz)	315	—	11
French Fries	1 reg (5 oz)	233	—	8
French Fries w/ Cheese	1 lg (7.7 oz)	219	—	20
Grilled Cheese Sandwich	1 (2.8 oz)	288	—	17
Grilled Chicken Sandwich w/o Dressing	1 (6.4 oz)	215	—	4
Hickory Burger	1 (5.1 oz)	314	—	16
Jalapeno Burger Double Meat & Cheese	1 (9.1 oz)	638	—	41
Mini Cheeseburger	1 (3.9 oz)	281	—	14
Mini Burger	1 (3.5 oz)	246	—	11
Onion Rings	1 lg (5 oz)	577	—	38
Onion Rings	1 reg (3.5 oz)	404	—	27
Regular Cheese Coney	1 (5 oz)	358	—	15
Regular Cheese Coney w/ Onions	1 (5.3 oz)	361	—	23

FOOD	PORTION	CALS.	SAT. FAT	FAT
Regular Hot Dog	1 (3.5 oz)	258	—	15
Steak Sandwich Breaded	1 (3.9 oz)	631	—	42
Super Sonic Burger w/ Mustard Double Meat & Cheese	1 (10.1 oz)	644	—	41
Super Sonic Burger w/ Mayo Double Meat & Cheese	1 (10.1 oz)	730	—	52
Tater Tots	1 serving (3 oz)	150	—	7
Tater Tots w/ Cheese	1 serving (3.6 oz)	220	—	13

SUBWAY

FOOD	PORTION	CALS.	SAT. FAT	FAT
Ham Sandwich Round	1 (4 in)	317	—	3
Roast Beef Sandwich Round	1 (4 in)	326	—	2
Roast Turkey Breast Salad	1 serving	154	—	7
Roast Turkey Breast Sub White Bread	1 (6 in)	312	—	8
Subway Club Salad	1 serving	165	—	7
Veggies & Cheese Sub Wheat Bread	1 (6 in)	258	—	6

T. J. CINNAMON'S

FOOD	PORTION	CALS.	SAT. FAT	FAT
Doughnuts Cake	2	454	—	22
Doughnuts Raised	2	352	—	22
Mini-Cinn Plain	1	75	—	5
Mini-Cinn With Icing	1	80	—	5
Original Gourmet Cinnamon Roll Plain	1	630	—	34
Original Gourmet Cinnamon Roll With Icing	1	686	—	34
Petite Cinnamon Roll Plain	1	185	—	10
Petite Cinnamon Roll With Icing	1	202	—	10
Sticky Bun Cinnamon Pecan	1	607	—	35
Sticky Bun Petite Cinnamon Pecan	1	255	—	15
Triple Chocolate Classic Roll Plain	1	412	—	28
Triple Chocolate Classic Roll With Icing	1	462	—	31

FOOD	PORTION	CALS.	SAT. FAT	FAT
TACO BELL				
Burrito Bean	1	381	—	14
Burrito Beef	1	431	—	21
Burrito Chicken	1	334	4	12
Burrito Combo	1	407	5	16
Burrito Supreme	1	503	8	22
Chilito	1	383	8	18
Cinnamon Twists	1 order	171	3	8
Green Sauce	1 oz	4	0	0
Guacamole	0.66 oz	34	0	2
Jalapeno Peppers	3.5 oz	20	0	0
MexiMelt Beef	1	266	8	15
MexiMelt Chicken	1	257	7	15
Mexican Pizza	1	575	11	37
Nacho Cheese Sauce	2 oz	105	3	8
Nachos	1	346	—	18
Nachos Bellgrande	1	649	12	35
Nachos Supreme	1	367	5	27
Pico De Gallo	1	6	—	0
Pintos 'N Cheese	1	190	4	9
Ranch Dressing	2.5 oz	236	5	25
Red Sauce	1 oz	10	0	0
Salsa	0.33 oz	18	0	0
Sour Cream	0.66 oz	46	2	4
Taco	1	183	5	11
Taco Salad	1	905	19	61
Taco Salad w/o Shell	1	484	14	31
Taco Sauce	1 pkg	2	0	0
Taco Sauce, Hot	1 pkg	3	0	0
Taco, Soft	1	225	5	12
Taco, Soft, Chicken	1	213	4	10
Taco, Soft, Supreme	1	272	8	16
Taco, Supreme	1	230	8	15
Tostada	1	243	4	11
TACO JOHN'S				
Bean Burrito	1	197	—	6
Beef Burrito	1	303	—	18
Chicken Burrito w/ Green Chili	1	344	—	16
Chicken Super Taco Salad w/ Dressing	1	507	—	27
Chicken Super Taco Salad w/o Dressing	1	377	—	15
Chimichanga	1	464	—	21

FOOD	PORTION	CALS.	SAT. FAT	FAT
Chimichanga w/ Chicken	1 serving	441	—	19
Combo Burrito	1	250	—	12
Mexican Rice	1 serving	340	—	8
Nachos	1 serving	468	—	25
Potato Olé	1 lg	414	—	6
Smothered Burrito w/ Green Chili	1	367	—	18
Smothered Burrito w/ Texas Chili	1	455	—	23
Softshell	1	224	—	13
Softshell w/ Chicken	1	180	—	8
Super Burrito	1	389	—	16
Super Burrito w/ Chicken	1	366	—	14
Super Nachos	1 serving	669	—	39
Super Taco Bravo	1	361	—	19
Super Taco Salad w/ 2 oz Dressing	1	558	—	32
Super Taco Salad w/o Dressing	1	428	—	20
Taco	1	178	—	13
Taco Bravo	1	319	—	14
Taco Burger	1	281	—	14
Taco Salad w/ 2 oz Dressing	1	359	—	24
Taco Salad w/o Dressing	1	228	—	13

TCBY

FOOD	PORTION	CALS.	SAT. FAT	FAT
Nonfat, All Flavors	1 kiddie size	88	—	tr
Nonfat, All Flavors	1 sm	162	—	tr
Nonfat, All Flavors	1 reg	226	—	tr
Nonfat, All Flavors	1 lg	289	—	tr
Nonfat, All Flavors	1 super	418	—	tr
Nonfat, All Flavors	1 giant	849	—	tr
Regular, All Flavors	1 kiddie size	104	—	2
Regular, All Flavors	1 sm	192	—	4
Regular, All Flavors	1 lg	341	—	8
Regular, All Flavors	1 super	494	—	11
Regular, All Flavors	1 giant	1027	—	24
Sugar Free, All Flavors	1 kiddie size	64	—	tr
Sugar Free, All Flavors	1 sm	118	—	tr
Sugar Free, All Flavors	1 reg	164	—	tr
Sugar Free, All Flavors	1 lg	210	—	tr
Sugar Free, All Flavors	1 super	304	—	tr
Sugar Free, All Flavors	1 giant	632	—	tr

FOOD	PORTION	CALS.	SAT. FAT	FAT
TGI FRIDAY'S				
Charbroiled Chicken Sandwich	1 (7.58 oz)	320	—	4
Garden Burger	1 (7.58 oz)	410	—	8
Herb Grilled Chicken	1 (17.72 oz)	550	—	12
Manicotti	1 serving (15.44 oz)	680	—	35
P&E Shrimp	1 serving (4.38 oz)	120	—	tr
P.C. Tuna	1 (16.33 oz)	280	—	7
Pea Salsa	1 (6.35 oz)	170	—	2
Spinach Salad	1 (8.67 oz)	240	—	11
Turkey Burger	1 (9.81 oz)	410	—	19
Vegetable Bagette	1 (16.1 oz)	440	—	11
Vegetable Medley	1 serving (13.8 oz)	140	—	3
UNO RESTAURANT				
DeepDish Pizza	1 serving	770	13	38
VILLAGE INN				
French Toast Cinnamon Raisin	1 serving	809	4	16
Fruit & Nut Pancakes Low Cholesterol	1 serving	936	2	19
Omelette Chicken & Cheese	1 serving	721	4	19
Omelette Fresh Veggie	1 serving	704	4	18
Omelette Mushroom & Cheese	1 serving	680	4	18
Turkey & Vegetable Scrambled Sensation	1 serving	726	4	19
WENDY'S				
BEVERAGES				
Coffee, Black	6 oz	2	0	0
Coffee, Decaffeinated Black	6 oz	2	0	0
Cola	8 oz	90	0	0
Hot Chocolate	6 oz	92	1	1
Lemonade	8 oz	90	0	0
Lemon-Lime	8 oz	90	0	0
Milk, 2%	8 oz	110	3	4
Tea, Hot	6 oz	0	0	0
Tea, Iced	12 oz	0	0	0

FOOD	PORTION	CALS.	SAT. FAT	FAT
CHILDREN'S MENU SELECTIONS				
Kid's Meal Cheeseburger	1 (4.3 oz)	310	5	13
Kid's Meal Hamburger	1 (4.3 oz)	270	3	9
DESSERTS				
Chocolate Chip Cookie	1 (2.2 oz)	280	4	13
Frosty Dairy Dessert	1 lg (20 fl oz)	570	9	17
Frosty Dairy Dessert	1 med (16 fl oz)	460	7	13
Frosty Dairy Dessert	1 sm (12 fl oz)	340	5	10
MAIN MENU SELECTIONS				
¼-lb Hamburger Patty (no bun)	1 (2.3 oz)	190	5	12
American Cheese	1 slice (0.6 oz)	70	4	6
American Cheese Jr.	1 slice (0.4 oz)	45	3	4
Bacon	1 strip (0.2 oz)	30	1	3
Baked Potato	1 lg (12 oz)	290	4	9
Baked Potato	1 sm (8 oz)	190	3	6
Baked Potato Bacon & Cheese	1 (13.3 oz)	530	4	18
Baked Potato Broccoli & Cheese	1 (14.4 oz)	460	3	14
Baked Potato Cheese	1 (13.4 oz)	560	8	23
Baked Potato Chili & Cheese	1 (4.8 oz)	610	9	24
Baked Potato Plain	1 (10 oz)	310	0	0
Baked Potato Sour Cream & Chives	1 (11 oz)	380	4	6
Big Bacon Classic	1 (10.1 oz)	640	13	36
Breaded Chicken Fillet, no bun	1 (3.5 oz)	220	2	10
Breaded Chicken Sandwich	1 (7.3 oz)	450	4	20
Cheddar Cheese Shredded	2 tbsp (0.6 oz)	70	3	6
Chicken Club Sandwich	1 (7.7 oz)	520	6	25
Chicken Nuggets	6 pieces (3.3 oz)	280	5	20
French Fries	1 Biggie (6 oz)	450	5	22
French Fries	1 med (4.8 oz)	360	4	17
French Fries	1 sm (3.2 oz)	240	3	12
Grilled Chicken Breast, no bun	1 (2.5 oz)	100	1	3
Grilled Chicken Sandwich	1 (6.2 oz)	290	2	7
Honey Mustard (Reduced Calorie)	1 tsp (0.2 oz)	25	0	2
Jr. Bacon Cheeseburger	1 (6 oz)	440	8	25
Jr. Cheeseburger	1 (4.5 oz)	320	5	13
Jr. Cheeseburger Deluxe	1 (6.3 oz)	390	7	20

FOOD	PORTION	CALS.	SAT. FAT	FAT
Jr. Hamburger	1 (4.1 oz)	270	3	9
Jr. Hamburger Patty, no bun	1 (1.3 oz)	90	3	6
Kaiser Bun	1 (2.4 oz)	190	1	3
Ketchup	1 tsp (0.2 fl oz)	10	0	0
Lettuce	1 leaf (0.5 oz)	0	0	0
Mayonnaise	1½ tsp	70	1	7
Mustard	½ tsp (0.2 oz)	5	0	0
Nuggets Sauce, Barbecue	1 pkg (1 oz)	50	0	0
Nuggets Sauce, Honey	1 pkg (0.5 oz)	45	0	0
Nuggets Sauce, Sweet & Sour	1 pkg (1 oz)	45	0	0
Nuggets Sauce, Sweet Mustard	1 pkg (1 oz)	50	0	1
Onion	4 rings (0.5 oz)	0	0	0
Pickles	4 slices	0	0	0
Plain Single	1 (4.7 oz)	350	6	15
Saltines	2 (0.2 oz)	25	1	0
Sandwich Bun	1 (2 oz)	160	1	3
Single w/ Everything	1 (7.7 oz)	440	7	23
Sour Cream	1 oz	60	4	6
Tomatoes	1 slice (0.9 oz)	5	0	0
Whipped Margarine	1 pkg (0.5 oz)	60	1	5
SALAD DRESSINGS				
Blue Cheese	2 tbsp (1 fl oz)	180	3	19
Blue Cheese Reduced Calorie Reduced Fat	2 tbsp (1 fl oz)	70	2	7
Celery Seed	2 tbsp (1 fl oz)	60	1	7
French	2 tbsp (1 fl oz)	120	2	11
French Fat Free	2 tbsp (1 fl oz)	35	0	0
French Sweet Red	2 tbsp (1 fl oz)	130	2	10
Hidden Valley Ranch	2 tbsp (1 fl oz)	90	2	10
Italian Caesar	2 tbsp (1 fl oz)	150	3	16
Italian Golden	2 tbsp (1 fl oz)	90	1	7
Italian Reduced Calorie Reduced Fat	2 tbsp (1 fl oz)	40	1	3
Salad Oil	1 tbsp (0.5 fl oz)	130	2	14
Thousand Island	2 tbsp (1 fl oz)	130	2	13
Wine Vinegar	1 tbsp (0.5 fl oz)	0	0	0
SALADS AND SALAD BARS				
Alfredo Sauce	¼ cup (1.4 oz)	30	0	2
Applesauce Chunky	2 tbsp (1.4 oz)	30	0	0
Bacon Bits	2 tbsp (0.5 oz)	40	1	2
Breadstick Sesame	1 (3 g)	15	0	0

FOOD	PORTION	CALS.	SAT. FAT	FAT
Broccoli	¼ cup (0.5 oz)	0	0	0
Cantaloupe	1 piece (1.6 oz)	15	0	0
Carrots	¼ cup (0.6 oz)	5	0	0
Cauliflower	¼ cup (0.6 oz)	0	0	0
Caesar Side Salad	1 (3.1 oz)	110	2	5
Cheddar Chips	2 tbsp (0.4 oz)	70	1	4
Cheese Sauce	1.4 cup (1.2 oz)	25	0	1
Cheese Shredded Imitation	2 tbsp (0.6 oz)	50	1	4
Chicken Salad	2 tbsp (1.2 oz)	70	1	5
Chives	1 tbsp (1 g)	0	0	0
Chow Mein Noodles	¼ cup (0.2 oz)	35	0	2
Cole Slaw	2 tbsp (1.3 oz)	45	0	3
Cottage Cheese	2 tbsp (1.1 oz)	30	1	2
Croutons	2 tbsp (0.2 oz)	30	0	1
Cucumbers	2 slices (0.5 oz)	0	0	0
Deluxe Garden Salad	1 (9.5 oz)	110	1	6
Eggs hard cooked	2 tbsp (0.9 oz)	40	1	3
Green Peas	2 tbsp (0.7 oz)	15	0	0
Green Peppers	2 pieces (0.3 oz)	8	0	0
Grilled Chicken Salad	1 (11.9 oz)	200	2	8
Honeydew Melon	1 piece (1.8 oz)	20	0	0
Jalapeno Peppers	1 tbsp (0.4 oz)	0	0	0
Lettuce Iceberg/Romaine	1 cup (2.6 oz)	10	0	0
Macaroni & Cheese	½ cup (3.2 oz)	130	3	6
Mushrooms	¼ cup (0.5 oz)	0	0	0
Olives Black	2 tbsp (0.5 oz)	15	0	2
Orange Sections	1 piece (1.1 oz)	10	0	0
Parmesan Cheese	2 tbsp (0.5 oz)	70	3	5
Pasta Salad	2 tbsp (1.2 oz)	35	0	0
Peaches Sliced	1 piece (1 oz)	15	0	0
Pepperoni Sliced	6 slices (0.2 oz)	30	1	3
Picante Sauce	2 tbsp (1 oz)	10	0	0
Pineapple Chunks	4 pieces (1.1 oz)	20	0	0
Potato Salad	2 tbsp (1.3 oz)	80	3	7
Pudding Chocolate	¼ cup (1.8 oz)	70	1	3
Pudding Vanilla	¼ cup (1.8 oz)	70	1	3
Red Onions	3 rings (0.5 oz)	0	0	0
Red Peppers Crushed	1 tbsp (0.2 oz)	15	0	1
Refried Beans	¼ cup (1.9 oz)	80	1	3
Rotini	½ cup (1.9 oz)	90	0	2
Seafood Salad	¼ cup (1.3 oz)	70	1	4
Side Salad	1 (5.4 oz)	60	1	3
Soft Breadstick	1 (1.5 oz)	130	1	3
Sour Topping	2 tbsp (1 oz)	60	5	5

FOOD	PORTION	CALS.	SAT. FAT	FAT
Spaghetti Meat Sauce	¼ cup (1.4 oz)	45	1	2
Spaghetti Sauce	1.4 cup (1.5 oz)	30	0	0
Spanish Rice	¼ cup (1.8 oz)	60	0	1
Strawberries	1 (0.9 oz)	10	0	0
Strawberry Banana Dessert	¼ cup (1.6 oz)	30	0	0
Sunflower Seeds & Raisins	2 tbsp (0.5 oz)	80	1	5
Taco Chips	8 (0.9 oz)	120	1	7
Taco Meat	2 tbsp (1.3 oz)	80	1	4
Taco Salad	1 (17.9 oz)	580	11	30
Taco Sauce	2 tbsp (0.8 oz)	10	0	0
Taco Shell	1 (0.4 oz)	60	1	4
Tomatoes Wedged	1 piece (0.9 oz)	5	0	0
Tortilla Flour	1 (1.2 oz)	110	1	3
Turkey Ham Diced	2 tbsp (0.8 oz)	50	1	4
Watermelon	1 piece (2.2 oz)	20	0	0

WHATABURGER
BAKED SELECTIONS

FOOD	PORTION	CALS.	SAT. FAT	FAT
Apple Turnover	1	215	—	11
Blueberry Muffin	1	239	—	8
Buttermilk Biscuit	1	280	—	13
Cookie Chocolate Chunk	1	247	—	16
Cookie Macadamia Nut	1	269	—	16
Cookie Oatmeal Raisin	1	222	—	4
Cookie Peanut Butter	1	262	—	14
Pecan Danish	1	270	—	16

BEVERAGES

FOOD	PORTION	CALS.	SAT. FAT	FAT
Coffee	1 sm	5	—	0
Coke Cherry	16 fl oz	151	—	0
Coke Classic	16 fl oz	141	—	0
Creamer	1 pkg	10	—	1
Diet Coke	16 fl oz	1	—	0
Dr. Pepper	16 fl oz	138	—	tr
Iced Tea	16 fl oz	3	—	0
Lemon Juice	1 pkg	1	—	0
Milk 2%	1 serving	113	—	4
Orange Juice	1 serving	77	—	tr
Root Beer	16 fl oz	158	—	0
Shake Chocolate	1 (12 fl oz)	364	—	9
Shake Strawberry	1 (12 fl oz)	352	—	9
Shake Vanilla	1 (12 fl oz)	325	—	10
Sprite	16 fl oz	141	—	0
Sugar	1 pkg	15	—	0
Sweet And Low	1 pkg	4	—	0

FOOD	PORTION	CALS.	SAT. FAT	FAT
BREAKFAST SELECTIONS				
Biscuit With Bacon	1	359	—	20
Biscuit With Egg And Cheese	1	434	—	26
Biscuit With Egg, Cheese And Bacon	1	511	—	33
Biscuit With Egg, Cheese And Sausage	1	601	—	42
Biscuit With Gravy	1	479	—	27
Biscuit With Sausage	1	446	—	29
Breakfast Platter With Bacon	1 serving	695	—	44
Breakfast Platter With Sausage	1 serving	785	—	53
Breakfast On A Bun	1	455	—	28
Breakfast On A Bun Bacon	1	365	—	19
Butter	1 pkg	36	—	4
Egg Omelette Sandwich	1	288	—	13
Grape Jelly	1 pkg	38	0	0
Hash Brown	1	150	—	9
Honey	1 pkg	27	0	0
Margarine	1 pkg	25	—	3
Pancake Syrup	1 pkg	169	0	0
Pancakes	3	259	—	6
Pancakes w/ Sausage	1 serving	426	—	21
Scrambled Eggs	2 eggs	189	—	15
Strawberry Jam	1 pkg	37	0	0
MAIN MENU SELECTIONS				
Bacon	1 slice	38	—	3
Baked Potato	1	310	—	tr
Baked Potato w/ Broccoli Cheese Topping	1	453	—	10
Baked Potato w/ Cheese Topping	1	510	—	16
Baked Potato w/ Mushroom Topping	1	360	—	2
Cheese Large	1 serving	89	—	7
Cheese Small	1 serving	46	—	4
Chicken Sandwich Grilled	1	442	—	14
Chicken Sandwich Grilled w/o Dressing	1	385	—	9
Club Crackers	1 pkg	31	—	1
Croutons	1 serving	29	—	1
Fajita Taco Beef	1	326	—	12

FOOD	PORTION	CALS.	SAT. FAT	FAT
Fajita Taco Chicken	1	272	—	7
French Fries	1 junior	221	—	12
French Fries	1 lg	442	—	24
French Fries	1 reg	332	—	18
Garden Salad w/o Dressing	1	56	—	1
Grilled Chicken Salad	1 serving	150	—	1
Jalapeno Pepper	1	3	—	tr
Justaburger	1	276	—	11
Onion Rings	1 lg	493	—	29
Onion Rings	1 reg	329	—	19
Picante Sauce	1 pkg	5	—	0
Sour Cream	1 serving (2 oz)	121	—	12
Steak Sandwich	1	387	—	12
Taquito Bacon	1 serving	335	—	16
Taquito Potato	1 serving	446	—	22
Taquito Sausage	1 serving	443	—	26
Turkey Sandwich Grilled	1	439	—	15
Whataburger	1	598	—	26
Whataburger Double Meat	1	823	—	42
Whataburger Jr.	1	300	—	12
Whatacatch	1	475	—	25
Whatachick'n Deluxe	1	573	—	27
Whatachick'n Sandwich	1	501	—	23
SALAD DRESSINGS				
French	1 pkg	249	—	20
Ranch	1 pkg	364	—	38
Thousand Island	1 pkg	280	—	27
Vinaigrette Lite	1 pkg	36	—	2

WHITE CASTLE

Bun Only	1	74	—	tr
Cheese Only	3 oz	31	—	2
Cheeseburger	1 (2.3 oz)	200	—	11
Chicken Sandwich	1	186	—	7
Fish Sandwich w/o Tartar	1	155	—	5
French Fries	1 reg	301	—	15
Hamburger	1 (2.1 oz)	161	—	8
Onion Rings	1 reg order	245	—	13
Sausage Sandwich	1	196	—	12
Sausage & Egg Sandwich	1	322	—	22

WINCHELL'S DONUTS

Apple Fritter	1	580	—	37
Cinnamon Crumb	1	240	—	11
Cinnamon Roll	1	360	—	21

FOOD	PORTION	CALS.	SAT. FAT	FAT
Glazed Jelly	1	300	—	13
Glazed Round	1	210	—	12
Glazed Twist	1	210	—	11
Iced Chocolate Bar	1	220	—	11
Iced Chocolate Cake	1	230	—	10
Iced Chocolate Devil's	1	240	—	12
Iced Chocolate French	1	220	—	13
Iced Chocolate Raised	1	210	—	10
Plain	1	200	—	11
Plain Donut Hole	1	50	—	3